Public Health

Public Health
The Development of a Discipline

VOLUME II

Twentieth Century Challenges

Edited by

Dona Schneider and David E. Lilienfeld

RUTGERS UNIVERSITY PRESS

New Brunswick, New Jersey, and London

Library of Congress Cataloging-in-Publication Data

Public health : the development of a discipline, volume 2, twentieth-century challenges/
edited by Dona Schneider and David E. Lilienfeld.
   p. ; cm.
  Includes bibliographical references and index.
  ISBN 978-0-8135-5008-4 (hardcover : alk. paper)— ISBN 978-0-8135-5009-1
  (pbk. : alk. paper)
  1. Public health—History. I. Schneider, Dona, 1946–   II. Lilienfeld, David E.
  [DNLM: 1. Public Health—history—Collected Works. WA 5 P9757 2008]
  RA424.P83 2008
  362.1—dc22   2007019970

A British Cataloging-in-Publication record for this book is available from the British
Library.

Visit our Web site: http://rutgerspress.rutgers.edu

CONTENTS

PART II
Diseases, Therapies, and Prevention

PART III
Improving Public Health

PREFACE

The works included in this volume were scanned, dictated, transcribed, or typed in from the originals. Several of the pieces chosen as selected readings have been reprinted in other venues, some more than once. A few of the selections have won awards and, where appropriate, we note this information for the reader in either the source statement following the selected reading or in the suggested readings at the end of the introductory sections to each chapter. Some of the selections are quite long or have complex tables, figures, or appendixes that we felt did not add to the reading. These works appear abridged, and we note this as well as where material has been removed in the text. We have to admit that there are some pieces we would have liked to have included in this anthology, but because of space or other technical issues, we could not include them.

The reader will find that all of the selected works in Volume II were published or translated into English and republished in the twentieth century. The selected readings are also mostly shorter than those in Volume I because journal space, the primary outlet for these types of publications, has become dear over time. The reader will occasionally find a typo that slipped by the editors of the original works. We have chosen to retain these and have identified them by [*sic*].

Each selected reading contains its references as they appeared in the original publication. Thus, the reader will note that citation format changes from piece to piece. In order to comply with copyright restrictions, we have limited our editorial comments about the readings to the selected readings section at the end of each chapter introduction. As with Volume I, we hope our efforts present the reader with an enjoyable experience with some of the key published works of the twentieth century—those that made a significant impact on our understanding of public health.

ACKNOWLEDGMENTS

The authors are indebted to Professors Manning Feinleib, Bernard Goldstein, Michael R. Greenberg, Gerald F. Pyle, and Warren Winkelstein, Jr. for supporting the publication of Volume II. Their suggestions helped us determine a logical structure to this work. We also thank the Rutgers University Press, especially Doreen Valentine, who encouraged us every step of the way. We would be remiss if we did not thank all of the reference librarians who made our searches an exciting and worthwhile experience, especially those toiling on our behalf at Rutgers University. The difficulties in putting together a work of this scope cannot be understated, and we thank the various journals whose works appear in this work for their help and understanding of the importance of this work. We thank our family members, who were tolerant of our time commitment to this project. And finally, we thank all the students who continue to inspire us, especially the many who gave us their input over the years. We hope this volume serves them well.

INTRODUCTION

We are slowly learning one of life's most important lessons: not just how to live longer, but also how to stay longer in good health with less dependence on others.

　　—World Health Report 1998. Life in the 21st Century. A Vision for All.
　　Report of the Director-General.
　　Geneva, Switzerland: World Health Organization. 1998.

In 1900, life expectancy for whites in the United States was about 50 years; for blacks it was about 35 years. In England and Wales, life expectancy in 1900 was about 45 years; in India it was about 23 years. A century later, life expectancy had risen across the globe, though unevenly. Those born in the United States, the United Kingdom, and most of Europe in the year 2000 could expect to live into their mid to upper seventies; those in India could expect to live to about 60 years of age. The longest life expectancy, averaging about 85 years, was estimated for those born in Andorra, a tiny country about 2.5 times the size of Washington, D.C., located in the Pyrenees Mountains between France and Spain. Other countries with high life expectancies in 2000 were Japan, Macau, San Marino, and Singapore. The shortest life expectancies in that year, averaging only about 35 years, were for those born in Angola, Liberia, Swaziland, Zambia, and Zimbabwe, countries stricken by war, famine, and human immunodeficiency virus/acquired immune deficiency syndrome (HIV/AIDS).

　　Why life expectancy rose more in some places than it did in others over the twentieth century can be explained by a few key factors, such as sanitation, political and economic stability, and the investments governments made in their own people, especially for education and health care. For example, the Brookings Institution lists 3 of the 10 most important achievements of the U.S. government in the twentieth century as being related directly to the public health of American citizens: 1) reducing disease (polio vaccination; targeting heart disease, cancer, and stroke; banning smoking; and preventing lead-based poisoning); 2) ensuring safe food and drinking water (Federal Insecticide, Fungicide, and Rodenticide Act of 1947; Poultry Products Inspection Act of 1957; Wholesome Meat and Poultry Acts of 1967 and 1968; Federal Environmental Pesticide Control Act of 1972; Safe Drinking Water Act of 1974; and the Food Quality Protection Act of 1996); and 3) increasing access to health care for older Americans (Medicare, 1965). Similarly, the Centers for Disease Control and Prevention (CDC) lists the 10 great public health achievements in the United States as 1) vaccination, 2) motor-vehicle safety, 3) safer workplaces, 4) control of infectious diseases, 5) decline in deaths from coronary heart disease and stroke, 6) safer and healthier foods, 7) healthier mothers and babies, 8) family planning, 9) fluoridation of drinking water, and 10) recognition of tobacco as a health hazard.

The World Health Organization (WHO) also helped improve global public health. That agency can take credit for the global eradication of smallpox and nearly global eradication of polio, two diseases that diminish life expectancy. Private foundations and organizations, too, played a role in improving both health and longevity of people in many regions of the world, particularly with regard to clean water access and education. National and local efforts dedicated to improving health for all by creating healthy nations, healthy cities, healthy communities, and healthy people all began in the twentieth century. Indeed, global awareness about the importance of public health for improving the quality of life for all people continues to grow.

Addressing all of the players and factors that contributed to the advancement of public health in the twentieth century is a challenge. As we began outlining Volume II, it soon became apparent that the format we used for Volume I of this series, which focused on the selected works of individuals who drove the development of public health from the Age of Hippocrates to the Progressive Era, was inadequate. The second volume would require the recognition of the technological advances, social movements, and the political and economic decisions that drove the field.

After several attempts at an organizational structure, we finally decided on separating the volume into three parts. Part I covers population health issues: the recognition of food and nutrition (or the lack thereof), tobacco, and dental caries as potential health risks; the emerging fields of environmental and occupational health; and concerns about the health of women, including maternal–child health. Part II contains six chapters that focus on major diseases, as well as their therapies and prevention. For example, tuberculosis has been a scourge of humankind for millennia. Indeed, the disease has been found in Egyptian mummies. For the year 2000, the WHO estimated that approximately 1.86 billion people across the globe had tuberculosis, and there were an additional 10-plus million being added to that figure annually. Thus, although we may talk of the demographic transition moving the primary causes of mortality from infectious to chronic diseases during the course of the twentieth century, it is clear that we have yet to contain tuberculosis, one of our oldest and most resistant infectious diseases. Other chapters in Part II cover the development of vaccines; our ability to find new and effective treatments for diseases; and progress on heart disease and stroke, cancer, and the HIV/ AIDS epidemic.

Part III includes the roles of organizations, research and technology, and global efforts to improve public health. There are chapters on medical and preventive care, as well as international efforts to stem select diseases or syndromes that decimate populations, such as infantile diarrhea. Finally, the appendixes contain some of the major documents affecting public health in the twentieth century. We hope these reference materials will continue to serve the reader for many years to come.

We would love to honor the work of each individual who contributed to the ability of public health to further develop as a discipline in the twentieth century, but we obviously cannot include them all. Therefore, we attempted to select readings for each chapter that complement each other and that point to new ideas, to new treatments or technologies, or to other broad contributions in public health. Whether these readings are "classics" will likely be challenged by some, but we feel they are significant works representing their times. We must also confess that we were unable to obtain copyright for some of the pieces that we felt should have been designated as selected readings. In those cases, we discuss the contribution of the authors in the introductions to the relevant chapters and refer the reader to the original works. Overall, however, we hope we have served the field well by outlining what we believe were some of the most important original works of public health in the twentieth century.

BIBLIOGRAPHY

Centers for Disease Control and Prevention. 1999. Ten great public health achievements—United States, 1900–1999. *MMWR* 48 (12): 241–43.

Light, PC. 2000. Government's greatest achievements of the past half century. Brookings Institution Reform Watch Brief #2. http://www.brookings.edu/comm/reformwatch/rw02.htm (accessed October 15, 2009).

World Health Organization Statistical Information System (WHOSIS). http://www.who.int/whosis/en/ (accessed October 15, 2009).

CHRONOLOGY

1900   Walter Reed reports that mosquitoes carry Yellow Fever.

Karl Landsteiner discovers ABO blood groups.

Bubonic plague strikes Sydney, Australia, and spreads across the territories; more than 300 people are infected and 100 die.

1900–09   Bubonic plague outbreaks occur across the American West, leaving the disease endemic in that region.

1901–05   In Uganda, 200,000 people die of African trypanosomiasis (sleeping sickness).

1902   The Eleventh International Sanitary Conference takes place in Paris.

The International Sanitary Bureau is established for the Americas. The name will later be changed to the Pan American Sanitary Bureau (1923). This organization is the predecessor of the Pan American Health Organization (1958).

1902–04   Cholera ravages the Philippines.

1902–07   African trypanosomiasis (sleeping sickness) strikes Gabon.

1903   Spain requires smallpox vaccination.

1904   The National Child Labor Committee is organized to monitor the effects of child labor on health and development.

Pneumonic plague strikes South Africa.

Bubonic plague occurs in Siam.

Smallpox breaks out in Brazil.

1904–07   Plague outbreaks continue across India, killing 6 million people.

1905   Antimosquito campaigns eliminate yellow fever from the Panama Canal Zone and the United States.

The Japanese Army suffers 200,000 cases of beriberi among its soldiers. The Japanese Navy experiences no cases, the result of better diets.

Bubonic plague strikes Burma.

New Zealand suffers a pertussis (whooping cough) epidemic.

Plague breaks out in Saigon, Viet Nam.

Yellow fever is eliminated from Brazil; outbreaks of the disease continue in Cuba.

Mary Mallon (Typhoid Mary) is arrested and detained in New York City, becoming the first known asymptomatic carrier of a contagious disease.

The American Public Health Association begins publishing the *American Journal of Public Hygiene*. It also publishes standards for examining milk.

London begins the continuous chlorination of public water supplies.

1906   Sand filtration for the disinfection of drinking water is employed in Philadelphia, Pennsylvania.

Ozone is used for water disinfection in Nice, France.

1907   The Bureau of Child Hygiene is established in New York City.

Basel, Switzerland, hosts the First International Conference on Infant Care.

A pertussis (whooping cough) epidemic strikes Samoa.

New York City experiences a polio epidemic.

The Office International d'Hygiène Publique (OIHP) is founded in Paris to oversee international rules regarding the quarantine of ships and ports to prevent the spread of disease. The agency grew from 12 primarily European members to more than 60 countries and colonies by 1914. Its epidemiological service was later incorporated into the World Health Organization.

The International Committee of the Red Cross (ICRC) creates the International Prisoners-of-War Agency for humanitarian purposes. The ICRC monitors compliance with the Geneva Conventions throughout World War I and vigorously denounces chemical warfare. During the course of the century, the agency will receive three Nobel Peace Prizes.

1907–12   Cholera outbreaks in Arabia kill 25,000 people.

1908   The U.S. Census adopts a standardized death certificate.

New York City establishes a Division of Child Health, directed by Josephine Baker.

Chicago, Illinois, becomes the first U.S. city to mandate pasteurization of milk.

Bubonic plague strikes Ecuador, Peru, Trinidad, and Venezuela, becoming endemic in the northwestern part of South America.

Smallpox in Brazil kills 9,000 people.

Cholera spreads across Persia, Russia, and Siberia.

Jersey City, New Jersey, becomes the first city in the United States to continuously chlorinate its public water supply.

1909   President Theodore Roosevelt hosts the First White House Conference on the Care of Dependent Children.

Organized prenatal care begins in Boston, Massachusetts.

The American Public Health Association publishes standards for examining air.

The Rockefeller Foundation is persuaded by Charles W. Stiles to create a commission to eradicate hookworm in the southern United States.

1910   The U.S. Bureau of Mines is created and begins to study "black lung."

An extensive cholera outbreak occurs in the Donets Basin of Russia. The Russian government requests aid from the Red Cross to stem the epidemic.

Cholera breaks out in the Balkans, Italy, and Portugal.

Pneumonic plague breaks out in Manchuria, killing 60,000 victims.

Bubonic plague breaks out in the East Indies and spreads to Java.

The Flexner Report for the Carnegie Foundation calls for radical reform in American medical education (See Volume I, Chapter 20).

1911   The Twelfth International Sanitary Conference takes place in Paris.

An International Plague Conference is held in Mukden, Manchuria, spurring creation of a Chinese public health system.

A major polio outbreak occurs in Sweden.

Bubonic plague breaks out in Morocco.

Cholera breaks out in Libya, Persia, and Tunisia.

A measles outbreak kills one-seventh of the population of Fiji.

Portugal launches a public health campaign against African trypanosomiasis (sleeping sickness) in West Africa, eradicating the disease by 1914.

Parliament passes the National Insurance Act, the first state medical insurance scheme in Britain.

1912   McCollum and Davis discover vitamin A (see Chapter 1).

Congress restructures the public health system, creating the U.S. Public Health Service from the Marine Hospital Service.

The Institute for Tropical Medicine is established in Puerto Rico.

The Mexican Federal Army is stricken with typhoid.

African trypanosomiasis (sleeping sickness) appears in Chad.

Bubonic plague breaks out in Cuba, Ecuador, Java, Kenya, Puerto Rico, and the Mekong Delta.

The National Organization of Public Health Nursing is established by Lillian Wald.

1912–13   The U.S. Children's Bureau is created (proposed by President Theodore Roosevelt and signed into law by President William H. Taft).

1913   British National Health Insurance goes into service.

Britain begins medical education reform.

The American Society for the Control of Cancer (later the American Cancer Society) is created with financial backing from John D. Rockefeller, Jr.

The U.S. Army becomes the first fighting force to be inoculated against typhoid. Britain quickly follows suit.

In Vienna, Austria, Béla Schick describes an intradermal test to determine whether a person has immunity to diphtheria.

The first state hospital opens in Kabul, Afghanistan.

1914   Manchester, England, opens the first modern sewage treatment plant to treat sludge with bacteria.

Joseph Goldberger identifies pellagra as a dietary deficiency (see Volume I, Chapter 21).

1915   The Welch-Rose *Report on Schools of Public Health* (Rockefeller Foundation) is released. The document outlines a model for the United States where schools of public health are developed in association with but independent from medical schools. This is in contrast to Britain and the European nations where public health is developed as a subdiscipline of medicine.

The United States establishes a National Birth Registry.

1916   Margaret Sanger founds the first American birth control clinic in Brooklyn, New York (see Volume I, Chapter 22).

Paralytic polio strikes New York City. Children are its primary victims.

1917   Chloramination is used for water disinfection in the Canadian provinces of Ottawa and Ontario, as well as in Denver, Colorado.

World War I breaks out. Recruiting efforts in the United States show the poor health status of American youth, generating interest in improving the health of children.

1918   The Spanish Flu (influenza A) or *La Grippe* strikes worldwide, killing 20 to 50-plus million people. The influenza pandemic is the worst epidemic in recorded human history, exceeding the mortality from the Black Death in the fourteenth century.

1919   Abel Wolman and Linn H. Enslow demonstrate that chlorine consumption varies with water characteristics and introduce a chlorination technique to address the problem (see Volume I, Chapter 24).

1919–20   Poland and the Union of Soviet Socialist Republics (USSR) struggle with more than two million cases of typhus.

1920   The American Medical Association passes a resolution opposing any government related insurance program.

1921   Congress passes the Maternity and Infancy Act (Shepard–Towner Act) with a goal of reducing infant mortality. The act gives matching grants-in-aid to related facilities and services such as nursing and education. It also provides for the inspection of "maternity homes."

Marie Stopes opens the first birth control clinic in London.

1922   The League of Nations bans white-lead interior paint, but the United States does not comply with the ban.

Dr. Ludwig Rajchman becomes the Secretary of the Health Committee and the Director of the Health Section under the newly established League of Nations Health Organization, which becomes the World Health Organization (WHO) in 1948.

Amelia Maggia, a watch dial painter with the U.S. Radium Corporation in Orange, New Jersey, dies of radiation poisoning

Elmer McCollum discovers Vitamin D, used for the treatment of rickets (see Chapter 1).

1922–23   Malaria epidemics strike Russia, with 10 million cases and 20,000 deaths.

1923   The first leaded gasoline goes on sale in Dayton, Ohio.

Diphtheria vaccine is developed.

1924   Five workers die at a Standard Oil (later Exxon) refinery from making tetraethyl lead gasoline additive under grossly unsafe conditions; the workers were reportedly "violently insane" at the time of their deaths.

1925   The U.S. Surgeon General holds a conference on leaded gasoline. Ethyl industry officials claim that no alternatives are possible (see Chapter 4).

1926   Pertussis (whooping cough) vaccine is introduced.

The Thirteenth International Sanitary Conference takes place in Paris. Smallpox, typhus, plague, cholera, and yellow fever are declared reportable to the IOHP.

1927   The Committee on the Cost of Medical Care (CCMC) is established to comprehensively study the economics of health care. Dr. I.S. Falk of the University of Chicago is hired to oversee the five-year research project, which will recommend basic public health services for the entire population but come to multiple conclusions about how to pay for it.

Five New Jersey women (The Radium Girls) file lawsuits against the U.S. Radium Corporation for negligence and dangerous working conditions. All five die of radiation-induced cancer within a few years after the suit is settled in 1928.

Bacille Calmette-Guérin vaccine is introduced for the prevention of tuberculosis.

Tetanus vaccine is introduced.

Vitamin C is isolated.

1928   The U.S. Public Health Service begins checking air pollution levels in eastern cities, reporting that sunlight is cut by 20 to 50 percent in New York City.

In Oxford, England, Alexander Fleming discovers penicillin.

1929   Blue Cross Insurance is founded.

1930   The National Institute of Health is established, building upon the existing U.S. Public Health Service's Hygienic Laboratory.

1932   The *British Medical Journal* says leaded gasoline is dangerous because it will create a "slow, subtle insidious saturation of the system by infinitesimal doses of lead extending over long periods of time."

1933   Pertussis vaccine is used for the first time in the United States.

1934   Francis Perkins, U.S. Secretary of Labor, establishes the Division of Labor Standards (forerunner of the Occupational Safety and Health Administration)

1934–35   Malaria strikes Ceylon, causing 3 million cases and 82,000 deaths.

1935   Congress passes the Social Security Act with grants to states for aid to dependent children, maternal and child welfare (Titles IV and V, respectively), and public health (Title VI).

Yellow fever vaccine is developed.

1936   Frances Perkins calls for a federal occupational safety and health law.

1936   The Walsh-Healey (Public Contracts) Act is passed requiring that all federal contracts be fulfilled in a healthful and safe working environment.

1938   The Garfield/Kaiser Prepaid Group Practice (forerunner of Kaiser Permanente) is founded in the United States.

Eddie Canter urges his radio listeners to send their spare change to the White House to be used in the fight against polio. The name "March of Dimes" is coined for this effort. President Franklin D. Roosevelt founds an agency of the same name.

The Fourteenth International Sanitary Conference takes place in Paris.

Malaria strikes Brazil, causing 100,000 cases of the disease and 14,000 deaths.

1939   Smog is so thick in St. Louis, Missouri, that lanterns are needed during daylight hours during the course of one week. The episode sparks intense reporting by the *St. Louis Post–Dispatch* which, in 1940, receives the first Pulitzer Prize for environmental reporting.

DDT begins being used with great success to control malaria and typhus among civilians and troops serving in World War II.

1940   The Center for Control of Malaria in War Areas (forerunner of the Centers for Disease Control) is founded.

The Kark Community-Oriented Primary Care Clinic is established in South Africa.

1941   St. Louis, Missouri, adopts the first smoke-control ordinance in the United States.

George Papanicolaou and Herbert Traut identify the diagnostic value of cervical smears in identifying carcinoma of the cervix.

In New York, Karl Landsteiner and Philip Levine discover Rh factor.

1942   Malaria strikes Lower Egypt, causing 100,000 cases and 14,000 deaths.

In England, Howard Florey is the first to use penicillin for clinical purposes; Wesley Spink of Minneapolis, Minnesota, is the first to use it in the United States.

Studies at the Orlando, Florida, laboratory of the Bureau of Entomology and Plant Quarantine demonstrate that DDT can be used against lice, mosquitoes, and houseflies. The insecticide is put into large-scale production and large stocks are ordered by the U.S. and British armies.

1943   Congress passes the Emergency Maternity and Infant Care Act to provide care for the wives and children of enlisted men.

Chloroquine is synthesized for the treatment of malaria.

Selman A. Waksman discovers streptomycin.

1943–49   The United Nations Relief and Rehabilitation Administration (UNRRA) is established for the relief of victims of World War II. UNRRA provides billions of U.S. dollars in aid, helping about 8 million refugees. Its functions were later transferred to the International Refugee Organization.

1944   The Public Health Service Act is passed to consolidate all legislation relating to public health services in the United States.

1945   Influenza vaccine is developed.

Fluoridation of water is introduced in the United States to prevent tooth decay.

The United Nations Conference in San Francisco approves the establishment of a new, autonomous international health organization.

1946   Congress passes the Hospital Survey and Construction Act (Hill–Burton), authorizing grants to the states for surveying and determining the need for hospitals and public-health centers, as well as for the planning and construction of additional facilities.

The Communicable Disease Center is founded in Atlanta, Georgia, (forerunner of the Centers for Disease Control and Prevention).

The International Health Conference in New York approves the Constitution of the World Health Organization.

The United Nations establishes the United Nations International Children's Emergency Fund.

1947   The Los Angeles Air Pollution Control District is formed, the first air pollution control bureau in the United States.

Congress passes the Federal Insecticide, Fungicide, and Rodenticide Act (FIFRA).

The World Health Organization creates the Epidemiological Information Service.

1947–1951   The United States creates the National Malaria Eradication Program, and the disease is declared eradicated as a public health problem by 1949.

1948   In Britain, the National Health Service is created.

The World Health Organization constitution goes into force on World Health Day (April 7).

Congress passes the Federal Water Pollution Control Act, authorizing comprehensive programs for reducing the pollution of interstate waters and improving the sanitary condition of surface and underground waters.

In Donora, Pennsylvania, 20 people die, 600 are hospitalized, and thousands more are stricken in a smog disaster.

In London, 600 deaths result from a "killer fog."

1949   Canadian complaints about Detroit, Michigan, pollution launch a Public Health Service study and spark the first U.S. conference on air pollution.

The United States is declared free of malaria as a public health problem.

The National Foundation for Cerebral Palsy is established in New York City.

1950   Arie Haagen-Smit identifies causes of smog in Los Angeles, California, as the interaction of hydrocarbons and oxides of nitrogen.

President Harry S. Truman calls for government and industry to join forces in a battle against smog.

In Poza Rica, Mexico, a killer smog caused by gas fumes from an oil refinery leaves 22 dead and hundreds hospitalized.

President Harry S. Truman convenes the Mid-Century White House Conference on the total well-being of children.

The World Health Organization undertakes mass tuberculosis immunization with the Bacille Calmette-Guérin vaccine to protect children from tuberculosis.

1952   A polio epidemic strikes the United States. More than 57,000 cases are reported, including 3,000 dead.

The Salk polio vaccine (killed virus version) is tested at the Watson Home for Crippled Children and the Polk State School, a mental retardation facility in Pennsylvania.

The worst of the London "killer fogs" kills 4,000 people. The fog is so bad that buses can run only with a guide walking ahead. All transportation except the subway comes to a halt.

The U.S. Congress passes the Coal Mine Safety Act.

The United Nations International Children's Emergency Fund launches a yaws control program, treating 300 million people in 50 countries and reducing global levels of the disease by more than 95 percent.

1953   A New York City smog incident kills between 170 and 260 people.

Tests show radioactive iodine in children's bodies in Utah—the legacy of atomic testing.

President Dwight D. Eisenhower establishes the U.S. Department of Health, Education, and Welfare.

1954   Heavy smog shuts down industry and schools in Los Angeles, California, for most of October.

Field trials of the Salk vaccine are sponsored by the National Foundation for Infantile Paralysis.

Japanese encephalitis vaccine is developed.

In Massachusetts, John Rock and George Pincus launch the first human trial of an oral contraceptive pill under the guise of a fertility study.

1955   An International Air Pollution Conference is held in New York City.

Excerpta Medica creates a section (17) for Public Health, Social Medicine, and Hygiene.

The Centers for Disease Control establishes the Polio Surveillance Program.

Injectable polio vaccine (IPV) is introduced.

The World Health Organization begins the Global Malaria Eradication Campaign to be based mainly on the spraying of DDT. The program results in the elimination of endemic malaria from Europe and Australia and a radical reduction of cases in less-developed countries.

1956   The National Library of Medicine is created.

A killer smog in London kills 1,000 people; Parliament passes the Clean Air Act.

The etiology of "Minamata disease" is identified as mercury poisoning from eating contaminated fish. By the mid 1970s, 67 people die and another 330 are permanently disabled from the disease. By the mid 1990s, more than 3,000 children in Minamata are born with birth defects related to mercury exposure.

1957   Congress passes the Poultry Products Inspection Act.

Canada passes the Hospital Insurance and Diagnostic Services Act requiring acute hospital services to be covered by a publicly funded insurance plan.

A vaccine against Adenovirus-4 and Adenovirus-7 is developed.

Albert Sabin develops a live, attenuated polio vaccine.

After a fire, Britain's Windscale Nuclear Complex (Sellafield) sends radioactive clouds into the atmosphere.

The Asian flu pandemic (influenza A) kills 100,000 people.

1958   Field trials show the Sabin oral polio vaccine (live, attenuated virus) is effective.

The March of Dimes organization shifts its focus to preventing birth defects.

Malaria strikes Ethiopia, causing 3 million cases and 150,000 deaths.

1959   California becomes the first state to impose automotive emissions standards.

The United Nations issues a declaration on the Rights of the Child.

1960   MEDLARS technology comes online in the United States at the National Library of Medicine.

James Watson, Francis Crick, Maurice Wilkins, Rosalind Franklin, Sydney Brenner, and others crack the genetic code.

Birth control pills are approved for use in the United States by the Food and Drug Administration.

1961   Robert Guthrie develops a screening test for phenylkenonuria, the first universal newborn screening test that could identify infants requiring dietary changes to prevent severe mental retardation.

1962   Oral polio vaccine is developed.

A measles epidemic occurs in Greenland.

Henry Kempe describes Battered Child Syndrome, creating recognition of child abuse in the United States.

Rachel Carson publishes *Silent Spring*, bringing the deleterious effects of DDT to light.

1962–65   A pandemic of German measles (rubella) affects 12.5 million people worldwide. In the United States alone, 30,000 babies suffered from deafness and blindness due to maternal rubella.

1963   After Hurricane Flora, Haiti suffers 75,000 cases of malaria due to disruption of mosquito control campaigns.

Measles vaccine is developed.

1964   The U.S. *Surgeon General's Report on Smoking* declares that "cigarette smoking is a health hazard of sufficient importance in the United States to warrant appropriate remedial action."

The Community Health Centers Program is funded by Congress as part of the War on Poverty.

1965   Congress adds Title XVIII (Medicare) and Title XIX (Medicaid) to the Social Security Act.

1965   Congress passes the Health Professions Educational Assistance Act.

1966   The United States establishes a Migrant Health Program, supporting more than 400 migrant clinics in the United States and Puerto Rico.

President Lyndon B. Johnson signs the Highway Safety Act and the National Traffic and Motor Vehicle Safety Act, regulating standards for highways and vehicles.

1967   Mumps vaccine is developed.

The Nineteenth World Health Assembly requests the Director-General of WHO to initiate a worldwide smallpox eradication program.

1967–68   Congress passes the Wholesome Meat and Poultry Acts.

1968   The Hong Kong flu pandemic kills 700,000 people.

A highly infectious respiratory disease, later identified as Legionnaire's disease, emerges in Pontiac, Michigan.

Canada passes the Medical Care Act.

Eunice Kennedy Shriver founds the Special Olympics.

1968–70   Sri Lanka suffers 1.5 million cases of malaria.

1970   Earth Day is celebrated for the first time.

Congress passes the Clean Air Act.

The U.S. Environmental Protection Agency is created.

The U.S. Occupational Health and Safety Administration is created.

Rubella vaccine is developed.

1971   The U.S. National Center for Health Statistics conducts the first National Health and Nutrition Examination Survey to capture the health status of Americans.

1972   The Centers for Disease Control assists Sierra Leone in fighting an outbreak of Lassa fever.

The Tuskegee syphilis study is exposed by the Associated Press and whistle-blowers inside the Public Health Service.

Congress passes the Federal Water Pollution Control Act (over President Richard Nixon's veto).

Congress passes the Federal Insecticide, Fungicide, and Rodenticide Act amendments to transfer responsibility from the U.S. Department of Agriculture to the Environmental Protection Agency.

Congress passes the Toxic Substances Control Act requiring testing for health and environmental effects prior to a chemical's manufacture or distribution.

The United States bans the use of DDT.

The United Nations Conference on the Human Environment convenes in Stockholm, Sweden.

Congress creates the Special Supplemental Food Program for Women, Infants, and Children.

The United States ends mandatory smallpox vaccination.

1973   Health Maintenance Organizations are created.

1974   The Lalonde Report, *A New Perspective on the Health of Canadians*, is released.

Congress passes the Clean Drinking Water Act.

Varicella (chicken pox) vaccine is developed.

1975   Congress passes the Hazardous Waste Transportation Act.

1976   A chemical explosion in Seveso, Italy, spreads dioxin, directly injuring about 30 people and causing chloracne, a severe skin disease, in more than 300 schoolchildren.

The Centers for Disease Control investigates two outbreaks of a previously unknown deadly hemorrhagic fever, later known as Ebola, in Zaire and Sudan.

Legionnaire's disease breaks out in Philadelphia, Pennsylvania. The organism, Legionella, is later linked to poorly maintained air conditioning systems.

1976–77   A malaria epidemic in India yields 7 million cases of the disease.

1977   The Allied Chemical Company and the State of Virginia settle a lawsuit for $5 million over extensive Kepone contamination of the James River.

The World Health Organization reports that the global eradication of smallpox is achieved.

Pneumococcal (pneumonia) vaccine is developed.

1977–78   Turkey suffers an epidemic of malaria with 270,000 cases.

1977–86   Typhoid outbreaks plague Chile.

1978   The International Conference on Primary Health Care, meeting in Alma-Ata, USSR, declares that "health, which is a state of complete physical, mental and social wellbeing, and not merely the absence of disease or infirmity, is a fundamental human right and that the attainment of the highest possible level of health is a most important world-wide social goal whose realization requires the action of many other social and economic sectors in addition to the health sector." It is the first international declaration underlining the importance of primary health care.

Meningitis vaccine is developed.

1979   *Healthy People: Surgeon General's Report on Health Promotion and Disease Prevention* is released.

China introduces the "one child" policy for family planning.

Afghanistan suffers a malaria epidemic.

1980   President Jimmy Carter announces the relocation of 700 families in the Love Canal area of Niagara Falls, New York, who had been exposed to toxic wastes deposited there by the Hooker Chemical Company.

Congress passes the Comprehensive Environmental Response, Compensation, and Liability Act (Superfund) directing the clean up of abandoned toxic waste dumps.

The National Academy of Sciences calls leaded gasoline the greatest source of atmospheric lead pollution.

1981   Acquired Immunodeficiency Syndrome (AIDS) is first described and quickly becomes epidemic.

Hepatitis B vaccine is developed.

1982   Dangerous levels of dioxin threaten the health of residents in Times Beach, Missouri, after the chemical was mixed with waste oil and sprayed on local unpaved roads to control dust. The federal government spends $33 million to buy the homes of 2,400 people in Times Beach, relocates the people, and demolishes the town.

The Centers for Disease Control issues an advisory about the risk of Reye's syndrome associated with the use of aspirin by children who have chickenpox or flu-like symptoms.

E. coli O157:H7 is identified in contaminated food and determined to be the cause of outbreaks of hemolytic uremic syndrome.

Borrelia burgdorferi bacterium is identified as the cause of Lyme disease.

1983   The first genetic disease is mapped (Huntington's disease).

1984   A Union Carbide fertilizer plant leaks methyl icocyanide in Bhopal, India. More than 2,000 die immediately and another 8,000 die of chronic effects.

The Canada Health Act is passed, requiring universal coverage for all insured persons (including all medically necessary physician and hospital services, without copayments).

1985   An ozone hole is confirmed over Antarctica. Warnings go out about sun exposure and skin cancer.

Haemophilus influenzae type b (HiB) vaccine is developed.

The First International AIDS Conference is held in Atlanta, Georgia.

1986   The Chernobyl nuclear disaster in Belarus causes 31 immediate deaths with mid-term deaths estimated around 4,200. Various agencies report a 10- to 200- fold increases in thyroid cancer.

A naturally occurring cloud of carbon dioxide gas boils out of Lake Nyos in Cameroon, killing 1,700 people.

The Second International AIDS Conference is held in Paris.

The World Health Organization, in its Ottawa Charter for Health Promotion, *Achieving Health For All*, declares that "Health promotion is the process of enabling people to increase control over, and to improve, their health." Health promotion is defined as building healthy public policy in the full range of administrative and legislative action; creating supportive environments via a socioecological approach to health; strengthening community action and democratic planning processes; developing personal skills via education; and reorienting health services toward health promotion in addition to curative services.

1987   The Montreal Protocol international agreement to phase out ozone-depleting chemicals is signed by 24 countries, including the United States, Japan, Canada, and the European Economic Community nations.

1988   *The Future of Public Health* (Institute of Medicine) is released, calling for the delineation of the mission of the public health service system and improved skills for public health practitioners.

The World Health Organization passes a resolution to eradicate polio by the year 2000.

The World Health Organization declares World AIDS Day.

1989   *U.S. Preventive Services Task Force: Guide to Clinical Preventive Services* is released.

The United Nations opens the Convention on the Rights of the Child. The convention finds that children have the right: to survival; to develop to the fullest; to protection from harmful influences, abuse, and exploitation; and to participate fully in family, cultural, and social life. As of 1996, the convention is ratified by 187 countries.

Hepatitis C is identified and later indicated as the most common cause of post-transfusion hepatitis worldwide.

1989–90   A flu epidemic in the United Kingdom kills 29,000 people.

1989–91   Outbreaks of measles occur in the United States, beginning in Maryland.

1990   Congress passes the Nutritional Labeling and Education Act.

President George H.W. Bush signs the Americans With Disabilities Act, the world's first civil rights law for persons with disabilities.

1992   The Environmental Protection Agency issues FIFRA rules to limit farm worker exposures to pesticides. An estimated 300,000 farm workers had been poisoned each year, about 1,000 of them fatally.

Hepatitis A vaccine is developed.

1993   The Health Plan Employer Data and Information Set is released.

1993–94   Tajikistan and Azerbaijan suffer malaria epidemics.

The Clinton Health Care Plan requiring each U.S. citizen and permanent resident to become enrolled in a qualified health plan is proposed and defeated.

1993–95   Northern Iraq and southern Turkey experience malaria epidemics.

1994   Congress passes the Food Quality Protection Act.

Polio is certified by the World Health Organization as eradicated in the Americas.

The U.S. Public Health Service recommends the use of azidothymidine (AZT) to reduce the perinatal transmission of AIDS.

Canada releases *Strategies for Population Health: Investing in the Health of Canadians*.

1995–96   Northern India suffers a malaria epidemic.

1995–96   Maryland becomes the first state to mandate a minimum inpatient length of stay for mothers and newborns, responding to public outrage about "drive-through deliveries."

1996   The National Congress of Medicine/Public Health Initiative is unveiled.

Congress passes the Newborns' and Mothers' Health Protection Act requiring health insurance plans that offer maternity coverage to pay for at least a 48-hour hospital stay following vaginal childbirth or a 96-hour stay following a cesarean section.

U.S. tobacco company Liggett is instructed to pay more than $10 million for the medical treatment of smokers.

Nelson Mandela officially launches the Kick Polio Out of Africa campaign.

Malaria strikes Botswana, Mozambique, South Africa, Swaziland, and Zimbabwe.

Creutzfeldt-Jakob disease is identified as being caused by the same agent (prion) that causes bovine spongiform encephalitis (Mad Cow disease). Mad Cow disease emerged in the 1980s and affected thousands of cattle in the United Kingdom and Europe.

1996–97   Switzerland experiences a measles epidemic with more than 300 cases.

1997   Title XXI (State Child Health Insurance Program) is added to the Social Security Act in the United States.

Bird flu virus (H5N1), an avian influenza A virus, infects 18 patients after close contact with poultry; 6 of the 18 patients die.

Epidemic typhoid fever breaks out in Dushanbe, Tajikistan.

1998   Lyme disease vaccine is developed.

Rotavirus vaccine is developed.

In the United States, the Birth Defects Prevention Act passes Congress with March of Dimes support.

A settlement between the tobacco industry and 46 states is reached, requiring the industry to cease targeting youth and to pay $246 billion to states as repayment for the costs they paid out for tobacco-related health care.

1998–2000 Lithuania experiences an epidemic of mumps with more than 11,000 cases.

1999   A polio outbreak occurs in Angola with more than 800 cases and 50 deaths.

2000   The European Union bans leaded gasoline as a public health hazard.

The Netherlands experiences a measles epidemic with more than 1,750 cases.

Francis S. Collins and J. Craig Venter announce completion of the analysis (mapping) of the human genome.

LIST OF ABBREVIATIONS

ACS	American Cancer Society
ADA	American Dental Association
ADI	acceptable daily intake
AFL-CIO	American Federation of Labor and Congress of Industrial Organizations
AIDS	acquired immune deficiency syndrome
ALCOA	Aluminum Company of America
AMA	American Medical Association
APHA	American Public Health Association
AZT	azidothymidine
BBC	British Broadcasting Company
BCG	Bacillus Calmette-Guérin
BCME	bischloromethyl ether
BMI	body mass index
BPA	bisphenol A
CABG	coronary artery bypass graft
CARDIA	Coronary Artery Risk Development in Young Adults
CAT or CT	computerized axial tomography
CDC	Centers for Disease Control and Prevention
CME	chloromethyl methyl ether
CMS	Centers for Medicare and Medicaid Services
CVD	cardiovascular disease
CWP	coal worker's pneumoconiosis
DALY	disability-adjusted life year
DBCP	dibromochloropropane
DES	diethylstilbestrol
DDT	dichlorodiphenyltrichloroethane
DMFT	decayed, missing, and filled teeth
EHR	electronic health record
EKG	electrocardiogram
ELISA	enzyme-linked immunosorbent assay
EMR	electronic medical record
EPA	Environmental Protection Agency
ESRD	end-stage renal disease
ETS	environmental tobacco smoke
FASEB	Federation of American Societies for Experimental Biology

FDA	Food and Drug Administration
FFQ	food frequency questionnaire
FGM	female genital mutilation
GBD	Global Burden of Disease study
GRID	gay-related immune deficiency
HAART	highly active antiretroviral therapy
HIE	Health Insurance Experiment
HIP	Health Insurance Plan of New York
HIV	human immunodeficiency virus
HMO	health maintenance organization
HPV	human papilloma virus
HRT	hormone replacement therapy
HSV	herpes simplex virus
HTLV	human T-cell lymphotropic virus
IARC	International Agency for Research on Cancer
IBFAN	International Baby Food Action Network
ICD	International Classification of Diseases system
ICRC	International Committee of the Red Cross
IDU	injection drug user
INFACT	Infant Formula Action Coalition
IOM	Institute of Medicine
IRB	Institutional Review Board
IUD	intrauterine device
IV	intravenous
JECFA	Joint Expert Committee on Food Additives
KS	Kaposi's sarcoma
KSOI	Kaposi's sarcoma and opportunistic infections
LAV	lymphadenopathy virus
MCLG	maximum contaminant level goal
MCO	managed care organization
MDR	multidrug resistant
MONICA	Monitoring of Trends and Determinants in Cardiovascular Disease Study
MRC	Medical Research Council
MRFIT	Multiple Risk Factor Intervention Trial
NCGIH	National Conference of Governmental Industrial Hygienists
NCI	National Cancer Institute
NFIP	National Foundation for Infantile Paralysis
NHANES	National Health and Nutrition Examination Survey
NHS	National Health Service
NICE	National Institute for Clinical Excellence
NIH	National Institutes of Health
NIOSH	National Institute for Occupational Safety and Health

NLM	National Library of Medicine
NMR	nuclear magnetic resonance
NRC	National Research Council
OC	oral contraceptive
OIHP	Office International d'Hygiène Publique
ORT	oral rehydration therapy
OSHA	Occupational Safety and Health Administration
PAD	peripheral artery disease
PCP	*Pneumocystis carinii* pneumonia
PET	positron emission tomography
PHS	Public Health Service
PKU	phenylketonuria
PM	particulate matter
PPD	protein purified derivative
PV	poliovirus
PVD	peripheral vascular disease
RCP	Royal College of Physicians
RQ	Rose Questionnaire
SGSH	Study Group on Smoking and Health
SMON	subacute myelo-opticoneuropathy
TB	tuberculosis
TLV	threshold limit value
TORCH	toxoplasmosis, rubella, cytomegalovirus, herpes simplex, and others
UN	United Nations
UNICEF	United Nations International Children's Emergency Fund
VA	Veterans Administration
WHA	World Health Assembly
WHI	Women's Health Initiative
WHO	World Health Organization

PART I

Population Health Issues

Health is a state of complete physical, mental and social well-being and not merely the absence of disease or infirmity.

The enjoyment of the highest attainable standard of health is one of the fundamental rights of every human being without distinction of race, religion, political belief, economic or social condition.

The health of all peoples is fundamental to the attainment of peace and security and is dependent upon the fullest co-operation of individuals and States.

The achievement of any State in the promotion and protection of health is of value to all.

—*Constitution of the World Health Organization*, Geneva, 1948

CHAPTER 1

FOOD AND NUTRITION

I do not like broccoli. And I haven't liked it since I was a little kid and my mother made me eat it. I'm President of the United States and I'm not going to eat any more broccoli!
>   —George H. W. Bush (b. 1924), President of the United States
>   Spoken at a news conference, August 27, 1989

Paradoxically coexisting with undernutrition, an escalating global epidemic of overweight and obesity—"globesity"—is taking over many parts of the world.
>   —World Health Organization
>   http://www.who.int/nutrition/topics/obesity/en/index.html
>   (accessed 15 May 2009)

SIGNIFICANT EFFORTS WERE MADE IN IMPROVING the quality of food and its nutritional value over the course of the twentieth century, in both developed and developing nations. These efforts included but were not limited to fortifying foods to prevent diseases such as goiter, rickets, beriberi, and pellagra. Many nations passed legislation that would improve food safety and guarantee the accurate labeling of food products. Yet as the century came to a close, problems related to the global distribution of food and its nutritional quality remained. Large numbers of people faced malnutrition, including under- and overnutritional states linked with increased rates of morbidity, mortality, and adverse birth outcomes. This chapter begins with a discussion of food safety, then moves to the discovery of vitamins and the practice of food fortification, and concludes with current concerns about the international trend toward obesity.

FOOD SAFETY

Merchants have undoubtedly added substances to food products and used other shortcuts to increase their profit margins throughout history (e.g., adding water to milk or wine; adding offal or sawdust to ground meat products or selling meat from diseased animals; adding alum to whiten flour; or adding lead or other minerals to food products to slow spoilage). Today, rapid urbanization and globalization increasingly separate consumers from the places where food is produced and processed. This situation encourages producers and processors from areas with lax or absent regulations to cut corners in an effort to increase profits. In the 1990s, for example, many countries banned importation of British beef when it was discovered that feeding animal wastes to cattle led to Mad Cow Disease. The United States had infectious disease outbreaks traced to raspberries from Guatemala; strawberries, scallions, and cantaloupes from Mexico; carrots from Peru; and coconut milk from Thailand, to name but a few. And as globalization took root, Chinese goods, such as pet foods tainted with melamine, toothpaste containing antifreeze, and toys festooned with colorful lead paints flooded Western markets. China also exported problematic foods intended for human consumption, including frozen catfish treated with banned antibiotics, scallops and sardines contaminated with pathogenic bacteria, and mushrooms containing illegal pesticide residues.

The first law to protect consumers from food adulteration was passed by the British Parliament in 1860, but it had no means of enforcement until it was replaced by the 1875 Sale of Food and Drugs Act. In the United States, consumer protection began with the Pure Food and Drug Act of 1906, passed under President Theodore Roosevelt. That act provided for federal inspection of meat (see Volume I, Chapter 19) and forbade the manufacture, sale, or transportation of adulterated food products or poisonous patent medicines. For example, the act prevented turpentine from being added to cough medicines but allowed addictive substances, such as caffeine and cocaine, to be added to products such as Coca-Cola, as long as the products were accurately labeled.

The field of bacteriology advanced in the late nineteenth century as did sanitation for removing and limiting exposure to wastes, refrigeration for holding foods and reducing spoilage, and rapid transportation for moving foods from farm to market. Food safety also advanced with an understanding of the importance of handwashing, the safer handling of foods, meat and milk inspection, the inspection of food processing plants and places of food service, and the appropriate use of pesticides. Despite these precautions and technological advances, foodborne diseases remain widespread, both in developed and developing countries. In 2005 alone, the WHO estimated that contaminated food and drinking water accounted for about 1.8 million deaths. Furthermore, the WHO estimates that about 30 percent of the populations of industrialized countries continue to suffer from foodborne illnesses in any given year. The CDC reports that about 76 million cases of foodborne disease occur annually resulting in 325,000 hospitalizations and 5,000 deaths among Americans. Clearly, foodborne illness remains a public health challenge.

Attempts to manipulate the food supply in order to improve profit margins remain a serious concern in both developed and developing countries. Changes in the means of production, for instance, can lead to dangerous outcomes for food safety. Bovine Spongiform Encephalopathy (BSE), or Mad Cow Disease, emerged in England in 1986, the result of adding the remains of sick animals to cattle feed in an effort to increase the levels of protein in the feed. Changes in the pattern of consumption of foods can also lead to serious health concerns. For example, Chinese consumers' demand for raw seafood led to an increase in the incidence of parasitic diseases, especially *Clonorchis sinensis*, or Chinese liver fluke, in that nation. In 2007, about 12 million people were estimated to have the parasite, which can cause hepatic distomiasis, a potentially fatal liver disorder.

Clean Milk

Milk has been a staple food for human beings for millennia. Rapid urbanization in the nineteenth century resulted in crowding and unhealthful local environments, along with increased maternal mortality and infant abandonment. In the absence of sufficient numbers of wet nurses, infants became increasingly dependent upon bovine milk for survival. The milk supply was often of poor quality, obtained from cows that were fed on distillery swill. Dairy conditions and the milk handlers themselves were largely unclean. To improve profits, milk was often adulterated with water, which was also contaminated.

At the beginning of the twentieth century, two competing ideas emerged to improve the quality of milk. The first was designed to enforce controls at the level of milk production. Proponents of the "clean milk" campaign wanted animals inspected for disease and dairies inspected for cleanliness. Clean milk would then be certified and sold at select locations or at licensed milk stations. Physicians endorsed certified (clean, raw) milk and recommended it for its healthful effects. The clean milk campaign was also supported by sanitarians, many of whom saw the advantage of clean environments as protecting the public's health.

The second idea for improving the quality of milk was endorsed by those who favored a technological solution. The burden of bacterial contamination could be reduced by pasteurization, and the result of the effort would be improvements in mortality and morbidity rates. This technological method was endorsed by Milton J. Rosenau, Director of the Hygienic Laboratory of the U.S. Public Health Service (PHS). Despite the fact that pasteurization did not force milk producers to clean up their production environments, Rosenau stated that it did kill germs and save lives.

In 1924, the first documented statewide milk sanitation program was created for Alabama. In an effort to promote their product, dairies jumped on the bandwagon with claims that pasteurized milk was safer than raw milk. These efforts were quite successful as by 1936, half of all milk in the United States was pasteurized. Today, all milk that is shipped between states must be pasteurized, according to the uniform sanitation standards set out in the Grade A Pasteurized Milk Ordinance of the U.S. Department of Agriculture. Despite the fact that the majority of U.S. milk and milk products are pasteurized, the demand for clean, raw milk as an alternative continues to persist, bolstered by claims that pasteurization destroys healthful proteins in the milk.

Pasteurization works, but it is an expensive fix for reducing diseases from tainted and contaminated milk. The ability to produce and hold clean milk for limited time periods without expensive processing is, however, still important for populations in many areas of the world. Studies show that despite the primitive conditions under which milking takes place in some locations, milk produced with minimal use of equipment and placed directly into clean storage vessels has far lower bacterial counts than milk produced under mechanized circumstances in developed countries. Pastoralists of Ethiopia, Kenya, and Tanzania, for example, burn select plant material to produce smoke in order to disinfect the vessels used to hold clean milk. In India, an initiative to produce clean milk provides stainless steel pails and filters to individual milk producers. The milk is then transferred to plastic cans with lids so it can be transported to dairies. In 2006, the Erode District Milk Producers Cooperative Union in India had 729 milk producing cooperatives, with 131 of them run by women. The expansion of these and other efforts to produce clean milk hold great promise for improving the safety of milk worldwide.

VITAMINS AND FOOD FORTIFICATION

Diseases linked to dietary deficiencies have been known for centuries, despite the fact that the actual nutrient lacking in the diet may not have been able to be identified. For example, sailors at sea for lengthy periods often developed scurvy, a disease characterized by weakness, joint pains, loose teeth, easy bleeding, and death. Sick seamen were treated with a variety of concoctions to try to cure the condition until it was finally determined that scurvy was preventable and often reversible by consuming even small amounts of citrus fruits (see Volume I, Chapter 3). A second dietary scourge, beriberi, is characterized by weakness and loss of feeling in the lower extremities, edema of the trunk, difficulty in breathing, and heart failure. This disease was described in early Chinese and Japanese medical treatises but was unknown in Europe until Western physicians encountered it in colonial South and East Asia. In 1803, Thomas Christie, a British army physician serving in Sri Lanka, noted that citrus fruits had no effect on beriberi. It would be another century before the breakthrough to prevent this disease would come to light.

As the fields of biology and chemistry advanced in the nineteenth century, scientists determined that fats, proteins, starches, and sugars provide energy to the body. They also determined that certain minerals were required for normal bodily function. In the 1890s, Christiaan Eijkman, a Dutch military physician stationed in Java, tested beriberi as an infectious agent by injecting blood from sick soldiers into chicks. Some of the chicks developed the characteristic leg weakness of beriberi, but Eijkman noted that the chicks were fed only cooked, unpolished white rice. When he added rice polishings back to the diet of the chicks, their leg weakness disappeared. Eijkman discussed these findings with Adolphe Vorderman, the medical director of prisons in Java. Vorderman compared the diets of inmates at various prisons on the island and found that where they were fed brown rice, the incidence of beriberi was less than 1 in 10,000. Where prisoners were fed mostly white rice, the incidence of beriberi was 1 in 39. This descriptive epidemiologic finding led others to seek the ingredient in rice polishings that could cure the disease.

Gerrit Grijins at the University of Utrecht, the Netherlands, confirmed Eijkman's results in his laboratory in 1896. Grijins concluded that there must be substances in food that are necessary to the proper neurologic functioning of the body. If the elements could be isolated and synthesized, new treatments for neurological diseases might be possible.

Casimir Funk, a Polish biochemist working at the Lister Institute in London, reported in 1910 that he had isolated the active factor in rice polishings and that it belonged to the chemical class of "amines" (i.e., amino acids). He coined the term *vitamine* for "vital amines." In rapid succession, multiple vitamins and other nutrients were discovered and synthesized throughout the twentieth century. Table 1 lists some of the investigators and their discoveries that contributed significantly to our knowledge of nutrition during the period.

Vitamin research is a highly complex field, inexorably linked to the study of physiology and metabolism. Vitamins and other nutrients are reduced to their molecular structures and studied in relation to normal growth, development, and reproduction. Today, the total sum of metabolites in a biological organism is called its metabolome. The Human Metabolome Project, led by David Wishart of the University of Alberta, Canada, completed the first draft of the human metabolome in 2007. The emerging field of nutrigenomics seeks to link genomics, transcriptomics, proteomics, and metabolomics to human nutrition.

Table 1 Twentieth-Century Breakthroughs in Vitamin Research

Year	Investigator(s)	Substance
1912	Casimir Funk	Discovered vitamin B_1 (thiamin, aneurine hydrochloride)
1912–14	Elmer V. McCollum and M. Davis	Discovered vitamin A (retinol)
1912	A. Hoist and T. Froelich	Discovered vitamin C
1913	Thomas Osborne and Lafayette Mendel	Discovered vitamin A (fat-soluble) in butter
1915–16	Elmer V. McCollum	Discovered vitamin B complex
1922	Edward Mellanby	Discovered vitamin D
1922	Herbert Evans and Katherine Bishop	Discovered vitamin E
1926	D.T. Smith and E.G. Hendrick	Discovered vitamin B_2 (riboflavin)
1928	Adolf Otto Reinhold Windaus	Received Nobel Prize for "research into the constitution of the sterols and their connection with the vitamins"
1929	Christiaan Eijkman	Received Nobel Prize for discovering "antineuritic vitamin" (thiamine)
1929	Sir Frederick Gowland Hopkins	Received Nobel Prize for discovering "growth stimulating vitamins"
1933	Lucy Willis	Discovered folic acid (folate, vitamin B_9)
1933	Roger J. Williams	Isolated vitamin B_5 (pantothenic acid)
1934	George Hoyt Whipple	Received Nobel Prize for discovering "liver therapy in cases of anaemia" (B_{12})
1934	George Richards Minot	Received Nobel Prize for discovering "liver therapy in cases of anaemia" (B_{12})
1934	William Parry Murphy	Received Nobel Prize for discovering "liver therapy in cases of anaemia" (B_{12})
1935	Tadeusz Reichstein	Synthesized vitamin C
1936	Max Tishler and Robert R. Williams	Synthesized vitamin B_2
1936	Paul Gyorgy	Discovered vitamin B_6 (pyridoxine)

Table 1 *(continued)*

Year	Investigator(s)	Substance
1937	Conrad Elvehjem	Discovered vitamin B_3 (niacin, nicotinic acid)
1937	Walter Norman Haworth	Received Nobel Prize for "investigations on carbohydrates and vitamin C"
1937	Paul Karrer	Received Nobel Prize for "investigations on carotenoids, flavins and vitamins A and B2"
1938	Albert von Szent-Györgyi Nagyrápolt	Received Nobel Prize for "discoveries in connection with the biological combustion processes, with special reference to vitamin C and the catalysis of fumaric acid"
1938	Richard Kuhn	Received Nobel Prize for "work on carotenoids and vitamins"
1947	Otto Isler	Synthesized vitamin A
1943	Henrik Carl Peter Dam	Received Nobel Prize for "discovery of vitamin K"
1943	Edward Doisy	Received Nobel Prize for "discovery of the chemical nature of vitamin K"
1957	Frederick Crane	Discovered coenzyme Q10
1971	Robert Burns Woodward	Synthesized vitamin B_{12}

Iodine and Goiter

Goiter, or enlargement of the thyroid gland, is a widespread problem in areas of the world where there is iodine deficiency primarily because the iodine has been leached out of soils subjected to severe glacial melt, intense rainfall, or flooding. The condition was successfully treated by the ancient Chinese, Greeks, and Romans by adding seaweed and sea sponges to the diets of populations living in areas where goiter was prevalent. As early as the sixteenth century, Paracelsus hypothesized that goiter was caused by a deficiency of minerals in drinking water. Even though the biology and chemistry of the disease were not yet understood in the nineteenth century, Switzerland required that all table salt be iodized as a preventive for goiter in 1840.

A series of research papers on goiter and its treatment in a variety of mostly farm animals rapidly confirmed that iodine was a successful treatment for the disease. In the endemic goiter belt of the upper Midwest region of the United States, physicians and research scientists began to consider whether these findings could be extrapolated to humans. If so, countless cases of goiter could be treated or prevented. For example, in 1921 physicians David Marine and O.P. Kimball reported that about 28 percent of Akron, Ohio, schoolchildren who did not have iodine added to their diet had goiter, whereas only 0.2 percent of those with trace amounts of iodine in their diets had the condition. They proposed giving iodine directly to patients.

Goiter was such a problem that draft boards seeking conscripts for World War I found up to 30 percent of eligible men in Michigan were disqualified for service due to the condition. To address the widespread problem, the Michigan State Medical Society formed an Iodized Salt Committee. The committee set up a study to evaluate the impact of iodized salt on goiter and found spectacular results, with goiter incidence inversely proportional to the iodine content of the local water supply. David Murray Cowie, a professor at the University of Michigan, and the Michigan Medical Society began to encourage salt manufacturers to adopt the Swiss process for iodation of their products. On May 1, 1924, iodized salt appeared on grocery shelves in Michigan for the first time. By that fall, iodized salt was distributed nationally. No ill effects have ever been documented from iodized table salt, and no federal regulations on its use have been formulated in the United States. Since 1972, however, salt that is not iodized but destined for sale in the United States must be labeled "This salt does not supply iodide, a necessary nutrient." The results of iodizing salt have been significant as the vast majority of the population of the Americas no longer suffers from goiter.

Goiter is not the only problem caused by iodine deficiency. Today we know that low levels of iodine can cause stillbirth and miscarriage, hypothyroidism, impaired growth, and mental and neurological disorders. These neurological conditions may manifest along a range of adverse outcomes, from poor school performance to the most severe form—cretinism. The WHO uses two measures to determine whether iodine deficiency is a public health problem for nations: total goiter prevalence (TGP) and median urinary iodine (UI). Using these measures, nearly two billion people in 54 countries had insufficient iodine intake in 2005; this included one-third of the world's school-age children. Iodized salt or providing foods enriched with iodized salt is important for improving the health of individuals in these iodine-deficient areas.

Enrichment of Flour

Changes in flour milling processes in the early twentieth century brought improved industrial efficiency and improved product texture, but the result was flour with only one-eleventh of the thiamin it had under the stone milling process. The new form of flour and the baked goods using it put consumers at risk for beriberi and pellagra. Pellagra was already a serious concern in the early 1900s in the American South (see Volume I, Chapter 21), where rates were particularly high. Additionally, the nation was coming out of the Great Depression during which nutritional deficiencies left their mark. The low number of men fit for military service caused concern about the nation's ability to mount a fighting force.

In Britain, flour was enriched with thiamin as soon as commercial synthesis became available. In 1936, the American Medical Association (AMA) Council on Foods and Nutrition recommended that cereal and flour products in the United States be enriched with B vitamins and iron. Health professionals picked up the cause, recommending enriched bread and flour as preventives against nutritional deficiency diseases. Bakers added high-vitamin yeast to breads and other bakery products and used increased marketing techniques to promote their improved wares. By 1942, however, only 40 percent of bread and flour was enriched in the United States. The problem was that the non-enriched, cheaper items were still available and households with limited means selected them in order to stretch their food budgets.

Change can come quickly when national security is threatened, and it did. In 1941, a resolution of the Food and Nutrition Board of the Institute of Medicine (IOM) encouraged consumption of enriched bread and flour. The U.S. Army decided that enriched products would result in a healthier civilian population, the source of badly needed military recruits. Both of these efforts spurred additional advertising to promote enriched products, but it was the signature of President Franklin D. Roosevelt on War Food Order No. 1 in 1943 that truly made the difference. His pen stroke made enriched bread the temporary law of the land. Today, although both enriched and regular flour are generally available, most households continue to consume enriched bread, flour, and other cereal products.

Vitamin D and Rickets

Vitamin D is required for absorption of dietary calcium in the gut. Adults with low levels of vitamin D can develop osteomalacia, a disease characterized by bone weakness and easy fracturing. Children with low levels of vitamin D can develop rickets, a disease characterized by bone pain or tenderness, dental problems, weak muscles, and growth problems, as well as skeletal deformities such as bowlegs and knock-knees. Infants and children living in high latitudes where sunlight is low, as well as children in countries where staying indoors during early childhood is the cultural norm, remain at risk for rickets. Children with vegetarian diets and infants with lactating mothers who have low levels of vitamin D may also be at increased risk.

In 1919, Edward Mellanby discovered that cod-liver oil could prevent rickets in puppies. Shortly after, S. J. Cowell found that irradiated milk was more effective than regular milk in stimulating bone calcification because it converts inactive ergosterol into vitamin D. Irradiated milk had a consumer following for a short period of time until 1932, when vitamin D was purified and isolated, thus allowing milk to be directly fortified. Today, milk and many cereal grains consumed in the United States are fortified with vitamin D, though other dairy products, such as cheese and ice cream, generally are not. Orange juice is now offered with both calcium and vitamin D supplementation. Canada routinely fortifies both milk and margarine with vitamin D. In contrast, the United Kingdom and the Netherlands do not fortify milk or milk products. Norway has limited vitamin D fortification of foods, and Japan has none. Instead, these nations recommend sensible sun exposure and a varied diet rich in oily fish.

Folic Acid

The most recent food fortification program in the United States was initiated in 1988 when folic acid was added to cereals and grain products. Folic acid is the synthesized form of folate, a naturally occurring, water-soluble B vitamin (B9) found in leafy green vegetables, nuts, berries, and some fruits. The story of folate begins in the 1930s in Mumbai, India, when Lucy Willis demonstrated that anemia in pregnant women could be corrected by giving the women brewer's yeast. The substance in brewer's yeast responsible for correcting the anemia was subsequently identified as folate. Folate was later isolated from spinach in 1941 and synthesized as folic acid by researchers at Lederle Laboratory in 1945.

Although folate did cure some anemias, it was also found to enhance the growth of tumor cells. This knowledge that folate affected rapidly dividing tissues led researchers to develop a new anti-cancer treatment (methotrexate) and to consider whether folate was critical in another situation where cells were rapidly dividing—fetal development. They found that low folate levels were one of the factors linked to malformations of the spinal cord (neural tube defects) in newborns. Clinical trials with prenatal vitamins containing folic acid demonstrated lowered rates of neural tube defects, leading the PHS and the IOM in 1992 to recommend that all women of reproductive age consume at least 400 micrograms of folic acid daily. Policymakers in both the United States and Canada passed legislation requiring that flour and uncooked cereal grains be fortified with folic acid by 1998. Studies monitoring the prevalence of neural tube defects in both countries reported a subsequent decline in these adverse birth outcomes but warned that the results could be due to factors other than folic acid fortification of the food supply. In addition, some warning flags have since been raised about too much folic acid intake. For example, high folic acid intake has been associated with increased cognitive decline in the elderly and with suppressed immune function in postmenopausal women.

MALNUTRITION

Malnutrition is a term encompassing both under- and overnutritional states. Undernutrition results from the inadequate intake of food, specifically protein, vitamins, or trace elements. Undernutrition may also occur where there is adequate food intake but the body cannot process it (malabsorption) or where the body has faced an excessive loss of nutrients due to dieting, purging, or diarrheal diseases. The main causes of undernutrition include drought, famine, economic struggles, and war. The United Nations (UN) World Food Program estimated that there were 854 million undernourished people in the world in 2003, mostly in developing nations. The UN also estimated that one in seven people do not get enough food for a healthy and active life; this makes hunger and malnutrition the number one health risk in the world (see United Nations Millenium Goals, Appendix G).

The converse of undernutrition, overnutrition results from consuming excess calories or specific nutrients. Some political scientists claim that overnutrition is the natural result of economic prosperity, a condition to be expected as the world succeeds in bringing the developing countries into the global arena with free trade. These social scientists are less concerned about the health effects of obesity than with the preservation of the social order, which tends to be more stable in times of economic prosperity.

From a public health perspective, overnutrition can result in overweight and obesity, both of which increase the risk for coronary heart disease, diabetes, hypertension, hyperlipidemia, osteoarthritis, and other chronic disorders. The speed with which obesity is spreading around the world has led some to question whether globalization is going to be the underlying cause of the world's next major epidemic. The UN has already coined the term *globesity* to describe its growing concern.

During the course of the twentieth century, efforts to improve food safety and knowledge about nutrition increased. We now know how to prevent beriberi, goiter, pellagra, rickets, and scurvy. We understand the importance of clean milk, as well as many of the nutritional functions of vitamins and trace elements. Clearly, food in developed nations is safer than a century ago, and the labeling of retail foods has improved. For example, in response to the knowledge that trans fats are a risk factor for heart disease, New York City changed its health code to ban the substance from restaurants as of October 2007. Not only New York City's restaurants but also many restaurants and food chains across the

United States now offer calorie counts on menus, some with codes in the margins that indicate that the food is heart healthy. Supermarkets offer organic as well as non-organic produce though organics are more expensive. Larger markets offer high-cost choices of fish (antibiotic free, wild caught), poultry (antibiotic free, free range), and meats (antibiotic free, grass fed). Smaller markets, however, usually carry only one choice, as do bodegas, convenience stores, food kiosks, and pushcarts. Providing more food choices to people in developed nations is unlikely to impact world hunger or globesity. On the other hand, it might change the rates of chronic disease in the subpopulations choosing to make the change. Only time will tell if offering more types of fortified foods, banning trans fats, and increasing the numbers of people choosing to eat organic foods and antibiotic-free meats will reduce obesity.

Obesity increases the costs of medical care because of its link to multiple chronically morbid conditions. It is rapidly becoming a problem for developing countries that are already suffering substantial rates of morbidity due to iron, iodine, and vitamin A nutritional deficiencies. The WHO estimated that in 2007, adjusting for ethnic differences, more than 1.7 billion people were overweight worldwide. The prevalence of adult obesity between 2003 and 2005 was 5 percent for people living in rural China, 23 percent for those living in Canada and England, 33 percent in the United States, 50 and 60 percent (for men and women, respectively) in Mexico, 75 percent in urban Samoa, and 80 percent for American Indians in Arizona.

With the prevalence of overweight and obesity rising at the current rate, the WHO estimates a global pandemic of diabetes with 366 million prevalent cases by 2030. The largest number of cases—as many as 228 million—are estimated for developing countries in Southeast Asia, the Western Pacific region, India, and China. Complications from diabetes are expected as well, especially increased rates of cardiovascular disease, hypertension, and kidney disease. The burden of these chronic diseases could be crippling for some nations, not only because of health care costs, but also because of loss of human capital and economic drain.

Selected Readings

The readings for this chapter begin with Elmer V. McCollum's retrospective on his life's work in nutritional research. McCollum describes the way fundamental nutritional research evolved during the early part of the twentieth century and the scientific collaborations that led to the discovery of micronutrient vitamins A and D. He reminds us that these discoveries led to ideas about food supplementation, treatments for eye diseases, and the virtual disappearance of rickets worldwide. McCollum also tips his hat to rats, creatures who contributed mightily to nutritional research in the laboratory.

Alfred Sommer, an American ophthalmologist, worked for the CDC's Epidemic Intelligence Service in the 1970s. Sommer was charged with finding a way to treat night blindness among populations with vitamin A-deficient diets. A large-scale randomized field trial was set up in Aceh, Indonesia, and Sommer's results were astonishing. When he gave vitamin A drops to children suffering from night blindness, not only did their eyesight return to normal, but they also had far lower mortality rates than did children who did not receive the drops. The second reading contains the results of that trial. However, Sommer's findings were challenged by experts who were skeptical. This led to another study in Nepal that confirmed Sommer's findings.

The last reading by Barry Popkin makes us consider the impact of globalization on nutrition, especially for those trapped in the lower socioeconomic strata of both developed and developing countries. The work is abridged in that tables and figures that are discussed in detail in the text have been removed to save space, but their removal does not hinder the impact of the work. There is, for example, a detailed discussion of the impact of the nutrition transition, moving populations from morbidity and mortality linked primarily to infectious conditions to those from primarily chronic ones. Popkin notes that there is a moral imperative to address undernutrition, but there is no similar perception that obesity and chronic disease will overwhelm medical resources in the near future. We must, he states, formulate methods to deal with dietary excess among the global poor.

BIBLIOGRAPHY

Andersson M, Takkouche B, Egli I, Allen HE, and de Benoist B. 2005. Current global iodine status and progress over the last decade toward the elimination of iodine deficiency. *Bull World Health Organ* 83 (7): 518–25.

Barclay AJG, Foster A, and Sommer A. 1987. Vitamin A supplements and mortality related to measles: a randomised clinical trial. *Brit Med J* 294:294–96.

Bishai D and Nalubola R. 2000. The history of food fortification in the United States: its relevance for current fortification efforts in developing countries. *Economic Development and Cultural Change* 51 (1): 37–53.

Block G. 1982. A review of validations of dietary assessment methods. *Am J Epid* 115:492–505.

Brush BE and Altland JK. 1952. Goiter prevention with iodized salt: results of a thirty-year study. *J Clin Endocrinol Metab* 12 (10): 1380–88.

Burks JD. 1911. Clean milk and public health. *Annals of the American Academy of Political and Social Science* 37 (2): 192–206.

Centers for Disease Control and Prevention. 1999. Achievements in Public Health, 1900–1999: Safer and healthier foods. *MMWR* 48 (40): 905–13.

Cheftel JC. 2005. Food and nutrition labelling in the European Union. *Food Chemistry* 93, doi:10.1016/j.foodchem.2004.11.041.

Council on Foods and Nutrition. 1969. Improvement of nutritive quality of foods. *JAMA* 205 (12): 160–61.

Craig W and Belkin M. 1925. The prevention and cure of rickets. *The Scientific Monthly* 20 (5): 541–50.

Delange F, de Benoist B, Pretell E, and Dunn JT. 2001. Iodine deficiency in the world: where do we stand at the turn of the century? *Thyroid* 1 (5): 7–47.

deOnis M. 2000. Measuring nutritional status in relation to mortality. *Bull World Health Organ* 78 (10): 1271–74.

Dunn JT. 2001. Correcting iodine deficiency is more than just spreading around a lot of iodine. *Thyroid* 11 (4): 363–64.

Food and Agriculture Organization of the United Nations (FAO). 2005. Understanding the Codex Alimentarius. Rome: FAO, World Health Organization. http://www.fao.org/docrep/008/y7867e/y7867e00.htm (accessed May 16, 2007).

Gómez F, Ramos Galvan R, Frenk S, Cravioto Muñoz J, Chávez R, and Vázques J. 1956. Mortality in second and third degree malnutrition. *J Trop Pediatr* 2 (September): 77–83.

Gowen JW, Murray JM, Gooch ME, and Ames FB. 1926. Rickets, ultra-violet light and milk (in Special Articles). New series, *Science* 63 (1621): 97–98.

Hawkes C. 2006. Uneven dietary development: linking the policies and processes of globalization with the nutrition transition, obesity, and diet-related chronic diseases. Review, *Globalization and Health* 2 (4), doi:10.1186/1744-8603-2-4.

Hess AF. 1921. Newer aspects of some nutritional disorders. *JAMA* 76:693–700.

Hess AF. 1932. The role of activated milk in the anti-rickets campaign. *Am J Public Health & The Nation's Health* 22 (12): 1215–19.

Horton S. 2006. The economics of food fortification. *J Nutr* 136:1068–71.

Keys A. 1980. *Seven Countries: A Multivariate Analysis of Death and Coronary Heart Disease.* Cambridge, MA: Harvard University Press.

Kohn LA. 1975. Goiter, iodine, and George W. Goler: the Rochester experiment. *Bull Hist Med* 49 (3): 389–99.

Lawrence M. 2005. Challenges in translating scientific evidence into mandatory food fortification policy: an antipodean case study of the folate-neural tube defect relationship. *Public Health Nutr* 8 (8), doi: 10.1079/PHN2005749.

Marine D and Kimball OP. 1921. The prevention of simple goiter in man. *J Am Med Assoc* 77 (14): 1068–70.

Marine D and Williams WW. 1908. The relation of iodin to the structure of the thyroid gland. *Arch Int Med* 1:349–84. Reprinted in *Nutr Rev* 33 (11) (1975): 338–40.

Markel H. 1987. When it rains it pours: endemic goiter, iodized salt, and David Murray Cowie, MD. *Am J Public Health* 77 (2): 219–29.

McCollum EV, Simmonds N, Kinney M, Shipley PG, and Park EA. 1922. Studies on experimental rickets. XVII. The effects of diets deficient in calcium and in fat-soluble A in modifying the histological structure of the bones. *Am J Hyg* 2:97–106. Reprinted in *Am J Epidemiol* 141 (4) (1995): 280–96. (See Sommer below.)

McCollum EV, Simmonds N, Becker JE, and Shipley PG. 1922. Studies of experimental rickets. XXI. An experimental demonstration of the existence of a vitamin which promotes calcium deposition. *J Biol Chem* 53:293–312. Reprinted in *Nutr Rev* 33(2) (1975): 48–50.

Mellanby E. 1919. An experimental investigation of rickets. *Lancet* 1:407–12. Reprinted in *Nutr Rev* 34 (11) (1976): 338–40.

Mitchell JM, Eiman J, Whipple DV, and Stokes J. 1932. Protective value for infants of various types of vitamin D fortified milk. *Am J Public Health* 22 (12): 1220–29.

Nestel P, Bouis HE, Meenakshi JV, and Pfeiffer W. 2006. Biofortification of staple food crops. *J Nutr* 136:1064–67.

Oakley GP. 1997. Let's increase folic acid fortification and include vitamin B-12. *Am J Clin Nutr* 65:1889–90.

Olin RM. 1924. Iodin deficiency and prevalence of simple goiter in Michigan. *J Am Med Assoc* 82 (17): 1328–32.

Park YK, McCowell MA, Hanson EA, and Yetley EA. 2001. History of cereal-grain fortification in the United States. *Nutrition Today* 36 (3): 124–37.

Pettifor JM. 2004. Nutritional rickets: deficiency of vitamin D, calcium, or both? *Am J Clin Nutr* Suppl. 80:1725S–9S.

Rafter GW. 1987. Elmer McCollum and the disappearance of rickets. *Perspect Biol Med* 30 (4): 527–34.

Romano PS, Waitzman NJ, Scheffler RM, and Pi RD. 1995. Folic acid fortification of grain: an economic analysis. *Am J Public Health* 85 (5): 667–76.

Shama T and Villalpando S. 2006. The role of enriched foods in infant and child nutrition. *Brit J Nutr* 96 (Suppl. 1), doi: 10.1079/BJN20061704.

Shipley PG, Park EA, McCollum EV, and Simmonds N. 1921. Studies on experimental rickets. VII. The relative effectiveness of cod-liver oil as contrasted with butter fat for protecting the body against insufficient calcium in the presence of normal phosphorus supply. *Am J Hyg* 1:512–25. Reprinted in *Nutr Rev* 42 (5) (1984): 192–94.

Slimani N, Deharveng G, Unwin I, Southgate DAT, Vignat J, Skeie G, et al. 2007. The EPIC nutrient database project (ENDB): a first attempt to standardize nutrient databases across the 10 European countries participating in the EPIC study. *Eur J Clin Nutr* 61: 1037–56.

Sommer A. 1995. Invited commentary on "Studies on experimental rickets. XVII. The effects of diets deficient in calcium and in fat-soluble A in modifying the histological structure of the bones." *Am J Epidemiol* 141 (4): 279.

Tice JA, Ross E, Coxson PG, Rosenberg I, Weinstein MC, Hunink MG, Goldman PA, Williams L, and Goldman L. 2001. Cost-effectiveness of vitamin therapy to lower plasma homocysteine levels for the prevention of coronary heart disease: effect of grain fortification and beyond. *JAMA* 286 (8): 936–43. For comments see Bostom AG. 2002. Letter. *JAMA*. 287 (2): 190 and author reply 191–92. Also see Sunder-Plassman G and Födinger M. 2002. Letter. *JAMA* 287 (2): 190 and author reply 191–92. Also see Pogach L. 2002. Letter. *JAMA* 287 (2): 191–92.

United States Department of Health, Education, and Welfare. 1980. Nutritional quality of foods; Addition of nutrients. Final policy statement. 21 CFR Part 103 [Docket No. 79N-0377]. Federal Register 45 (18) (January 25): 6314–24.

Wald G. 1935. Vitamin A in eye tissues. *J Gen Physiol* 18:905–15. Reprinted in Nutr Rev 43 (8) (1985): 244–46.

Waserman MJ. 1972. Henry L. Coit and the certified milk movement in the development of modern pediatrics. *Bull Hist Med* 46 (4): 359–90.

Weart EL. 1929. The conquest of goiter. *North American Review* 228 (3): 359–66.

West KP Jr., Katz J, Shrestha SR, LeClerq SC, Khatrv SK, Pradhan EK, Adhikari R, Wu LS, Pokhrel RP, and Sommer A. 1995. Mortality of infants <6 mo of age supplemented with vitamin A: a randomized, double-masked trial in Nepal. *Am J Clin Nutr* 62:143–48.

The Paths to the Discovery of Vitamins A and D
(1967)

Elmer Verner McCollum
Professor Emeritus of Biochemistry
Johns Hopkins University, Baltimore, Maryland

In 1907, on completing my studies at Yale, I was, by the standards of the period prepared to undertake investigations in organic and biological chemistry. I wanted an academic position. The only opportunity I found was an instructorship in Agricultural Chemistry in the College of Agriculture at the University of Wisconsin. I was to work principally in the Experiment Station under the direction of Professor E. B. Hart. The project was to find the cause or causes of the malnutrition manifested by cows which had been restricted through most of their period of growth to rations derived solely from single plant sources, viz., the wheat, oat, and corn (maize) plant. Malnutrition was severe in the wheat-fed cows. They were inferior in appearance, had become blind, and delivered very premature, undersized, dead calves. The oat-fed cows looked better, their eyes appeared normal, and though they carried their calves to term, none survived longer than a few hours. In marked contrast, the corn-fed cows were in fine condition and produced vigorous calves. Chemical analysis had shown that the rations were of equivalent nutritive value. Obviously the chemical method of analysis was unreliable as a guide to nutritive values.

I had never analyzed a food, nor conducted an animal experiment. I set to work to educate myself by reading books, journal articles and bulletins. After consultation with Professor Hart, I began to make extensive analyses of the blood, urine, milk and feces of the calves in hopes that the data secured might furnish a clue to the cause or causes of their contrasting condition.

The sources of information available to me afforded no assistance for the solution of my problem. I decided to examine all abstracts of scientific publications in recent decades relating to the chemistry of plant and animal substances, physiology, and nutrition studies with men and animals to seek facts or suggestions as to what I may do next. These were available in Maly's *Jahres-Bericht Uber die Fortschritte der Thier-Chemie*. There were 37 volumes covering the publications from 1870 to 1907. I bought the file, and of evenings leafed the pages of every volume, studying all abstracts with care. My knowledge of biochemistry was greatly enlarged. While thus engaged my mind was alert to discover ideas which suggested philosophic insight.

In the volume for 1880 I found a description of the experiments of N. Lunin, a Russian student of the distinguished Professor C. von Bunge at Dorpat. Lunin restricted mice to a diet of isolated, purified protein (casein), carbohydrates, fats and an inorganic salt mixture made in imitation of the ash of milk. The mice failed rapidly and all were dead within 21 days. Mice, to which he gave only milk, were in good condition and were lively at 60 days. He concluded that milk contained unidentified nutrients not hitherto suspected. In other volumes I found descriptions of similar experiments with "purified" food-stuffs described by 13 other investigators. All reported that their animals, mostly mice, failed rapidly and died when confined to such diets. I took notes on the studies, and concluded that the most important problem in nutrition was to discover what was lacking in diets containing only "purified" constituents.

Another result of this study of the experiments of earlier biochemists was the discovery that no one had attempted to investigate the degree of completeness of individual natural food substances such as leaf, seed, tuber, root or fruit, as sole source of essential nutrients for an animal. Such an inquiry would be the simplest possible type of nutrition investigation. If in any case the animals failed nutritionally it should be possible to systematically study the problem of what was lacking by supplementing the food with single or multiple known substances . . . If this approach was not successful the addition of very small amounts of one or another natural food, should reveal where the missing unidentified nutrient was to be found. From this reasoning the thought occurred that animal feeding studies with two-source diets, one constituent small, the other large, should reveal which foods made good the deficiencies of each other. Similar studies, I concluded, should be made using single type animal derivatives— muscle, liver, kidney, etc. Nothing in this type of study had ever been attempted. Reflecting on these ideas, I saw a vista of great promise for revealing new knowledge of the biochemistry of nutrition.

It also occurred to me that experiments should be made with small animals. They grew to maturity in a short time, reproduced, reared young, and had a short life-span. They ate little, so one could afford to do the necessary chemical work on the diets. The life history of the animals could be observed.

While engaged in these speculations I became convinced that the project we were engaged in with cows, fed highly complex chemical rations could not lead to the discovery of anything of importance and that I was wasting my time.

I was in a predicament, because Professor Hart was elated by his cow experiment and it had been given wide publicity. Animal husbandrymen were enthusiastically discussing it. The discovery of what was wrong with the wheat ration would reflect great credit on us. But I was 28 years old. It was imperative that I accomplish something of scientific worth to gain advancement and establish myself as a productive scientist. It was dishonest for me to continue accumulating analytical data which I considered worthless, so it was imperative that I divulge my thoughts and take the consequences.

Professor Hart was astonished and offended at my pronouncement on the cow project. He was contemptuous of my suggestion that we turn to the rat as an experimental animal. I was at fault in wanting to abandon so soon the project on which I had agreed to work. Our interview was brief and stormy.

Two days later I told about my speculations to Emeritus Professor Stephen M. Babcock. He responded enthusiastically, saying that mine was the best suggestion he had ever heard of for a study of foods and nutrition. He took me to the office of Dean H. L. Russell and asked me to tell him of my ideas. Dr. Russell's answer was an emphatic "no." The rat was a farm pest and it would never do to spend Federal and State funds on experiments with rats. Dr. Babcock was the most honored man in the College of Agriculture, and because he insisted that he wanted to know what could be learned from my plan, I was meekly permitted to set up my rat colony. No formal project was made of my enterprise, and no funds were allocated for its support.

I made cages out of boxes in which supplies came to the laboratory. I needed quarter-inch wire netting for one side, and placed on Professor Hart's a desk a requisition for two dollars' worth. He declined to sign it and I bought it out of my $1,200 annual salary. I caught wild rats and tried to use them, but they were so frightened and ferocious that I discarded them and bought, at my own cost, a dozen albino rats from which I built up my colony.

The ingredients of my diets were prepared identically while doing analytical work on the cows, but I cared for my rats outside of regular work hours. Starting with enthusiasm I soon realized that although most of my projected experiments would be terminated in a short time because of failure of the little rats to survive on my "purified" diets, much time would be required to complete the several hundred tests on formulas I had devised. It would take several years to accumulate sufficient data to enable me to make any important conclusions. I doubted I should be permitted to continue so long without justifying myself by results.

In July 1909, I had the good fortune to have Miss Marguerite Davis asked me to take her as a student in biochemistry. She had just graduated at the University of California at Berkeley, and had come to Madison to live with her father. I gave her a place in the laboratory and assigned some exercises, and from time to time stopped to talk with her. Before long I told her what I was trying to do with my rat colony. She was enthusiastic about the project and volunteered to take care of the rats. I at once began to teach her rat housekeeping, and began the construction of more cages. Before long we were carrying on 10 or more times as many experiments as I alone could manage. It was due to her interest and loyalty to the enterprise that we made important discoveries.

It had been proposed that certain foreign rations which failed to give satisfactory results were deficient in certain organic phosphorylated compounds, e.g., phosphoproteins, lecithin, cephalin or nucleic acids. I was able to demonstrate that rats could synthesize all such compounds using inorganic phosphates as [a] source of phosphorus—an important discovery at that time.

At the outset of my rat experiments I was aware of the great differences in the amino acid make-up of different proteins, as had been shown by chemists. Hopkins, in 1906 had demonstrated the indispensability of tryptophan. More than a year after I started work with rats and the "purified" diet, Osborne and Mendel began work with rats to study the comparative values of proteins of widely different chemical composition. They included in their diets a single isolated protein and 28.3% of dried whey from which lactalbumin had been removed by coagulation. This supplied sufficient of all identified nutrients to make their growth studies successful. They interpreted their results without considering unidentified dietary essentials. They dramatized the significance of individual amino acids, confirming the differences shown by chemists.

Our first highly important discovery was that a certain diet which I supposed to contain only "purified" substances, was able to support growth and apparent well-being for a few weeks when either butter fat or the fat of egg yolk were included, but when the fat was supplied by lard or olive oil, the rats soon failed nutritionally and manifested an eye condition characterized by swollen lids, ulceration of the cornea, and destruction of the eye. We called this nutrient fat-soluble A. It is now known as vitamin A. Later I was to learn that the diet, which contained commercial milk sugar, was inadequate to support life when the sugar was recrystallized. Furthermore the mother liquor from crystallization of lactose was of significant value in improving the condition of the little rats. It became evident that we had proven that there was a water-soluble as well as a fat-soluble unidentified essential nutrient. This we confirmed in our studies of the dietary deficiencies of polished rice. At the outset of our studies I was not acquainted with the work of Eijkman and of Grijns on the experimental production of polyneuritis in birds by restricting them to a diet of polished rice. But the "toxicity" theory of Eijkman and the "deficiency" theory of Grijns had been debated by medical writers for two decades. We independently discovered what I believed at the time to be the antiberi-beri substance.

The discovery of a fat-soluble indispensable nutrient (vitamin A) aroused great interest among the biochemists and physiologists. Hitherto all fats had been considered as sources of energy only and were believed to be alike on an equal caloric basis. We described the eye conditions and published pictures of rats exhibiting the disorder. We extended our studies and found that fats from liver and kidney, and ether extract of the leaf of a plant supplied the new nutrient. The earliest study of the pathological changes in the eye condition was made in my laboratory by Dr. S. Mori, a Japanese ophthalmologist, who saw pictures of our rat's eyes in the new deficiency state, and spent a year making histological studies of the eye, the lachrymal, harderian and mibomian glands. I prepared for him rats in several stages of deficiency for vitamin A, and he concluded that keratinization of epithelial cells, of whatever type of specialization as to function, was the primary cause of the pathological manifestations of the eyes. Keratinization destroyed the function of the tear glands, with consequent stagnation of tears in the conjunctival sac. This permitted overgrowth of the eye and inner surfaces of the eyelids by microorganisms, ulceration of the cornea and destruction of the eye.

That liver fats contained the new nutrient soon brought to light that a condition long known as night blindness was cured by eating liver. In ancient Egypt a household remedy for night blindness was eating liver of a black cock. In Newfoundland, where night blindness was common in 1912, the belief prevailed that fishermen whose eyes were exposed to the glare of sunlight on water, who could not see in twilight or darkness, were cured by eating the liver of a sea gull. Within a few years it emerged that vitamin A is essential for regeneration of light sensitive visual purple of the retina. The discovery of vitamin A induced an increasing number of scientists to attempt its isolation, chemical identification and synthesis. Its functions other than those relating to the eye invited inquiry by biochemists, physiologists and pathologists. After half a century it is still a prominent subject for investigation.

Examination of the photographs which we published showed that by the end of 1916, when we had completed application of what I called a biological method for an analysis of a foodstuff, we had produced several kinds of dietary deficiency diseases. We had completed over 1,600 experiments. The kinds of information secured about the dietary properties of single seeds, tubers, root vegetables, alfalfa leaf, wheat germs, refined wheat flour and cornmeal, constituted an array of information of an entirely new kind. We had also shown as a source of nutrients the superiority of liver and kidney over muscle, and the extent to which gelatin supplied amino acids which were not optimally abundant in the protein mixture in several seeds.

Among the effects produced by certain of our diets, were strongly contrasting appearance of the rats, loss of hair on different parts of the body, scaliness of the skin and in others dermatitis. Abnormalities of body form, posture, stunted size, sudden decline and death of rats which had grow well for a time; in some, fertility was decreased; some were sterile; others gave birth to dead or of living, but nonviable young, etc. Many had the eye disorder already mentioned.

It was evident to me that here was pathology of several types which was caused by deficiencies or excesses, or unfavorable quantitative relations among the nutrients already known. My approach to this study was that of a chemist, and I was keenly aware of my inability to interpret the meaning of symptoms. I carried with me photographs of rats with contrasting symptoms and showed them to physicians, pathologists and veterinarians. I explained the nature of the faults in certain diets, but in most cases the defects in the diets were a mystery. None of the people contacted were interested and they gave me little or no assistance.

My hope at the outset that my comprehensive project for studying the properties of foods might assist in explaining the cause of the malnutrition of the wheat-fed cows, was realized. When we discovered that the leaf of the plant is a far superior source of essential nutrients than the seed, reflection brought to memory that we had not fed the leaf of wheat to the cows. We did not grow wheat on the experiment station farm except in plots for testing varieties for their performance in the short Wisconsin summer. We had purchased wheat, wheat gluten and wheat straw secured from neighboring farmers. In threshing, the whirring teeth of the cylinder beat the wheat leaves to bits too small to be picked up with a pitchfork, so when the farmers brought us straw, they left the leaves on the farm. The two most serious deficiencies in the wheat plant rations were calcium and vitamin A.

Our experiments were described in a series of papers in scientific journals and attracted much favorable comment. As evidence of this, an invitation was extended to me to give a lecture before the Harvey Society in New York on January 17, 1917, on "The Supplementary Relations Among Our Common Food-stuffs." The following day Professor William H. Howell offered me the professorship in chemistry at the newly established School of Hygiene and Public Health at the Johns Hopkins University. I accepted and moved my rat colony to Baltimore, leaving about 100 behind, which formed the basis of the colony with which Professor Hart and his associates accomplished highly meritorious investigations. Our work led to the setting up of rat colonies in other institutions. The rat became highly popular as a subject for nutrition studies.

At the Johns Hopkins Medical School I was fortunate in securing excellent collaboration of Drs. Edwards A. Park and Paul G. Shipley which resulted in the discovery of a second fat-soluble vitamin, whose function was directing bone growth along normal lines even when the diet was of unfavorable composition. We had observed little rats on a certain diet to exhibit deformity of the thorax characterized by buckling of the ribs at the costochondral junctions, and nodes due to callous formation at spontaneous fractures. The condition resembled the so-called "pigeon breast" seen in human rickets. I believed that the condition was experimentally induced rickets. Dr. John Howland, Pediatrician-in-Chief, asked me if I thought anyone had ever produced rickets experimentally in an animal. I showed our deformed rats to him and he confirmed my belief that the condition was rickets. We arranged a collaborative research. Drs. Park and Shipley were to describe the histology of bones of such animals as I should prepare with a view to finding the nature of the dietary defect. Two technicians were employed to cut sections and differentially stain the region of growing bones. I at once set about planning a series of more than 300 modifications of the incidentally discovered rickets-producing diet. Little rats restricted to these formulas were prepared with a view to studying how growing bones responded to a long series of diets which induced one or another kind of malnutrition. Many diets were devised after listening to descriptions of the histological details of bone sections, such as abnormalities in appearance of cartilage as it changed from resting to vesicular type, distribution of blood capillaries, presence or absence of bone trabeculae, and presence or absence of osteoid tissue, etc. After hearing such comment, I studied the diet and planned another intended to accentuate or to alleviate certain tendencies of growing bones to deviate from normal. In this way we learned how to induce severe and acute rickets in a short time. One, diet 3413, was exactly suitable for preparing little rats for testing their response to an anti-rachitic agent, and served as a method of quantitative assay of any substance for its potency in preventing or curing rickets. We thus clearly demonstrated the existence of a hitherto unknown nutrient of great significance in directing the processes of bone growth.

In 1918, Mellanby had tentatively concluded that the protective power of certain fats and oils against rickets might be assigned to vitamin A. To examine this question we treated a sample of cod liver oil, which not only prevented or cured rickets, but also prevented or cured the eye disease due to vitamin A deficiency, by passing heated air bubbles through it to destroy vitamin A. This treated oil was still effective in preventing or curing rickets. We called the new nutrient vitamin D. This discovery was announced in 1922. Owing to the high reputation of Dr. Park, the medical profession immediately began to prescribe a source of vitamin D for infants and children. This rapidly led to the virtual disappearance of rickets in children throughout the world.

Employing our "line-test" in rats fed diet 3413 we confirmed the observation of others that sunlight which had not passed through glass, had anti-rachitic effects. Bills subjected many liver oils of fishes to this assay method, and discovered the extremely high potency of the liver oil of tuna. Steenbock, using a rickets-producing diet, discovered that irradiation of certain foods conferred on them anti-rachitic properties.

The rat has had a long history of evil deeds, including the nourishing and distribution of rat fleas, which transmitted the bubonic plague. It has been the agent of rat-bite fever and has caused immense destruction of young poultry, and of feed grains about farmyards. Its past is a history of evil not equaled by any other animal. But its introduction as a subject for nutrition investigation, gave it the opportunity to contribute enormously to human welfare. When placed in carefully designed situations where its physiological status depended on its response to diets, faulty in one or another respect, it has answered more questions about essential nutrients and their roles in metabolism, than has any other animal. Caged and used intelligently the rat has at last conferred very great benefits on mankind.

SOURCE

McCollum EV. 1967. The paths to the discovery of vitamins A and D. *J Nutr* 91 (2), Suppl. 1: 11–16. Reprinted in *Nutr Rev* 44 (7) (1986): 242–4. Copyright 1986 by *Journal of Nutrition*. Reprinted with permission of American Society for Nutrition.

Impact of Vitamin A Supplementation on Childhood Mortality

(1986)

A Randomised Controlled Community Trial

Alfred Sommer, Edi Djunaedi, A.A. Loeden, Ignatius Tarwotjo, Keith P. West, Jr., Robert Tilden, Lisa Mele, And the ACEH Study Group

International Center for Epidemiologic and Preventive Ophthalmology, Dana Center of the Wilmer Institute and School of Public Health, Johns Hopkins University, Baltimore, Maryland; Directorate of Nutrition and National Center for Health Research and Development, Ministry of Health, Government of Indonesia; and Helen Keller International, New York, USA

SUMMARY—450 villages in northern Sumatra were randomly assigned to either participate in a vitamin A supplementation scheme (n = 229) or serve for 1 year as a control (n = 221). 25,939 preschool children were examined at baseline and again 11 to 13 months later. Capsules containing 200,000 IU vitamin A were distributed to preschool children aged over 1 year by local volunteers 1 to 3 months after baseline enumeration and again 6 months later. Among children aged 12–71 months at baseline, mortality in control villages (75/10,231, 7.3 per 1,000) was 49% greater than in those where supplements were given (53/10,919, 4.9 per 1,000) (p < 0.05). The impact of vitamin A supplementation seemed to be greater in boys than in girls. These results support earlier observations linking mild vitamin A deficiency to increased mortality and suggest that supplements given to vitamin A deficient populations may decrease mortality by as much as 34%.

Introduction

A longitudinal observational study in rural central Java indicated that children with ocular signs of mild vitamin A deficiency were more likely than neighbourhood controls to die, that mortality was directly related to severity of vitamin A deficiency, and that poor survival was probably attributable, at least partly, to high rates of respiratory disease and diarrhoea.[1-3] We report here the results of a randomised, controlled, community trial of vitamin A prophylaxis in northern Sumatra.

Subjects and Methods

The study was carried out in Aceh Province, which is at the northern tip of Sumatra where xerophthalmia is prevalent.[4,5] The population is ethnically distinct from that of Java, where the earlier observational study had been conducted.[1-3]

For political and administrative reasons a cluster sampling scheme was employed. The sampling frame consisted of 2,048 villages in Aceh Utara and Pidie, two contiguous rural kabupatens (districts) chosen because they had no current or planned development projects or vitamin A supplementation schemes. From a random start, 450 villages were systematically selected for the study; these were then randomised for capsule distribution after the baseline examination (programme villages, n = 229) or after the follow-up examination (control villages, n = 221). 18 villages from among those still in the sampling frame were substituted for adjacent villages found to have started vitamin A supplementation before the baseline survey.

All members of the two study teams, each consisting of an ophthalmologist (team leader), a nurse, an anthropometrist, a dietary interviewer, five enumerators, and a driver, all fluent in the local dialect received a month's classroom, hospital, and field training. The enumerators, responsible for collecting demographic data, were unaware that mortality was a research question. Standardisation exercises were done before and regularly throughout the study. First, each village was visited to identify households containing children aged 0–5 years and to mark their dwellings. Within 2 days the village was visited by the full team. Enumerators visited every house containing preschool children, collected socioeconomic, demographic, and medical data, and rounded up children at a central point for their clinical examination. Dates of birth were ascertained by reference to local events charted on the Muslim calendar and then translated to their roman equivalent by the use of a specially prepared conversion table. Eyes were examined with a focused light and 2X loupes and diagnoses were made according to standard diagnostic criteria.[5,6] Parents were carefully questioned about the presence of nightblindness.[5,7] They were also asked about a history of diarrhoea (4 or more loose, watery stools per day), of fever or cough lasting at least 24h in the previous 7 days, and of "ever having" measles.

Recumbent length (if less than 24 months old) or standing height (if 24 months or older) to the nearest 0.1 cm, and weight (using a calibrated Salter scale) to the nearest 0.1 kg, were measured on a 10% subsample of all study children.

All children with active xerophthalmia at baseline examination received at least one large dose of vitamin A and were referred to the local health unit. They were excluded from the analyses of subsequent morbidity and mortality. All children received vitamin A at the follow-up examination 9–13 months later.

Teams first visited villages between September, 1982, and August, 1983, and follow-up visits were made by the same team in the same sequence 9–13 months later. The variation in follow-up time resulted from attempts to minimise the potential confounding influence of the Muslim fasting month and post-fasting holidays.

Standard capsules (supplied by UNICEF) were given to every child aged 1–5 years in programme villages, by a local volunteer trained to do so. The capsule nipple was snipped off and the contents (200,000 IU vitamin A and 40 IU vitamin E) were expressed into the child's mouth. This volunteer kept a list of children treated and issued the household with a distribution card. The first dose was given 1–3 months after the baseline examination and the second 6–8 months later. A distribution monitor visited each village 2–4 weeks after the scheduled distribution and interviewed 10% of eligible households. If coverage was less than 80% the local distributor was encouraged to reach children previously missed.

All data were collected on precoded forms, entered onto diskettes, and shipped to the data management facility at the International Center for Epidemiologic and Preventive Ophthalmology, Johns Hopkins University, where the information was processed with the SIR data management package run on an IBM 4341 computer. Statistical analyses were made with SIR, SAS, and GLIM software. Statistical tests for significance and development of confidence intervals were adjusted for clustering associated with randomization by village rather than by individual, and for the small number of events expected and observed in any one village by applying poisson regression with extra-poisson variation, to account for natural variability in mortality among villages.[8,9] Two-tailed tests were used.

The study was designed to examine overall differences between non-infant preschool-age children in programme versus control villages, on the assumption that mortality would be reduced by at least 20% and allowing for an alpha error of 0.05 and a beta error of 0.2 (1-tailed). Stratified subgroup analyses are, strictly speaking, inappropriate, and, because of the small numbers, not very reliable.

Although Indonesian government regulations proscribe administration of vitamin A prophylactically to infants, a considerable proportion of them received capsules nonetheless, so the impact on infant mortality was also examined.

All study procedures were approved by a steering committee consisting of representatives of the Indonesian Center for Nutrition Research, the directorate of Community Health Services, the provincial health authorities, Johns Hopkins University, and Helen Keller International.

Results

29,236 preschool-aged children were enumerated at baseline. Follow-up information was available on 89.0% of the programme children and 88.4% of the controls. The age and sex distribution of children lacking follow-up was identical in the two groups.

Baseline Characteristics

Of the 25,939 children with baseline and follow-up information, details of the initial ocular examination are available for 91.9% of programme children and 90.5% of controls. Active xerophthalmia was more prevalent in controls than in the programme group (2.25 versus 1.88%), but the difference was not significant and was accounted for almost entirely by the males (table I). Xerophthalmia was more prevalent among males

Table I   Baseline Prevalence of Active Xerophthalmia

—	No. of patients with:		
	Nightblindness* **(XN)**	**Bitot's spots*** **(X1B)**	**Active xerophthalmia*** **(XN, X1B, X3)**
Total†			
Programme (n = 12,281)	136 *(1.11%)*	143 *(1.16%)*	231 *(1.88%)*
Control (n = 11,378)	150 *(1.32%)*	164 *(1.44%)*	256 *(2.25%)*
Males			
Programme (n = 6,043)	69 *(1.14%)*	72 *(1.19%)*	120 *(1.99%)*
Control (n = 5,583)	88 *(1.58%)*	102 *(1.83%)*	150 *(2.69%)*
Females			
Programme (n = 5,881)	66 *(1.12%)*	69 *(1.17%)*	108 *(1.84%)*
Control (n = 5,494)	61 *(1.11%)*	59 *(1.07%)*	103 *(1.87%)*

*Prevalence rates for XN and X1B are not mutually exclusive. For "active xerophthalmia" an individual was counted only once. There were only 6 patients with corneal ulceration (X3), 3 in each group. Conjunctival and corneal xerosis were excluded as being potentially less reliable.[6]

† Includes 357 programme and 301 control children whose sex was unknown.

Table II   Age and Sex Distribution on Non-Xerophthalmic Children

—	Programme	Control
Total*	12,991 *(100%)*	112,209 *(100%)*
Sex†		
Male	6,365 *(50%)*	5,975 *(50%)*
Female	6,243 *(50%)*	5,888 *(50%)*
Total	12,608 *(100%)*	11,863 *(100%)*
Baseline age (months)		
<12	2,074 *(16.0%)*	1,979 *(16.2%)*
12–23	1,979 *(15.2%)*	1,941 *(15.9%)*
24–35	2,086 *(16.1%)*	2,072 *(17.0%)*
36–47	2,274 *(17.5%)*	2,016 *(16.5%)*
48–59	1,887 *(14.5%)*	1,724 *(14.2%)*
60–71	2,686 *(20.7%)*	2,465 *(20.2%)*
Total	12,986 *(100.0 %)*	12,197 *(100.0%)*
*Includes infants, as well as children on whom age and/or sex are unavailable.		
†Sex not known for some children.		

than females, especially among controls. Xerophthalmia prevalence was negligible during the first 2 years of life (less than 0.5%).

The age and sex distributions of the non-xerophthalmia children in the two groups were similar (table II). The disproportionate number of children purported to be in the 6th year of life probably includes children really in their 5th and 7th years, as has been noted previously.[5] Programme and control children were also similar for most other baseline demographic and socioeconomic variables, including occupation of the head of the household, maternal education, source of drinking water, distance to the nearest elementary school, and distance to the nearest health centre.

The two groups were also similar in most health variables such as recent history of fever or cough or of ever having had measles; relative risks of these variables for the two groups differed by less than 5% (table III) except for diarrhoea, a recent history being 23% commoner among control than programme children ($p = <0.05$), with the greatest excess in girls. Recent diarrhoea was commonest during the 2nd year of life, when the frequency was 9.8% in programme villages and 10.7% in control villages. Thereafter it steadily declined. The most objective baseline health variable

Table III Baseline Morbidity Variables

—	Programme		Control		Relative risk compared with that for control
	Total no.	% positive	Total no.	% positive	
Cough*	12,781	31.2	11,555	32.7	1.05
Fever*	12,781	45.7	11,555	46.7	1.02
Measles†	11,753	22.3	10,059	21.7	0.97
Diarrhoea*	12,781	7.1	11,555	8.7	1.23

*Present in past seven days. Data missing on 210 programme children and 654 controls.

†Any time in past. Smaller denominator because of change in question shortly after survey began.

Table IV Baseline Anthropometry

—	Programme (n = 1,382)	Control (n = 1,271
Height for age (% of median)*		
<85†	8.2%	8.9%
85–89	23.9%	27.6%
90–94	43.0%	37.8%
≥95	24.9%	25.7%
Weight for height (% of median)*		
<80	3.0%	3.7%
80–89	38.3%	35.6%
≥90	58.6%	60.7%

*Median NCHS standards.[11] Represents 10% subsample of children.

† Less than 1.5% of children in either group were below 80% of median.

was nutritional status. Anthropometric indices were similar for the two groups, both total and sex-specific (table IV).[10]

In 99% of children in the two study groups, the interval between baseline and follow-up examination was at least 11 months, and for 59%, at least 12 months. This interval did not vary among age-sex-specific categories by more than ±2%.

Vitamin A Distribution Level

Of our three methods of monitoring for capsule administration only inter-rogation of the child's guardian(s) proved feasible. Report forms provided by the local distributors were largely illegible, and most cards issued to households were faded, torn, or lost.

Over 93% of preschool children (12–71 months at baseline) living in programme villages received at least one large dose of vitamin A be-tween baseline and follow-up examinations; 78% received two doses (table V). In every age-group coverage of boys and girls differed by less than 1%.

In theory, only two-thirds of the infants were eligible for one capsule and less than one-quarter for two. Surprisingly, 82% received at least one capsule and almost 62% both. This discrepancy may reflect disregard of normal government guidelines or of small differences in age.

Only 1% of control subjects received any capsule, presumably obtained at the health centres by children presenting with xerophthalmia.

Table V   Number* Reported to Have Received Vitamin A Capsules During Follow-Up

Age (months) at baseline	Programme villages		Control villages	
	At least 1 capsule	2 capsules	At least 1 capsule	2 capsules
12–23	1,899 (93.1)	1,854 (77.7)	1,707 (0.7)	1,895 (0.2)
24–35	2,007 (93.3)	1,946 (78.1)	1,792 (1.2)	2,010 (0.1)
36–47	2,192 (94.0)	2,130 (78.7)	1,771 (1.3)	1,956 (0.2)
48–59	1,806 (93.5)	1,765 (78.4)	1,509 (0.7)	1,683 (0.1)
60–71	2,593 (92.4)	2,528 (77.5)	2,121 (1.2)	2,400 (0.2)
Total	10,497 (93.2)	10,223 (78.1)	8,900 (1.1)	9,944 (0.2)
<12	1,968 (82.4)	1,879 (61.8)	1,728 (1.1)	1914 (0.1)
Respondent uncertain about capsules	259	259	130	130
Information unavailable	260	623	1,438	208

*Number of those for whom information was complete (age not known for 7 other programme children and 13 other controls).

Numbers in parentheses are percentages.

Impact on Xerophthalmia and Mortality

The prevalence of active xerophthalmia in programme villages declined from 1.9% at baseline to 0.3% at follow-up and that in the control villages declined from 2.3% to 1.2%. These changes meant that the risk of xerophthalmia in control villages relative to that in programme villages rose from 1.2 at baseline to 4.0 at follow-up (p < 0.05). Sex-specific prevalence rates followed a similar pattern.

During the follow-up period 75 preschool study children from control villages and 53 from programme villages died, giving mortality rates of 7.4 and 4.9 per 1,000, respectively (p < 0.05, two-tailed) (table VI). The relative risk of dying in control versus programme villages was therefore 1.51 (95% confidence limits 1.03, 2.28), equivalent to a reduction in mortality in programme villages of 34%. Infants in control villages had a mortality rate 21% greater than those in programme villages.

To compare age/sex/study group-specific mortality, children were classed as preschool children and infants (table VI). Both infant and preschool control boys died 70% more frequently than did those in the programme villages. The relative risk of death for boys in control versus programme villages was 1.69 (95% confidence limits 1.14, 2.51). Excess mortality was less pronounced among control girls, in whom it was limited to preschool children.

To examine further the effect of large doses of vitamin A on mortality, cumulative sex-specific mortality rates for preschool children were calculated every month after baseline examination (see accompanying figure). Boys and girls show similar patterns: mortality in control villages was initially the same as (females) or lower (males) than that in programme villages; with time, mortality in control villages gradually exceeded mortality in programme villages, a trend which was more pronounced in boys; by the end of the follow-up period, 2–4 months after the second dose of vitamin A, cumulative mortality had reached a plateau in programme villages, but it continued to climb in control villages. The pattern among infant boys mimicked that of preschool boys. Cumulative mortality among infant girls in control villages was virtually indistinguishable from that in programme villages.

Discussion

Mortality rates have been reported to be higher in malnourished children in hospital with xerophthalmia than in those with normal eyes.[11,12] However, another study has shown that in children admitted to hospital for xerophthalmia, severe malnutrition was the most important factor associated with mortality.[5] Interpretation of these studies is hindered by

Table VI Age And Sex-Specific Mortality During Follow-Up

Baseline age (months)	Programme villages		Control villages		
	Proportion dying	Rate per 1,000	Proportion dying	Rate per 1,000	RR
Both sexes					
12–23	19/1,979	9.6	22/1,941	11.3	1.17
24–35	14/2,086	6.7	25/2,072	12.1	1.81
36–47	11/2,274	4.8	8/2,016	4.0	0.83
48–59	5/1,887	2.6	7/1,724	4.1	1.58
60–71	4/2,686	1.5	13/2,465	5.3	3.53
Total preschool*	53/10,917	4.9	75/10,230	7.4	1.51 (1.03, 2.28)[‡]
Infants (<12)	48/2,074	23.1	55/1,979	27.8	1.21 (0.73, 1.97)[‡]
Total* (0–71)	101/12,991	7.8	130/12,209	10.6	1.36 (1.01, 1.85)[‡]
Males[†]					
0–11	18/1,014	17.8	29/970	29.9	1.68
12–71	28/5,348	5.2	44/4,998	8.8	1.69
Total (0–71)	46/6,362	7.2	73/5,968	12.2	1.69 (1.14, 2.51)[‡]
Females[†]					
0–11	28/994	28.2	25/942	26.5	0.94
12–71	23/5,245	4.4	27/4,933	5.5	1.25
Total (0–71)	51/6,239	8.2	52/5,875	8.9	1.09 (0.71, 1.71)[‡]

*Includes children with age unknown.

[†]Excludes children for whom age and/or sex are unknown.

[‡]95% confidence limits.

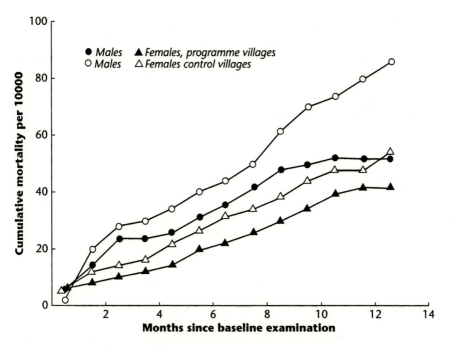

Cumulative sex-specific mortality at monthly intervals after baseline examination for preschool children (aged 12–71 months at baseline examination).

First dose given during months 1–3; second a mean of 6 months later.

Males—denominator for first 12 months in programme villages, 5,351 (no further deaths); in control villages, 5,005 initially, 3,046 during the last month.

Females—denominator for first 12 months in programme villages, 5,249 (no further deaths); in control villages, 4,946 initially and 2,978 during the last month.

the biases inherent in family motivation and hospital admission criteria, and the impact intensive therapy has on mortality.

In a longitudinal study of 4,000 preschool-aged Javanese children we found that children with mild xerophthalmia (night blindness, Bitot's spots, or the two conditions together—a ranking shown to be closely correlated with serum vitamin A levels[5,7]) died at four times the rate for their non-xerophthalmic peers; the excess mortality was related to the severity of the xerophthalmia; and this "dose-related" risk was independent of the child's general nutritional status.[1,2] The shape of the dose-response curve suggested that subclinical vitamin A deficiency (i.e., in the absence of detectable xerophthalmia) was also associated with increased mortality. Follow-up of surviving children revealed that respiratory and diarrhoeal diseases were 2–4 times more likely to have developed in those who had been xerophthalmic than in their non-xerophthalmic peers.[3] Again, vitamin A status seemed to be more important than anthropometric status in predicting morbidity.

The present study was thus undertaken, partly to determine whether supplements of vitamin A given to preschool children (12–71 months of age) would reduce their mortality by at least 15%. Ideally all "treatment" children would have received at least the recommended daily allowance. But this would have required a special, impracticable delivery system. Instead we opted for the regular Indonesian government scheme of twice-a-year administration of UNICEF-supplied capsules by trained local volunteers, although we realised that it did not cover infants. The Government of Indonesia would not condone the use of placebos but field-workers collecting demographic data were unaware that mortality was a research issue.

Strict randomisation of the 450 study villages seemed to have worked reasonably well. The populations were similar in most baseline characteristics investigated except for xerophthalmia and history of recent diarrhoea, which were slightly more prevalent among the controls. The differences between programme and control populations in mortality were out of proportion to their baseline differences; the baseline difference in diarrhoeal history was greatest for females, whereas excess mortality was greatest for males; and the most objective, quantifiable baseline indices of health status, weight-for-height and height-for-age, were virtually identical in the two groups on both an age and sex specific basis.

There was no evidence during the course of the study of differences in economic or medical initiatives in the study area, though clearly the vitamin A status throughout the province was improving as shown by a substantial reduction in prevalence of xerophthalmia between the 1978 nationwide survey and the baseline examination in the present study. The reduction in prevalence of xerophthalmia in control villages during our study may have been part of the general spontaneous improvement, which is the reason for having controls.[5,6] The mortality rates in this study were also lower than previously recorded for Java,[13] where rates seem to be falling, and more closely resemble those of neighbouring "medium" infant mortality rate countries (e.g., Philippines, Malaysia, Thailand), where the median mortality in preschool-aged children is 3 per 1,000.[14]

Results were strongly positive, even in this "intent-to-treat" analysis. Xerophthalmia prevalence among preschool children living in programme villages declined by 85%, a result similar to those obtained in other carefully conducted pilot trials,[3,15–17] and it confirms the high distribution rate of capsules reported. Preschool control children died 1.5 times more frequently than did programme children (95% confidence limits 1.03, 2.28), equivalent to a 34% reduction in non-infant mortality among residents of programme villages. To control for baseline differences in prevalence of xerophthalmia and history of recent diarrhoea between programme and control villages, the proportion of children with xerophthalmia or recent history of diarrhoea at baseline was included as a covariate (predictor variable) in the analysis. Mortality results (relative risks and their confidence limits) were nearly identical when either xerophthalmia alone or when both xerophthalmia and diarrhoea were included in the analysis.

Although the study was not designed to investigate subgroups, and the numbers concerned preclude definite conclusions, they provide additional evidence consistent with the beneficial impact of vitamin A supplementation: mortality among controls was greater at almost every age, including the first year of life; the difference in cumulative mortality increased with time, even though male and female controls had initial mortality rates that were the same as or lower than those in programme villages; the impact was greatest among boys, in whom vitamin A deficiency is generally far more prevalent;[5,17-20] and among boys, the time-related mortality pattern corresponded with the expected temporal impact of capsule distribution. This internal consistency and agreement with previous studies is more important than the size of the p value or width of the confidence limits, which are direct consequences of the enormous sample size required.

These results are especially encouraging for the following reasons: capsule distribution was less than universal and probably missed those who needed it most;[21] single large dose supplementation maintains raised serum vitamin A levels for only 1–3 months;[22] distribution did not start until 1–3 months after enumeration; xerophthalmic controls took vitamin A at health centres; and those in whom the greatest impact might have been expected (children xerophthalmic at baseline) were treated and dropped from the analysis.

How vitamin A reduces mortality remains uncertain. Vitamin A deficiency is associated with changes in surface epithelium and these may disrupt normal barrier function, support bacterial growth (as seen on the conjunctiva[23] and presumably the bladder[24]), and obstruct smaller branches of the tracheobronchial tree. Abnormalities in systemic immune competence associated with vitamin A deficiency may also be as important in contributing to mortality; in animals at least, vitamin A deficiency interferes with humoral and especially cell-mediated immunity.[25-27] Limited data suggest similar effects in man.[28] High doses of vitamin A given to otherwise normal animals have been reported to produce a non-specific, adjuvant-like increase in resistance to infection.[29] The response to the high doses given in our study was unlikely to be due to non-specific changes. The children came from a vitamin A deficient population,[5,7] and the impact was sustained. The rise in blood retinyl ester levels after one large dose of vitamin A given to deficient patients do not last for more than 8–12 weeks;[22,30] and holo-retinol-binding-protein levels rise, but not above normal levels.[30,31]

The presence of the study teams was unlikely to have influenced the results of our study because the only difference between programme and control villages in their interaction with study personnel consisted of at most two contacts in 12 months with the local vitamin A distributor in treatment areas. This distributor was neither trained nor instructed to undertake any other intervention.

Vitamin A status probably modulates the incidence and severity of disease caused by a variety of pathogenic organisms. The impact that vitamin A supplementation will have on mortality will therefore depend upon a constellation of factors, including the prevalence and severity of vitamin A deficiency; the frequency of exposure to pathogenic organisms, size of the inoculum, and their virulence; and the presence and degree of other adverse influences with which the young child must contend (e.g., malnutrition, parasitic load). The results of the study reported here and those done in Java[1-3] confirm the importance that vitamin A deficiency in childhood has on mortality in Indonesia and show the impact that supplementation can have on child survival.

This study was carried out under cooperative agreement DSAN·CA·0267 with the Office of Nutrition, United States Agency for International Development, with additional financial assistance from Hoffman-La Roche, P. T. Vicks, Ford Foundation, UNICEF, and the Asian Foundation for the Prevention of Blindness.

SOURCE

Sommer A, Djunaedi E, Loeden A A, Tarawotjo I, West KP Jr., Tilden R, Mele L, and the Aceh Study Group. 1986. Impact of vitamin A supplementation on childhood mortality. *Lancet* 327 (8491): 1169–73. Copyright 1986 by *Lancet*. Reprinted with permission of Elsevier.

The Nutrition Transition in Low-Income Countries: An Emerging Crisis
(1994, Abridged)

Barry M. Popkin, Ph.D.

Scientists have long recognized the importance of the demographics and epidemiologic transitions in higher income countries. Only recently has it become understood that similar sets of proxy-based changes are occurring in lower income countries. What has not been recognized is that concurrent changes in nutrition are also occurring, with equally important implications for resource allocation in many low-income countries. Several major changes seem to be emerging, leading to a marked shift in the structure of diet and the distribution of body composition in many regions of the world: a rapid reduction in fertility and aging of the population, rapid urbanization, the epidemiologic transition, and economic changes affecting populations in different and uneven ways. These changes vary significantly over time. In general, we find the problems with under- and overnutrition often coexist, reflecting the trend in which an increasing proportion of people consume the types of diets associated with a number of chronic diseases. This is occurring more rapidly than previously seen in higher income countries, or even in Japan and Korea. Examples from Thailand, China, and Brazil provide evidence of the changes and trends in dietary intake, physical activity, and body composition patterns.

There is little need to present the health concerns that motivate this work. Diet excess and deficit and under- and overnutrition have significant impacts on health and survival. Most work in low-income countries has focused on undernutrition and its effects on survival and mortality in development. As populations age and countries move through epidemiologic, demographic, and nutrition transitions, there is a clear need to understand the expanding literature which links nutrition and chronic disease patterns.[1, 2] It is crucial that lower income countries facing rapid dietary change learn from the lessons of higher income countries and try to direct the nutrition transitions in more healthy directions. (While it is assumed by most epidemiologists and health researchers that improvements in diet are associated with increased life expectancy and improve functioning, Harper[3] questions the validity of the effect of improved diet on life expectancy in the United States and other higher income countries.)

I proceed from the premise that it is crucial to understand past dietary patterns and their antecedents. Human diet and nutritional status have undergone a sequence of major shifts between each characteristic phase, defined as a broad pattern of food use and corresponding nutrition-related disease. Over the past three centuries, the pace of dietary change appears to have accelerated to varying degrees in different regions of the world. Additionally, dietary and body composition changes are paralleled by major changes in health outcomes as well as by demographic and socioeconomic changes. The patterns of change in low-income countries described here suggest that the rates of change occurring in the structure of diet, physical activity, and obesity are greater in these countries than ever experienced before. Thus, this component of the nutrition transition represents a crisis demanding both recognition and action. This paper uses data from nationwide surveys in several countries that have experienced rapid economic change and will examine an emerging issue of international importance: the rapid shift in the structure of diet in low-income countries and the coexisting problems of under- and overnutrition.

Patterns of the Nutrition Transition

As noted, large shifts have occurred in the composition of diet. These dietary changes are reflected in nutrition outcomes, such as changes in body size and composition. Modern societies seem to be converging on a dietary pattern which is high in saturated fat, sugar, and refined foods and low in fiber (the "Western" diet). At its most basic level, these changes represent a simple imitation of the Western diet and there is little evidence yet to indicate what else is involved. The nature and pace of the change vary significantly and there are important differences in the food pattern changes; nevertheless, the net effect on nutrient intake and nutritional status are similar.

Concurrent changes in demographic and epidemiologic outcomes are linked with the nutrition transition. Figure 1 presents the broad historical sweep of changes in these demographic, health, and nutrition factors and how they are intertwined [Not shown here, Ed.]. There are extant theories of change which address the demographic and epidemiologic transitions. One relates to the *demographic transition*—the shift from a pattern of high fertility and high mortality to low fertility and low mortality (typical of modern and industrialized nations). Even more directly relevant is the *epidemiologic transition*, first described by Omran in 1971.[4] The epidemiologic transition describes the shift from a pattern in which pestilence, famine, and poor sanitation lead to a high prevalence of infectious diseases and malnutrition to a pattern in which the prevalence of chronic and degenerative diseases is high. Another pattern of "delayed" degenerative diseases has been more recently formulated by Olshansky and Ault.[5] Accompanying this progression is a major shift in age-specific mortality patterns and life expectancy. The concept of demographic and epidemiologic transition share a focus on the ways in which populations move from one pattern to the next.

It is useful to consider briefly the nutrition transition within its detailed historical context. The nutrition transition has been described in five broad patterns: (1) collecting food, (2) famine, (3) receding famine, (4) degenerative disease, and (5) behavioral change (Table 1) [Not shown here, Ed.]. These patterns are not restricted to particular periods of human history. For convenience, the patterns are outlined in the past tense as historical development; however, earlier patterns are not restricted to the periods in which they first arose but continue to characterize certain geographic and socioeconomic subpopulations.

Pattern 1: Collection of Food

The diet of people during the hunter-gatherer period was high in carbohydrates and fiber, low in fat (particularly saturated fat), and high in biologically available iron.[6, 7] The wild animal meat consumed had a polyunsaturated content significantly higher than in modern domesticated animal meat.[8] These early humans were relatively tall but had short life expectancies, possibly due to high rates of infectious disease.[9]

Pattern 2: Famine

The diet became less varied and subject to episodic periods of extreme food shortage. These dietary changes are thought to be associated with nutritional stress and a reduction in stature, estimated by some at about 4 inches.[9, 10] During the later phases of this pattern, social stratification began to appear, and dietary variation according to gender and social status increased.[11] The pattern of famine (as with each of the other patterns) was manifested heterogeneously over time and space. Some civilizations were more successful than others in alleviating famine and chronic hunger, particularly for their more privileged citizens.[12, 13] This pattern of famine accompanied the development of agriculture (the first "agricultural revolution"); however, the causal relationship between the agricultural revolution and changes in nutrition is widely debated. Famines continued well into the 18th century in parts of Europe and still continue in some parts of the world. Over the past decade, famine has become limited mainly to subSaharan and southern Africa.

Pattern 3: Receding Famine

The consumption of fruits and vegetables and animal protein increased, and starches became less important dietary staples. Many earlier civilizations made great progress in reducing chronic hunger and famines, but it is only in the last third of this millennium that widespread changes have led to marked dietary shifts.

Pattern 4: Degenerative Disease

A diet high in total fat, cholesterol, sugar, and other refined carbohydrates and low in polyunsaturated fatty acids and fiber accompanied by a sedentary life-style is characteristic of many high-income societies (and some segments of the population in lower income societies). This results in increased prevalence of obesity and contributes to the degenerative diseases of Omran's final epidemiologic stage.[4]

Pattern 5: Behavioral Change

Consumption patterns resemble more the pattern of collecting food (Pattern 1) rather than that of degenerative disease (Pattern 4). Increased intake of fruits and vegetables, complex carbohydrates, and reduced intake of refined foods, meats, and dairy products are features of this pattern. This "new" dietary pattern appears to be emerging as a result of changes in diet associated with the desire to prevent degenerative diseases and prolong life. These changes have been instituted in some countries by consumers and in other countries by a combination of government policy and consumer behavior. It remains to be seen if these changes will result in a large-scale transition in diet structure and body composition.[14–16] These new changes are also associated with a renewed understanding of physical activity and fitness in promoting health. If both changes occur, they may be very important in our goal of enhancing successful aging, by reducing the period between the age at which a person suffers permanent infirmity and the age at death.[17, 18]

To date, most behavioral change has resulted from changes in consumer preference, usually linked to concerns about health. However, recent changes in food policy and education efforts in Norway have been based on systematic policy changes. China is also trying to adopt a similar national approach to address the problems of dietary excess.

Examples of These Transitions

The progress of dietary change throughout the world does not necessarily replicate the pattern of nutritional change that has occurred in high-income countries. To understand the nutrition transition in this century, we would like to have information on individual dietary intake and body composition for many populations surveyed over long periods of time. Unfortunately, there are significant information constraints, so we must patch together food balance sheets and other crude sources of information with surveys conducted on limited population subgroups. It is hoped that as we understand more about dietary nutrition patterns, we will be able to explore the causal relationships among these factors.

Western High-Income Model

The pattern of change in the United States appears to be one that has been followed by European countries during the past century. This is a more gradual shift in the structure of the diet. Over the first half of the 20th century, sugar intake rose rapidly, grain consumption decreased, and meat and dairy product consumption rose.[19] During the last 30–40 years, the increase in sugar consumption has slowed markedly, and consumption of meat, dairy products, and eggs has decreased.[20] There has been a concomitant increase in stature, body size, and obesity.

Dietary changes observed during the past decade provide evidence that in some subpopulations of the United States, a pattern of health-conscious behavioral change has begun. Among better educated groups, increased consumption of low-fat and high-fiber foods is evident.[15] From a nutritional perspective, however, the changes are not all positive. For instance, an increase in the consumption of high-fat mixed-grain dishes and desserts offsets the decrease in fat intake in the diet of elderly Americans.[16] Among lower income Americans there is no evidence of positive dietary shifts. The combination of minimal dietary change and reduced physical activity among lower income groups may be part of the reason why lower income persons, particularly Hispanics and blacks, have a higher proportion of obesity than higher income groups.[21–23] This pattern occurs in children as well as adults.

In other high-income countries such as Canada, France, Germany, and Great Britain, the supply of fat-free foods has increased. Only in several Scandinavian countries, Canada, and the United Kingdom has the per capita consumption of animal fat declined. The increases in obesity prevalence in these countries are also significant.[24–26]

The only Western countries that have attempted to change this trend at the national level are Norway and Finland.[27] Among European countries, Norway has most markedly reduced the proportion of energy obtained from animal fats, from 29% in 1961 to 23% in 1988. Reductions in total fat (41–35%) was <sic> observed between 1975 and 1989, with equally significant declines in saturated fat.[27, 28]

Japanese and Korean Accelerated Model

Following World War II, energy intake in Japan increased slowly, peeking between 1970 and 1975, while intake of animal products and fat increased continuously from 1946 to 1987. During this period, daily per capita consumption of animal products increased by 257 grams; daily per capita total fat consumption increased by 341%; and the proportion of energy from that increased from 8.7% to 24.8%.[29] Although there appear to be marked cohort differences whereby younger Japanese consume a Western-style diet, while older persons cling to the more traditional pattern, little systematic analysis has been conducted on Japanese dietary trends.

Obesity is increasing rapidly among the Japanese. Moreover, there is evidence that obesity among the Japanese is associated with greater visceral fat mass[30,31] and a much higher risk of coronary heart disease at lower levels of body mass index (BMI).

South Korea is another Asian country that achieved remarkably rapid growth during the last three or four decades, and it appears to be undergoing a change in dietary structure similar to that of Japan.[32,33] Trends in the South Korean diet for the last three decades include a marked decline in the per capita consumption of greens and a large increase in the per capita consumption of fish, meat, and milk. Rising consumption of animal products, particularly in the last decade, is reflected in an increased proportion of energy obtained from animal fat. By the late 1980s, Koreans had a total fat intake as a proportion of energy intake of only 15%. Japan had reached this level in 1965 and by 1987 was at 25%. The South Korean diet might be expected to undergo rapid change in a similar manner, resulting in a shift in disease patterns comparable to those experienced by Japan.

An important element for these as well as other East Asian countries is not a change in the average diet, but the change in the composition of the diet. Increasingly larger segments of the population are consuming high-fat diets and have reduced their physical activity, leading to an increase in obesity patterns and risk factors for a number of chronic diseases. Although we present detailed descriptions of dietary, physical activity, and body composition patterns in China, such data are not available at the national level for most countries.

Rapidly Growing Asian Countries

The larger countries in Asia are experiencing an economic and demographic transformation, which is reflected in food consumption patterns. The food balance data presented in Figure 2 [Not shown here, Ed.] illustrate the proportional change in food available for consumption from 1980 to 1990 in four rapidly growing Asian countries. In each case, the change in energy intake has been small, but there have been large changes in consumption of animal products, sugar, and fats. Clearly, these countries are moving along somewhat different paths toward a diet associated with a degenerative disease pattern. The foods differ among each country, leading one to expect that the resultant long-term health implications will also vary.

China

Information comes from the China Health and Nutrition Surveys (CHNS), based on patterns of dietary intake for adults surveyed in 1989 and 1991. The data include an average of three 24-hour dietary recalls, direct measurement of height and weight, and detailed interview to determine physical activity and household and individual income.[22]

Dietary change has been very rapid in China. Over the past decade, China has achieved overall dietary adequacy and has seen a marked change in dietary structure. While the traditional Chinese diet was felt to be low in fat, we now find only a small proportion of the population consuming this traditional low-fat pattern, with an increasing proportion consuming more than 30% of their energy from fat. This high-fat diet was significantly more common in urban and higher income populations than in rural and lower income ones (Table 2) [Not shown here, Ed.]. At the same time, there were decreases in the proportion of adults consuming a low-fat diet among all income groups.

Associated with this change in diet has been a marked change in physical activity pattern. For example, in 1991, urban residents in all income groups were likely to have adopted a more sedentary pattern that in 1989 (Table 3) [Not shown here, Ed.]. In contrast, this pattern was not noted in the rural areas. In fact, low-income rural residents showed a significant change from low and moderate activity patterns toward a high activity pattern. When coupled with the dietary intake changes, it is clear that one would expect an increase in obesity in the urban sample and possibly an increase in undernutrition among the low-income rural residents. The net effect has been a significant change in adult body composition. We define under- and overweight according to BMIs below 18.5 and above 25. The proportions of adults aged 20–45 years in different weight categories grouped by household income level appear in Table 4 [Not shown, Ed.]. During 1989–1991, a decline in the proportion underweight was observed among the middle- and high-income tertiles, with an increase in underweight noted in the lowest income territorial, particularly among the low-income men. The increase in proportion underweight among low-income adults (+2.2%) is particularly noteworthy.

During the same period, there was an increase in proportion of overweight in all groups except for the low-income women. The largest increase in proportion overweight was observed among the middle-income women (+4.7%) and a high-income men (+4.6%). As already noted, changes in physical activity and diet were significantly associated with changes in BMI; thus, polarization of nutritional problems is emerging in China. Increasingly it appears that earlier equal distribution of nutritional problems is being replaced by problems of excess and deficit among the rich and poor, respectively.

Thailand

Thailand is undergoing an economic transition, which began about 5 years after China's and is proceeding at a slower pace. There are new increases in obesity noted in Bangkok and other urban areas as well. Such changes are comparable to those seen in China. A longitudinal study done in a small urban area of southern Thailand revealed an unexpectedly large proportion of obese persons: 12.7% of 1,156 children ages 6–12 years old.[34] One large study of 2,703 men and 792 women living in urban areas found that 25.5% of the men and 21.4% of the women had BMIs ≥25.0.[35] In the last decade, Thailand has experienced a rapid increase in the consumption of energy from fat and a comparable if not larger decline in the proportion of fat from complex carbohydrates.

There is currently no large population-based study of diet in obesity encompassing all economic groups elsewhere in South or Southeast Asia, so it is difficult to understand these trends.[36] Large community-based surveys in India indicate that people from higher socioeconomic status (SES) backgrounds have the prevalence of coronary heart disease three to four times higher than the rate for the lower SES groups.[36–38] The same surveys in New Delhi provide some indirect evidence.[36] These surveys showed that higher income persons consumed a diet averaging greater than 32% of energy from fat, while lower income persons consumed a diet with 17% of energy from fat.[38] A study of a large random sample of adults in New Delhi suggests that between 30 and 40% of the adults in various SES categories were obese.[37] Other small surveys produce evidence that higher income groups consume a diet much higher in saturated fat than the 32% reported above. In addition, there is a trend toward increasing prevalence of diabetes mellitus, and Gopalan feels that despite the lack of definitive survey results, obesity is becoming increasingly prevalent in India.[36]

Modernization has been associated with an even higher prevalence of obesity in the South Pacific islands, particularly among urban residents.[24,39,40] High rates of obesity is are seen in Fiji, Kiribati, and Vanatu, mirroring the rates found among Native American groups in the United States.[12] Changes in diet, physical activity, and obesity have been associated with urban residence and modernization in these islands.[40] These changes, along with increases in diabetes and coronary heart disease in the South Pacific island populations, have given rise to a series of hypotheses regarding the evolutionary adaptation to reduced energy, which causes rapid increases in fat tissue during times of dietary excess (the thrifty gene hypothesis).[41] As life-styles change, the level of obesity associated with the risk of chronic disease has also changed, as noted both in longitudinal studies in the South Pacific islands and in a series of studies done in migrant communities.[41-44]

How inevitable is the transition toward a high prevalence of obesity in Asia? Among large populations in Asia, too little is known yet to understand whether the pattern of body composition found in the small islands in the South Pacific will occur in the larger countries of Asia. However, the rapid increase in diabetes rates in China and other Asian countries, and the dietary and physical activity patterns and obesity information presented above provide some evidence of a similar trend.

Another unique challenge facing the Asian countries of China, Thailand, Indonesia, and several smaller countries (e.g., Sri Lanka) is population aging, largely driven by rapid reductions in the birth rate.[45] Many of these countries will experience a doubling or tripling of the proportion of the population aged 65 and older between 1990 and 2025.[46,47] An increase of elderly one-person female households is also expected. The unique nutritional demands of aging Asian populations deserve special consideration.[36] For instance, there is an increased concern about the frailty and health of this older Asian population. Their low calcium intake coupled with the effects of repeated births is expected to lead to poor bone health and excessive fractures associated with osteoporosis.

Latin American Pattern

In Central and South America and the Caribbean, information is available to document the pace and nature of the transition in diet and body composition. In Brazil, national surveys suggest a rapid change in body composition. However, more detailed measures of household and individual dietary data are needed to provide a careful tracking of this trend. In addition, the present data do not allow us to look at the differential trends for different socio-economic and geographic groupings in the detail needed to see if the types of bipolar changes seen in the China data occur here.

The problems of dietary excess have begun to dominate the higher income Central and South American countries and most of the Caribbean. At the national level, few countries have a security problem, and problems of household dietary deficit and individual malnutrition are rapidly being reduced among the low-income populations. The United Nations Administrative Committee on Coordination/Subcommittee on Nutrition has developed a set of remarkable case studies on these trends. One of the best is by Lunes and Monteiro[48] for Brazil, in which they show a remarkable decline in the proportion of malnourished children. Sichieri et al.[49] show this same pattern for adults. In this region, where patterns of dietary change have been much slower, we have begun to face the problem of obesity and other problems of dietary excess among not only the rich, but also the poor.[33]

Two very large nationally representative surveys were conducted in Brazil in 1974–1975 and 1989, each of which collected weight and height data along with other socioeconomic data.[49] In Brazil, obesity is greater in urban areas and in the more economically advanced southern region. Overall, income increases have been associated with greater obesity. More importantly, Brazilian women experience a prevalence of obesity comparable to that of women in the United States, although the obesity prevalence for Brazilian men remains lower than that of men in the United States.

There has been no large increase in the proportion of obese Brazilians between the two studies' time points.[49] Unlike China, we do not see equally important increases in undernutrition among the poor; in fact there have been significant declines in undernutrition among all income groups.[48] In contrast to China, the situation in many areas of Brazil approximates that of the United States, where the poor suffer more from problems of dietary excess than do the rich, with noncommunicable diseases and mortality from cardiovascular and other diseases greater among the poor. Figure 3 [Not shown, Ed.] shows a negative relationship among income, obesity, and hypertension in a medium-sized city in southern Brazil.[50,51] Between 1974–1975 and 1989 the proportionate and absolute increases in obesity were much greater for lower income populations.[52] In a survey of 4,241 people in Santiago, Chile, similar situations have been reported.[53]

In the Caribbean, adult obesity and high rates of morbidity and mortality from chronic degenerative diseases have begun to predominate. For example, in most countries of the English-speaking Caribbean more than half of adult females and a quarter of adult males are obese, with weight for height greater than 120% of the ideal body weight.[54] When BMI is used as a measurement of obesity, the rates also approximate those of the United States.[55] The structure of the diet has shifted in a manner comparable to the high-income Western country model.[54]

Africa and the Near East

A number of national food consumption surveys in urban Africa have shown large increases in the consumption of refined foods and fats.[56]

In most African countries, changes in dietary structure have been small. Nevertheless, despite the low levels of economic development, shifts in diet have begun to appear. Cote d'Ivoire, Mozambique, Algeria, and Libya have begun to show increases of fat in the overall food supply. This change is most rapid in the higher income Libya, where at the aggregate level more than 30% of energy is derived from fat, with about 10% from animal fat. In African countries, the rapidity of diet-related health changes in subpopulations independent of socioeconomic change is striking. For example, in 1930 there was virtually no incidence of diabetes in Kenya (two patients per year). By the late 1970s, diabetes had become common, despite the absence of socioeconomic change that has accompanied such increases in chronic diseases in the higher income countries.[56]

The most detailed information on the nutrition transition comes from South Africa.[57-59] A variety of small studies conducted over the past five decades combined with two larger studies indicate that the transition to a Western diet has occurred in rural and urban areas. The shift has been from a traditional high-carbohydrate diet with minimal refined foods to the Western diet. The authors of one detailed survey of adults in Cape Town provide evidence of the shift in the structure of the diet since a prior survey was undertaken in 1940.[57,58,60] In addition, they show that the level of obesity among females was very high. On the average this population consumed 26% of its energy from fat. More marked was the shift in the structure of diet associated with the proportion of time that each person had spent living in an urban environment.[59] The proportion of carbohydrate decreased considerably, and the proportion of fat and saturated fat increased with increased exposure to the urban environment (Figure 4) [Not shown, Ed.]. There was an equally significant and important increase in both the proportion and level of saturated and monounsaturated fat among the sample associated with urbanization. The proportion of protein from animal products increased while that from plant sources decreased proportionally to the time spent living in urban areas.

A similar shift in the structure of diet was associated with the long-term trend in diet for urban residents. Bourne et al.[57] compared the diet composition of adults in 1990 with the diet in 1940, which confirmed a 14% reduction in carbohydrate intake as a proportion of energy and an increase of 63% in fat intake over this 50-year time span. Compared to the post-World War II transition in East Asia, this represents a slower, but equally important shift. More than 44% of the black females in the sample had a BMI above 30, while only 7.9% of males were in this high-risk group. It is also interesting to note that growth retardation and wasting coexisting with obesity among preschoolers has also been observed.[61]

Government and Nutrition Professional Responses: What Can't Be Done?

The Nutrition Profession

The nutrition and health communities must consider how best to respond to this emerging crisis. One of the more interesting paradoxes is that nutrition professionals working in lower income countries have traditionally focused their interests on problems of poverty in undernutrition, which also represent important and difficult topics. It will be important not to magnify artificially the problems of deficit or distort resource allocation, which might actually hurt the poor who are beginning to suffer from problems of dietary excess.

It is possible to create a joint set of messages which will address the concerns of both under- and overnutrition. It is becoming clear that there are common underlying concerns that can unite nutritionists to lobby for selected common objectives. Good examples are the promotion of breast-feeding and increased consumption of β-carotene.

While problems of under- and overnutrition compete at any point for funding, it is important to emphasize the relationship of nutrition to the development of chronic disease. A failure to articulate the role of nutrition and coronary heart disease, cancer, and other problems associated with dietary excess will lead to an increased likelihood that tertiary interventions will dominate the available resources, and primary prevention will take a back seat. For example, the 1993 World Development Report[62] focused on a range of interventions for addressing problems of deficit and excess. While problems of undernutrition were discussed extensively, issues of dietary excess were largely ignored. The result was a cataloging of chronic-disease-related interventions which focus almost entirely on medical interventions and exclude the role of food and nutrition policies and other educational interventions related to nutrition.

Of potentially equal importance is the need for us to align with the medical profession and others who express great concern for problems of overnutrition. We should begin to promote one unified diet, rather than one special diet for malnourished and poor populations and other diets for higher income groups.

The other side of this issue is the need to adjust our understanding and prioritization of scarce nutrition resources to changes in actual need. Professionals and programs focused on problems of dietary deficiencies must be adjusted as the nature of the problem changes, or those who are actually in need may be hurt. Chile is an important example. The problems and needs of Chile have undergone a significant shift. Today, only a small segment of the population suffers from problems of malnutrition, and problems of overnutrition predominate. Assistance to this population at risk requires a new set of more targeted programs and a new surveillance procedure. Although fewer resources may be needed, they should be directed at the most needy population. One controversial approach to prevent malnutrition proposed in Chile is to target food program resources to those preschoolers who are at or below minus one standard deviation of the growth curve for weight or height for age. The previous reference point was minus two standard deviation units. Many have also voiced concern about the continued use of free milk for infants and preschoolers, because this practice is clearly a disincentive to breastfeeding, and there is minimal evidence that there is a clear undernutrition rationale for the distribution of milk.

Chile is at a middle level of development. It is undergoing a transition now that will occur in other countries over the next several decades. The types of programs noted above provide resources to a larger population, but there is considerable concern that these strategies will result in the use of scarce resources for those less in need rather than the development of a more targeted focus on those who are truly undernourished. Provision of other resources for newly emerging nutrition problems must also be a priority. Most importantly, this allows us to return to a crucial theme, namely that as long as nutritionists focus solely on problems of undernutrition, the problems of overnutrition and diseases will be left to higher cost medical interventions.

The economic transition in China will require a new set of solutions. In the past, China has not had poverty alleviation programs per se. Instead, economic development was viewed as the engine to eliminate poverty. For much of the population, this has worked admirably. At the same time, information presented here documents that there is an emerging low-income population for whom the problems of undernutrition are worsening. This may require a new array of poverty alleviation initiatives and targeted assistance to help poor households take advantage of the tremendous economic and social changes shaping China.

How nutrition ultimately adjusts to these rapid changes in the lower income world will to a large extent affect its role. There is a considerable need to develop a set of cost-effective programs and policies to address the problems of dietary excess. Yet, until experimentation and evaluation are undertaken, we have little to offer that will provide low-cost preventive solutions to problems that higher income countries have not yet successfully tackled. The efforts in the Scandinavian countries, China, and the United States provide a starting point for possible strategies.

Program and Policy Arsenal

Ideally, we would like to have a set of options for addressing problems of dietary excess similar to those for dietary deficiency, and then be able to combine them to fit the needs of each country. We are at far too early a stage in the process and there are too few countries which have yet to address the problems of excess. In fact, we are still in the stage whereby we do not even fully understand this transition.[63]

The first country to merge health and agricultural concerns systematically into an effective nutrition policy was Norway. Norway began an effort to reduce dietary fat intake in the 1960s and developed the Norwegian National Nutrition Policy in 1976, formally linking economic and agricultural policy with nutrition and health.[14,27,28] The results are impressive: Norway has stimulated research such as breeding cows for lower fat milk; denied consumer price subsidies when import prices of sugars soared in the mid-1970s; increased consumer subsidies for skim milk more than for whole milk, for poultry more than for pork, and for fish more than for beef; and implemented a set of producer subsidies to favor fish production over beef production.[28] The results have been dramatic and include a large increase in the consumption of reduced-fat milk, rapid increase in the consumption of poultry, and increase in consumption of margarine. Millo[27] hypothesizes that a systematic nutrition information policy directed at producers, governmental and private organizations, and consumers (along with significant agricultural policy changes) has been a key factor in the dietary changes in Norway during the past decade.

The Norwegian model used wide-scale national debate in conjunction with several coordinating bodies to lead the changes in legislation and regulations and education policy. A Norwegian government white paper prepared in 1975 was followed by a series of changes. The National Nutrition Council had been established much earlier, in 1946. The major breakthrough was the creation of a national expert committee, which established and publicized the linkage between diet and coronary heart disease. This initiated a series of national meetings and attempts to implement new dietary guidelines. The Ministry of Agriculture's development of the White Paper in 1975 led to the significant shift in government policy.[27,28]

The first low-income country to address problems of overnutrition appears to be China. In 1993, the Chinese government organized the National Commission for Food Reform and Development. The State Council[64] issued the first document that addressed future food production and marketing in terms of its significance to nutritional well-being. In effect, they issued the first dietary guidelines for China. These guidelines focus on food and production to eliminate undernutrition, and also on "diseases of affluence," or dietary excess and obesity. Public education and other activities during this past year have focused on retaining the current intake levels of fruits and vegetables and decreasing the proportion of high-fat relative to low-fat sources of protein. These guidelines explicitly attempt to increase seafood, poultry, and soybean production and consumption. The guidelines point out the many difficulties faced by the Chinese since large pockets of undernutrition exist, but they do provide a clear policy base for the development and implementation of food and nutrition policy to shift the composition of the diet. What is unique about this proclamation is the Ministry of Agriculture's recognition of the need to achieve a more balanced diet for the Chinese people and the role that the nutrition community is taking in this activity.

The Future

The biggest difficulty faced by nutritionists focusing on obesity and excess is that they are not offered the moral imperative enjoyed by their colleagues. There is no equivalent enthusiasm in attacking obesity in terms of drawing the attention and sympathy of the public. Moreover, in most low-income countries, the stigma against obesity is absent; in fact, obesity is often viewed as a symbol of beauty and status in unaware countries.[65] Humanitarian assistance that is partly driven by appeals to prevent starvation will be unable to obtain similar resources to address problems of dietary excess among the poor in lower income countries. Too often, society views obesity as a problem of idleness and personal failure and not one of public policy. Moreover, there is a need to examine these changes in dietary trends and learn whether they are inevitable, or simply representative of modernization. At the same time, it is important to consider that the poor people in lower income countries will be hurt in the long run if we do not begin to develop solutions for addressing their emerging problems now. The true challenge will be in generating approaches that inform and elicit public response and in forcing the nutrition profession to face and confront the problem.

We are a long way from understanding the effectiveness of an array of food price policy, regulations, and other tools in addressing the problems of nutrition transition. Aside from the Scandinavian countries, few countries have systematically tackled these problems over the past two decades, and the Chinese experience is too recent to enable us to draw any conclusions. This is not a reason to argue for inaction, but rather to imply that solutions will not be easily found, and must be accompanied by adequate evaluation. While it will be difficult for many agencies and professionals who have focused their careers on the problems of hunger and deficit to deal now with these newly emerging issues, it is very important that we begin to work out methodologies and programs to manage the problems of dietary excess in the poor.

Acknowledgments. Preparation of this review was supported in part by grants from the U.S. National Institutes of Health (P01HD28076-01).

SOURCE

Popkin B. 1994. The Nutrition Transition in Low-Income Countries: An Emerging Crisis. *Nutr Rev* 52 (9): 285–98. Copyright 1994 by Nutrition Reviews. Reprinted with permission of Wiley-Blackwell Publishing.

CHAPTER 2

TOBACCO

To cease smoking is the easiest thing I ever did. I ought to know because I've done it a thousand times.

    —Samuel L. Clemens, "Mark Twain" (1835–1910),
    American humorist

The cigarette has a violent action in the nerve centers, producing degeneration of the brain, which is quite rapid among boys. Unlike most narcotics, this degeneration is permanent and uncontrollable. I employ no person who smokes cigarettes.

    —Thomas A. Edison (1847–1941)
    Written in a letter to Henry Ford, 1914

JAMES ALBERT BONSACK'S SEPTEMBER 4, 1880, invention of the cigarette rolling machine sparked little interest from the era's large tobacco companies. Yet one chief executive officer, James Buchanan Duke of W. Duke and Sons, understood the machine's potential; he purchased a number of them. Within a decade, Duke's trust, the American Tobacco Company, defined the American industry. Assured a plentiful supply of product after buying the Bonsack patent, Duke focused on marketing. His success is writ in the ascending global mortality statistics for tobacco-related diseases: lung cancer, bladder cancer, laryngeal cancer, chronic obstructive pulmonary disease, and cardiovascular disease, among others.

The story of tobacco and its public health consequences encapsulates the twentieth century's major themes: capitalism, advertising, government regulation of hazardous products, the first campaign against cigarette smoking (by the Nazis), and a powerful growth stimulus for the health care industry. The insights gained about creating consumer desire flowed into society.

The industry's impact in the United States was supremely felt in one state, North Carolina, where tobacco meant agricultural wealth, political power, and industrial might. The tobacco marketing juggernaut converted two Southern cities, Winston-Salem and Raleigh, into globally known brand names. As Kentucky was known for bourbon, Maine for lobsters, and Iowa for corn, so North

Carolina was known for tobacco. North Carolina, a Confederate state during the American Civil War, was left destitute at that war's end. Tobacco offered North Carolina and its neighbor states a path toward economic survival. As American tobacco reached across both the Pacific and Atlantic Oceans and south of the Rio Grande River into Latin America, North Carolina felt tobacco's impact the most. And James Duke was squarely in the middle of that impact. Oil money built the University of Chicago, railroad money built Stanford and Johns Hopkins Universities, and tobacco money built Duke University, Wake Forest University's Bowman Gray School of Medicine, and Duke Power Company. But tobacco's greatest impact was on the public's health in both the developing and the developed worlds.

The Tobacco Industry: Marketing Cigarettes

Tobacco has been associated with the New World since Columbus's first voyages. Europeans, noting that Native Americans burned tobacco leaves for medicinal and other cultural purposes, began farming tobacco as a lucrative export commodity. The tobacco's harshness, however, restricted its use to snuff, chewing tobacco, and pipe smoking. As the United States industrialized, charcoal became widely available. Use of charcoal allowed tobacco curing at higher temperatures, resulting in a bright-yellow leaf ("flue-cured bright tobacco"). When burned, these leaves produced a milder smoke, full of nicotine and amenable to deep inhalation. Thus, innovation in curing resulted in the delivery of addictive nicotine deep into the lungs.

Cigarettes had not much mattered to the industry until the Bonsack machine appeared. Automated production decreased the cost of manufacturing a cigarette even as it increased by orders of magnitude the quantity of cigarettes available for sale. Duke bankrolled the Bonsack machine's development and cut a deal with Bonsack for a kickback on each machine Duke's competitors bought. Understanding the economies of scale afforded by the Bonsack machine, Duke appreciated the necessity of marketing to create a consumer base for his company's products. He moved his company's headquarters to New York City, the emerging center of the U.S. consumer-led economy. Understanding young men as the core market for cigarettes, Duke added trading cards featuring scantily clad women to the packages of cigarettes. He also advertised his products with an intensity not hitherto seen in American commerce. His innovations included new corporate structures, as the growth of Duke's company gave him leverage with his competitors to form a new entity: the trust.

The Tobacco Trust, formed around Duke's American Tobacco Company in 1890, grew into the third largest company in the United States, surpassed only

Men vs Women on tobacco

by Standard Oil and U.S. Steel. Indeed, John Rockefeller took his cue in forming the Standard Oil Trust from Duke's Tobacco Trust. However, President Theodore Roosevelt had the Tobacco Trust prosecuted as a violation of the Sherman Anti-Trust Act. In 1911, on the same day the United States Supreme Court ordered the dissolution of the Standard Oil Trust, it did the same for the Tobacco Trust, the American Tobacco Company. Duke, convinced the United States cigarette market was saturated, turned his attention to electricity generation. Forming Duke Power, he lost all interest in the tobacco industry that he had been instrumental in creating.

As Duke exited the American tobacco industry, national brands emerged. In 1913, the only nonmember of the Tobacco Trust, R.J. Reynolds Company, brought Camel cigarettes to the national marketplace. Camel brought hegemony to the commercial tobacco marketplace similar to what Duke brought to the corporate tobacco world. As the United States entered World War I, Camel was the only national cigarette brand. World War I was a bonanza for cigarette manufacturers. Young soldiers with little to do in the trenches tried cigarettes (included in their rations) to pass the time. Similarly, the advertising push by Reynolds expanded the domestic market even further. In 1918, thinking Camel's market share secure, Reynolds cut back on Camel's advertising support. Seizing the opportunity, both Liggett & Myers's Chesterfield and American Tobacco Company's Lucky Strike brands began Camel-like advertising campaigns. By the mid-1920s, these "Big Three" dominated (at more than 80 percent) the American market, with Camel alone sustaining a 45 percent share.

During the 1920s, 16 states tried to control the promotion and sale of cigarettes, but all such legislation was short-lived. Brands jostled for market position with advertising campaigns seeking to ensnare the young, persuade existing smokers to change brands, and tap into new markets. For example, in the mid-1920s, Philip Morris introduced Marlboro as a brand for women with the motto "Mild as May." The faltering brand was withdrawn from the marketplace just before World War II. Lorillard fared better in its introduction of Old Gold in the 1920s. Old Gold's market share was in the single digits for the next two decades, but it was still the fourth leading cigarette brand in the United States. In the early 1930s (hardly an auspicious time for new consumer products), Philip Morris introduced a brand of the same name. A blitz of advertising (a dwarf dressed as a bellhop bellowed, "Call for Philip Morris!") coupled with new technology to maintain tobacco leaves' moisture established Philip Morris cigarettes as the fifth leading brand in the marketplace. During World War II, free cigarettes were issued to American soldiers. When the soldiers returned to civilian life, a ready-made population of cigarette consumers continued smoking, addicted to the nicotine delivered by their cigarettes.

As the postwar era unfolded, the United States emerged as an economic powerhouse, responsible for one-quarter of global gross national product (GNP). Cigarettes became the most advertised products in the United States, followed by automobiles. Yet all was not well with tobacco. Public concerns were aroused by articles in *Reader's Digest* about smoking's health effects. In response, the tobacco industry introduced filtered cigarettes. For instance, in 1952 Kent cigarettes with filters made of asbestos were introduced. In 1954, Reynolds countered by putting filters onto its new brand, Winston. During the next decade, assisted by American Tobacco's fumbled marketing efforts, Winston became the best-selling cigarette in the United States by sponsoring a race of the National Association for Stock Car Auto Racing (NASCAR), the Winston Cup. In 1956, Reynolds introduced Salem filtered mentholated cigarettes (the menthol suppressed the cough reflex induced by smoke inhalation). Philip Morris, however, perceived filters as problematic—a feature of feminine cigarettes. The market for cigarettes was predominantly male, and it would be decades before women caught up with men in their smoking habits. Better, Philip Morris reasoned, to take a feminine brand with a filter and masculinize it. The "Mild as May" Marlboro brand fit the bill.

In the mid-1950s, Philip Morris reintroduced Marlboro as a premium cigarette for men. Repositioning the brand required considerable advertising support. The marketing campaign, led by the Marlboro Man, worked and solidly established Marlboro as the leading brand by the end of the decade. To improve market share, Philip Morris ordered marketing surveys and identified what caught the public's attention: a cowboy theme. Philip Morris executives ordered TV ads featuring a cowboy. One of these had movie music from *The Magnificent Seven* in the background and a voice-over stating, "Come to where the flavor is. Come to Marlboro Country." There was immediate agreement that the ads were exactly what the product needed. The ensuing marketing campaign is acclaimed as the one of the best ever implemented. The 1960s closed with Marlboro as the best-selling brand not only in the United States but also globally. It has never relinquished that position.

The women's liberation movement helped bring cigarettes to the female market. With the rise of women in the workforce during World War II, cigarette smoking among women increased. This uptrend continued with the feminist movement, and cigarette manufacturers responded by launching brands targeting women. Philip Morris introduced Virginia Slims, marketed with the tagline, "You've come a long way, baby." In the 1970s, Virginia Slims began sponsoring women's professional tennis just as women's tennis professionals Billy Jean King and Chris Evert emerged as major sports celebrities. Soon after, women's lung cancer rates and those of other smoking-related diseases began climbing toward those of their male counterparts.

Public Health Consequences

The consideration that tobacco might be linked to cancers of the respiratory tract dates back to the 1700s when English physician John Hill associated the use of snuff with nasal cancer and German physician Samuel Thomas van Sommering suggested pipe smoking as a cause of cancer of the lip. In 1858, French surgeon Étienne-Frédéric Bouisson observed that 63 of his 68 patients with cancer of the mouth were pipe smokers. In 1885, President Ulysses S. Grant died from throat cancer attributed to his cigar smoking. All of these observations, however, predate the widespread use of cigarettes and the meteoric rise of lung cancer.

In the 1800s, miners in Schneeberg, Germany, were observed to be at increased risk for lung cancer, but this was presumably due to their exposure to radon gas in the mines. It was noteworthy at that time because lung cancer was a rare malignancy. Indeed, the renowned German pathologist Rudolph Virchow reported only one case of lung cancer in his 3,390 autopsies of deceased cancer patients in Würzburg from 1852 to 1855. In the United States, future cancer researcher Alton Ochsner wrote that as a medical student in 1919 he was called to see a rare case of lung cancer in the operating room. By 1923, however, the increasing occurrence of lung cancer was reported at the annual meeting of Germany's Pathology Association.

One of the early experimental investigators into the relationship between tobacco and health was Professor A. H. Roffo from the Institute of Experimental Medicine for the Study and Treatment of Cancer in Buenos Aires. Roffo's animal experiments in the 1930s (see selected reading) suggested that tobacco, when burned, led to the creation of carcinogens. Some epidemiologic data on tobacco smoking and cancer was collected before World War II, but almost none was directed at cigarette smoking. In fact, only one country waged war against cigarette smoking before World War II—the Third Reich. The Nazis fervently believed that cigarettes were a sign of moral weakness and thus sought to discourage youth from smoking. As soon as the party came into power in 1933, schools began to discuss the dangers of tobacco. Nazi scientists examined smoking from a medical perspective and discovered what American and British researchers would find two decades later: cigarette smoking caused lung cancer and other adverse health outcomes. Because Nazi science was distrusted in both Western Europe and North America, the results of the research were dismissed. This rejection of scientific results haunts Europe to this day; Socialists came to view cigarette smoking as a political statement, a demonstration of antifascist sentiment. Unfortunately, this rejection remains one of the explanations for the persistence of cigarette smoking in Europe, even into the twenty-first century.

Interest in the health effects of tobacco focused on cancer until 1940, the year when English, Willius, and Berkson reported a clear association between smoking and coronary heart disease among 2,000 subjects at the Mayo Clinic. Could the same agent cause different diseases in different organ systems? This idea went against conventional wisdom that held an agent caused one disease only. Shortly afterward, scientists at the National Cancer Institute (NCI) noted an elevated rate of lung cancer in cities and proposed air pollution as a possible explanation. Cigarette smoking was not explicitly suggested as a cause, perhaps because cigarette smoke was considered a component of air pollution. In 1950, five case-control studies of lung cancer and cigarette smoking were published, and all identified an association between smoking and lung cancer. Three of the five studies (Wynder and Graham, Levin et al., and Doll and Hill) are frequently cited as the seminal investigations regarding smoking and lung cancer.

During the late 1940s, Ernst Wynder, a medical student at Washington University in St. Louis was doing a summer internship in New York City. While attending the autopsy of a decedent with lung cancer, he noted that the medical chart lacked mention of smoking. Wynder asked the widow if her deceased husband smoked, and she reported that he had been a two-pack-a-day smoker. That caused Wynder to wonder whether underreporting was a cause of the lack of association between cigarette smoking and lung cancer. He continued interviewing lung cancer cases and controls about their smoking habits but was unable to finish his project before returning to school. Back at Washington University, Wynder approached Evarts Graham, chief of surgery, to get permission to continue interviews with patients on his service. Graham, the first American surgeon to successfully remove a lung, consented despite the fact that he was both a heavy smoker and a skeptic about a smoking-lung cancer relationship. Wynder's data, however, showed a striking relationship. The surgeon and his student promptly drafted a report of the findings and submitted it to the *Journal of the American Medical Association* (later *JAMA*). The journal faced two problems if it rejected the paper: First, Graham was a major figure in the American medical community and rejection of his paper was politically problematic. Also, the journal had just rejected a similar paper written by Levin and colleagues. Levin had reported similar results. How could the journal accept Graham's paper and not Levin's?

In the mid-1930s, Mortin L. Levin was a house officer at Baltimore's Sinai Hospital when he was selected for epidemiology training at the Johns Hopkins University School of Hygiene and Public Health. Later, Levin took a position as an epidemiologist at the Roswell Park Memorial Institute in Buffalo, New York, where he studied the viral etiology of cancer. By the late 1930s, with experimental evidence mounting (for example, Roffo's work), Levin shifted his perspective. In 1940, he directed the Roswell Park staff to begin interviewing all new admissions about their smoking status. Before the end of the decade, Levin had sufficient data to show an association between smoking and lung cancer. He submitted his results to the *Journal of the American Medical Association*, but it rejected his paper. At the time, Levin was serving as Director of the Commission on Chronic Illnesses, based in Chicago. The commission's office was in the same building as the journal, which allowed Levin the opportunity to visit the editor and assure him of the soundness of the analyses. In turn, the editor gave him a copy of the Wynder-Graham manuscript. Levin urged the editor to publish both papers, which he did in the May 27, 1950, issue.

In 1947, British public health officials became concerned about the increasing lung cancer mortality rate. The Medical Research Council (MRC) began studies into the role of air pollution, as well as experimental studies. An explicit inquiry into cigarette smoking was also begun under the direction of Austin Bradford Hill, an MRC statistical consultant from the London School of Hygiene and Tropical Health. Hill developed the study design and assigned a young postdoctoral student, Richard Doll, to conduct it. By 1950, the study was complete and showed a strong relationship between smoking and lung cancer. The Doll–Hill report appeared in the *British Medical Journal* four months after the *Journal of the American Medical Association* published the Wynder-Graham and Levin et al. study results.

The mounting evidence left two questions unanswered. First, could smoking actually transform cells into a malignancy? Roffo's data had been discounted because his experiments used temperatures that were far higher than would be present in a burning cigarette. Second, all five of the epidemiologic studies from 1950 were of a case-control design and had weaknesses. For instance, Wynder had asked the cases "Do you smoke?" and the controls "You don't smoke, do you?" The difference in question structure could have biased the results. The only way to address the issue of bias would be to use a prospective cohort study in which people were selected by smoking status and followed forward in time for disease. Three such studies were conducted during the 1950s, those by Doll and Hill (the Doctors Study), Hammond and Horn (the American Cancer Society Study), and Dorn (the Veteran's Administration [VA] Life Insurance Study).

The first of these studies was designed by Hill, who recognized that physicians might be an especially cooperative group of subjects. As the study was beginning, however, English physicians began changing their smoking habits in response to new health risk information. Hill turned the study over to Doll, who monitored the decline in cancer risk associated with declines in smoking. This natural experiment continued for the next half century and clearly demonstrated the positive effect of smoking cessation.

At the American Cancer Society (ACS), the director of research, E. Cuyler Hammond, and his associate director, Daniel Horn, thought of using ACS's many local fundraisers to constitute cohorts of smokers and nonsmokers who could be followed by their local chapters. Within three years, the relationship between smoking and lung cancer was evident in the ACS data. The ACS Study would, in time, follow 188,000 people to determine which causes of death were increased among smokers.

The last of the major cohort studies was Harold F. Dorn's VA Life Insurance Study. Dorn, like Hammond and Hill, had trained as a demographer before becoming an epidemiologist. The idea of using a population of government employees in a cohort study of cancer etiology had been suggested as early as 1940. Dorn modified the idea, ascertaining the smoking habits of men who had purchased life insurance from the VA. Then, using the death certificates presented with each claim, he determined the occurrence of lung cancer among the smokers and nonsmokers. The Dorn study was the largest of the cohort studies (293,658 people) and had the added benefit of being conducted by the NCI, a government agency. Anyone choosing to attack the study risked appearing to attack the U.S. government, a dangerous proposition in 1950.

The principal findings of all three cohort studies showed a strong statistical relationship between smoking and lung cancer. The tobacco industry's response was to dismiss the findings as statistical gibberish. Some leading biostatisticians, such as R.A. Fisher and Joseph Berkson, argued that the proclivity for selection bias precluded making a causal inference. Other biostatisticians suggested revising the basic postulates for causal reasoning. However, none of the discussion elements diminished the conclusion that smoking was a cause of lung cancer.

In 1957, the NCI and the National Heart Institute, the two government agencies most connected with smoking research, joined with their nongovernmental counterparts, the ACS and the American Heart Association, to sponsor the seven-member Study Group on Smoking and Health (SGSH) to review the available data on smoking and lung cancer. The group's 1957 publication established the relationship between smoking and lung cancer "beyond a reasonable doubt." Yet the U.S. PHS was unwilling to place warnings on cigarette packs, and the NCI's director opined that smoking less than two packs of cigarettes a day probably did not have health consequences. The general public, lacking an understanding of the data, assumed that anyone smoking less than two packs a day was safe. People continued to puff away.

The timidity shown by the PHS generally and the NCI in particular spurred some SGSH members to assemble the scientific data in an effort to convince the medical community about the hazards of smoking. Their work was summarized in a 1959 publication (one of the selected readings) that provided a capstone for the 1950s epidemiologic work on the tobacco-health relationship. In the United Kingdom, the Royal College of Physicians (RCP) created its own review committee and also concluded that the evidence was sufficient to view smoking as a cause of lung cancer. At the same time, the U.S. Surgeon General assembled a group of distinguished scientists to conduct a similar review. Vetted by the tobacco industry, the membership of the surgeon general's committee explicitly excluded all SGSH members and included two committee members (Leonard Schuman, an epidemiologist, and William Cochran, a statistician) who were cigarette smokers. After reviewing 7,000 papers and consulting with 150 experts, the committee issued its report on January 11, 1964. Its verdict was unequivocal: smoking caused lung cancer and other diseases. At a news conference discussing the results, Schuman and Cochran appeared with lit cigarettes and an ashtray between them. In front of reporters, both took their cigarettes and snubbed them out. The photo taken of this action was prominent on the front page of newspapers throughout the United States. The war against smoking had begun. The next year, the U.S. Presidential Commission on Heart Disease, Cancer, and Stroke recommended banning cigarette advertising on electronic media. It also recommended placing warnings about the health effects of smoking on all cigarette packages. Both recommendations eventually became law.

Over the next decade, the relationship between cigarette smoking and other diseases became apparent (bladder cancer, chronic obstructive lung disease, hypertension, and myocardial infarction). Tobacco smoke was also found to act synergistically with asbestos in causing lung cancer and with oral contraceptives in causing pulmonary embolism. Exposure to environmental tobacco smoke (ETS) also became a concern. For instance, Takeshi Hirayama identified cohorts of nonsmoking Japanese women and noted whether their spouses smoked. In 1981, he reported that the women living with spouses who smoked had an elevated risk of lung cancer, despite the fact that they did not smoke. Subsequent studies replicated the finding and sparked considerable concern about nonsmoking individuals who were occupationally exposed to ETS. Pressure grew to reduce such exposure, and smoking was banned on airplanes flying over the United States. As more studies linked ETS to a variety of conditions, such as pediatric asthma, bans on smoking in the workplace and in common public spaces were implemented.

During the late 1970s and early 1980s, plaintiff attorneys turned their attention to the American tobacco industry, filing lawsuits on behalf of smokers who held the industry responsible for their diseases. Joining these suits were several states, who claimed that the industry was responsible for hundreds of billions of dollars in health care for which the states had paid. A plethora of documents that showed that the tobacco industry perpetrated a monumental cover-up of research linking smoking and disease were made public. The industry had engaged in disinformation and corruption of the American academic medical research community for more than half a century. Yet even as the tobacco industry was negotiating to settle these law suits, it was casting its gaze on the developing world for future profits and beginning to target people under age 16 to entice them into becoming smokers. The "Cool Joe Camel" campaign from the early 1990s is an exemplar of these efforts. As the twentieth century closed, the industry was incented to counter its prior efforts at seducing youth into smoking as part of the developing lawsuit settlements.

The negative impact of tobacco on global public health continues to grow. Unlike the United States, the United Kingdom, and select other countries, most nations control the sale of tobacco through government ownership of tobacco companies and/or the cigarette retail distribution system. The profits afforded by cigarette sales provide little incentive for governments to wean their populations from smoking. For example, China today earns almost 10 percent of its national tax income from smokers. Thus, smoking continues to expand in the developing world even as public health efforts to contain it have yet to succeed in the developed one.

Tobacco exemplifies the twentieth century in a variety of ways. For instance, it was the most successful product of a consumer-led economy fostered by advertising and brand promotion. It also allowed corporate structures to create and support the expansion of national and global brands. In tobacco, one finds the economic and political history of twentieth-century America, as the United States broke up one monopoly (the Tobacco Trust, as part of the Square Deal), subsidized tobacco growth (a by-product of the New Deal), and subsidized the treatment of tobacco-related illnesses such as lung cancer (provided by Medicare, as part of the Great Society). Epidemiologic efforts in the United States and Europe have focused on tobacco for more than half a century, spurring the creation of the modern public health enterprise with its focus on chronic diseases. Through its addictive properties, both chemical and financial, tobacco continues to sow fatal effects throughout the world. It is moving from being the grim reaper in the developed world to being a scourge in the developing one. Yet smoking prevalence rates continue to rise as all too many are dying for a smoke.

Selected Readings

The three selected readings cover the development of our modern understanding of the health consequences of cigarette smoking, the focus of public health efforts for almost a century. The first reading is one of the initial papers on experimental demonstrations of the carcinogenicity of tobacco smoke. During the 1920s, Roffo's clinical observations associated cigarette smoking with respiratory tract cancers. By the early 1930s, Roffo was administering components of cigarette smoke onto rabbit ears. Using this technique, he isolated the carcinogenic component of the smoke as the polycyclic aromatic hydrocarbons, not the nicotine or inorganic components, and published his results in the German medical literature. This limited his audience to some physicians and some in the tobacco industry and kept the results from most consumers. Roffo's findings were the subject of disdain by some in the tobacco industry, and British researchers assessing the possible role of cigarette smoking in the increasing lung cancer mortality rate later incorrectly discounted them.

The second reading is the 1959 review paper by Cornfield and colleagues. It summarized the available evidence on smoking and lung cancer for the medical community for the first time, and it raised sufficient interest in the issue so as to lead the RCP to convene its own committee on the matter. The work is abridged in that we have removed one figure and the appendixes. We felt that the figure on percent of necropsies is adequately discussed in the text, and as the appendixes are statistical proofs written in mathematical notation, their removal did not detract from the paper. This particular reading is important in that its conclusion—that the evidence relating smoking to lung cancer was compelling—helped change the American medical community's view of cigarette smoking from being a bad habit to being a lethal addiction.

Takeshi Hirayama's 1981 paper on cancer mortality in nonsmoking women living with smoking husbands is a politically important paper. Hirayama showed conclusively that passive smoking (exposure to ETS) is a distinct risk for the development of lung cancer. From this work came efforts by widespread lobbying groups to implement nonsmoking policies in public places. In 1987, the U.S. Congress banned smoking on U.S. airline flights of two hours or under; this extended to all airline flights within the United States and to all U.S. air carrier flights regardless of destination in 1998. At century's end, antismoking campaigns were in full swing worldwide with more than 80 countries and hundreds of global cities issuing smoking bans for public places.

BIBLIOGRAPHY

Barnes DE, Hanauer P, Slade J, Bero LA, and Glantz SA. 1995. Environmental tobacco smoke. The Brown and Williamson documents. *JAMA* 274 (3): 248–53.

Berkson J. 1955. The statistical study of association between smoking and lung cancer. Proc Staff Meet, Mayo Clinic 30:319–48.

Bero L, Barnes DE, Hanauer P, Slade J, and Glantz SA. 1995. Lawyer control of the tobacco industry's external research program. The Brown and Williamson documents. *JAMA* 274 (3): 241–47. Erratum in: *JAMA* 277 (11): 885.

Brandt AM. *The Cigarette Century: The Rise, Fall, and Deadly Persistence of the Product That Defined America.* 2007. New York: Basic Books.

Centers for Disease Control and Prevention. 1999. Achievements in Public Health, 1900–1999: Tobacco use—United States, 1900-1999. *MMWR* 48 (43): 986–93.

Dockery DW and Trichopoulos D. 1997. Risk of lung cancer from environmental exposures to tobacco smoke (in Review Papers). Harvard-Teikyo Program Special Issue, *Cancer Causes & Control* 8(3): 333–45.

Doll R and Hill AB. 1950. Smoking and carcinoma of the lung. *Brit Med J* 2:739–48.

Doll R and Hill AB. 1956. Lung cancer and other causes of death in relation to smoking: A second report on the mortality of British doctors. *Brit Med J* 2:1072–81.

Doll R and Peto R. 1976. Mortality in relation to smoking: 20 years' observations on male British doctors. *Brit Med J* 2:1525–36.

Dorn HF. Morbidity and mortality from cancer of the lung in the United States. 1953. *Acta Unio Int Contra Cancrum* 9 (3): 552–61.

English JP, Willius FA, and Berkson J. 1940. Tobacco and coronary disease. *J Am Med Assoc* 35:556–58.

Environmental Protection Agency. 1992. Respiratory Health Effects of Passive Smoking: Lung Cancer and Other Disorders (EPA/600/6-90/006F). Washington, DC: Environmental Protection Agency, Office on Air and Radiation.

Fisher RA. 1958. Cancer and smoking. *Nature* 182:596.

Gellhorn A. 1958. Carcinogenesis and tobacco tar. *Cancer* 18:510–17.

Giovino GA, Henningfield JE, Tomar SL, Escobedo LG, and Slade J. 1995. Epidemiology of tobacco use and dependence. *Epidemiologic Reviews* 17:48–65.

Glantz SA, Barnes DE, Bero L, Hanauer P, and Slade J. 1995. Looking through a keyhole at the tobacco industry. The Brown and Williamson documents. *JAMA* 1274 (3): 219–24.

Hanauer P, Slade J, Barnes DE, Bero L, and Glantz SA. 1995. Lawyer control of internal scientific research to protect against products liability lawsuits. The Brown and Williamson documents. *JAMA* 274 (3): 234–40.

Kluger R. 1996. *Ashes to Ashes: America's Hundred-Year Cigarette War, the Public Health, and the Unabashed Triumph of Philip Morris.* New York: Alfred A. Knopf.

Levin ML, Goldstein H, and Gerhardt PR. 1950. Cancer and tobacco smoking; a preliminary report. *J Am Med Assoc* 143 (4): 336–38.

MacDermot HE. 1951. Tobacco and pulmonary cancer (editorial). *Can Med Assoc J* 65:266–67.

Mattson ME, Boyd G, Byar D, Brown C, Callahan JF, Corle D, Cullen JW, Greenblatt J, Haley NJ, Hammond K, Lewtas J, and Reeves W. 1989. Passive smoking on commercial airline flights. *JAMA* 261 (6): 867–72.

Nishino Y, Tsubono Y, Tsuji I, Komatsu S, Kanemura S, Nakatsuka H, Fukao A, Satoh H, and Hisamichi S. 2001. Passive smoking at home and cancer risk: A population-based prospective study in Japanese nonsmoking women (in research papers). *Cancer Causes & Control* 12 (9): 797–802.

Ochsner A. 1973. Corner of history: My first recognition of the relationship of smoking and lung cancer. *Prev Med* 2:611–14.

Peace LR. 1985. A time correlation between cigarette smoking and lung cancer. *The Statistician* 34 (40): 371–81.

Pirkle JL, Flegal KM, Bennert JT, Brody DJ, Etzel RA, and Maurer KR. 1996. Exposure of the U.S. population to environmental tobacco smoke. *JAMA* 275 (16): 1233–40.

Slade J, Bero LA, Hanauer P, Barnes DE, and Glantz SA. 1995. Nicotine and addiction. The Brown and Williamson documents. *JAMA* 274 (3): 225–33.

U.S. Public Health Service. 1964. Smoking and health. Report of the Advisory Committee to the Surgeon General of the Public Health Service (PHS 1103). U.S. Department of Health, Education, and Welfare, Public Health Service, Centers for Disease Control, Atlanta, GA.

Ware JH, Dockery DW, Spiro A III, Speizer FE, and Ferris BG Jr. 1984. Passive smoking, gas cooking, and respiratory health of children living in six cities. *Am Rev Respir Dis* 129:366–74.

Wright AA and Katz IT. 2007. Tobacco tightrope—balancing disease prevention and economic development in China. *N Engl J Med* 356 (15): 1493–95.

Wynder EL and Hoffman D. 1963. Experimental aspects of tobacco carcinogenesis. *Chest* 44:337–44.

The Carcinogenic Effects of Tobacco
(1940)

A summary of numerous experiments carried out at the Cancer Institute in Buenos Aires which provide evidence for the carcinogenic effect of tobacco smoking.

Professor Dr. A.H. Roffo

Even a cursory glance at the cancer statistics for all countries shows the currently well known fact that, while the numbers of cases of cancers other than throat cancer have either only slowly increased or decreased (even if only temporarily or to a very small extent), *disturbingly, the number of cases of lung cancer has increased.*

We observed this trend several years ago in our clinic before we could confirm it statistically and it coincided with another observation: *that lung and throat cancer are extraordinarily rare among women.* A third statistically proven fact was that *95% of patients with lung or throat cancer were heavy smokers.* The fact that the bad habit of tobacco smoking has not yet been taken up by women in our society explains why this cancer is so infrequent among them; furthermore, the few cases of throat cancer that we have observed among women in our institute all involved heavy smokers. Here are some statistics from our work which illustrate these conclusions: [see table I on next page, Ed.]

These observations made the carcinogenic effect of tobacco fairly obvious. However, this hypothesis was based on clinical observations, and needed to be proved experimentally.

Over the past few years we have provided such proof through a series of experimental studies and present a short overview here.

In March 1930, my article "Experimental tobacco leukoplakia" appeared (1). (Based on our clinical observations, we believe that leukoplakia is a clear precancerous form). The rabbits used in the experiments were exposed to tobacco smoke, since previous experiments had already shown that nicotine or whole tobacco extract did not have a cancer-producing effect.

The animals were divided into three groups. The gums of the rabbits in two of the groups (2) were first modified by being treated with cholesterol. The gums of all the animals were then exposed to tobacco smoke for 3 minutes per day by means of a water pump. The result was the clear

Table I Deaths Due to Cancer among the "Smoker's Highway"

1926	148
1927	200
1928	207
1932	335
1933	397
1934	496
1935	468
1936	498
1937	513

Table II Statistical Excerpt Showing Cancer Deaths According to Site and Sex

	1932		1933		1934		1935	
	M.	F.	M.	F.	M.	F.	M.	F.
Throat	115	1	119	5	105	3	126	7
Lung	150	30	187	51	188	48	196	57
Monatschrift f. Krebsbekfg., 1940, issue 5.								

formation of leukoplakia, whereby the lesions appeared earlier among the animals treated with cholesterol.

In July of the same year (1930), I published the results of other experiments under the title "Carcinoma and rabbits classified tobacco" (3).

To make the experimental conditions as similar as possible to those of the smoker, we extracted three products from the tobacco smoke:

1. An aqueous solution obtained by passing the tobacco smoke through cold water;

2. A product obtained from the nicotine solution produced by ether-chloroform extraction of the first solution above;

3. A product resulting from the distillation of the residue.

The experimental animals were divided into three groups of 10 rabbits and the interior surface of each of their ears was painted, respectively, with one of the above test solutions every second day. Before being thus painted, the interior of the ears of each animal was first sprayed with a 5% aqueous solution of cholesterol.

In the first group, treated with the first solution, one animal showed signs of carcinoma after eight months and died one month later. An additional 7 animals in this group died from chronic poisoning.

We did not observe any tumors in the second and third groups, however, some of the animals died of chronic poisoning.

Pursuing a line of thinking provoked by this work, we conducted a further series of experiments whereby we exposed the interior surface of the rabbits' ears to whole tobacco smoke. One rabbit developed lesions after three years, the product of a prolific simple neoplastic process. This is described in detail in the publication "The development of carcinoma in a smoking rabbit" (4) (1931).

These last two studies prove the carcinogenic effect of the combustion products of tobacco and the harmless effect of nicotine with respect to cancer formation.

We have also observed clinically that bladder cancer, which is very widespread, occurs almost exclusively among men, which we believe is related to tobacco smoking. We were able to confirm this experimentally and published our findings in September 1931 in "The role of tobacco in bladder cancer" (5).

In August 1936, my fundamental work in this area appeared in our *Bulletin* under the title "Tobacco as the carcinogenic agent" (6). Therein, after summarizing our previous clinical and laboratory results, I described a new series of experiments and their results.

This time we did not use tobacco smoke or its products. Instead, using *fractional distillation*, we separated three *products* from the tobacco itself.

The *first product* was obtained at a temperature of 100° C.

The *second product* was obtained by gradually increasing the temperature from 120° C to 350° C.

The *third product* was obtained by further heating the residue; like the second product, it is a viscous, black-brown tar, only somewhat thicker and darker.

Using another series of 30 rabbits, we painted the interior surface of the ears of each group with one of these three products.

We found the following results:

1. The first product caused no lesions.

2. The second product yielded lesions in about 98% of rabbits. Already after 7 months small papillomas appeared on the painted areas in some of the animals and later became carcinogenic.

3. The third product also yielded the same kind of lesions but fewer, so that the last two products resulted, on average, in cancers in about 95% of the rabbits.

This makes it completely clear that, 1) tobacco is highly carcinogenic, and 2) that this is a property of the tobacco tar obtained from distillation at temperatures of 350° C and higher. 3) Nicotine does not play a role in this respect because it decomposes below 100° C and there are only rarely traces of it even in the first product. 4) Chemical and spectrographic analyses of tobacco lead us to believe that it contains the same or similar substances as the hydrocarbons obtained by distillation of coal, particularly as the effect of the tobacco tar is the same as that of coal tar.

Reinforcing and expanding the results presented here is the work done at our institute and published by A. E. Roffo (jr.) in September 1937 as "Spectrographic analysis of the derivatives directly distilled from tobacco" (7). The analysis was done on a variety of tobacco types (German, Italian, Turkish, Egyptian, Havana [from the Argentinean province of Corrientes], Kentucky and chewing tobacco). The tobacco was heated in closed retorts: a) to 100° C, b) from 100° C to 350° C, and c) then fractionally distilled from 85° C to 320° C. In all three cases, absorption bands appeared in the same region of the ultraviolet spectrum as those of carcinogenic hydrocarbons. This provided spectrographic evidence that the hydrocarbons distilled from the tobacco tar of the types listed above contained condensed benzene nuclei.

In our work "Blond tobacco as a carcinogenic substance" (8) (1938)[1], we painted the ears of our test animals with the tar distilled from blond tobacco with the following results:

1. Blond tobacco not only produced a larger amount of tar than the dark tobacco but also was much more toxic. For these two reasons, blond tobacco is much more harmful than dark tobacco.

2. Blond tobacco tar has exactly the same carcinogenic effect as that obtained from dark tobacco.

I ascribed the carcinogenic effect of the tar from this tobacco to the presence of substances containing condensed benzene nuclei belonging to the aromatic hydrocarbon series, as already mentioned. We have studied the ultraviolet absorption; even with very diluted solutions, bands appear at 3,870 Å, which correspond to the absorption spectrum of the hydrocarbons mentioned above. In addition, the substance is characterized by a

---

1 Ds. Mschr. 1939, issue 3, p. 75. Schriftw.

strong fluorescence ranging from dark blue to violet, corresponding to 1:2 benzopyrene, 1:2 benzanthracene and 1:2:5:6-dibenzanthracene.

In conclusion, we would like to mention that the experimental results attributing strong carcinogenic properties to light tobacco also highlight the necessity of taking preventive measures against cancer by stemming tobacco use, particularly among women, who have recently begun smoking blond tobacco in particular.

In September 1938, I published the results of other experiments which proved, as the title itself states, "The carcinogenic component of various tobacco tars" (9). I have *summarized* the results of this experimental research as follows:

1. The tars of 9 different types of tobacco all have carcinogenic effects; some types cause a very high percentage of tumors—up to 100%.
2. All have carcinogenic effects; however, the intensity depends on plant variety.
3. The carcinogenic effect is strongest in the Turkish, Egyptian, Kentucky and chewing tobaccos; these are followed by other tobacco types, which nevertheless cause cancer in more than 50% of the test animals.
4. The development of lesions occurred in the same way in all animals: hyperkeratosis → papilloma → squamous cell carcinoma.
5. To achieve these results, painting tar on the inner surface of the ear of a rabbit every second day is enough; 100 to 150 ml tar is needed for a complete carcinoma to occur.
6. A carcinogenic property of tobacco tar and coal tar, which we proved experimentally, indicates the necessity of tackling cancer preventatively by actively supporting the fight against smoking.

If only 100 grams of tar is needed to cause various carcinogenic tumors in rabbits within 9 to 10 months, it is easy to imagine the risk to an average smoker who smokes one kilo of tobacco per month, or the equivalent of approximately 70 ml of tar. In other words, 840 ml of tar annually or 8 liters of tar in 10 years coat the mucous membranes of the mouth, larynx, throat, and lungs, which are biologically less resistant than rabbit skin.

Our most recent publication, from last year (1939), entitled "Carcinogenic benzopyrene from tobacco tar" (10), pursued the already mentioned task of isolating the actual carcinogenic component in tobacco tar. We succeeded in obtaining a distillation product from tobacco tar, having the spectrographic characteristics and fluorescence of 1:2 benzopyrene. Furthermore, we proved in our animal experiments that:

1. This product is highly carcinogenic; it causes carcinomas which are invasive, metastatic and aggressive;

2. The majority of the animals died within 1 to 2 years of starting the experiment;

3. The first lesions appeared earlier than those caused by tobacco tar in its crude form;

4. Based on these experimental results, we believe that the strong carcinogenic effect of crude tobacco tar, which consists of numerous substances, is due to the tobacco benzopyrene.

[Mschr. Krebsbekpfg. 1940, issue 5.]

In conclusion I would like to repeat that the numerous animal experiments conducted at our institute have proved the carcinogenic effect of tobacco and of the tobacco benzopyrene contained in the tobacco tar. A direct consequence of this is the need to energetically campaign against the bad habit of smoking (Lickint, Dresden) as a preventative measure against cancer.

Our experiments also provide an answer to the frequently asked question as to why all smokers do not die of cancer: the second factor necessary for the development of cancer is the genetic predisposition to it, which, fortunately, is not present in all people just as it is not present in all animals. The genetic predisposition can be influenced by many things and as soon as the condition has been met, a smoker dies of cancer.

SOURCE

Roffo AH. 1940. Krebserzeugende Tabakwirkung. [The Carcinogenic Effects of Tobacco]. *Monatsschrift für Krebsbekämpfung* 8 (5): 97–102. Reprinted with English translation in 2006 by the *Bulletin of the World Health Organization* 84 (6): 497–502. English translation reprinted by permission of WHO Press.

Smoking and Lung Cancer: Recent Evidence and a Discussion of Some Questions[1]
(1959, Abridged)

Jerome Cornfield,[2,3] William Haenszel,[4] E. Cuyler Hammond,[5] Abraham M. Lilienfeld,[2] Michael B. Shimkin,[4] *and* Ernst L.Wynder[6]

Summary

This report reviews some of the more recent epidemiologic and experimental findings on the relationship of tobacco smoking to lung cancer, and discusses some criticisms directed against the conclusion that tobacco smoking, especially cigarettes, has a causal role in the increase in bronchogenic carcinoma. The magnitude of the excess lung-cancer risk among cigarette smokers is so great that the results cannot be interpreted as arising from an indirect association of cigarette smoking with some other agent or characteristic, since this hypothetical agent would have to be at least as strongly associated with lung cancer as cigarette use; no such agent has been found or suggested. The consistency of all the epidemiologic and experimental evidence also supports the conclusion of a causal relationship with cigarette smoking, while there are serious inconsistencies in reconciling the evidence with other hypotheses which have been advanced. Unquestionably there are areas where more research is necessary, and, of course, no single cause accounts for all lung cancer. The information already available, however, is sufficient for planning and activating public health measures. —J. Nat. Cancer Inst. 22: 173–203, 1959.

In 1957 a Study Group (75), appointed by the National Cancer Institute, the National Heart Institute, the American Cancer Society, and the American Heart Association, examined the scientific evidence on the effects of tobacco smoking on health and arrived at the following conclusion:

> "The sum total of scientific evidence establishes beyond reasonable doubt that cigarette smoking is a causative factor in the rapidly increasing incidence of human epidermoid carcinoma of the lung."

1 Received for publication October 15, 1958.
2 School of Hygiene and Public Health, Johns Hopkins University, Baltimore, MD.
3 Department of Biostatistics, paper # 323.
4 National Cancer Institute, Public Service, U.S. Department of Health, Education, and Welfare, Bethesda, MD.
5 American Cancer Society, Inc., New York, NY.
6 Sloan-Kettering Institute for Cancer Research, New York, NY.

Concurrently, a report from the Medical Research Council (57) of Great Britain appeared which also drew the inference of a causal relationship between smoking and lung cancer from the statistical, clinical, and laboratory evidence available by midyear 1957.

The consideration of the accumulated scientific evidence has led to the acceptance of a similar viewpoint by responsible public health officials in Great Britain, the Netherlands, Norway, and the United States. This consensus of scientific and public health opinion does not mean that all problems regarding smoking and lung cancer have now been solved or that valid questions and reservations about some aspects of the subject do not remain. An excellent collection of primary references and opinions expressing both "sides" of the question was issued by a committee of the House of Representatives (42) which sought to examine the claims of filter-tip cigarette advertisements.

The general acceptance of the cigarette–lung-cancer relationship has not decreased research interests but has accelerated research in this and in such related fields as respiratory physiology and environmental carcinogens, and on the effect of tobacco smoke in a wide range of physiological and pathological reactions.

The result is that considerably more information has been published or has become available through other media. Included in the recent scientific evidence are the following:

1) Additional retrospective studies (68, 69, 73) on men with lung cancer and on matched controls have appeared. All show an association between cigarette smoking and epidermoid-undifferentiated lung cancer.

2) Additional retrospective studies on women (34, 73) also show the association.

3) The first results of a third large prospective study (20), which included 200,000 United States veterans who were observed for 30 months, duplicate closely the reported findings of the Hammond-Horn (38) and the Doll-Hill (18) studies.

4) Analyses by Kreyberg and others (19, 46) substantiate that, epidemiologically, primary lung cancer must be divided into epidermoid-undifferentiated and adenocarcinoma. The latter is much less related to smoking and, so far as is known at present, to other carcinogenic inhalants.

5) Additional findings have become available on the impingement of tobacco-smoke particles in the bronchi of animals, ciliary paralysis, and penetration of unidentified fluorescent materials into the bronchial cells (40, 41, 45).

6) Additional data have been published (2, 12) on the more frequent occurrence of hyperplastic and metaplastic changes in the lungs of smokers as compared with the lungs of nonsmokers. Hyperplastic and metaplastic changes have been produced in bronchi of dogs exposed to direct contact with tobacco "tars" (62) and in bronchi of mice exposed to tobacco smoke (48).

7) Additional confirmations have been obtained on the induction of cancer of the skin in mice painted with tobacco-smoke condensates (7, 23, 28, 61, 63).

8) Progress continues on the isolation and identification of chemical constituents in tobacco smoke, including compounds of the carcinogenic polycyclic type (53, 61, 77, 84, 85).

The growing and consistent body of evidence has had no noticeable effect upon the viewpoint of a small but important group of individuals who would deny a causal role of cigarette smoking and cancer of the lung. Among these critics are Little (52) and Harnett (39), spokesmen for the American tobacco industry. Berkson (3, 4) has been critical of many aspects of the statistical studies, and his reservations are, in part, also evident in papers by Neyman (60) and Arkin (1). More general objections by Fisher (25, 26), Greene (31), Hueper (43), Macdonald (54), Rigdon (64), and Rosenblatt (67) have been published.

We have reviewed the criticisms that have been made regarding the cigarette–lung-cancer relationship in the light of new evidence. In this review we have several objectives: a) to point out recorded facts that directly answer some of the criticisms; b) to define more precisely some inadequacies of information, with the hope that this will lead to further research. The particular references we have used were selected because in our opinion the criticism was well stated; it is not our intention to reply to any specific publication or to any specific critic. Our view is that all valid questions should be answered. However, some questions may not be relevant, or there may be no information presently available for an answer. In the latter case, we believe that a distinction should be made between data that are unavailable and data that have been found to be contradictory.

For convenience, we have divided the criticisms and answers into five major topics, as follows: (I) Mortality and population data; (II) Retrospective and prospective studies; (III) Studies on pathogenesis; (IV) Other laboratory investigations; and (V) Interpretation.

I. Mortality and Population Data

The rising death rate from lung cancer in all countries that have suffi-ciently detailed mortality statistics is the most striking neoplastic phenom-enon of this century. That this increase is a fact and not a spurious result of statistical classification is now commonly accepted. An entirely con-trary view is held by only a few persons (64), though there are dissenting opinions (29, 43) regarding the extent and time relationship of this re-corded increase.

Obviously, the case for the etiologic role of cigarette smoking would be seriously compromised if it could be demonstrated that the lung-cancer rate over the past half century had been stationary, particularly after 1920 when much of the rise in cigarette consumption, instead of other forms of tobacco, occurred (59).

In a recent review, Ringdon and Kirchoff (65) document that primary lung cancer was first recognized as an entity during the early part of the 19th century, and that its occurrence has increased steadily since then, as manifested by the recorded relative frequency with which it was recog-nized in the clinic and at necropsy. This is undoubtedly correct but does not constitute evidence against a true increase in the incidence of the dis-ease during the whole, or a more recent part, of the last 100 years.

Hueper (43), accepting a true increase in the incidence of lung cancer, regards an increase dating back to 1900, or before the widespread use of cigarettes, as evidence against the cigarette–lung-cancer relationship. His contention would have crucial import only if it were maintained that ciga-rette smoking is the sole cause of lung cancer.

The vital statistics and the necropsy data that support the presumption of a real increase in lung-cancer risk certainly apply to the years after 1920. Because of the uncertainties associated with changes in diagnostic accuracy, no firm conclusions can be reached on whether the *rate* of in-crease in lung-cancer mortality has, in truth, accelerated since 1920.

Effect of Aging

Rosenblatt (67) has raised a question about the effect of the aging popula-tion on the lung-cancer rate. This particular point has been investigated by the use of age-adjusted rates. Dunn (22) has noted that only one sixth of the over-all increase in lung-cancer mortality among males in the United States (from 4 to 24 deaths per 100,000 males between 1930 and 1951) could be attributed to an aging population. Similar findings (16) have been presented for England and Wales where observations on lung-cancer mortality date back to 1900; the 1953 mortality rate for both sexes, 34 per 100,000 population, was 43 times the corresponding 1900 rate, 0.8

per 100,000 population. Allowance for increased average age of the population could account for only half this rise in lung-cancer mortality, with a 24-fold difference between 1900 and 1953.

Also, an aging population does not affect the age-specific death rates and cannot account for the phenomenon of increasingly higher lung-cancer mortality at all ages throughout the lifespan, which has occurred among successively younger groups of males born in the United States and England and Wales since 1850. A similar but less pronounced "cohort displacement" has been shown for females.

Diagnostic Factors

Little (52) and others (64) have raised the important question on whether better diagnostic measures and more complete reporting have resulted in a spurious increase in the recorded attack rate. Several special features of the increase in lung-cancer mortality would be difficult to account for on diagnostic grounds. These include the continuous rising ratio of male to female deaths, the increasing lung-cancer mortality rate among successively younger cohorts, and the magnitude of the current, continuing, increase in lung-cancer mortality (16). By 1955, among white males, 50 to 64 years of age, in the United States, more deaths were attributed to lung cancer than to all other respiratory diseases combined.

Gilliam (29) has made a careful study of the potential effect of improved diagnosis on the course of the lung-cancer death rate. Even assuming that 2 percent of the deaths certified in past years as tuberculosis or other respiratory disease were really due to lung cancer, he concluded that ". . . all of the increase in mortality attributed to cancer of the lung since 1914 in United States white males and females cannot be accounted for by erroneous death certification to other respiratory diseases without unquestionable assumptions of age and sex differences in diagnostic error." His computations reduced the respective 26-fold and sevenfold increase in lung-cancer mortality among males and females, between 1914 and 1915, to the more modestly estimated dimensions of fourfold and 30 percent, respectively. These estimates are certainly the lower bound on the magnitude of the true rate of increase during this period.

The Copenhagen Tuberculosis Station data, examined by Clemmesen et al. (14), provide the greatest measure of control on the diagnostic improvement factor. In a tuberculosis referral service, used extensively by local physicians, where diagnostic standards and procedures including systematic bronchoscopy remained virtually unchanged between 1941 and 1950, the lung-cancer prevalence rate among male examinees increased at a rate comparable to that recorded by the Danish cancer registry for the total male population. This can be regarded as evidence that the reported increase in Danish incidence is not due to diagnostic changes.

Necropsy Data

Most necropsy data agree with mortality data on the increase in lung-cancer risk. To establish this point we referred to a necropsy series summarized by Steiner (72), and returned to the original sources for evidence on the nature of changes over time. Since an existing compilation was chosen, the results do not represent a culling of autopsy series for data favorable to the thesis. The findings from 13 series are summarized in text-figure 1 [Not shown, Ed.] as the proportion of lung cancers in relation to all necropsies. The relative frequency in terms of total tumors or total carcinomas yielded results which would lead to substantially the same inferences.

Mortality and necropsy data have their own virtues and weaknesses. Death certificates provide a complete report of deaths, but do not emphasize a high quality of diagnostic evidence, while the reverse holds true for necropsies. However, since both approaches lead to the same inferences, neither great variation in the quality of diagnostic evidence nor the unrepresentative nature of some of the necropsy observations can be viewed as plausible interpretations of the results. The alternative conclusion of a real increase in lung-cancer risk remains.

Urban-Rural Differences

Emphasis has been placed on the alleged incompatibility of the excess lung-cancer mortality, among urban residents, with the cigarette-smoking hypothesis (43, 44, 54). Mortality data from several countries indicates strongly that lung-cancer rates are much higher in cities than in rural areas, and the observation that urban males in general have higher lung-cancer mortality than rural males is undoubtedly correct. The assertion of Macdonald (54) that ". . . country people smoke as much, if not more, than do city people . . ." is not borne out by the facts (35). Nevertheless, the evidence indicates that adjustment for smoking history could account for only a fraction of this urban-rural difference (33).

However, this does not establish the converse proposition that control of residence history in the analysis of collected data would account for the excess lung-cancer risk among cigarette smokers. Evidence now in hand weighs strongly against this last assertion. Stocks and Campbell (74), in their report on lung-cancer mortality among persons in Liverpool, the suburban environs, and rural towns in North Wales, showed that heavy smokers have higher lung-cancer rates when urban and rural males were studied separately. Mills and Porter (58) reported similar findings in Ohio. These results agree with the experience of the Hammond-Horn (38) study, which revealed markedly higher death rates from bronchogenic carcinoma among smokers regardless of whether they lived in cities or in rural areas. No contradictory observations are known to us.

Sex Differences

The sex disparity in lung-cancer mortality has also been cited (25, 54) as grounds for discarding the cigarette-smoking hypothesis. In this connection it should be noted that persons advocating this line of argument have minimized sex differences in smoking habits to a degree not supported by available facts. A survey of smoking habits in a cross section of the United States population (35) demonstrated that men, on the average, have been smoking for longer periods than women. The sex differences in tobacco use were especially pronounced at ages over 55, when most lung-cancer deaths occur; 0.6 percent of United States females in this age group have been reported as current users of more than 1 pack of cigarettes daily compared to 6.9 percent of United States males. British data (76) also revealed much lower tobacco consumption among females, particularly in the years before World War II.

The present data contrasting the experience by sex would appear to support the cigarette-smoking hypothesis rather than discredit it. When differences in smoking habits are considered, it is possible to reduce the observed fivefold excess lung-cancer mortality among males to the 40 percent excess mortality which prevails in many other causes of death (33). One intriguing finding from these studies is that the estimated death rates for female nonsmokers agree closely with the death rates derived from retrospective studies on male nonsmokers (34).

Evidence for Other Etiologic Factors

Etiologic factors of industrial origin, such as exposure to chromates and coal gas, are well established (16). Excess lung-cancer risks among such groups as asbestos workers who develop asbestosis, appear likely (16). One epidemiologic study (11) of British, World War I, veterans exposed to mustard gas and/or with a wartime history of influenza reveals virtually no excess lung cancer risk among these groups.

The existence of other important lung cancer effects associated with such characteristics as socioeconomic class cannot be questioned. Cohart (15) found that the poorest economic class had a 40 percent higher lung-cancer incidence than the remaining population of New Haven, Connecticut. Results from the 10-city morbidity survey (21) have revealed a sharp gradient in lung-cancer incidence, by income class, for white males, which is consistent with Cohart's findings. Since cigarette smoking is not inversely related to socioeconomic status, we can agree with Cohart ". . . that important environmental factors other than cigarette smoking exist that contribute to the causation of lung cancer." These and other findings are convincing evidence for multiple causes of lung cancer. It is obviously untenable to regard smoking of tobacco as the sole cause of lung cancer.

Two points should be made: The population exposed to established industrial carcinogens is small, and these agents cannot account for the increasing lung-cancer risk in the remainder of the population. Also, the effects associated with socioeconomic class and related characteristics are smaller than those noted for smoking history, and the smoking–class differences cannot be accounted for in terms of these other effects.

Special Population Groups

Haag and Hanmer (32) reported that employees in nine processing plants of the American Tobacco Company, with an above-average proportion of smokers, had a lower mortality than the general population of Virginia and North Carolina for all causes and for cancer and cardiovascular diseases, but no higher mortality for respiratory cancer and coronary disease. They concluded: "The existence of such a population makes it evident that cigarette smoking *per se* is not necessarily or invariably associated with a higher risk of lung cancer or cardiovascular diseases or with diminished longevity."

The group studied by Haag and Hanmer was too small to yield significant results on respiratory cancer. Moreover, a major flaw in the conclusion has been pointed out by Case (10). It is well known that mortality comparisons cannot be drawn directly between employee groups and the general population, since the death rates for many groups of employed persons are lower than death rates for the general population with age, sex, and race taken into consideration. This is true because there is a strong tendency to exclude from employment those persons who have acute or chronic diseases or who are seriously disabled from any cause and those employees who develop permanent disabilities from disease or other causes are usually discharged, retired, or dropped from the list of regular employees. Reasons of this nature undoubtedly account for the deficit in deaths from all causes noted in the group of employees under consideration.

A different picture is provided by the Society of Actuaries (71) who made a study for 1946 through 1954. The death claims for employees of the tobacco industry were reported to be slightly higher than, and the permanent disability claims were reported to be over three times as high as, those for employees in nonrated industries as a whole. This latter comparison indicates that the basic assumption of the Haag and Hanmer study is incorrect. Also, interpretation of group comparisons in this field should account separately for the experience of smokers and nonsmokers. We hope that Haag and Hanmer will supplement the report to provide data for smokers and nonsmokers in the study population.

II. Retrospective and Prospective Studies

The association between smoking and lung cancer has now been investigated and reported by at least 21 independent groups of investigators in 8 different countries, who employed what is known as the retrospective method (16, 34, 68, 69, 73, 75). In these studies, patients with lung cancer, or their relatives, were questioned about their smoking history and other past events, and the answers compared with those of individuals without lung cancer who were selected as controls. Although these 21 studies have certain features in common, they varied greatly in the methods of selecting the groups, the methods of interview, and other important aspects.

The association between smoking and lung cancer was further investigated in two countries by three independent groups (18, 20, 38), using the prospective method. In these studies, large groups were questioned on smoking habits and other characteristics, and the groups were observed for several years for data on mortality and causes of death. The three prospective studies also varied in several important details including the type of subjects, the selection of subjects, and the method of obtaining information on smoking habits.

In each of the studies, an association was found between smoking and lung cancer. In every investigation where the type of smoking was considered, a higher degree of association was found between lung cancer and cigarette smoking than between lung cancer and pipe or cigar smoking. In every instance where amount of smoking was considered, it was found that the degree of association with lung cancer increased as the amount of smoking increased. When ex-cigarette smokers were compared with current cigarette smokers, it was found that lung-cancer death rates were higher among current cigarette smokers than among ex-cigarette smokers.

A number of investigators (3, 36, 54) have criticized the retrospective method but, for the most part, the specific points of criticism apply only to some of the studies and not to others. Some features of the three prospective studies on smoking have been criticized. Again, certain of the points of criticism apply to one or another of the three prospective studies but not to all three. Specifically, doubts raised as to the validity of the early findings of the prospective studies have been eliminated by the persistence of the findings in the later phases of the same studies.

The validity of the findings on these extensive investigations has been questioned in regard to two major aspects: 1) the methods of selection of the study groups, and 2) the accuracy of information regarding smoking habits in the diagnosis of lung cancer.

Selection of Study Groups

Neyman (60) pointed out that a study based on a survey of a population at some given instant in time may yield misleading results. Suppose that a study is made on a day when all patients with lung cancer and a group of people without lung cancer are questioned about their smoking habits. If smokers with lung cancer live longer than nonsmokers with lung cancer, there would be a higher proportion of smokers in the lung-cancer group than in the control group—this would follow without questioning the proposition on which the model is based. However, only two of the retrospective studies were conducted in a way approximating an "instantaneous survey" procedure, so that this criticism does not apply to most of the studies. Furthermore, this difficulty is completely avoided in prospective studies.

Berkson (3) indicated that people with two specific complaints are more likely to be hospitalized than people with only one of these complaints. If a retrospective study were conducted exclusively on hospital patients an association would be found between these two specific complaints, even if there were no association between the same two complaints in the general population. This would influence the results if smokers with lung cancer are more likely to be hospitalized than nonsmokers with lung cancer. However, Berkson showed that this difficulty is trivial if a high percentage of people with either one of these two conditions is hospitalized, which is the situation with lung-cancer patients. Furthermore, one retrospective study (74) included all lung-cancer patients who were in the study area, including those not hospitalized; another retrospective study (82) was based on individuals who died of lung cancer and other diseases regardless of whether they had been hospitalized or not. This difficulty does not arise in prospective studies.

In all but one of the 21 retrospective studies, the procedure was to compare the smoking habits of lung-cancer patients with the smoking habits of the control group who did not have lung cancer. Hammond (36), Berkson (3), and others have pointed out the grave danger of bias if the control group is not selected in such a way as to represent (in respect to smoking habits) the general population which includes the lung-cancer patients. Subsequent events have proved that this criticism is well-founded, though the direction of the bias in the studies turned out to yield an underestimate of the degree of association between cigarette smoking and lung cancer. The reason was that in most of the retrospective studies the control group consisted of patients with diseases other than lung cancer. The choice of such a control group is tantamount to assuming that there is no association between smoking and diseases which resulted in hospitalization of the control subjects. This was an incorrect assumption since other studies have indicated an association between smoking and a number of diseases, such as coronary artery disease, thromboangiitis obliterans, and cancer of the buccal cavity.

Doll and Hill (17), recognizing the possibility of bias in a control group selected from hospital patients, attained an additional control group by ascertaining the smoking habits of the general population in a random sample of the area in which their hospital was located. The largest percentage of smokers (particularly heavy smokers) was found in the lung-cancer group, the smallest percentage of smokers was found in the general population sample, and an intermediate percentage of smokers was found in a hospital-control group. Similar results have been reported in a recent study of women (34).

Berkson (3) pointed out that the criticisms in regard to selection bias in the retrospective studies are also applicable to the earlier findings in a prospective study. Suppose that, in selecting subjects for a prospective study, sick smokers are overrepresented in relation to well smokers and/or well nonsmokers are overrepresented in relation to sick nonsmokers. In this event, during the earlier period after selection, the death rate of the smokers in the study would be higher than the death rate of the nonsmokers in the study, even if death rates were unrelated to smoking habits of the general population. If smoking is unrelated to death from lung cancer (or other causes), the death rate in the smokers would tend to equalize with that of the nonsmokers as the study progressed. Thus, the bias would diminish with time, and the relationship due to such bias would disappear. This general principle is well known to actuaries and is one of the cornerstones of the life insurance business.

Hammond and Horn (38), recognizing this possible difficulty, excluded from the study all persons who were obviously ill at the time of selection. As expected, the total death rate of the study population was low and very few deaths from lung cancer occurred during the first 8 months after selection. The total death rate, and particularly the death rate from lung cancer, rose considerably in the subsequent 3 years. What is more important, the observed association between cigarette smoking and lung cancer was considerably higher in the latter part than in the early part of the study, and the association between cigarette smoking and total death rates was also somewhat greater in the latter part of the study. This showed that the original bias in the selection of the subjects was slight and that it yielded an underestimate of the degree of association between smoking and death rates.

This particular problem was not encountered in the prospective studies of Doll and Hill (18) who could observe the death rates of all physicians in Great Britain (nonresponders as well as responders to the smoking questionnaire). The prospective study of Dorn (20) also had a defined population of veterans holding insurance policies, and nonresponders were observed as well as responders. Moreover, these two studies also showed that higher mortality from lung cancer among smokers was more evident during the later period than in the earlier period of observation. Thus, in the course of time, there was no disappearance of any selection bias factors that may have been introduced into the original study groups.

The subjects for the Hammond and Horn prospective study (38) were selected by volunteer workers with specific instructions on how it should be done. Mainland and Herrera (55) have suggested that the volunteer workers may have introduced a bias in the way they selected the subjects. The foregoing evidence of persistence and accentuation of the differences between smokers and nonsmokers, in time, effectively counters purposeful, as well as unknown, sources of such selection.

Accuracy of Information

Berkson (3, 4) has remarked that the two major variables considered in all these studies—the ascertainment of smoking habits and the diagnosis of disease—are both subject to considerable error. The accuracy of diagnosis is not a major problem in retrospective studies because the investigator can restrict his study to those patients whose diagnosis of lung cancer has been thoroughly confirmed. This feature has been taken into consideration in several retrospective studies. It is more a problem in prospective studies since all deaths that occur must be included, and certainly some of the diagnoses will be uncertain. However, in all three prospective studies, the *total death rate* was found to be higher in cigarette smokers than in nonsmokers and found to increase with the amount of cigarette smoking. If some of the excess deaths associated with cigarette smoking and ascribed to lung cancer were actually due to some other disease, then it means that: a) the association between cigarette smoking and lung cancer was somewhat overestimated, but b) the association between smoking and some other disease was somewhat underestimated. The reverse would be true if some of the excess deaths associated with cigarette smoking and ascribed to diseases other than lung cancer were actually due to lung cancer. Hammond and Horn (38) found that the association with cigarette smoking was greater for patients with a well-established diagnosis of lung cancer than for patients with less convincing evidence for a diagnosis of lung cancer. This suggests that inaccuracies in diagnoses resulted somewhat in an underestimate of the degree of association between smoking and lung cancer.

The study on physicians, by Doll and Hill (18), in which presumably the clinical and pathologic evidence of the cause of death would be somewhat more than in the general population considered by Hammond and Horn and by Dorn, yields the most identical risks to lung cancer by smoking class.

In regard to information about smoking, Finkner *et al.* (24) have made a thorough study of the accuracy of replies to questionnaires on smoking habits. Their results indicate that replies are not completely accurate but that most of the errors are relatively minor—very few heavy smokers are classified as light smokers. Random and independent errors simply tend to diminish the apparent degree of association between two variables. A national survey of smoking habits in the United States (35) yielded results on tobacco consumption that were consistent with figures on tobacco production and taxation.

On two occasions several years apart, Hammond and Horn (38) and Dorn (20) questioned a proportion of their subjects. The results indicated close reproducibility in the answers.

Hammond (36) and others (54) have questioned the reliability of the retrospective method on the grounds that the illness may bias the responses given by the patient or his family when they are questioned about smoking habits, and the knowledge of the diagnosis may bias the interviewer. This possible difficulty was minimized in several of the 21 retrospective studies on smoking in relation to lung cancer. For example, in a study conducted by Levin (49), all patients admitted to a hospital during the course of several years were questioned about their smoking habits *before* a diagnosis was made. Only a small proportion later turned out to have lung cancer, though many had lung disease symptoms or lung diseases other than lung cancer. Doll and Hill (18) also showed that patients whose diagnosis of lung cancer was subsequently established to be erroneous had smoking histories characteristic of the control rather than of the lung-cancer group. Furthermore, a larger percentage of cigarette smokers have been found among patients with epidermoid carcinoma of the lungs than among patients with adenocarcinoma of the lungs (34, 46, 79). This would hardly have resulted from bias either on the part of the patient or on the part of the interviewer.

Multiple Variables

Arkin (1), Little (52), Macdonald (54), and others have criticized the studies of cigarette–lung-cancer relationship on the grounds that only smoking habits were really investigated, and that numerous other possible variables were not considered.

This criticism may seem especially appropriate in view of the accepted fact that no single etiologic factor has been proposed for any neoplastic disease. The criticism may also be valid in relation to any one of the retrospective and prospective studies. However, in the aggregate, quite a number of other variables have been specifically investigated or can be inferentially derived. Of course, all studies considered the basic factors of age and sex; some dealt with geographic distribution (74), occupation (8), urban or rural residence (74), marital and parous states (34), and some other habits such as coffee consumption (34).

The Doll and Hill (18) prospective study was confined to a single professional group, physicians. Thus there can be no great variation attributable to occupation or socioeconomic status. Stocks and Campbell (74) put particular emphasis on the study of air pollution and occupational exposure and included a number of other factors in addition to smoking. It is evident, in the Hammond-Horn (38) study and other investigations, that there is a consistent relationship between urban residence and a higher mortality due to lung cancer. The important fact is that in all studies, when other variables are held constant, cigarette smoking retains its high association with lung cancer.

The only factors that may show a higher correlation with lung cancer than heavy cigarette smoking are such occupations as those of the Schneeberg miners and manufacturers of chromate (16). We are not acquainted with actual studies of these and related occupation groups in which cigarette and other tobacco consumption is also considered. Such studies, we suggest, would be useful additions to our knowledge of other etiologic agents and the interplay between multiple causes in human pulmonary cancer.

III. Studies on Pathogenesis

Inhalation of Smoke

If cigarette smoking produces cancer of the lungs as a result of direct contact between tobacco smoke and the bronchial mucosa, smokers who inhale cigarette smoke should be exposed to higher concentrations of the carcinogens than noninhalers and therefore have a higher risk to the development of lung cancer. The retrospective study of Doll and Hill (17), however, elicited no difference between patients with lung cancer and the controls in the proportion of smokers who stated that they inhaled. Fisher (25), Hueper (43), and Macdonald (54) have emphasized this point as contradictory to the smoking–lung-cancer relationship, and, of course, it is. Unfortunately, this particular finding was not reinvestigated in a prospective study of Doll and Hill (18).

Three authors, Lickint (50), Breslow *et al.* (8), and Schwartz and Denoix (68), however, *did* find the relative risk of lung cancer to be greater among inhalers than among noninhalers when age, type, and amount of smoking were held constant. It must be admitted that there is no clear explanation of the contradiction posed by the Doll-Hill (17) findings, though a number of plausible hypotheses could be advanced. More experimental work is required, including some objective definition and measurement of the depth and length of inhalation.

Hammond (37) has recently queried male smokers about their inhalation practices. He found that very few pipe and cigar smokers inhale; that most men inhale who smoke only cigarettes; and that there are proportionally fewer inhalers among men who smoke both cigars and cigarettes than among men who smoke only cigarettes. These findings are compatible with the view that differences in inhaling account for the fact that the lung-cancer death rate of cigar and pipe smokers is less than the lung-cancer death rate of cigarette smokers; and that the lung-cancer death rate of men who smoke both cigars and cigarettes is somewhat lower than the lung-cancer death rate of men who smoke only cigarettes.

Upper-Respiratory Cancer

Rosenblatt (67) has drawn attention to the fact that increased consumption of cigarettes has not been accompanied by an increase in the upper-respiratory cancer similar to that noted in cancer of the lung and bronchus. Hueper (43) has also expressed doubts about the causative role of cigarette smoking on the basis that cigarette smoking is not associated with cancer of the oral cavity or of the fingers, which are often stained with tobacco tar.

The premise that a carcinogen should act equally on different tissues is not supported by experimental or clinical evidence (70). Carcinogens, which produced liver tumors in animals, may be noncarcinogenic when applied to the skin. Coal soot, accepted as etiologically related to carcinoma of the scrotum in chimney sweeps, does not increase the risk to cancer of the penis. There is no *a priori* reason why a carcinogen that produces bronchogenic cancer in man should also produce neoplastic changes in the nasopharynx or in other sites. It is an intriguing fact, deserving further research, that carcinoma of the trachea is a rarity, whereas carcinoma of the bronchus is common among individuals exposed to chromates, as well as among chronic cigarette smokers.

Several studies have established the association of all types of tobacco smoking, including cigarettes, with cancer of the oral cavity (81). However, the *relative* risk of developing cancer of the mouth is greater for cigar and pipe smokers than for cigarette smokers. The risk of laryngeal cancer is increased by smoking and an equal risk exists among cigarettes, cigar, and pipe smokers (80). The per capita consumption of cigars and pipe tobacco has decreased since 1920, while cigarette smoking has increased (59).

These associations contrast sharply with the findings on lung cancer, which have consistently shown that cigarette smokers have much higher risks than either cigar or pipe smokers. Since 1920 the increase in tobacco consumption has been primarily due to the rise in cigarette consumption (59), and the stabler rates for intra-oral and laryngeal cancer, while the lung-cancer rates have increased steeply, can be considered compatible with the causal role of cigarette smoking in lung cancer.

Effect of Tobacco Smoke on Bronchial Mucosa

Statements by Hartnett (39), Macdonald (54), and others (3, 52) implied that the relationship of cigarette smoking and lung cancer is based exclusively on "statistics" and lacked "experimental" evidence. The differentiation between various methods of scientific inquiry escapes us as being a valid basis for the acceptance or the rejection of facts. Nevertheless it is true that historically the retrospective studies on lung cancer preceded the intensive interest in laboratory investigations stimulated by the statistical findings.

Hilding (40) has shown experimentally that exposure to cigarette smoke inhibited ciliary action in the isolated bronchial epithelium of cows. Kotin and Falk (45) obtained essentially the same results in experiments on rats and rabbits. Hilding (41) further showed that inhibition of ciliary action interfered with the mechanism whereby foreign material is ordinarily removed from the surface of the bronchial epithelium. In addition, he found that foreign material deposited on the surface tended to accumulate in an area where the cilia have been destroyed. Auerbach *et al.* (2) found that the small areas of the bronchial epithelium where columnar cells were absent appeared more frequently in smokers than in nonsmokers. Chang (12) found that cilia were shorter, on an average, in the bronchial epithelium of smokers than in that of nonsmokers.

Auerbach and his associates (2) studied the microscopic appearance of the bronchial epithelium of patients who died of lung cancer and patients who died of other diseases. Each of these two groups of patients were classified according to whether they were nonsmokers, light smokers, or heavy cigarette smokers. Among the cancer patients there were no non-smokers. Approximately 208 sections from all parts of the tracheo-bronchial tree from each patient were examined. Many areas of basal-cell hyperplasia, squamous metaplasia, and marked atypism with loss of co-lumnar epithelium were found in the tracheo-bronchial tree of men who had died of lung cancer. Almost as many such lesions were found in heavy cigarette smokers who had died of other diseases; somewhat less were found in light cigarette smokers; and much less in nonsmokers. Chang (12) has reported similar findings in the bronchial epithelium of smokers com-pared with nonsmokers.

The chief criticism of Auerbach's study has concerned terminology. Following the definition previously set forth by Black and Ackerman (5), Auerbach *et al.* used the term "carcinoma-*in-situ*" to describe certain lesions with marked atypical changes and loss of columnar epithelium. Whether this is an appropriate term may be questioned, but it is not rel-evant to the validity of the findings. Certainly there are no data to indi-cate what proportion of these morphologically abnormal areas would progress to invasive carcinoma.

The recent findings of Auerbach *et al.* and Chang have been repro-duced experimentally in animals. Rockey and his associates (66) applied tobacco "tar" directly to the bronchial mucosa of dogs. Within 3 to 6 weeks, the tar-treated surface became granular and later developed wart-like elevations. Upon microscopic examination, hyperplasia, transitional metaplasia, and squamous metaplasia were found in these areas. Leuchten-berger *et al.* (48) exposed mice to cigarette smoke for periods up to 200 days. The bronchial epithelium was then examined microscopically. Bron-chitis, basal-cell hyperplasia, and atypical basal-cell hyperplasia were found in the majority of the animals, and squamous metaplasia in a few. Further work and longer periods of observation are necessary to establish whether some of these lesions would progress to frank neoplasia.

IV. Other Laboratory Investigations

Skin Cancer in Rodents

One of the links in the total evidence for the causal relationship of ciga-rette smoking and lung cancer is the demonstration that tobacco-smoke condensates (usually referred to as "tars") have the biologic property of evoking carcinoma in certain laboratory animals, particularly mice. The production of skin cancer in mice, following repeated, long-term applica-tions of tobacco tar, has now been reported from at least six different laboratories (7, 23, 28, 61, 63, 83). It is undeniable that some investigators did not obtain positive results, perhaps because the dose and other experi-mental conditions were different, or because the complex tobacco tars probably varied widely in their composition. The negative results of Passey *et al.* (62) have been quoted by Hueper (43) and others, but a more recent experiment by Passey (63) with Swiss strain mice did lead to the appearance of at least two carcinomas after repeated applications of tobacco-smoke condensate.

Little (52) indicated that ". . . the extrapolation to human lung of results obtained by painting of or interjection into the skin of mice is decidedly questionable." Direct extrapolation from one species to another is, of course, not justified. Nevertheless, results in animals are fully consistent with the epidemiologic findings in man. A quotation from Kotin (44) is appropriate: "The chemical demonstration of carcinogenic agents in the environment and their successful use for the production of tumors in experimental animals do not prove or even especially strongly suggest a like relationship in the instance of man. When, however, a demonstrable parallelism exists between epidemiologic data and laboratory findings, greater significance accrues to both. Medical history is replete with examples in which laboratory findings have been proved ultimately to have their counterpart in the healing experience. Exceptions have been very few."

Greene (31), while discounting the significance of the induction of skin carcinoma in Swiss mice because of the constitutionally "high differential susceptibility" of the strain, believes that the failure to induce neoplasms in embryonic transplants exposed to tobacco tar is more important evidence. Greene's interesting technique does produce positive results when fewer chemicals such as benzo[a]pyrene are used, and this chemical has been recovered from some samples of tobacco-smoke condensates. We are not acquainted with reports of neoplasms arising in embryonic tissue that has been exposed *in vitro* to coal tar, another crude mixture that contains carcinogens.

The high frequency of carcinoma induction reported by Wynder *et al.* (83) has not been achieved by other investigators, who reported that no more than 20 percent of animals, and usually considerably less, developed carcinoma of the skin. The presence of cocarcinogenic materials in tobacco-smoke condensates has been demonstrated by Gellhorn (28) and by Bock and Moore (7). To the mouse data are now added the data on the induction of skin cancer in some rabbits painted with tobacco-smoke condensate (30); this condensate, when combined with a killed suspension of tubercle bacilli, and introduced into a bronchus, produced a carcinoma of the bronchus in one rat (6).

Since malignant neoplasms have been obtained in several strains of mice, and a few neoplasms have been produced in rabbits and rats, the issue of strain or species limitation to the reaction is more difficult to maintain. It is, of course, a fact that many agents shown to be carcinogenic to the skin of mice had not been proved carcinogenic to man. In most instances there is simply no experience with such agents in man, so that lack of proof really represents lack of data, pro and con.

The Problem of Dosage

Little (52) has further questioned the applicability of animal data to man, as follows: "Tobacco smoke or smoke condensate has failed to produce cancer even on the skin of susceptible strains of mice when applied in the quantity and at an exposure rate that would simulate conditions of human smoking."

The differences in species, tissues, and conditions between the induction of neoplasms on the skin of mice and in the bronchi of man preclude fine comparisons of dose and time relationships.

Bronchogenic Cancer in Animals

The pulmonary adenomatous tumor in mice, rats, and guinea pigs cannot be compared with the bronchogenic carcinoma in man (70). Until a few years ago, the experimental induction of epidermoid carcinoma had been achieved only in a few mice by passing strings impregnated with carcinogenic hydrocarbons through the lung. Epidermoid carcinoma of the lung was consistently produced in rats by beryllium (78), by carcinogenic hydrocarbons introduced as fixed pellets into bronchi of rats (47), and by inhalation of radioactive particles (13).

Little (52) has noted that ". . . prolonged exposure of the lungs of rodents to massive doses of cigarette smoke has failed to produce bronchogenic cancer." This remains true at the time of this report, although it can be questioned whether any animal receives as large a dose of cigarette smoke through indirect exposure as a human being does by voluntary deep inhalation. Therefore the failure may be a technical one, which may be solved by further experimentation. The early results of Leuchtenberger *et al.* (48) suggested that this may be achieved.

Carcinogens in Tobacco

The isolation and identification of specific chemical constituents in tobacco smoke, which are carcinogenic for the pulmonary tissue of man, is an important area for research.

It has been clear for some time that combustion or pyrolysis of most organic material, including tobacco, will form higher aromatic polycyclics of established carcinogenic activity (85). A number of higher polycyclics have been identified and isolated (53, 61, 77, 84). These materials include benzo[e]pyrene, benzo[a]pyrene, dibenz[a,h]anthracene, chrysene, and, most recently, a newly established carcinogen, 3,4-benzfluoranthene. Whether these compounds are equally involved in human pulmonary carcinogenesis is, of course, conjectural.

Little (52) has implied that a specific constituent must be found to account for the biologic activity of tobacco smoke. This is not necessary. The situation is similar to the establishment of the carcinogenic activity of tar, which was accepted before the isolation of benzo[a]pyrene by Kennaway and his coworkers. In this instance, also, benzo[a]pyrene is most probably not the only carcinogen in a complex mixture called tar, and there are strong indications that some noncarcinogenic components in tar may have cocarcinogenic effects.

V. Interpretation

Three interpretations of the observed association of lung cancer and cigarette smoking are possible: 1) that cigarette smoking "causes" lung cancer, either (a) through the direct carcinogenic action of smoke on human bronchial epithelium or (b) by a more indirect mode of action such as making the individual susceptible to some other specific carcinogenic agent in the environment; 2) that lung cancer "causes" cigarette smoking, perhaps because a precancerous condition sets up a process which leads to a craving for tobacco; 3) that cigarette smoking and lung cancer both have a common cause, usually specified as a special constitutional makeup, perhaps genetic in origin, which predisposes certain individuals to lung cancer and also makes them cigarette smokers.

The second hypothesis was advanced by Fisher (26), apparently for the sake of logical completeness, and it is not clear whether it is intended to be regarded as a serious possibility. Since we know of no evidence to support the view that the bronchogenic carcinoma diagnosed after age 50 began before age 18, the median age at which cigarette smokers begin smoking, we shall not discuss it further.

The Constitutional Hypothesis

The first hypothesis may be referred to as the *causal* hypothesis and the third as the *constitutional* hypothesis. Nothing short of a series of independently conducted, controlled, experiments on human subjects, continued for 30 to 60 years, could provide a clear-cut and unequivocal choice between them. We nevertheless argue that evidence, in addition to that associating an increased mortality from lung cancer with cigarette smoking, is entirely consistent with the causal hypothesis but inconsistent, in many respects, with the constitutional hypothesis, so that even in the absence of controlled experimentation on human beings the weight of evidence is for the one and against the other.

The difficulties with the constitutional hypothesis include the following considerations: (a) changes in lung-cancer mortality over the last century;

(b) the carcinogenicity of tobacco tars for experimental animals; (c) the existence of a large effect from pipe and cigar smoke on cancer of the buccal cavity and larynx but not on cancer of the lung; (d) the reduced lung-cancer mortality among discontinued cigarette smokers. No one of these considerations is perhaps sufficient by itself to counter the constitutional hypothesis *ad hoc* modification of which can accommodate each additional piece of evidence. The point is reached, however, when a continuously modified hypothesis becomes difficult to entertain seriously.

Changes in Mortality

Mortality from lung cancer has increased continuously in the last 50 years, and considerably more for males than females. Such an increase can be explained either as the result of an environmental change (to which males are more exposed or more sensitive than females, if both are equally exposed) or as the result of a sex-linked mutation. The constitutional hypothesis must be modified in the light of this increase, since an unchanging constitutional make-up cannot by itself explain the increase in mortality. Proponents of the constitutional hypothesis have not indicated the type of modification they would consider. Three suggest themselves to us: 1) differences in constitutional make-up are genetic in origin, but rather than predisposing one to lung cancer, they make one sensitive to some new environmental agent (other than tobacco), which does induce lung cancer; 2) differences in constitutional make-up are not genetic but are the result of differential exposure to some new environmental agents, which both predisposes to lung cancer and creates a craving for cigarette smoke; 3) the mutation has led to a greater susceptibility to lung cancer and a preference for cigarette smoke.

In the first two situations the effect of the postulated constitutional make-up would be mediated through an environmental agent. The modified hypothesis thus requires the existence of an environmental agent other than tobacco, exposure to which would be at least as highly correlated with lung-cancer mortality as exposure to cigarettes, and which also would be highly correlated with cigarette consumption. No such agent has yet been found or suggested. In view of the magnitude of the increase in mortality from lung cancer, the third situation would require a mutation rate exceeding anything previously observed.

Experimental Carcinogenesis with Tobacco Tar

Condensed tobacco smoke contains substances that are carcinogenic for mouse and rabbit skin. It does not necessarily follow that these substances are also carcinogenic for human lungs nor does it follow that they are not. However, the constitutional hypothesis asserts that they are not; and that it is simply a coincidence that these materials which are carcinogenic for experimental animals are also associated with a higher lung-cancer mortality in man.

Types of Tobacco and Cancer Site

A greatly increased lung-cancer risk is associated with increased cigarette consumption but not with increased consumption of pipe and cigar tobacco. Studies on cancer of the buccal cavity and larynx, however, have demonstrated a considerably higher risk among smokers, irrespective of the form of tobacco use. Only two ways of modifying the constitutional hypothesis to take account of this evidence occur to us: 1) there are two different constitutional make-ups, one of which predisposes to cigarettes but not to pipe and cigar consumption and to cancer of the lung, and the other predisposes to cancer of the buccal cavity and larynx but not of the lung and to tobacco consumption in any form. 2) Constitutional make-up predisposes to cigarette consumption and lung cancer only, but tobacco smoke, whether from cigarettes, cigars, or pipes, is carcinogenic for the mucosa of the buccal cavity and the larynx but not for the bronchial epithelium.

Mortality among Discontinued Smokers

Mortality from lung cancer among discontinued cigarette smokers is less than that among those continuing to smoke (18, 38); the magnitude of the reduction depending on amount previously smoked and the length of the discontinuance. The hypothetical constitutional factor which predisposes to lung cancer and cigarette smoking cannot therefore be a constant characteristic of an individual over his lifetime but must decrease in force at some time in life, thus resulting in the cessation of cigarette smoking and a concomitant, but not closely related, reduction in the lung-cancer risk. Furthermore, since cigarette smoking is rarely begun after age 35 (35), it must be inferred that the constitutional factor cannot increase in force with the passage of time, even though it may decrease.

In summary, the constitutional hypothesis does not provide a satisfactory explanation of all the evidence. It is natural, therefore, to inquire about the positive findings which support it. Even those who regard this hypothesis with favor would agree, we believe, that supporting evidence is quite scanty.

There are a number of characteristics in which cigarette smokers are known to differ from nonsmokers and presumably more will be discovered. Thus, cigarette smokers consume more alcohol, more black coffee, change jobs more often, engage more in athletics, and are more likely to have had a least one parent with hypertension or coronary artery disease (34, 51, 56). Discontinued cigarette smokers are weaned at a later age than those continuing to smoke (56). Recently, Fisher (27) reported that 51 monozygotic twins resembled each other more in their smoking habits than 33 dizygotic twins, thus suggesting a genetic determinant.

Two somewhat obvious, but necessary, comments on results of this type are in order: 1) The demonstration that a characteristic is related to smoking status does not by itself create a presumption that it is a common cause. It must also be shown to be related to the development of lung cancer among subgroups of individuals with the same smoking status. Alcohol and coffee fail to meet this test, while none of the other characteristics related to smoking status have been investigated from this point of view. 2) There is a quantitative question. Cigarette smokers have a ninefold greater risk of developing lung cancer than nonsmokers, while over-two-pack-a-day smokers have at least a 60-fold greater risk. Any characteristic proposed as a measure of the postulated common cause to both smoking status and lung-cancer risk must therefore be at least ninefold more prevalent among cigarette smokers than among nonsmokers and at least 60-fold more prevalent among two-pack-a-day smokers. No such characteristic has yet been produced despite diligent research.

These comments on the quantitative aspects of association apply also to the relationship of certain characteristics with lung cancer. Thus, a possible genetic basis to lung cancer has been suggested to some by the association between gastric cancer and blood group. The difference, in risk of developing gastric cancer, between blood groups A and O, however, is 20 percent, while the only study of lung cancer and blood groups (9) with which we are familiar shows a difference of 27 percent (and is not quite significant at the $P = 0.01$ level).[7] Such differences are suggestive for further work, but cannot be considered as casting much light on differences of magnitude, ninefold to 60-fold.

Measures of Differences

The comments in the last two paragraphs have utilized a relative measure of differences in lung-cancer risk. Since Berkson (4) has argued that a relative measure is inappropriate in the investigation of smoking in mortality, we now discuss the use of relative and absolute measures of differences in risk. When an agent has an apparent effect on several diseases, the ranking of the diseases by the magnitude of the effect will depend on whether an absolute or a relative measure is used. Thus, in Dorn's study (20) of American veterans there were 187 lung-cancer deaths among ciga-

---

7 Our attention has been called to a summary of three additional studies, which reported no association between ABO blood groups and lung cancer, by: Roberts, J. A. F.: Blood groups and susceptibility to disease. Brit. J. Prev. & Social Med. 11: 107–125, 1957.

rette smokers compared with an expectation of 20 deaths, based on the rates for nonsmokers. This yields a mortality ratio of 9.35 as a relative measure and an excess of 167 deaths as an absolute measure. For cardiovascular diseases there were 1,780 deaths among cigarette smokers compared to an expectation of 1,165. This gives a relative measure of 1.53 and an absolute measure of 615 deaths. Relatively, cigarettes have a much larger effect on lung cancer than on cardiovascular disease, while the reverse is true if an absolute measure is used.

Both the absolute and relative measures serve a purpose. The relative measure is helpful in 1) appraising the possible noncausal nature of an agent having an apparent effect; 2) appraising the importance of an agent with respect to other possible agents inducing the same effect; and 3) properly reflecting the effects of disease misclassification or further refinement of classification. The absolute measure would be important in appraising the public health significance of an effect known to be causal.

The first justification for use of the relative measure can be stated more precisely, as follows:

> If an agent, A, with no causal effect upon the risk of a disease, nevertheless, because of the positive correlation with some other causal agent, B, shows an apparent risk, r, for those exposed to A, relative to those not so exposed, then the prevalence of B, among those exposed to A, relative to the prevalence among those not so exposed, must be greater than r.

Thus, if cigarette smokers have 9 times the risk of nonsmokers for developing lung cancer, and this is not because cigarette smoke is a causal agent, but only because cigarette smokers produce hormone X, then the proportion of hormone-X-producers among cigarette smokers must be at least 9 times greater than that of nonsmokers. If the relative prevalence of hormone-X-producers is considerably less than ninefold, then hormone X cannot account for the magnitude of the apparent effect (Appendix A) [Not shown, Ed.].

The second reason for using a relative measure may be phrased as follows:

> If two uncorrelated agents, A and B, each increase the risk of a disease, and if the risk of the disease in the absence of either agent is small (in a sense to be defined), then the apparent relative risk for A, r, is less than the risk for A in the absence of B.

The presence of other real causes thus reduces the apparent relative risk. If, for example, the relative risk of developing either disease I or disease II on exposure to A is the same in the absence of other causes, and if disease I, but not disease II, also has agent B present, then the apparent relative risk of developing disease I on exposure to A will be less than that for disease II (Appendix B) [Not shown, Ed.].

The third reason for using a relative measure is:

If a causal agent A increases the risk for disease I and has no effect on the risk for disease II, then the relative risk of developing disease I, alone, is greater than the relative risk of developing disease I and II combined, while the absolute measure is unaffected.

Thus, in the Hammond-Horn study, the association of cigarette smoking and lung cancer was higher when only patients with a well-substantiated diagnosis of lung cancer were considered, and was lower when the group included questionable diagnoses. Using the relative risk reveals the stronger association of cigarette smoking for epidermoid-undifferentiated carcinoma than for adenocarcinoma. The absolute measure would not differentiate between the risk for these subgroups.

The Causal Hypothesis

We turn now to a consideration of some of the contradictions in the causal hypothesis, alleged by various authors. Fisher (25) has stated:

When the sexes are compared it is found that lung cancer has been increasing more rapidly in men relatively to women . . . But it is notorious, and conspicuous in the memory of the most of us, that over the last 50 years the increase of smoking among women has been great, and that among men (even if positive) certainly small. The theory that increasing smoking is 'the cause' of the change in apparent incidence of lung cancer is not even tenable in the face of this contrast.

The available statistics do not confirm Fisher's statement. According to the Tobacco Manufacturer's Standing Committee (76) male per capita consumption of cigarette tobacco in Great Britain increased from 1.9 pounds in 1906 to 8 pounds in 1956. Female per capita consumption increased from essentially zero, in 1906, to 3.1 pounds in 1956. Far from making the causal hypothesis untenable, these results are entirely consistent with it, and constitute, in fact, one of the links in the chain of evidence implicating cigarettes.

The fact that cigarette smoking was associated with a higher mortality not only from lung cancer but from many other causes of death was originally considered as a contradiction by Arkin (1). Commenting on the first Hammond-Horn report, he wrote:

It would thus appear that cigarette smoking is one of the causes of all ills and contributes to the over-all death rate, remembering that this rate includes such causes as accident, homicide, etc. It seems quite clear that cigarette smoking is a symptom, not a cause. It is possible—even though this is a conjecture—that the type of person who is careful of his health is less likely to be a cigarette smoker and that the cigarette smoker is likely to be the person who generally takes greater health risks.

Both the later Hammond-Horn (38) report in the study of the American veterans (20) show no difference between cigarette and noncigarette smokers in mortality from accidents, violence, and suicide. If nonsmokers are biologically self-protective, it is only with respect to nonaccidental causes of death.

Berkson (4) has also pointed to the multiple findings in both the Hammond-Horn and the Doll-Hill results and concluded that the observed associations may have some other explanation than a causal one. He suggests three: 1) "The observed associations are 'spurious'. . . . 2) The observed associations have a constitutional basis. Persons who are nonsmokers, or relatively light smokers, are the kind of people who are biologically self-protective, and biologically this is correlated with robustness in meeting mortal stress from disease generally. 3) Smoking increases the 'rate of living' (Pearl), and smokers at a given age are, biologically, at an age older than their chronological age."

One might ask why the finding of an association with a number of diseases, rather than just one, is necessarily contradictory and must be regarded as supporting the constitutional hypothesis. Arkin (1) supplied no answer, while the relevant statements of Berkson (4) on this point were:

For myself, I find it quite incredible that smoking should cause all of these diseases.

When an investigation set up to test the theory, suggested by evidence previously obtained, that smoking causes lung cancer, turns out to indicate that smoking causes or provokes a whole gamut of diseases, inevitably it raises the suspicion that something is amiss.

It is not logical to take such a set of results [e.g., an association of smoking with a 'wide variety of diseases'] as confirming the theory that tobacco smoke contains carcinogenic substances which, by contrast with the pulmonary tissues, initiate cancerous changes at the site of contact.

We see nothing inherently contradictory nor inconsistent in the suggestion that one agent can be responsible for more than one disease, nor are we lacking in precedents. The Great Fog of London in 1952 increased the death rate for a number of causes, particularly respiratory and coronary disease, but no one has given this as a reason for doubting the causal role of the Fog. Tobacco smoke, too, is a complex substance and consists of many different combustion products. It would be more "incredible" to find that these hundreds of chemical products all had the same effect than to find the contrary. A universe in which cause and effect always have a one-to-one correspondence with each other would be easier to understand, but it obviously is not the kind we inhabit.

The apparent multiple effects of tobacco do raise a question with respect to the mode of action, however, and since this question is related to another alleged contradiction—the apparent lack of an inhalation effect—we shall discuss them together. What mode of action, it has been asked, can one postulate to explain these diverse attacks? Two remarks are in order: 1) The evidence that tobacco is a causal agent in the development of other diseases seems weaker than the evidence for lung cancer simply because the effects are smaller. While we would not exclude the possibility that cigarettes play a causal role in, for instance, the development of arteriosclerotic-coronary heart disease, the possibility that a common third factor will be discovered, which explains a 70 percent elevation in risk from coronary heart disease among cigarette smokers, is less remote than the possibility that the ninefold risk for lung cancer will be so explained. 2) Accepting, for the sake of discussion, the causal role of cigarettes for any disease showing an elevated mortality ratio, no matter how small, the presence of other causes will be manifested in a lower mortality ratio. Thus, even if cigarette consumption causes an elevation of 70 percent in mortality from coronary heart disease, other causes of great importance must also be present, as is manifested by the high mortality from this disease among nonsmokers. The existence of a small number of nonsmokers who develop lung cancer is a definite indication, by the same token, that cigarettes are not an absolutely necessary condition and that there are other causes of lung cancer.

If tobacco smoke does have multiple effects, each of these effects must be studied separately because of the complex nature of the agent. To postulate in advance that a single mode of action will be found to characterize them all is an unwarranted oversimplification. It is generally accepted, for example, that tobacco smoke causes thromboangiitis obliterans in susceptible humans by interfering with the peripheral circulation, and that it causes tumors when painted on the backs of susceptible mice because of the presence of carcinogens in the tars. The *a priori* postulation of a single mode of action for these two effects is no substitute for detailed study of each.

As to the possible mode of action of tobacco smoke in inducing lung cancer, the evidence at this writing suggests direct action of substances in tobacco smoke on susceptible tissues with which they are in contact.

Aside from background knowledge derived from experimental carcinogenesis which suggests this explanation, the following evidence favors it:
1) Cigarette smoke, which is usually drawn into the lungs, is associated
with mortality from lung cancer, while smoke from pipes and cigars,
which is usually not inhaled, is not. 2) For sites with which smoke is in
direct contact, whether or not inhaled, particularly buccal cavity and
larynx, the type of tobacco used makes less difference in incidence. 3) In
experimental carcinogenesis, which uses tobacco tars, tumors have appeared at the sight of application, and their incidence has not been seriously dependent on the type of tobacco used. 4) The relative risk of lung
cancer is higher among cigarette smokers who inhale than among those
smoking the same number of cigarettes per day, but who do not inhale.

Several critics (26, 43, 54) have stressed the failure of Doll and Hill (17),
in their preliminary report, to find the difference in risk between inhalers
and noninhalers, but this finding was contradicted in three of the studies
(8, 50, 68). Further work on this point is desirable, but would be more convincing if a more objective measure were found of the amount of smoke to
which human bronchial epithelium is exposed in the course of smoking a
cigarette.

Why, it is sometimes asked, do most heavy cigarette smokers fail to
develop lung cancer if cigarettes are in fact a causal agent? We have no
answer to this question. But neither can we say why most of the Lübeck
babies who were exposed to massive doses of virulent tubercle bacilli failed
to develop tuberculosis. This is not a reason, however, for doubting the
causal role of the bacilli in the development of the disease.

One cannot discuss the mode of action of tobacco without becoming
aware of the necessity of vastly expanded research in the field. The idea
that the subject of tobacco in mortality is a closed one is not one we share.
As in other fields of science, new findings lead to new questions, and new
experimental techniques will continue to cast further light on old ones.
This does not imply that judgment must be suspended until all the evidence is in, or that there are hierarchies of evidence, only some types of
which are acceptable. The doctrine that one must never assess what has
already been learned until the last possible piece of evidence would be a
novel one for science.

It would be desirable to have a set of findings on the subject of smoking and lung cancer so clear-cut and unequivocal that they were self-
interpreting. The findings now available on tobacco, as in most other fields
of science, particularly biologic science, do not meet this ideal. Nevertheless, if the findings had been made on a new agent, to which hundreds of
millions of adults were not already addicted, and on one which did not
support a large industry, skilled in the arts of mass persuasion, the evidence for the hazardous nature of the agent would be generally regarded

as beyond dispute. In the light of all the evidence on tobacco, and after careful consideration of all the criticisms of this evidence that have been made, we find ourselves unable to agree with the proposition that cigarette smoking is a harmless habit with no important effects on health or longevity. The concern shown by medical and public health authorities with the increasing diffusion to ever younger groups of an agent that is a health hazard seems to us to be well founded.

[Appendixes A and B portray mathematical proofs and have been deleted here to save space, Ed.]

Source

Cornfield J, Haenszel W, Hammond EC, Lilienfeld AM, Shimkin MB, Wynder EL. 1959. Smoking and lung cancer: Recent evidence and a discussion of some questions. *J Nat Cancer Inst* 22:173–203. Reprinted with permission of Oxford University Press.

Non-smoking Wives of Heavy Smokers Have a Higher Risk of Lung Cancer: A Study from Japan
(1984)

Takeshi Hirayama

Abstract

In a study in 29 health centre districts in Japan, 91,540 non-smoking wives aged 40 and above were followed up for 14 years (1966–79), and standardised mortality rates for lung cancer were assessed according to the smoking habits of their husbands. Wives of heavy smokers were found to have a higher risk of developing lung cancer and a dose-response relation was observed. The relation between the husband's smoking and the wife's risk of developing lung cancer showed a similar pattern when analysed by age and occupation of the husband. The risk was particularly great in agricultural families when the husbands were aged 40–59 at enrolment. The husbands' smoking habit did not affect their wives' risk of dying from other disease such as stomach cancer, cervical cancer, and ischaemic heart disease. The risk of developing emphysema and asthma seemed to be higher in nonsmoking wives of heavy smokers but the effect was not statistically significant.

The husband's drinking habit seemed to have no effect on any causes of death in their wives, including lung cancer.

These results indicate the possible importance of passive or indirect smoking as one of the causal factors of lung cancer. They also appear to explain the long-standing riddle of why many women develop lung cancer although they themselves are non-smokers. These results also cast doubt on the practice of assessing the relative risk of developing lung cancer in smokers by comparing them with non-smokers.

Introduction

The possible consequences to the health of non-smokers of long-term exposure to cigarette smoke (passive smoking) should be studied thoroughly because the side-stream and secondhand smoke of cigarettes contain various toxic substances, including carcinogens.[1][2] The need for such a study increased by the report of small-airways dysfunction in non-smokers chronically exposed to tobacco smoke.[3]

The effect of passive smoking on lung cancer was studied by following 91,540 non-smoking housewives aged 40 and above and measuring their risk of developing lung cancer according to the smoking habits of their husbands.

Methods

To study the consequences to health of such factors as cigarette smoking, alcohol drinking, occupation, and marital status, a prospective population study has been in progress in 29 health centre districts in six prefectures in Japan since the autumn of 1965. In total 265,118 adults (122,261 men and 142,857 women) aged 40 years and over, 91–99% of the census population, were interviewed and followed by establishing a record linkage system between the risk-factor records, a residence list obtained by special yearly census, and death certificates.

Since the effect of direct smoking of cigarettes in this study has already been reported,[4-7] my study focused on the effect of husbands' smoking on the risk of lung cancer in their non-smoking wives. Such observation was possible since detailed questions about lifestyle, including smoking habits, were asked of husbands and wives independently at the start of this study. No subjective bias was therefore conceivable.

A total of 346 deaths from lung cancer in women were recorded during 14 years of follow-up (1966–79). Of these women 245 were married, and 174 of these were also non-smokers. These cases occurred among 91,540 non-smoking married women whose husbands' smoking habits were studied. The risk of lung cancer was carefully measured, taking into consideration possible confounding variables.

Results

Wives of heavy smokers were found to have a higher risk of developing lung cancer than wives of non-smokers and a statistically significant dose-response relationship was observed (Mantel-extension χ test result being 3.299; two-tailed p=0.00097). Age-occupation standardised annual mortality rates for lung cancer were 8.7/100,000 (32 out of 21,895) when husbands were non-smokers or occasional smokers, 14.0 (86 out of 44,184) when husbands were ex-smokers or daily smokers of 1–19 cigarettes, and 18.1 (56 out of 25,146) when husbands were daily smokers of 20 or more cigarettes. These figures gave risk ratios of 1.00, 1.61, and 2.08 respectively. A similar trend was observed in age and occupation groups of husbands (table I).

The relation between the husband's smoking habit and the wife's risk of developing lung cancer was particularly significant in agricultural families when the husband was aged 40–59 at enrolment (Mantel-extension chi being 2.597 or two-tailed p=0.0094); lung cancer risk ratios were 1.00, 3.17, and 4.57 when husbands were non-smokers or occasional smokers, ex-smokers or smokers of 1–19 cigarettes daily, and smokers of 20 or more cigarettes daily respectively (table II).

Table I Standardised Mortality for Lung Cancer in Women by Age, Occupation, and Smoking Habit of the Husband (patient herself a non-smoker)

Husband's smoking habit:	Non-smoker	Ex-smoker or 1–19/day	≥20/day
Husband's age: 40–59 years			
Population of wives	14,020	30,676	20,584
No. of deaths from lung cancer	11	40	36
Occupation-standardised mortality/100,000	5.64	9.34	13.14
Husband's age: ≥60 years			
Population of wives	7,875	13,508	4,877
No. of deaths from lung cancer	21	46	20
Occupation-standardised mortality/100,000	15.79	24.44	29.60
Standardised risk ratio for all ages	1.00	1.61	2.08
Husband working in agriculture			
Population of wives	10,406	20,044	9,391
No. of deaths from lung cancer	17	52	24
Occupation-standardised mortality/100,000	9.54	17.02	18.40
Husband working elsewhere			
Population of wives	11,489	24,140	16,070
No. of deaths from lung cancer	15	34	32
Occupation-standardised mortality/100,000	9.13	10.46	17.70
Standardised risk ratio for all ages	1.00	1.43	1.90

Table II   Mortality for Lung Cancer in Women by Occupation and by Smoking Habit of Husband among Men Aged 40–59 (patient herself a non-smoker)

Husband's smoking habit:	Non-smoker	Ex-smoker or 1–19/day	≥20/day
Agricultural workers:			
Population of wives	5,999	12,753	7,150
No. of deaths from lung cancer	3	20	16
Mortality/100,000	3.48	11.03	15.92
Other workers:			
Population of wives	8,021	17,923	13,434
No. of deaths from lung cancer	8	20	20
Mortality/100,000	7.15	8.09	11.05
Standardised risk ratio for all occupations	1.00	1.67	2.36

The husbands' smoking habits seemed to have no effect on their wives' risk of developing other major cancers, such as cancers of the stomach (n=716) and of the cervix (n=250) or ischaemic heart disease (0=406). The risk of developing emphysema and asthma seemed to be higher among the non-smoking wives of smokers, but the effect was not statistically significant (table III).

Other characteristics of the husbands, such as their alcohol drinking habits did not affect mortality from lung cancer in their wives. The relative risk ratios of death from lung cancer were 1.00. 1.13, and 1.18 (p=0.396) respectively when husbands were non-drinkers, occasional or rare drinkers, and daily drinkers. Similar results were found with other causes of death (table IV).

Finally, the effect of passive smoking was compared with the effect of direct smoking. The effect of passive smoking was around one-half to one-third that of direct smoking. The relative risk of developing lung cancer by passive smoking was about 1.8 compared with about 3.8 in direct smokers (fig 1).

Discussion

The possible effect of passive smoking was studied by following many non-smoking wives whose husbands had various smoking habits and

Table III   Age-Occupation Standardised Risk Ratio for Selected Causes of Death in Women by Smoking Habit of the Husband (patient herself a non-smoker)

Cause of death	Husband's smoking habit			
	Non-smoker	Ex-smoker or 1–19/day	≥20/day	p value
Lung cancer (n = 174)	1.00	1.61	2.08	0.001
Emphysema, asthma (n = 66)	1.00	1.29	1.49	0.474
Cancer of the cervix (n = 250)	1.00	1.15	1.14	0.249
Stomach cancer (n = 716)	1.00	1.02	0.99	0.720
Ischemic heart disease (n = 406)	1.00	0.97	1.03	0.393

Table IV   Age-Standardised Risk Ratio for Selected Causes of Death in Women by Alcohol-drinking Habits of the Husband

Cause of death	Husband's drinking habit			
	Non-drinker	Occasional or rare drinker	Daily drinker	p value
Lung cancer (n = 174)	1.00	1.13	1.18	0.396
Emphysema, asthma (n = 66)	1.00	0.92	1.39	0.292
Cancer of the cervix (n = 250)	1.00	0.84	0.89	0.514
Stomach cancer (n = 716)	1.00	0.88	0.95	0.285
Ischaemic heart disease (n = 406)	1.00	1.09	0.93	0.567

measuring their risk of developing lung cancer. Continued exposure to their husbands' smoking increased mortality from lung cancer in non-smokers up to twofold. The extent of the increase in the risk of developing cancer reached as high as 4.6 for non-smoking wives of agricultural workers aged 40–59 who smoked 20 or more cigarettes a day.

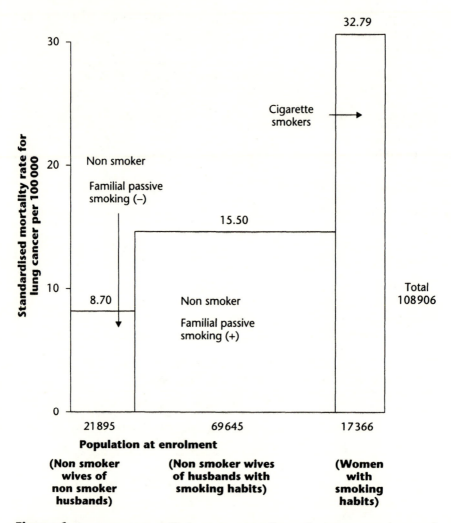

Figure 1 Lung cancer mortality in women according to the presence or absence of direct and familial indirect smoking.

The fact that there was a statistically significant relation (two-tailed p=0.00097) between the amount the husbands smoked and the mortality of their non-smoking wives from lung cancer suggests that these findings were not the result of chance. To determine whether such an effect was limited to lung cancer, similar studies were conducted with other causes of death. Although there seemed to be a relation between husbands' smoking habits and deaths from emphysema and asthma in their wives, the effect of passive smoking was strongest with lung cancer. Passive smoking did not seem to increase the risk of developing stomach cancer, cervical cancer, or ischaemic heart disease. We found that smoking was the only

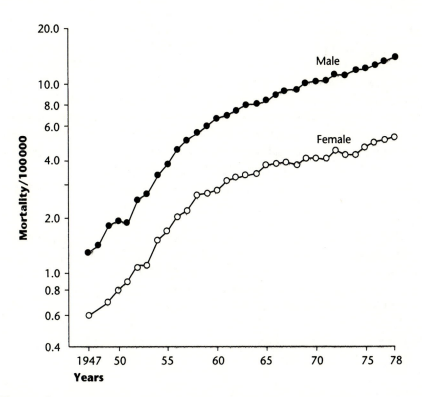

Figure 2 Age-adjusted mortality for lung cancer in Japan (1947–78).

habit of the husbands to affect wives' mortality. The absence of an effect of husbands' drinking habits on mortality in their wives was shown as an example.

The most important confounding variables would have been urban factors. Similar observations were therefore made for agricultural families and for non-agricultural families, and a similar dose-response relation was observed in both groups. The effect of passive smoking was most striking in younger couples in agricultural families, relative risk reaching 4.6, probably because of the lesser extent of the exposure of passive smoking outside the family in the case of rural residents. That the rate for non-smoking wives with husbands who were heavy smokers in urban families was lower than that in rural families is puzzling but probably reflects a longer period of mutual contact of couples in rural families. In urban families some couples meet only for a short period in the day.

Finally, the effects of passive smoking were compared with the effects of direct smoking. The results clearly indicated that the effect of passive smoking is about one-half to one-third that of direct smoking in terms of mortality ratio or relative risk. In terms of attributable risk, however, the effect of passive smoking on lung cancer in women must be much more important than that of direct smoking (fig 1), especially in countries such as Japan where 73% of men but only 15% of women smoke. Therefore, although the relative risk of indirect smoking was smaller than that of direct smoking, the absolute excess deaths from lung cancer due to passive smoking must be important because of the large size of the exposed group.

The age-adjusted mortality rates for lung cancer have been sharply increasing both for men and for women in Japan (fig 2). As only a fraction of Japanese women with lung cancer smoke cigarettes, the reasons why their mortality from lung cancer parallels that in men have been unclear. The present study appears to explain at least a part of this long-standing riddle.

This observation also questions the validity of the conventional method of assessing the relative risk of developing lung cancer in smokers by comparing them with non-smokers. This study shows that non-smokers are not a homogenous group and should be subdivided according to the extent of previous exposure to indirect or passive smoking.

This work was supported by Grants-in-Aid for Cancer Research from the Ministry of Health and Welfare.

SOURCE

Hirayama T. 1984. Cancer mortality in nonsmoking women with smoking husbands based on a large-scale cohort study in Japan. *Prev Med* 13 (6): 680–90. Copyright 1983 *Preventive Medicine*. Reprinted with permission of Elsevier.

CHAPTER 3

DENTAL HEALTH

Every tooth in a man's head is more valuable than a diamond.
　　—Miguel de Cervantes, *Don Quixote*, 1605

Even as our Nation's health has progressed, dental caries or tooth decay remains the most prevalent chronic childhood disease.
　　—Michael K. Simpson (b. 1950), U.S. Congressman and dentist

LEGEND HAS IT THAT GEORGE WASHINGTON had a set of wooden dentures, but this is apparently not so. Multiple sources report that although the first U.S. president did have several sets of dentures, they were made of metals, ivory, and various types of reshaped teeth (cow, elk, and perhaps human). Washington was fortunate to be able to afford dental care, such as it was in his day. His wealth made luxury items such as dentures available to him in the eighteenth century, a time when tooth loss from dental caries and periodontal disease was rampant. Dental appliances of the time were often made by craftsmen such as Paul Revere, the famous silversmith. Indeed, Revere advertised his services for creating these status symbols in a Boston newspaper.

Washington is only one example of how dental problems have always plagued humankind. Skulls of Cro-Magnon, for instance, show evidence of both dental diseases and dental injuries. Phoenician, Etruscan, and other archeological sites have unearthed early dental appliances, especially crowns and bridgework. Primitive toothbrushes have been found in ancient Chinese, Hindu, and Islamic archeological sites, showing that some cultural practices for dental hygiene go back a very long time. The Egyptians even had physicians who specialized in diseases of the teeth, providing both diagnosis and treatment. The works of Hippocrates make several references to the diseases of teeth and gums and show that extraction was widely accepted. For instance, in *De Affectionibus* we find: "In cases of toothache, if the tooth is decayed and loose it must be extracted."

Dental surgery flowered in Arabia during the Middle Ages, when Islamic physicians created specialized surgical instruments to deal with dental abscesses, caries, and extractions. In Europe, barber surgeons provided dental extraction and manual decay removal services, along with haircuts, blood letting, and the routine application of leeches. The French are credited with being the first to use both gold leaf and soft lead (later amalgam) for filling holes in teeth after decay was manually removed using a hand drill. This was perhaps as early as the fifteenth century. But all of these advances could not halt the rampage of dental caries that spread across the globe as expanding world trade allowed cane sugar to become widely available. Dental diseases were a particular problem at court, where the consumption of sweets became the norm. Queen Elizabeth I, for example, was known for her black teeth, a sign of significant dental caries.

Early dental surgery was painful, and the search for painless dentistry in the nineteenth century pushed many to experiment with nitrous oxide, ether, and chloroform. Unfortunately, all of these agents had drawbacks, and demonstrations of their effectiveness sometimes ended badly, even with the death of the patient. The invention of early x-ray technology to find infections and decay that were not visible to the naked eye may also have improved diagnostic abilities for those treating dental disease, but many of these exposures were clearly dangerous to the patient. Technology, then, provided little relief from dental diseases before the twentieth century. The realization that fluoride could prevent dental caries made the most significant impact on dental public health.

During the course of the early nineteenth century, scientists developed sensitive chemical analyses that could detect fluorine and fluorides. Because only very small amounts of these substances were detected in bones and teeth, there were serious disagreements about whether their presence was essential or simply coincidental. Although the majority of scientists held the latter position, animal experiments led a few scientists to strongly believe that fluoride was essential for the development of healthy bones and teeth. In 1874, for instance, Carl Erhardt, a physician in Emmendingen, Germany, who had done fluoride experiments on dogs, recommended potassium fluoride for tooth preservation. Erhardt noted that fluoride pastilles had already been introduced for dental health purposes in England. In that same year, Alvaro Reynoso, a Cuban who had spent many years conducting scientific experiments in France, filed U.S. Patent 146,781 for a fluoride-containing elixir or syrup. Reynoso recommended the syrup particularly for infants as their bones and teeth were just forming. The use of fluoride for dental health remained controversial, however, until the twentieth century.

THE ROLE OF FLUORIDE IN DENTAL PUBLIC HEALTH

The story of how fluoride became a tool of public health begins in Colorado in 1901. In that year, Frederick S. McKay, a recent graduate of the University of

Pennsylvania Dental School, opened a practice in Colorado Springs. McKay noted white and brown spots on the enamel of his dental patients, a condition that concerned him but seemed to be purely cosmetic. McKay brought his concerns to the El Paso County Odontological Society, but its members seemed particularly apathetic to the issue. Because of his insistence, the society launched an investigation of "Colorado brown stain" or "mottled enamel" by sending letters to a sample of practicing Rocky Mountain dentists to see if there were other geographic areas so affected. There was little response.

In 1905, McKay moved to St. Louis, Missouri, where he specialized in orthodontia. Returning to Colorado for health reasons in 1908, McKay persuaded the Colorado Springs Dental Society to investigate Colorado brown stain. With the permission of the local school board and armed with some minor financial support from the society, McKay and a colleague, Isaac Burton, went from desk to desk in the local schools, examining 2,945 children and noting the condition and degree of staining of their teeth. The dentists then correlated this information with birthplace, places of residence, and the age at which the child had moved to Colorado Springs. They obtained this information from parental questionnaires that they matched to each child examined. This massive effort by McKay and Burton determined that 87.5 percent of Colorado Springs schoolchildren had some degree of Colorado brown stain or "mottling" on their teeth. Of those affected, all were natives of the Pikes Peak region. The etiology of the condition, however, remained a puzzle.

Members of the Colorado State Dental Society wrote to the dean of the Northwestern University Dental School in Chicago, G.V. Black, about Colorado brown stain and the results of the study. Black requested some teeth for examination and then traveled to Colorado Springs in 1909 to observe the condition firsthand. During the next six years, armed with Grant No.1 from the newly created Dental Research Fund of the American Dental Association (ADA), McKay and Black were able to determine that 1) Colorado brown stain resulted from developmental imperfections and was not a problem for those who already had calcified teeth; and 2) teeth afflicted by Colorado brown stain were uncharacteristically resistant to decay. Although unable to pinpoint the etiology of the condition, Black's interest in it prompted professional awareness of tooth mottling.

In 1923, McKay was contacted by the parents of children in Oakley, Idaho, who noted the appearance of brown stains on their children's teeth. Parents reported that the stains began to appear shortly after a new well began supplying water to the town. McKay recommended that the water source be changed, and within a few years, secondary teeth emerged in the same children, this time without the brown stains. Armed with this clue that something in the water could be the cause of the mottling, McKay wrote to the PHS in 1926 to request that the agency do water analysis for various districts afflicted by mottled tooth enamel. His letter was bounced from department to department but received little support.

Around the same time, F.L. Robertson, a dentist practicing about five miles from Bauxite, Arkansas, reported to the Arkansas State Board of Health that his patients had brown stains on their teeth. In response, the Arkansas State Board of Health asked the PHS to make a study of mottled enamel in Bauxite. Lack of response from the PHS led Luther Branting, superintendent of the Aluminum Company of America (ALCOA), the mining company in Bauxite, to contact McKay in 1927. McKay urged Grover Kempf, of the PHS Bureau of Child Hygiene, to conduct a survey of mottling among children in the Bauxite region. Although the survey was done, no results were released in order to protect the identity of both the community and ALCOA. McKay broke rank and released the results in a paper he read at a meeting of the New York Section of the International Association for Dental Research in 1930. He confirmed that 100 percent of people living in Bauxite were afflicted with mottled tooth enamel.

Hoping to show that the aluminum mining industry was not the culprit causing mottled tooth enamel, ALCOA began a water testing program at its state-of-the-art laboratories in Pittsburgh. In 1930, H.V. Churchill, ALCOA chief chemist, ordered a spectrographic analysis of the well water in Bauxite and was surprised to find high concentrations of fluoride (13.7 parts per million [ppm]). Although fluoride is almost universally found in soil and water, it is generally found in concentrations less than 1.0 ppm. Churchill then received additional samples of well water for spectral analysis from McKay, who obtained them from geographic areas where mottled tooth enamel was prevalent. These samples also contained high levels of fluoride, implying there might be a causal link to the condition.

Churchill and McKay's findings led to the creation of the Dental Hygiene Unit at the National Institutes of Health (NIH) in 1931. Headed by H. Trendley Dean, the unit was charged with investigating the link between fluoride and mottled tooth enamel. By 1938, Dean was able to report on the geographic distribution of endemic fluorosis in the United States; the report estimated 345 geographic areas in 25 different states. Of these, 86 percent of the endemic regions were located west of the Mississippi River and 27 percent were located in Texas, primarily in the West Texas Panhandle region. Dean also reported endemic dental fluorosis in Argentina (known as *dientes veteados*); North Africa, especially Tunisia, Algiers, and Morocco (known as *le darmous*); the southeastern archipelago of Japan and parts of China; the northwestern part of the Punjab and parts of Madras, India; as well as the Azores, Canada, England, Italy, and Mexico.

By 1942, the Dental Hygiene Unit was able to report the "ideal" level of fluoride in drinking water that would substantially reduce decay without leaving the population with mottled tooth enamel (now called "fluorosis"). Researchers in the unit were able to identify this level by creating an ordinal classification scheme to describe the degree of tooth mottling (the Fluorosis Index: mild, moderate, or severe) and the amount of dental caries (measured as the number of decayed, missing, and filled teeth [DMFT]) observed during a dental examination. They could then correlate that information to the amount of fluoride in regional drinking water samples. The unit launched two major studies using this classification scheme. The first examined children's teeth and fluoride in the water supply in 26 states. The second, a confirmatory study, analyzed teeth and water in 21 cities. Both studies determined that the optimum fluoride concentration in a community water supply that would minimize both children's dental caries and dental fluorosis was 1.0 ppm. This information set the stage for the first field trial that would add fluoride to a public water supply, an effort not without controversy.

Fluoridation of Public Water Supplies

Nutritional studies conducted on rats by Gerald J. Cox at the Mellon Institute (ALCOA's industrial research lab) in Pittsburgh during the 1930s led Cox to conclude that fluorine is "one factor" in the development of caries-resistant teeth. In 1939, Cox became the first person to call for the addition of fluoride to community water supplies. In 1943, David B. Ast, the director of Dental Health at the New York State Department of Health, published a study designed to test the hypothesis that fluorine in community water could reduce dental caries. Four pairs of communities were eager to test the hypothesis. On January 25, 1945, Grand Rapids, Michigan, became the first community in the world to fluoridate its water supply. The control community for this field trial was Muskegon, Michigan, which decided to withdraw from the trial and in 1951 began a water fluoridation program of its own. The other three pairs of cities participating in the fluorine–caries study were Newburgh, New York (fluoridation began in May 1945) and Kingston, New York (no fluoride); Brantford, Ontario, Canada (fluoridation began in June 1945) and Sarnia, Ontario, Canada (no fluoride); and Evanston, Illinois (fluoridation began in February 1947) and Oak Park, Illinois (no fluoride). Results from these and other trials eventually placed the optimum fluoride concentration for reducing dental caries without inducing fluorosis between 0.7 and 1.2 ppm, depending upon climate.

Adding fluoride to community water supplies was, and remains, a controversial practice. Most of the controversy focuses on the fact that community water fluoridation is an imposed involuntary risk with potentially unforeseen health risks. In the mid twentieth century, Christian Scientists who claimed that water fluoridation was forced medication made strident arguments against it. Members of the John Birch Society claimed that fluoridation was a communist plot intended to poison American water supplies. Indeed, antifluoride groups remain active worldwide today. Yet despite strong antifluoridation sentiment, at the beginning of the twentieth century more than 60 percent of Americans were served by fluoridated water, as well as 40 percent of Canadians and 10 percent of United Kingdom residents. By 2008, the entire populations of New Zealand and Australia were served by fluoridated public water, as well as the majority of the population of the Republic of Ireland. In South America, about 70 percent of the population of Chile and 45 percent of those in Brazil were also so served.

Water is not the only way that fluoride has been made available to populations in an effort to improve dental public health. In 1992, the WHO Expert Committee Report on Advances in Oral Health confirmed that salt and milk were appropriate vehicles for implementing population-based fluoridation programs. Colombia, Costa Rica, France, Jamaica, and Switzerland, for example, add fluoride to table salt rather than to their potable water supplies. Fluoridated milk trials for schoolchildren have been ongoing in Bulgaria, Chile, China, Hungary, Peru, Russia, Thailand, the United Kingdom, and New Orleans, Louisiana. Although providing fluoride in salt and milk addresses the issue of making the risk from exposure to fluoride voluntary, controversy about the health effects continues.

Fluoride in Toothpastes, Tooth Powders, and Mouth Rinses

During the course of the twentieth century, multiple patents were issued in France, Germany, the United Kingdom, and the United States for toothpastes and tooth powders that contain various forms of fluoride. Toothpastes in collapsible tubes became popular around the time of World War I, including varieties that included fluoride, but these products were not approved by the ADA. Around 1950, Procter and Gamble, in cooperation with the University of Indiana, instituted a research program on the effectiveness of toothpaste containing fluoride. In 1955, the company launched its first fluoridated toothpaste, Crest. By 1961, research was sufficient to sway the conservative ADA. In that year Procter and Gamble received the following endorsement from the ADA, and the company continues to use it for advertising purposes even today: "Crest has been shown to be an effective anticaries (decay preventative) dentifrice that can be of significant value when used in a conscientiously applied program of oral hygiene and regular professional care." This endorsement spurred most other large U.S. manufacturers of toothpaste to provide products with fluoride as an option for consumers.

In 1994, the WHO Technical Report Series No. 846 on fluorides and oral health recommended the use of fluoridated toothpastes in developing countries. The use of fluoridated toothpastes, powders, and mouth rinses has become common worldwide, though there is some preference for "natural" toothpastes among populations who harbor lingering concerns about too much fluoride or the potentially harmful effects of any fluoride. In the United States, these concerns were addressed by the National Research Council (NRC) in 1993 and again in 2006. The first NRC report noted that although the decline in dental caries in the United States was an important health advance that could be ascribed primarily to fluoridated water and dental products, intake from multiple sources containing fluoride could be toxic, especially for infants fed with formula reconstituted with fluoridated water and children who ingest a large number of fluoride-containing soft drinks. That report also called for more research on fluoride in relation to bone fractures and osteosarcoma, a malignant form of bone cancer. The second NRC report, released in 2006, determined that the maximum contaminant level goal (MCLG) of 4 milligrams per liter of fluoride was probably too high to protect infants and children, as well as adults who consume more than 2 liters of water per day (i.e., athletes, dieters, outdoor workers, and people with diabetes insipidus). The 2006 report concluded that the MCLG should be lowered. At the time of this writing, the Environmental Protection Agency had not moved to change the standards.

DENTAL SEALANTS

Contemporaneous with the advent of fluoridated water, toothpastes, and mouth rinses, bonding technologies that allowed resins to be attached to the chewing surfaces of teeth were developed in the 1950s and 1960s. These resins, or dental sealants, were painted over the pits and fissures of the grinding teeth so that they could not harbor food and bacteria that cause decay. As about 80 percent of children's caries were located on these tooth surfaces, sealing the pits and fissures on molars was considered a practical way to improve children's dental health. As with fluoride, there were many who considered putting any foreign substances into children's bodies against the laws of nature. To address these concerns, in 1983 the NIH issued a *Consensus Conference Statement on Dental Sealants* indicating that the practice was safe. The conference stated: "Practitioners, dental health agency directors, and dental educators are urged to incorporate the appropriate use of sealants into their practices and programs." Two years later, the ADA Council of Dental Research recommended that sealants be universally applied to children's molar teeth within three or four years of eruption.

In 1996, a Spanish study raised concerns that dental sealants contained bisphenol A (BPA), a hormone-mimicking compound that can leach into saliva from the plastic resin. Almost immediately, manufacturing processes of sealants were changed and quality controls were implemented to remove BPA. Studies on the newly formulated sealants showed no detectable BPA and no adverse health outcomes. As a result, sealants that are tested and reveal no detectable BPA carry ADA approval.

From 1999 to 2002, the National Health and Nutrition Examination Survey (NHANES) determined the prevalence of the use of dental sealants among U.S. children ages 6 to 19 years at about 32 percent. Some regions of Canada offer free dental sealants to schoolchildren, although the uptake is apparently low. The use of dental sealants is reportedly increasing in Germany, Greece, and the United Kingdom, where studies have shown a decrease in DMFT among teenagers.

CHANGING DIETS

Reducing dietary sugar is the most important factor in preventing dental caries. Xylitol, a five-carbon sugar alcohol (penitol), is a naturally occurring substance that can be used effectively in place of sugar. Although it is found in berries, fruit, vegetables, and mushrooms, xylitol is best commercially extracted from birch trees or corn. The U.S. Food and Drug Administration (FDA) approved xylitol as safe for dietary use in 1963, but it had diabetics in mind, not children. The FDA commissioned a safety review of the substance by the Federation of American Societies for Experimental Biology (FASEB) in 1986, a review it again passed. During the same period, the European Union's Scientific Committee for Food found xylitol "acceptable" for dietary uses. The WHO's Joint Expert Committee on Food Additives (JECFA) reviewed xylitol safety in 1977, 1978, 1983, and 1996. That body of experts found no concerns about the safety of xylitol and set the sweetener's Acceptable Daily Intake (ADI) as "not specified," the safest of its food additive categories.

While the excessive use of xylitol can produce a laxative effect in some people, its judicious use is unquestionably helpful in improving dental health. Indeed, numerous controlled clinical trials and field trials of xylitol chewing gum in a variety of places around the world have demonstrated that replacing sugar with the sweetener dramatically reduces the incidence of dental caries among children. In Finland, for example, a school-based program showed that chewing xylitol gum daily was equal to a pit and fissure sealant program for preventing dental caries. So successful was that effort that in 1998 a national sample of Finnish schoolchildren showed that 45 percent of boys and 63 percent of girls chewed xylitol-based chewing gum daily as part of their dental health regimen. Studies in Australia, Belize, Canada, Estonia, Hungary, Kuwait, the Netherlands, Norway, Polynesia, the United States, and the Soviet Union also showed positive results.

Xylitol works for preventing dental caries because oral microflora (*Streptococcus mutans*) cannot ferment it to create the conditions necessary for cavities to develop. There is evidence that this anticariogenic process continues even after xylitol exposure ends and that pregnant mothers who use xylitol transfer the protection to their children during the first few years of life. Official endorsements for the use of xylitol by national health and/or dental associations include Finland (1988), Sweden (1989), Norway (1990), the United Kingdom (1992), Iceland (1993), Ireland (1993), Estonia (1995), the Netherlands (1996), and Switzerland (1997). Gum, candy, ice pops, and other foodstuffs made with xylitol and sold in the United States now carry the FDA-approved labeling of "does not promote tooth decay." Additionally, the ADA has recognized xylitol as "useful as part of a comprehensive program including proper dental hygiene" for improving oral health.

During the course of the twentieth century, many developed nations reduced their national burden of dental caries and tooth loss, particularly for children and adolescents, through the use of fluoridated water, salt, and milk; the use of fluoridated dentifrices; improvements in dental hygiene; and/or nutritional changes that reduced the intake of sugar. For instance, WHO data show that the number of DMFT for 12-year-olds decreased in Australia (9.3 in 1958; 0.8 in 1998), Finland (7.5 in 1975; 1.1 in 1997), Norway (12.0 in 1940; 1.5 in 1999), Switzerland (9.6 in 1961–1963; 0.8 in 1996), the United Kingdom (3.1 in 1983; 1.1 in 1996–1997), and the United States (7.6 in 1946; 1.4 in 1998). Developing countries, on the other hand, had mixed results. Those with an increase in sugar in their diets fared poorly in the number of DMFT for 12-year-olds: Chile (2.8 in 1960; 4.1 in 1996), Democratic Republic of the Congo (0.1 in 1971; 0.4–1.1 in 1987), Jordan (0.2 in 1962; 3.3 in 1995), and the Philippines (1.4 in 1967; 4.6 in 1998). Others, however, had significant successes: French Polynesia went from 6.5 in 1989 to 3.2 in 1994 after a dietary change replacing sugar with xylitol, and Mexico went from 5.3 in 1975 to 2.5 in 1997 after the introduction of fluoridated salt.

Nutritional status remains a key factor for dental health. In addition to excess sugar in the diet, we know that lack of vitamins A and D, as well as protein-energy malnutrition, cause developing teeth to be more susceptible to decay. In populations where dietary sugars are restricted, dental caries remain low despite undernutrition. On the other hand, in populations where sugar intake is high, undernutrition exacerbates the risk of caries. Additionally, vitamin C deficiency may result in periodontitis (inflammation of the gums, tooth socket bone, and periodontal ligament that holds the tooth in the socket), a condition linked to tooth loss (see Volume I, Chapter 3 for a discussion of James Lind and scurvy).

Challenges to dental public health remain in terms of improving dental hygiene, access to preventive and restorative dental services, and dental research. In the latter part of the twentieth century, research determined links between dental health and atherosclerosis (the underlying factor in cardiovascular and cerebrovascular diseases), low birth weight, and health complications for people with diabetes and the human immunodeficiency virus (HIV). These health issues are on the rise globally, and as such, further understanding of the links to dental health is becoming vitally important. There have been efforts to develop a vaccine against *S. mutans* as a preventive for dental caries, but such a vaccine has yet to show results in clinical trials. In the meantime, fluoride, xylitol, and dental sealants, as well as improved efforts at oral hygiene and access to preventive and restorative dental care remain important public health tools for ensuring the health of populations.

SELECTED READINGS

The first reading on dental public health is by Frederick S. McKay and G.V. Black in 1915. McKay is credited with being the first to report mottled teeth as an endemic condition in a regional population. Black encouraged him to test his hypothesis about mottled teeth being resistant to decay. This collaborative descriptive study validated McKay's observations and set off a search for the cause of the mottling. Eventually, it led to the understanding of the role of fluoride in caries prevention. It appears here abridged, missing only the photographs of mottled teeth included in the original.

The second reading, by David B. Ast and Edward R. Schlesinger, describes the results of the 10-year controlled trial of water fluoridation in the communities of Newburgh and Kingston, New York, from 1945 to 1955. The work is abridged in that it is missing one figure that was not possible to reproduce. We do not believe the bar graph contained in the figure is essential, as the results are discussed in the text. The authors conclude that fluoridation of a community water supply is not only effective for preventing dental caries, but it is also a safe public health practice, a statement that continues to be challenged in some circles today.

The last reading, by K.G. König, reviews the effects of diet on oral health. It is also abridged, missing only a few figures that are discussed in detail in the text. König, a dental researcher from the Netherlands and an expert on international dental public health, concludes that oral health risks do not necessitate dietary recommendations in addition to, or other than, those required for maintenance of general health. Of particular interest is the epidemiological evidence presented that draws distinctions between the rates of disease in developed and developing countries and their links with oral health.

BIBLIOGRAPHY

Ast DB. 1943. The caries–fluorine hypothesis and a suggested study to test its application. *Public Health Rep* 58:857–79.

Britten RH and Perrott GSJ. 1941. Summary of physical findings on men drafted in world war. *Public Health Rep* 56:41–62.

Brown LJ, Beazoglou T, and Heffley D. 1994. Estimated savings in U.S. dental expenditures, 1979–89. *Public Health Rep* 109:195–203.

Brunelle JA and Carlos JP. 1990. Recent trends in dental caries in U.S. children and the effect of water fluoridation. *J Dent Res* 69:723–27.

Burt BA. 1978. Influences for change in the dental health status of populations: An historical perspective. *J Public Health Dent* 38:272–88.

Centers for Disease Control. 1999. Achievements in Public Health, 1900–1999: Fluoridation of drinking water to prevent dental caries. *MMWR* 48 (41): 933–40.

Churchill HV. 1931. Occurrence of fluorides in some waters of the United States. *Ind Eng Chem* 23:996–98.

Cox GJ. 1939. New knowledge of fluorine in relation to dental caries. *J Am Water Works Assn* 31:1926–30.

Dean HT. 1938. Endemic fluorosis and its relation to dental caries. *Public Health Rep* 53:1443–52.

Dean HT. 1942. The investigation of physiological effects by the epidemiological method. In *Fluorine and Dental Health*, ed F.R. Moulton. Washington, DC: American Association for the Advancement of Science.

Dean HT, Jay P, Arnold FA Jr., and Elvove E. 1941. Domestic water and dental caries. II. A study of 2,832 white children, aged 12–14 years, of 8 suburban Chicago communities, including *Lactobacillus acidophilus* studies of 1,761 children. *Public Health Rep* 56:761–92.

Hodge HC. 1986. Evaluation of some objections to water fluoridation. In Fluorides and Dental Caries, 3rd ed., ed E. Newbrun, 221–55. Springfield, Ill.: Charles C Thomas.

Horowitz HS. 1996. The effectiveness of community water fluoridation in the United States. *J Public Health Dent* 56:253–58.

Hujoel PP, Drangsholt M, Spiekerman C, and DeRouen TA. 2000. Periodontal disease and coronary heart disease risk. JAMA 284 (11): 1406–10.

Klein H. 1941. Dental status and dental needs of young adult males, rejectable, or acceptable for military service, according to Selective Service dental requirements. *Public Health Rep* 56:1369–87.

Klein H, Palmer CE, and Knutson JW. 1938. Studies on dental caries. I. Dental status and dental needs of elementary school children. *Public Health Rep* 53:751–65.

Ly KA, Milgrom P, and Rothen M. 2006. Xylitol, sweeteners, and dental caries. *Pediatric Dentistry* 28 (2): 154–64.

Mattila KJ. 1993. Dental infections as a risk factor for acute myocardial infarction. *Eur Heart J* 14 (Suppl. K): 51–53.

McKay FS. 1928. Relation of mottled enamel to caries. *J Am Dent Assoc* 15:1429–37.

McKay FS. 1942. Mottled enamel: Early history and its unique features. In: *Fluorine and Dental Health*, ed F.R. Moulton. Washington, DC: American Association for the Advancement of Science.

National Research Council. 1993. *Health Effects of Ingested Fluoride.* Washington, DC: National Academy Press.

National Research Council. 2006. *Fluoride in Drinking Water.* Washington, DC: National Academy Press.

Pelton WJ, Dunbar JB, McMillan RS, Moller P, and Wolff AE. 1969. *The Epidemiology of Oral Health.* Cambridge, MA: Harvard University Press.

Public Health Service. 1962. *Public Health Service Drinking Water Standards–Revised 1962 (PHS 956).* Washington, DC: U.S. Department of Health, Education, and Welfare.

Rayman S. 2007. Transcultural barriers and cultural competence in dental hygiene practice. *J Contemp Dent Pract* 8 (4): 43–51.

Riley JC, Lennon MA, and Ellwood RP. 1999. The effect of water fluoridation and social inequalities on dental caries in 5-year-old children. *Int J Epidemiol* 28:300–305.

Soderling E, Isokangas P, Pienihakkinen K, Tenovuo J, and Alanen P. 2001. Influence of maternal xylitol consumption on mother-child transmission of mutans streptococci: 6-year follow-up. *Caries Res* 35 (3): 173–77.

U.S. Department of Health and Human Services. 2003. *A National Call to Action to Promote Oral Health: A Public-Private Partnership Under the Leadership of the Office of the Surgeon General* (NIH 03–5303). Washington, DC: U.S. Government Printing Office.

Weintraub JA. 1989. The effectiveness of pit and fissure sealants. *J Public Health Dent* 49 (5 Spec No): 317–30.

Weintraub JA and Burt BA. 1987. Prevention of dental caries by the use of pit-and-fissure sealants. *J Public Health Policy* 8 (4): 542–60.

Wu T, Trevisan M, Genco RJ, Dorn JP, Falkner KL, and Sempos CT. 2000. Periodontal disease and risk of cerebrovascular disease: The first national health and nutrition examination survey and its follow-up study. *Arch Intern Med* 160 (18): 2749–55.

An Investigation of Mottled Teeth
(1916, Abridged)
An Endemic Developmental Imperfection of the Enamel of the Teeth, Heretofore Unknown in the Literature of Dentistry

By Frederick S. McKay, D.D.S., Colorado Springs, Colorado, in collaboration with G.V. Black, M.D., D.D.S., Sc.D., LL.D.

I.

It is the purpose of this paper to describe an investigation into the occurrence and prevalence of a lesion of the enamel that until recently published by Dr. G.V. Black (Dental Cosmos, January 1960, vol. lviii, No. 1) has never before been described either accurately or comprehensively.* The term "mottled enamel" was applied to it by the writer somewhat empirically, but has become probably the accepted designation, having been suggested by the appearance of the teeth.

The remarkable thing about the lesion is that it is practically, if not absolutely limited in its distribution, in any large way, to certain well-defined geographical areas, in which it occurs in the teeth of only those individuals who were either actually born and lived continuously in any of these areas during the years of enamel formation; or in those who, although being born elsewhere, were brought into such districts for a continuous residence during the years of enamel formation. These circumstances indicate that we are dealing with a developmental dystrophy, and the term "endemic" is applied because the lesion is peculiar to a district or particular locality or class of persons—natives and those coming to the locality in early childhood.

An endemic disease is one constantly present to a greater or lesser degree in any place, and the investigation of this condition has left no doubt that a high percentage of those persons who conform to the conditions just set forth will exhibit mottled enamel upon the permanent teeth when they erupt. This seems to be a law pretty definitely determined, as will

---

* The histo-pathology of this lesion has been fully dealt with in a companion-paper by Dr. Black (as above noted), and Dr. McKay confines himself in this paper to a description of the clinical and other features and a detailed account of the investigation.

later be shown, as applied to all of such districts as can properly be termed "afflicted," "susceptible," or "endemic."

Macroscopical Description of Mottled Enamel and Brown Stain

Normal enamel is a dense, homogeneous structure, in which the enamel rods are closely bound to each other and in turn into columns by a structureless calcified material, variously termed the "cementing" or "interprismatic" substance.

Mottled enamel is characterized by minute white flecks, or yellow or brown spots or areas, scattered irregularly or streaked over the surface of a tooth, or it may be a condition where the entire tooth surface is of a dead paper-white, like the color of a china dish. In many cases the surface of the tooth is dotted with irregular, shallow pits which are usually darkly discolored because of the lodgment therein of débris. Such are spoken of as the "pitted" variety.

Any, or all, of the teeth may be mottled, or certain groups only according to circumstances which are discussed elsewhere in this paper, and also in Dr. Black's paper; or the area of some teeth, either above or below a certain point, may be mottled, and the rest of the enamel of such teeth [may] be practically normal.

In some slightly marked cases the white areas are found only on the points of the cusps, the rest of the enamel in the teeth being normal. The teeth present this appearance upon eruption, and the pits are present, when present at all, at the time. Perhaps the most frequent location for the pits is near the points of the cusps on the bicuspid teeth. Upper and lower teeth seem equally liable to mottling, and upon all surfaces, although as a rule the labial and buccal surfaces have the most pronounced markings. If there is any difference, the upper teeth are most affected. Mottled enamel, in my experience, has never been found upon the temporary teeth. In examining children in afflicted districts at ages when the permanent incisors and first molars have erupted, but the temporary molars are still in place, the contrast in the enamel on these two varieties of teeth is most pronounced. The white mottled enamel on the permanent teeth exhibits a marked contrast with the normal enamel on the temporary teeth, which has the customary almost bluish tinge. In explanation of this it is to be remembered that the temporary teeth are formed largely before birth, in an environment closely shielded against outside influences, with the nutritive supply dialyzed through placental osmosis.

This mottled condition, in itself, does not seem to increase the susceptibility of the teeth to decay, which is perhaps contrary to what might be expected, because the enamel surface is much more corrugated and rougher than normal enamel. It is recognized, however, by dental practitioners dealing with this sort of enamel, that, caries having occurred, it is difficult at times to find enamel sufficiently dense in which to lay cavity margins.

However, there is an associated phase of the lesion—the "brown stain"—and in this feature we come upon the serious and distressing part of the problem.

It has been pointed out in Dr. Black's paper that the initial or fundamental lesion is the failure of the cementing substance between the enamel rods, and it is the deposit of some sort of brown pigmented substance, termed by Black "brownin," in these otherwise empty spaces that produces the "brown stain." In only approximately 40 per cent of cases of mottled enamel is any of this substance deposited, but this occurs in all grades of intensity, from the faintest spots or tinge up to almost an ebony black. It is a most distressing and remarkable fact, also, that the discoloration is almost invariably located in the most conspicuous place—the labial surfaces of the upper incisors and cuspids. Rarely is it found upon the lower front teeth, and still more rarely upon the lingual surfaces of either uppers or lowers.

In its usual manifestation the stain is located upon the incisal half of the surface, and as a rule the central incisors will have the most, the lateral incisors somewhat less, and the cuspids still less and perhaps none at all. On the central incisors they may be about the middle of the labial surface; somewhat lower down on the lateral incisors, and just on the points of the cuspids. It is extremely erratic in its distribution, although in general following the plan just outlined. I can recall distinctly only one case in which the molars were thus marked, this occurring in one of the Arizona districts; but cases have been seen in which the entire denture, including the third molars, was of a dirty, smoky appearance. The bicuspids are not often discolored in any typical way.

The same rule that applies to the freedom of the temporary teeth from mottled enamel, holds good regarding their immunity from the brown stain. Never, to my knowledge, has this been observed in the temporary teeth.

Because of the lack of any previously published description or records of such a condition, dental practitioners in afflicted districts could only theorize in casting about for possible causes; and what was no doubt the first systematic endeavor to investigate this lesion was undertaken by the Colorado Springs Dental Society soon after its organization in 1902. At that time it was generally supposed that a limited area of territory, measured by a comparatively short radius of miles, was the only area afflicted, and as a first step toward defining its limits, a series of letters was addressed to dentists practicing in various portions of the Rocky Mountain region.

The answers received brought very little information of value, and the matter of further investigation was allowed to rest for the next six years.

It is a curious fact that the earlier thought was directed toward, or confined to that phase of the lesion which was spoken of as the brown stain; and this is easily accounted for by its conspicuousness, being located as it is, almost without exception, upon the labial surfaces of the upper incisors. The white spotted or opaque appearance of the enamel of the entire denture seemed hardly to have been noticed, or at least it was rarely spoke of in discussions.

Early in the investigation it was recognized that it was only those persons who were born and reared in afflicted territory, and those who came during infancy or early childhood, who had the lesion, and inasmuch as our western communities were not old enough to have raised many adult natives, the lesion became associated principally with children.

In 1908 the work of investigation was commenced in an organized way, and the first work that seemed necessary was to locate other communities that were similarly afflicted, with the hope of finding some condition common to such localities that might be studied as the possible cause, and gradually to map out, as time went on, the entire area of distribution. This work has been steadily carried on up to the present time, a detailed account of the examination of the various districts will be given later in the paper.

Specimens

One particularly difficult feature of the research has been to obtain specimens for examination, either histological or chemical, because of the lesion being found only in the permanent teeth; and so in appealing for aid to those having special knowledge along these lines, it has been hard to provide material from which studies could be made.

Theories as to Etiology

Some years ago, almost before any data had been collected, correspondence was opened with Drs. R.R. Andrews, Kirk, and Broomell. Broomell replied that he believed the food supply was the place to look for the cause. In correspondence with Andrews, in 1908, the following opinions were elicited from him:

"If the stain is within the enamel substance it must have formed there while the enamel was forming; that is, some unusual chemical combination may be formed with the lime salts and the blood, and this abnormal substance may cause the stain by being deposited with the lime salts in the ameloblast, where it is elaborated into a pigmented structure. I am free to confess I have never seen just such a condition. If the stain is formed within, the color would be all over the whole surface, I think, and not in a certain location. Any unusual chemical combination must act on all of the forming tissue. There are certain organisms that etch the surface to quite a depth, and then die, and leave their characteristic stain, and if the application of iodin caused a dark dry stain, I should think it was caused by dead organisms."

In later correspondence, after examining a specimen which was sent him, he says:

"It (the stain) was not there when the tooth was forming, but is a stain that *penetrated* [italics mine] after the tooth was erupted. This I feel pretty sure of. I have never seen a stain penetrate the enamel so deeply before."

Kirk called attention to the articles of J. Leon Williams on the histology and development of the enamel, which ran through several issues of the *Cosmos* in 1896, in which it is shown that during the period of calcification the forming enamel lies in close conjunction with the capillary loops, and suggested that a rise in temperature at that period might cause a stasis in the blood vessels, terminating in rupture with infiltration of the blood into the forming enamel, and thus account for the stain.

The attention of Dr. G.V. Black was directed to this lesion early in 1908 by Drs. G.Y. Wilson and Isaac Burton, and his sympathetic interest was at once aroused. A statement of the condition was sent him by the writer soon afterward, and his reply was that there must be some error, as it was difficult for him to believe that there could be a dental lesion that would uniformly afflict any large portion of the natives of any given locality and remain unmentioned in the dental literature. Further correspondence resulted in his coming to study the condition in the field, during the summer of 1909.

It will be realized from the illustrations how extremely disfiguring a pronounced case would be to an afflicted individual, and time and again had the practitioners in these afflicted districts been appealed to for relief, only to be forced to confess their utter helplessness in removing these imperfections.

It was with commendable hesitation that the operation of excising the crowns of these disfigured teeth and replacing by porcelain substitutes was resorted to, but in extreme cases this was insisted upon by parents and patients themselves, and in this way some material was finally obtained and sent to Dr. Black for sectioning for histological examination. These studies are fully described by him in his paper recently published. In further preparation for Dr. Black's study, an examination of the public school children in one city was made during the spring of 1909 by Dr. Isaac Burton and the writer, in order that the exact condition might be known.

The method of conducting the examination was as follows: Cards were printed, of which a sample is here shown [Not shown, Ed.]. These cards were distributed in each schoolroom previous to the examination, to be filled in by the pupils, with the aid of the parents when necessary. They were then returned to the teachers and redistributed to the pupils upon the day of the examination. The examiners went to each child, from desk to desk, and noted the condition of the teeth on the lines "Mottled" and "Stained." The entire school system was gone through—excepting the lowest primary grade, as these children as a rule had no permanent teeth. Twenty-nine hundred and forty-five children were thus examined in one city.

In this way was established for the first time any definite idea of the prevalence of this lesion among the natives of any community. In the city examined, L_____, the percentage of native children afflicted was found to be a 87.5.

Appearance

The accompanying series of illustrations [Figures not shown, Ed.] has been gathered with the view of conveying, as far as possible, an adequate idea of the various phases which this lesion assumes.

Fig. 1 illustrates the case in which the surface is irregularly speckled or mottled. In this case very little of the brown stain is present, but the enamel is very much mottled and somewhat pitted, as shown on the point of the cuspids. The entire denture is of this character. This person is a native of L_____, which community is described later in the paper.

Fig. 2 illustrates a pronounced case of the pitted variety, in which the teeth are of a dirty or smoky color, and the pits are very much darkened. In severe cases these pits often become the seat of caries, hence are a distinct menace, it having occurred in several pits in this illustration. This case is very badly disfigured. The darkening of the pits somewhat overshadows the brown stain, which is present to some extent, and the enamel is very rough. We see the opaque white appearance of the lower incisors, upon some of which are the brown marks, which is quite unusual upon the surfaces. The enamel of the entire denture is of this character. He is a native of L_____.

Fig. 3 shows just the slightest tinge of brown upon the central incisors, the left one having the most. The enamel of all the teeth is white, but the lower incisors are not stained. The pitted appearance of the right first bicuspid is just shown in the photograph. This child is a native of L_____.

In Fig. 4 we see the opaque whiteness of the enamel as before described and upon the prominent mesio-labial surface angles up the central advisers are brown spots. The lateral incisors have just a trace at the mesio-labial corners. Many cases show just such a symmetrical location of the brown spots occurring at the same corresponding places on teeth of the same class. The entire denture is of this opaque white appearance, and the bicuspids and molars are pitted somewhat. This child is a native of L_____.

The location of the brown stain in Fig. 5 is at the extreme labio-incisal edge of the central incisors, just at the incisal edge, and does not extend over onto the lingual surfaces of the teeth. The writer has never seen a case where the stain continued over the incisal edge from the labial surface on to the lingual. The lateral incisors and the lowers are not stained, but the mottled character of the enamel is well shown. The entire denture is mottled, and the bicuspids and molars are pitted. The child is a native of L_____.

Figs. 6, 7, and 8 are typical cases made from ordinary black-and-white negatives. They all show marked symmetry in the distribution of the stain. The children are all natives of L_____.

In Fig. 9 we have a more pronounced stain, which is located somewhat symmetrically upon the central incisors. No other teeth are thus marked, but the opaque whiteness of the enamel is noticeable. The entire denture is of this character. The child is a native of L_____.

Fig. 10 shows a darker discoloration than any previous case, it being almost black upon the central incisors and symmetrically arranged. The labio-incisal edges of the lateral incisors are also stained. This case is one of those rare ones that show the stain upon the lower incisors. The opaque whiteness of the uppers is well shown, and the mottled appearance of the lowers. A pit is noticed at the point of the left cuspid. The boy is a native of L_____.

Fig. 11 is badly pitted and stained, although the lowers show only the mottling. The boy is a native of L_____.

Fig. 12 shows a very pronounced case in which the stain occupies almost the whole labial face of the upper central incisors and a part of the lateral incisors. Here also we see a slight stain on some of the lowers. It is curious that when the stain does occur on the lowers, it is never so pronounced as upon the uppers. This girl is a native of L_____.

Fig. 13 shows a symmetrical location of the stain on the upper central incisors almost in the form of a band across from mesial to distal. The laterals are also stained, but the lower teeth have escaped. These latter show the mottled appearance, with pitting of the cuspids.

Fig. 14 is a side view of the preceding case, and illustrates the pitted appearance of the teeth. The boy is a native of L_____.

During the early part of this investigation the opinion was current that the brown discoloration was present at the time of the eruption of the teeth, but since close observation has been made enough young cases have been watched to lead us to the conclusion that while the teeth erupt in the mottled condition, the brown color does not make its appearance until some considerable period afterward.

It is a fact that in the very large number of partly erupted teeth observed, there is very little distinct recollection of the stain being present upon such teeth.

Fig. 15 shows a case in which I am positive that the child, who has been under constant observation during the past two years or more for orthodontic treatment, has been subject to a very gradual appearance of the brown discoloration—at this time comparatively faint spots being visible upon the upper central incisors, more upon the left than upon the right. This case can also be used as evidence tending to show that advantages of wealth, as reflected in the care and quality of food, are not factors contributing toward immunity if nativity has occurred in an afflicted district.

All through this investigation it has been a common experience to find a confusion in associating a lesion with the various forms assumed in what have been commonly known as "atrophies" of the teeth. The distinction is sharply drawn between the two by Black in his paper, but an opportunity is afforded by Fig. 16 to illustrate the two lesions in combination in the same individual.

In some thousands of individuals examined, many of whom presented "atrophy" alone, and a multitude, of course, mottled enamel alone, this illustration and the one to follow (Figs. 16 and 17) are two out of a total of four cases that I can recall in which the two lesions are associated.

A peculiarity about these two is that they are twins, a boy and a girl, and I can get no history beyond the fact that they both were exceedingly delicate children and reared with difficultly. A moment's study of these illustrations will be of interest. It will be noted that the "atrophy" marks upon the upper central incisors are pronounced and typical, and that the brown stain is absent, as usual, upon these latter teeth—which seems to signify that these two lesions have an etiology entirely apart and distinct. The mottling of the enamel is also more apparent upon the upper incisors; in fact, the enamel upon the lowers appears quite normal.

Much the same description can be applied to both cases, but Fig. 17 gives an opportunity to contrast the usual location of the brown stain with the ordinary superficial discolorations such as are frequently found near the gingival margins of the incisors. We note again the similarity of the "atrophy" marks on uppers and lowers, but with the absence of the brown stain upon the lowers. The mottled appearance is also pronounced upon the uppers and the lowers as well. I consider these two illustrations (Figs. 16 and 17) as among the most interesting in my collection.

Fig. 18 serves admirably to illustrate the symmetrical distribution of the stain upon the upper central and lateral incisors. The absence of stain upon the lowers is to be noticed. The case is typical in many ways.

Fig. 19 is extremely interesting, inasmuch as the subject is a colored person and the case very typical.

I will call attention to the general mottled condition of the upper and lower teeth, the pitted cusp of the lower first bicuspid on the right side (which condition is present upon other teeth, but not shown in the illustration), and chiefly to the irregular distribution of the stain upon the upper central incisors, and the symmetrical staining of the upper lateral incisors. The lowers are not stained.

This case effectually disposes of the question of nationality in its bearing upon this lesion, and emphasizes that its acquisition disregards nationality, social status, and condition of physical health—in fact, all other circumstances except the one essential, namely, residence in an endemic district during the enamel formation

SOURCE

McKay FS, Black GV. 1916. An investigation of mottled teeth: An endemic developmental imperfection of the enamel of the teeth, heretofore unknown in the literature of dentistry. *Dental Cosmos* 58:477–84.

The Conclusion of a Ten-Year Study of Water Fluoridation
(1956, Abridged)

David B. Ast, D.D.S., M.P.H., F.A.P.H.A. and Edward R. Schlesinger, M.D., M.P.H., F.A.P.H.A.*

Here in capsule form is a resumé of the Newburgh-Kingston Caries-Fluorine Study after a decade, with some additional information on the safety of water fluoridation.

In areas where the potable water supplies contain fluoride ion at optimum concentration at the source, the dental caries experience of children who ingest these water fluorides during the years of tooth development is about 60 per cent less than among children in areas with fluoride-deficient water supplies.[1] Adults who have used such water supplies continuously enjoy the dental benefits obtained during childhood.[2]

Controlled water fluoridation for the prevention of dental caries, i.e., the addition of fluoride compounds in optimum concentration to fluoride-deficient supplies, has been studied since 1945 in three different areas. These studies have demonstrated that dental caries can be effectively reduced through controlled water fluoridation to the same extent as observed in areas where water contains the fluoride at the source. A recent review[3] presented the DMF (decayed, missing, or filled teeth) rates for six- to 10-year-old children after nine years of fluoride experience in Grand Rapids, Mich., Newburgh, N.Y., and Brantford, Ontario, and compared these data with those in Aurora, Ill., which uses a water supply with naturally occurring fluoride at 1.2 ppm F. At ages six to nine the rates in all four communities were found to be quite comparable and at age 10 the rates for the three communities fluoridating their water supplies approached the expectancy level noted in Aurora.

One of the most comprehensive of the studies, the Newburgh-Kingston Caries-Fluorine Study has recently issued its final report based on 10 years of fluoridation experience. The report, consisting of three definitive papers dealing with the history of the study and its pediatric and dental aspects, and the fourth paper dealing with fluoride metabolism, was presented before the New York Institute of Clinical Oral Pathology on De-

---

* Dr. Ast is director, Bureau of Dental Health, and Dr. Schlesinger is associate director, Division of Medical Services, New York State Department of Health, Albany, N.Y.

cember 12, 1955. These papers appear in the March, 1956, issue of the *Journal of the American Dental Association*.[4-7]

Prior to the initiation of controlled water fluoridation programs in 1945 extensive epidemiological investigations[8a,b] had demonstrated (1) the occurrence of the defect of tooth enamel which discolored and, in extreme cases, caused pitting of the enamel; (2) the discovery that the stain or mottled enamel was caused by the ingestion of water-borne fluorides during the years of enamel calcification; (3) the direct relationship of the degree of mottling to the fluoride content of the water; (4) an inverse relationship of dental caries to fluorosed or mottled teeth; and (5) that where the water supply contained approximately 1.0 ppm F, the residents enjoyed considerable protection against dental caries without the hazard of disfiguring mottled enamel.

Cox and his coworkers[9] in 1939 suggested that the addition of fluorides to food and water to bring the fluoride content up to the optimal level could prevent dental caries if ingested during the years of tooth development. Ast[10] in 1942 outlined a plan to test the caries-fluorine hypothesis. He suggested a study of two comparable communities with fluoride-deficient water supplies, one of which should have its water supply supplemented with sodium fluoride to bring its fluoride content up to 1.0 ppm and the second to serve as a control.

This plan was considered by the New York State Department of Health. In 1944, a Technical Advisory Committee on the Fluoridation of Water Supplies was appointed to study the proposal. The committee was also asked to recommend the types of medical and dental examinations which should be made to determine the efficacy and safety of water fluoridation. After a careful review of the literature and the objectives of the study, the committee recommended that a long-range study be undertaken. The cities of Newburgh and Kingston, each with a population of approximately 30,000, situated about 35 miles apart on the west bank of the Hudson River and using fluoride-deficient water supplies, were asked to participate in a 10-year study. Newburgh agreed to serve as the study area and to have its water supply supplemented with sodium fluoride to bring its fluoride content up to 1.0–1.2 ppm. Kingston agreed to serve as the control and continue to use its water supply with approximately 0.1 ppm F.

In June, 1944, base line pediatric and dental examinations were begun and on May 2, 1945, Newburgh's water supply was fluoridated. This process has been in continuous operation since that date. The base line data showed that the children aged six to 12 in both cities have a similar dental caries experience. The Kingston rate was 20.2 DMF teeth per 100 permanent teeth and the Newburgh rate was 20.6. Periodic progress reports have demonstrated a downward trend in the dental caries experience among the children in Newburgh. In Kingston the caries rates have remained relatively unchanged.

In June, 1955, clinical and intraoral dental roentgenographic examinations were completed after 10 years of fluoride experience. In Newburgh 1,519 children aged six to 14 and 109 aged 16 who had had continuous residence there throughout the period of fluoridation were examined. The Kingston children examined included 2,021 aged six to 14 and 119 aged 16. The clinical examinations were made in both cities by the staff senior dentist and the roentgenograms were taken by the staff senior dentist and dental hygienist. The films were developed and sent to the Dental Bureau office in Albany. There statisticians randomized the film series so that the interpreters did not know whether they were reading Newburgh or Kingston films.

The children aged six through nine years in Newburgh had used fluoridated water throughout their lives. The 10- to 12-year-old children, who were under two years of age in 1945, had used fluoridated water during the partial calcification of the crowns of the first permanent molars and throughout the calcification of the second permanent crowns. The 13- to 14-year-old children were three to four years old in 1945. These children started drinking fluoridated water after the calcification of the crowns of the first molar teeth but prior to the eruption of these teeth, and throughout the period of calcification of the crowns of the second molars. The 16-year-old children were six years of age when fluoridation was started. At that time their first permanent molars were beginning to erupt into the mouth and the crowns of their second molars were almost fully calcified.

The DMF rate for the six- to nine-year-old children in Newburgh was 58 per cent lower than that for the Kingston children. The 10- to 12-year-old children in Newburgh had a DMF rate 53 per cent lower. At ages 13 to 14 the DMF rate was 48 per cent lower, and at age 16 it was 41 per cent lower, than the rates in Kingston (Table 1).

The first permanent molar is frequently referred to as the keystone of the dental arch and warrants special consideration because of its strategic position in the mouth. This tooth, because of its morphology and the early age at which it erupts into the mouth, frequently succumbs to dental caries early in life. It is therefore significant to note that among the six- to nine-year-old children in Newburgh the DMF rate for first permanent molars was 53 per cent lower than that for the Kingston children in the same age group. The DMF rate in Newburgh at ages 10 to 12 was 30 per cent lower, at ages 13 to 14 it was 14 per cent lower, and at age 16 it was 4 per cent lower, than in Kingston (Figure 1) [Not shown, Ed.].

Of even greater significance is the observation that the children in Newburgh at age six to nine had 68 per cent fewer untreated carious first

Table 1 DMF* Teeth per 100 Children Ages 6–16, Based on Clinical and Roentgenographic Examinations, Newburgh [†] and Kingston, N.Y., 1954–55

Age[‡]	Number of children with permanent teeth		Number of DMF teeth		DMF teeth per 100 children with permanent teeth**		
	Newburgh	Kingston	Newburgh	Kingston	Newburgh	Kingston	Per cent difference K–N
6–9[§]	708	913	672	2,134	98.4	233.7	–57.9
10–12	521	640	1,711	4,471	328.1	698.6	–53.0
13–14	263	441	1,579	5,161	610.1	1,170.3	–47.9
16	109	119	1,063	1,962	975.2	1,648.7	–40.9

* DMF includes permanent teeth decayed, missing (lost subsequent to eruption), or filled.

† Sodium fluoride added to Newburgh's water supply beginning May 2, 1945.

‡ Age at last birthday at time of examination.

** Adjusted to age distribution of children examined in Kingston who had permanent teeth in the 1954–1955 examination.

§ Newburgh children of this age group exposed to fluoridated water from time of birth.

molars and 88 per cent fewer first molars lost than did the Kingston children of the same ages. The 10- to 12-year-old children in Newburgh had a rate 45 per cent lower for untreated carious and 78 per cent lower for missing first molars. At ages 13 to 14 the differences were 26 per cent for untreated caries and 42 per cent for missing first molars, and at age 16 the differences were 41 per cent for untreated caries and 32 per cent for missing first molars (Table 2).

Another significant observation was that ingested fluorides afford selective protection to the proximal (adjacent) surfaces of the teeth in comparison with the occlusal (biting) surfaces. This is highly important because the proximal surfaces present difficulties in both caries detection and correction. Frequently caries on the proximal surface of the tooth requires the cutting of much sound tooth structure in order to place an adequate filling in the tooth. At each of the age levels studied the per cents of differentiable carious proximal surfaces among the Kingston children was about three times greater than that noted in the Newburgh children.

At ages six through nine all of the deciduous cuspids and deciduous molars are normally present in the mouth. If any of these teeth are missing it may reasonably be presumed that they were lost because of caries. Among the six- to nine-year-old children in Newburgh 22.5 per cent had all these teeth present and caries free, as compared with 4.7 per cent of the Kingston children (Table 3).

Dean's[11] epidemiological studies of endemic dental fluorosis demonstrated that there was no disfiguring dental fluorosis at the level of about 1.0 ppm F. Unfortunately, the term mottled enamel or dental fluorosis is applied to all degrees of this condition. In its more severe forms it does produce discoloring stains and possibly pitting of the enamel. However, in the milder forms of fluorosis the enamel of the tooth has a high luster which enhances the beauty of the tooth rather than disfigures it. The detection of the early signs of dental fluorosis requires an examiner who has had extensive experience in areas of endemic fluorosis. The average dental practitioner would in all probability not detect the earliest signs of mottling.

In order to determine whether the children of Newburgh showed any signs of dental fluorosis a specially trained officer of the Public Health Service with long experience in the detection of the mildest of such lesions was requested to make the examinations. He examined 621 children aged seven to 14 in Newburgh, of whom 438 had resided there continuously since the start of fluoridation. In Kingston 612 children of the same ages were examined. In addition to dental fluorosis, examinations were made for enamel opacities due to causes other than ingested fluorides. These other enamel opacities are generally developmental hypoplasias. They usually appear as circular white or colored patches and most of them are obvious even to the untrained eye.

Table 2 Status of Erupted First Permanent Molars in Children Ages 6–16, Based on Clinical and Roentgenographic Examinations, Newburgh* and Kingston, N.Y., 1954–55

Age‡	Caries-free		DMF**		Filled		Untreated caries		Missing	
	Newburgh	Kingston	Newburgh	Kingston	Newburgh	Kingston	Newburgh	Kingston	Newburgh	Kingston
6–9§	74.9	46.7	25.1	53.3	14.2	17.8	10.6	33.2	0.3	2.4
10–12	36.8	10.0	63.2	90.0	40.2	41.3	20.5	37.1	2.5	11.6
13–14	19.3	5.9	80.7	94.1	43.9	40.5	27.0	36.7	9.8	16.9
16	8.5	4.8	91.5	95.2	55.0	36.6	20.9	35.5	15.6	23.1

Per cent of erupted first permanent molars†

* Sodium fluoride added to Newburgh's water supply beginning May 2, 1945.

† Adjusted to the first permanent molar population in the Kingston 1954–55 examination.

‡ Age at last birthday at time of examination.

** DMF includes permanent teeth decayed, missing (lost subsequent to eruption), or filled.

§ Newburgh children of this age group exposed to fluoridated water from time of birth.

Table 3 Number and Per Cent of Children Age 6–9 with Caries-Free Deciduous Cuspids, First and Second Deciduous Molars, Based on Clinical and Roentgenographic Examinations, Kingston and Newburgh,* N.Y., 1954–55

Age†	Number of children examined		Number of children with all 12 teeth present and caries free		Per cent children with all 12 teeth present and caries-free	
	Kingston	Newburgh	Kingston	Newburgh	Kingston	Newburgh
6	216	184	24	68	11.1	37.0
7	255	208	12	58	4.7	27.9
8	277	213	5	53	1.8	24.9
9	192	129	3	13	1.6	10.1
Total	940	734	44	192	4.7	26.2
Adjusted rate‡					4.7	25.5

* Sodium fluoride added to Newburgh's water supply beginning May 2, 1945.

† Age at last birthday at time of examination. Newburgh children of these ages exposed to fluoridated water from time of birth.

‡ Adjusted to the age distribution of Kingston children in the 1954–55 examination.

Among the 438 children with continuous residence in Newburgh, 46 had questionable fluorosis, 26 had very mild, and six had mild fluorosis. There were no cases of moderate or severe mottling and in no instance was there any disfiguring discoloration. Thirty-six of the Newburgh children examined had nonfluoride opacities. Of the 612 children examined in Kingston, 115 had nonfluoride opacities. The relatively infrequent occurrence of nonfluoride enamel opacities in Newburgh compared with Kingston tends to confirm a previous report[12] that ingested water fluorides at the recommended concentration appear to reduce the occurrence of hypoplastic spots on the teeth.

The same groups of children examined for enamel opacities were also examined for evidence of gingivitis. A positive score was recorded only for flagrant gingivitis, thus making it possible to place greater emphasis on advanced disease and minimize examiner bias. There was slight, but significantly, more gingivitis observed among the Kingston children than among those in Newburgh.

The final report on the pediatric findings of the Newburgh-Kingston study pointed out that all the scientific evidence available at the time the study was first proposed indicated the safety of drinking water containing about 1.0 ppm F at the source. There was no reason at that time to believe that fluorides, when added to the drinking water as part of the water treatment process, would act in any way differently from fluorides already present. Nevertheless, it was considered desirable to test this remote possibility under the carefully controlled conditions established for the long-term Newburgh-Kingston study.

Closely similar groups of children were studied in Newburgh and Kingston. In the final year of the study 500 of the children enrolled in Newburgh and 405 in Kingston were examined in the study clinic. The points of concentration in the examination were those related to possible systemic effects of fluoride ingestion as manifested by changes in growth and development or in abnormalities on the physical, laboratory, and roentgenographic examinations. Each child was given a general medical examination by a qualified pediatrician. Height and weight were measured. Roentgenograms were taken of the right hand, both knees, and the lumbar spine. Bone density and bone age (maturation of the skeleton) were estimated by independent observers who were not aware of the city of origin of the individual roentgenograms. Laboratory examinations, including hemoglobin level, total leucocyte [sic] count, and routine urinalysis were also made. No differences of medical significance could be found between the groups of children in the two cities. This indicated the absence of any findings suggestive of systemic effects from the drinking of fluoridated water during the period of most rapid growth. In addition, special detailed studies on the eyes and ears were performed in a smaller group of children; these included determination of visual acuity, visual fields, and hearing levels. The results of these special examinations were well within the range of expected prevalence of the conditions studied.

Reference was made to another recently published paper [13] which presented further evidence for the absence of systemic effects from fluoridated water. The purpose of this study was to determine whether any irritative effects on the kidneys follow prolonged use of fluoridated water. The quantitative excretion of albumin, red blood cells, and casts in 12-hour urine specimens in 12-year-old boys, using a modified Addis technic [sic], was determined in the two cities. The differences in results between the groups in the two cities tended to favor the Newburgh children, but no medical significance could be attributed to any of the differences.

The review of current knowledge of the metabolism of fluorides, particularly in the human body, applied this information in estimating the factors of safety and water fluoridation. Knowledge of blood fluoride levels, of the rate and mechanism of urinary excretion of fluoride, and the magnitude and mechanism of bone deposition increases our understanding of some important biological effects of toxic doses of fluorides, such as acute fluoride poisoning, crippling fluorosis, osteosclerosis, and mottled enamel.

The blood fluoride level in experimental animals given lethal doses of fluoride rises to a peak in a half hour to an hour, falls rapidly within two to three hours, and returns to its normal level within 24 hours. The blood does not tend to accumulate fluoride, although the blood fluoride level in persons drinking fluoridated water is somewhat higher than in persons drinking fluoride-deficient water.

When human beings ingest small amounts of fluoride a significant fraction is probably excreted in the urine. It is probable that when human beings ingest small amounts of fluoride equivalent to that of fluoridated water over a period of years, the daily urinary excretion is greater than half of the amount absorbed each day. The extraordinarily rapid and efficient urinary excretion of fluoride is attributable to a somewhat lower resorption of fluoride in the kidney tubules than is characteristic of chloride.

The other mechanism for removal of fluoride from the blood is by deposition in the bones, the amount of fluoride present in the hard tissues probably being directly dependent on the amount of fluoride taken into the body day after day. The mechanism of fluoride deposition is simple, the fluoride ion replacing the hydroxyl groups of the surface of the bone crystals. There is no indication that any notable biological disadvantage results from this. Fluoride deposition in bone is a reversible process.

With regard to acute fluoride poisoning there is at least a 2,500-fold factor of safety and water fluoridation. The mechanics of water fluoridation are such that it is impossible to produce acute fluoride poisoning either by accident or intent.

Crippling fluorosis, characterized by stiffening in the back due to calcification of the broad ligaments of the back, occurs with the daily intake of 20 to 80 milligrams of fluoride or more for 10 to 20 years. Since five gallons of fluoridated water at 1 ppm F contain 20 milligrams, it is obvious that crippling fluorosis can never be produced by drinking fluoridated water. The earliest evidence of osteosclerosis, a hypercalcification detectable by roentgen examination, does not occur within intake of fluoride below eight to 10 times the level of fluoridated water.

The evidence with respect to heart disease, kidney disease, cancer, and possible influence of fluoride on the thyroid is also reviewed. Ample statistics are available to indicate no influence of fluoride intake on any of these at the levels found in any water supplies in the United States. Studies on experimental animals with the use of radioactive fluoride show that the thyroid gland does not concentrate fluoride as it does iodide. The presence of renal impairment in experimental animals and human beings with long-standing kidney disease appears not to affect excretion of fluoride by the kidneys.

A comprehensive analysis of the Newburgh-Kingston Caries-Fluorine Study after 10 years of experience, added to the wealth of evidence previously reported, demonstrates conclusively two important facts—fluoridation is effective in reducing dental caries and it is a safe public health practice.

SOURCE

Ast DB and Schlesinger ER 1956. The conclusion of a ten-year study of water fluoridation. *Am J Pub Health* 46:265–71. Copyright 1956 by *American Journal of Public Health*. Reprinted with permission of American Public Health Association.

Diet and Oral Health
(2000, Abridged)

K.G. König
Nijmegen, The Netherlands

This review paper looks at the effects of diet on oral health and is concerned mainly with the effects of localised attacks on the dental hard tissues. In analysing the epidemiological evidence, the paper draws distinctions between the rates of disease entities in developed and developing countries. The author concludes that oral health risks do not necessitate dietary recommendations in addition to, or other than, those required for maintenance of general health. The paper indicates an increasing need for evidence-based, individual tailor-made counselling [sic] and for specific programmes directed towards defined, high-risk groups or populations whose oral health problems have been carefully studied and identified.

General remark. The author has cited several passages from an earlier publication by König K G and Navia J M: Nutritional role of sugars in oral health. *Am J Clin Nutr* 1995 62(suppl): 275S–283S. In this article also *Figures 2–4* have been published, however, copyright for these is held by S. Karger Publishers, Basel, publisher of the *Journal of Caries Research*.

Diet and Nutrition in Relation to Oral Health and Disease

A review of nutritional influences on oral health requires consideration of three groups of oral tissues with different structure, morphology metabolism and pathologic response:

- the hard tissues of the teeth (with implications for dental health)
- the supporting structures of teeth (with implications for periodontal health)
- the oral mucosa (with implications for mucosal health).

Dental and periodontal health will be dealt with in more detail than mucosal health because of the high prevalence of pathology of hard tissues and periodontal structures.

Nutritional Systemic vs. Dietary Local Effects

In the relation of nutritional factors to oral health, there is a peculiarity to be considered regarding the dental hard tissues. Once formed, tooth enamel is no longer subject to systemic nutritional influences, however, it is subject to dynamic exchange of ions as well as organic molecules and particles with its oral environment. The role of nutrition in general on the growth, development and maintenance of oral tissues has been discussed in a wide context[1] and two major groups of effects are clear: one systemic/nutritional and the other local and dietary.

The main result of nutrition is the systemic effect of the absorbed nutrients on growth, development and maintenance of tissues and organs and their specific functions. Local dietary side effects are of great practical importance in the oral cavity. Dental enamel after eruption is particularly subject to local side effects from whatever may enter the mouth. Dietary components not only provide essential nutrients for tissues of the host, but also for bacteria in the oral cavity which use them as substrates if readily available. Besides 'indirect side effects' of e.g. bacterially metabolised sugars and of amino acids, there are 'direct side effects' of nutrients exerted by their ion content, (erosive) acidity and physical properties.

Pre-eruptive vs. Post-erected Influences

It is important in a discussion of oral health and its relation to nutritional factors that we differentiate between formative nutritional and post-eruptive local influences. The effect of nutrition on formation is in general constructive. In contrast, the influence of diet and its local side effects are more likely to be damaging than stabilising: the mouth is the port of entry for all food and drink, regularly accepting either very cold, hot, aggressive and/or very hard components eliciting enormous mechanical forces. Since the tissues lining the oral cavity are part of the surface of our body, they are colonised by numerous species of micro-organisms interacting with the food passing, and/or with the underlying structures.

If integrity is maintained, it will be the result of the continuous interaction of protective and destructive influences. The difficulty is that nutritive as well as local dietary protective and destructive factors both act on the same tissues and their respective effects cannot be differentiated readily and assessed separately. The fact that formative influences are effective in an early distinct period of development, and destructive influences usually do not start before exposure and functioning, does not solve the difficulty. A well-known example of this is the question of the mechanism of effective water-borne fluoride. When fluoride in drinking water in the US was first discovered to be the cause of mottling of teeth, and later was identified to be the protective factor against caries, the conclusion was rapidly drawn: Fluoride does have an effect on teeth during formation that shows as mottling after eruption; therefore, the other effect we see later on, that is fewer and smaller carious lesions, will likewise be due to the pre-eruptive deposition of fluoride. It took decades before the paramount importance of life-long topical fluoride availability was clearly recognised and dental science agreed that pre-eruptive administration of fluoride was less important. In 1990 the epidemiologic results of the US survey completed in 1987 were published[2]. The authors describe the findings in large representative samples of 5- to 17-year-old individuals residing life-long in areas with or without fluoridated drinking water. The difference in caries experience between people from non-fluoridated areas compared with those from fluoridated areas (50–60 per cent less with optimum concentration of fluoride in all pioneering fluoridation studies between 1945 and 1970) had fallen off to an average of 18 per cent; in certain regions the difference was much lower, and in region III, around and south of the Great Lakes, it was even slightly reversed: mean DMFS under life-long exposure to fluoridated water 2.86, vs. no exposure to fluoridated water with DMFS 2.69. The authors comment that 'because of the multifactorial etiology of caries, it is doubtful that an unequivocal explanation for this trend can be found, though there can be little argument that the ubiquity of fluoride in the environment has been a dominant factor.' The most plausible explanation, by our present knowledge, is the increasing popularity of personal oral hygiene and the use of fluoride toothpaste. The same conclusion was drawn from observations after the fluoridation of drinking water had been stopped in Tiel (The Netherlands[3]) and Kuopio (Finland[4]). These studies as well as the US samples illustrate the fact that systemic fluoride may not be necessary, at least for the permanent dentition, if local fluoride (mainly in toothpaste) is available from eruption of teeth onwards.

Special Position of Enamel among the Oral Structures

With respect to the tissues of bone, periodontium, mucosa, salivary glands, dentine and pulp, development and life-long integrity as well as functioning are associated with systemic molecular and cellular reactions to variables associated with nutrition and medication, some of them interacting with oral factors and bacterial antigens. Tooth enamel, in contrast, is subject to systemic influences on its development before eruption only; after eruption it interacts exclusively with local (topical) environmental factors.

Because of the importance of local effects in controlling demineralisation of teeth and inflammation of periodontal structures, which are the major risks to oral health, this review deals with side effects of diet rather than with metabolic nutritional aspects. In any event, nutritional advice during development is the field of the medical practitioner, and not of the dentist. For the maintenance of periodontal and mucosal health, systemic nutritional factors are more relevant than for maintenance of tooth structures, but even in this case, absence of local bacterial and cytotoxic irritants requires much more attention than to systemic nutritional factors.

Dental Health and Caries Risk Factors

Caries is a bacterial plaque-dependent disease that is characterised by an intermittent demineralisation of enamel, dentine and/or cementum. Oral micro-organisms, when organised in voluminous masses as in dental plaque on tooth surfaces, hydrolyze starches and metabolise sugars to form weak acids (mainly lactic acid) which slowly and intermittently demineralise the hard tissue underneath.

This utilisation of some food components such as sugars by bacteria is a local side effect in the mouth during food passage, in contrast to the systemic effect of carbohydrates as a source of energy for the host. Carious demineralisation is the result of a side effect, namely acid formation from sugars in the bacterial plaque on the teeth. The sugars and other carbohydrates *per se* exert no direct damaging effect on the teeth. During sleep and when no food is available, the acidogenic plaque bacteria can (slowly) metabolise and survive on a minimum supply of substrate derived from carbohydrate side chains of salivary mucins. At these low concentrations, no cariogenic amounts of acid are formed. However, oral acidogenic bacteria can handle substrate concentrations of a very large range from very low to very high, and to high concentrations of sugars they react with acid formation immediately.

For quite sometime in the early phases of acid attack on our dental tissues, the demineralisation is a diffusion-controlled process resulting in an increase in pore volume only, without disintegration of the mineralised tissues; supply and access of saliva are important for remineralisation between acid attacks because saliva contains buffering systems, and transports mineral and fluoride ions to the tooth-environment interface.

Both processes, that is, the attacks resulting in demineralisation and remineralisation resulting in repair, are modified by a number of variables. The most important factor on the side of attack is presence of plaque, its thickness and bacterial composition; there is a good reason for not listing carbohydrates such as sugars in the first place: if there is no mature plaque present, that is there are no more than thin layers of bacteria, no appreciable amount of acid is formed. This had been shown by Stephan and Miller[5] who measured acid formation on the teeth after rinsing with sugar solutions. They found plaque pH drops when thick plaque was present, whereas after removal of the plaque no dangerous acidity could be detected on a clean surface (*Figure 1*) [Not shown, Ed.]. The same phenomenon was reported from a number of laboratories were pH telemetry is used to measure the acidogenic potential of carbohydrate-containing foodstuffs: if the experimenter does not let plaque grow for at least two days, no acid formation can be observed[6].

Dietary Sugars and Caries Experience, and the Role of Eating Habits in the Development of Dental Caries

An association between intake of sugars and dental caries was first studied experimentally in the early 1950s on inmates of the Vipeholm asylum in Sweden[7]. Analysis of later (mostly not controlled, but epidemiological) studies conducted in the 1960s and 1970s confirmed this relationship[8]. The Vipeholm Study was the first to reveal the distinction between the effects of amount of sugars eaten, versus the frequency of sugar intake. The experiment showed that restriction of sugar intake to four main meals daily did not significantly increase the (low) baseline caries activity, even if large amounts of sugar (300g/day) were given. On the other hand, when 8 or 24 between-meal sugar-containing snacks were given daily, caries incidence rose dramatically. The reason is that plaque bacteria after exposure to sugar produced acid only for about 0.5h (*Figure 1*) [Not shown, Ed.]. Consequently, the total demineralisation time is 2h per day if 4 meals are taken, but 12h if 24 sugar exposures occur. With increasing frequency therefore the caries risk increases.

However, it is necessary to analyse and consider the conditions under which the Vipeholm Study[7] was conducted: the 436 Vipeholm inmates exposed to the various experimental dietary regimes consisted of mentally retarded, severely handicapped subjects who were unable to perform any oral hygiene technique. There were no dental hygienists available at that time to do regular professional cleaning, and cariostatic fluoride was not available; a similar condition prevailed in normal populations even in developed countries up until the seventies, because regular oral hygiene was only performed by a minority, and toothbrushing was particularly unpopular among children at school age, on which nearly all the caries epidemiology was done.

This has changed conspicuously during the last 20 years, starting and being observed first in hygiene-conscious populations such as in the US, Scandinavia, Switzerland and The Netherlands where toothbrushing among children became a habit, keeping plaque accumulation low.

Modern Caries Epidemiology vs. Findings in the Pre-hygiene Era

It has been mentioned in the theoretical part of this paper and shown in *Figure 1* [Not shown, Ed.] that sugars do not give rise to production of dangerous amounts of acid in the oral cavity when plaque is absent or only present in thin layers. Therefore, it is feasible to separate modern epidemiological research from early findings accumulated in the pre-hygiene era. This is the more important because during the same time span in which oral hygiene practice developed, the sale of toothpastes containing fluoride in caries-inhibiting concentrations rose from zero up to more than 90 per cent in the countries mentioned above.

Findings Based on Single Cross-sectional Sampling and Short Observations

Walker and Cleaton-Jones[9] without ignoring the caries risk associated with intake of sugars, have identified a number of situations in caries epidemiology reported in the literature where sugar intake alone does not explain the caries status of the consumers. A study of diet, oral hygiene and dental caries in 457 Canadian children has not revealed meaningful correlations between independent and dependent variables[10].

There have been many attempts to study in humans the specific relationship between sugar intake, dietary and nutritional parameters and dental caries, but three studies conducted using English[11], American[12], and Canadian[13] children deserve special consideration. The English study involved 405 children who had an initial age of 11.6 years and were followed for two years. Evaluation of the data indicated that the average consumption was 118g of sugar per day (43kg/year) which also accounted for 21 per cent of the total energy intake. Sugar intake explained only 4 per cent of the variance in caries increment and 94 per cent of the variance remained unexplained by the factors under consideration in the study. The authors believe that a large proportion of the variance was due to methodological inaccuracies, such as those related to dietary assessment, and a large intra-subject variability that could mask the true relationship. While this may be the case, other aetiological factors such as saliva, plaque, fluoride/oral hygiene practices should not be dismissed lightly. In that study, frequency of sugar consumption, although significant, had a much lower correlation value (+0.099) with caries than the weight of sugary foods consumed (+0.143).

The study done in the US was a longer, three-year investigation of 499 children aged 11–15 years in a nonfluoridated community in the state of Michigan. These American children consumed on the average 142g of sugar per day (51kg/year) and sugars accounted for 26.5 per cent of their total daily energy intake. In this study, pit and fissure caries were not found to be correlated with any aspect of sugar consumption, but increments in approximal caries were observed to be related to dietary sugar intake parameters. While children who consumed a high proportion of their energy intake of sugar had the higher increments of approximal caries, there was no relationship between the caries scores and the average frequency of eating during the day or the average number of sugary snacks consumed between meals. Results of the study did not differ much from those obtained in the study done in England, and suggested that while sugar continues to be a clear aetiologic component of the carious process and a high frequency of sugar consumption increases the risk of the disease, the dietary behaviour of the populations in these two sites was not sufficiently caries-promoting to make a major difference in their caries experience.

A third study was done in Canada, using 232, 11-year-old students to evaluate the association between dietary patterns and dental caries. Nutritional data were collected using a quality index based on the eating frequency recommended in food guides and divided into eight levels (with 1 being the worst nutrition and 8 being the rank given to the group that best complied with nutritional recommendations). They also considered the frequency of sugary food consumption in real time in between meals. Results of the study indicated that the nutritional status of these children was compromised; almost 50 per cent of the children had a nutritional quality level of 3 and only 8.2 per cent of the subjects had a quality level of 5, which is the minimal recommendation of Canada's Food Guide for the use of the four essential food groups. While there was a trend towards a decreased caries increment with improved nutritional quality of the diet, analysis of variance did not show statistical significance for this trend. Furthermore, no significant association was observed between frequency of consumption of sugary foods and increments in caries.

It is obvious that while dietary sugars are a determinant of caries risk, they are not the only factor in the aetiology of the disease. This understanding is highlighted in studies done with special populations such as mentally retarded children[14] where again, the frequent consumption of candy did not seem to be a significant determinant of caries, but rather, poor oral hygiene status appeared to be a more important caries risk factor. Similar conclusions concerning the importance of hygiene *vs.* diet were reached in a study[15] evaluating oral health of Latin-American preschool children living in Malmö: children with a sound gingiva due to good oral hygiene had only 1.1 tooth surfaces either carious or restored with fillings, while those with gingival inflammation due to poor oral hygiene had 6.2 surfaces carious or still. Another study[16] examining the oral health status of Greek immigrant (GI) children in comparison with Swedish (S) and rural Greek (G) children, illustrated the complexity inherent in the evaluation of determinants of oral health. The carbohydrate content of the diet consumed by these three groups was about the same, however, children in the G group had only 15 per cent caries free primary teeth, as well as a higher incidence of decayed and filled tooth surfaces in primary and permanent teeth than the other two groups. There was also a similar distribution of mutans streptococci and lactobacilli in the three groups, and this indicates a potential risk for any of the children, if other caries conducive conditions are increased. The availability of health services for children living in Sweden (S and GI) was made evident by the increased use of toothbrushes and improved oral hygiene of these groups compared to children in the G group and this could have been an important determinant of their oral health status.

Gibson and Williams[17] have published the results of a careful re-evaluation and advanced statistical analysis of the data collected in a representative sample of 1,450 pre-school children. They have been studied in the course of the British National Diet and Nutrition Survey (NDNS) conducted in 1992/93. The original report published in 1995 included the statement that 'overall, the benefits of frequent brushing of teeth did not appear to outweigh the damaging effect of frequent sugar consumption'[18]. The results of the recent multivariate analysis[17] applying three series of stepwise logistic regression models do not support this conclusion. Besides revealing age and social class as strong predictors of caries experience, the influence of toothbrushing frequency was also highly significant (probability of error $P < 0.001$). Based on the lacking or weak association of caries with eating sugar and sugary foods, the authors conclude with the 'hypothesis that regular brushing (twice a day) with a fluoride toothpaste may have greater impact on caries and young children than restricting sugary foods.'

In the Netherlands the caries experience of Turkish and Moroccan children is significantly higher than that of native ones of the same age. A comparative study of the dietary habits of 8-year-old immigrant and native children[19] revealed that an inferior nutrition can be ruled out as the cause of higher caries rates in Turkish and Moroccan children; it was found that the latter consumed much less potentially cariogenic sugary food, snacks and drinks, as well as more vegetables than the native children with significantly lower caries experience. In *Table 1* the dietary findings are presented together with percentages of caries free children from another sample, 6-year-old low-SES native (NL), Turkish and Moroccan children examined in The Hague and one year later.

Secular Trends Found by Sampling over Long Periods of Time

While most dental epidemiological results are based on a study of single cross-sectional samples or on observation periods not longer than a few years, there are also a number of observations over time, covering secular changes in caries prevalence over some decades. One of the pioneers in discovering secular changes in the prevalence of caries, R. L. Glass, in 1981 published a classic paper on epidemiologic findings between 1958 and 1978 in two non-fluoridated Massachusetts towns[21]. He seems to have been the

Table 1 Percentages of 6-Year Old Children with Intact Dentition (from Truin et al., 1990[20]) and Eating Habits of Samples from the Same Populations (Meulmeester, 1988[19]); Average Consumption (g/day) of Foods and Snacks Possibly Relevant as Determinants of Oral Health/Ill Health

	NL (low SES)	Turkish	Moroccan
% caries-free children	43	20	22
Bread	149	128	142
Vegetables	68	109	110
Cheese	19	24	16
Sweet pastry	25	9	12
Sweet beverages	256	80	121
Sweets	21	13	10
Jam	17	11	11

first to suggest that the decrease of caries experience could be due to increasing use of fluoride-containing toothpastes, and increased awareness of the importance of oral health.

Other series of observations, although published later, have been dug up from old records and were in addition based on a continuation of examinations by epidemiologists working in the same area and according to the same traditions. For instance, reductions in availability and intake of sugar as was seen in Europe during the war, were accompanied by a decrease in caries prevalence in populations involved in such dietary changes, that these effects were not permanent—they disappeared when the imposed drastic dietary changes were reversed. Caries experience of individuals who had to reduce their sugar intake during the war years showed that there was no long lasting beneficial effect when they were exposed once more to a caries-challenging situation during the post-war period[22].

It is obvious that both severe sugar restriction and optimum fluoride availability will decrease caries prevalence. The relative effect of the two inhibitory factors can be judged considering percentages of caries-free children in Basel, Switzerland, subsequently under pre-war, wartime, and post-war sugar supplies (*Figure 2*[23]) [Not shown, Ed.]. Before and during the first year of the war—with an unlimited sugar supply, poor oral hygiene and no fluoride available—the percentage of caries-free, 7-year-old children did not exceed 2–3 per cent.

Wartime restrictions reduced sugar supply from about 40 to 16kg/person/year, with a resulting increase in the number of caries-free children to about 15 per cent. This improvement of oral health tended to disappear when sugar became again freely available after the war. At that time the war-time improvement seemed impressive, but it was dwarfed by the up-coming modern preventive tools. Fluoride tablets and fluoride toothpaste became gradually available, oral hygiene lessons at school were intro-duced, and water fluoridation started in 1962: although sugar consump-tion rose rapidly after the war and has varied around 45kg *per capita* during the last 40 years, by 1989 the number of caries free schoolchildren 7 to 15 years of age had risen to 65 per cent, and the DMFT index of 12-year-olds had decreased to 1.0[23].

The Netherlands is one of the industrialised countries where caries prevalence within the last 25 years has decreased rapidly[20, 24, 25]. An aver-age DMFT of 1 in 12-year-old children was reached in the mid 1990s. The percentage of caries free children is still increasing although sugar con-sumption was still more than 90 per cent of that which it was in 1965 (38.5kg/p.p./per year in 1985 and in 1992[24, 25]; *Figure 3*) [Not shown, Ed.]. Fluoridation of drinking water stopped after a Supreme Court decision in 1973, but as a consequence of the publicity around this event many people became aware of the great importance of individual self-care. The most plausible explanation for the decreasing caries prevalence in the Nether-lands seems to be a combination of factors, the most important being the improved personal hygiene habits. Most children are now clinically plaque-free and are using a fluoride-containing toothpaste; some, especially high-SES children get occasional topical fluoride applications. In addition, more than 50 per cent of the chewing gum sold, contains xylitol and/or sorbitol in place of sucrose (see below).

There are some countries where between 1982 and 1985 sugar con-sumption has increased, but where nevertheless regular epidemiological monitoring of caries data has shown that the caries prevalence continued to decrease: these are Sweden[26], Norway[27], and New Zealand[24]. The situ-ation is illustrated in *Figure 4* [Not shown, Ed.].

A Secular Change in the Association between Sugar Consumption and Caries

When Sreebny in 1984 published his analysis of the sugar-caries relation-ship, he had based it on caries data in deciduous dentitions from 23 coun-tries and on data in permanent dentitions from 47 countries[8]. He found that every 20g of increased sugar consumed per person per year resulted in 0.5 DMFT increase for 5- to 6-year-old children, and an increase of 1 DMFT for 12-year-olds. Since, then, much has changed.

In his analysis of the secular trends published in 1990, Marthaler[28], shortly after Walker and Cleaton-Jones[9], came to the confirmatory conclusion that in many highly developed industrialised countries there was a 'lack of correlation between the decline of caries prevalence and average sugar consumption.' This is a comforting statement, however, there are still high-risk populations who force us to keep alert. These are found in developing countries, or in some populations (mostly ethnic minority groups) even in the highly developed 'low-caries countries.' Appropriate alertness does not mean that we should continue issuing the same general recommendations for everybody as in past decades when the high caries experience of nearly 100 per cent of the people was clearly sugar dependent. A specific analysis of risk factor(s) per race group is necessary, and a specific package of preventive measures should be composed.

Cariogenicity of Diets Rich in Carbohydrates Other than Sucrose

Up to this section caries data have been presented as populations feeding on diets containing sucrose as the preponderant carbohydrate, although these diets eaten in highly developed countries also contain a great variety of sugars other than sucrose and also high-molecular-weight carbohydrates. Because of the special situations in developing countries, it seems appropriate also to consider constellations in which the cariogenic potential of certain foodstuffs can be isolated because they are the ones preponderantly, or even solely used.

Milk

Lactose has repeatedly been reported to stand out among the major dietary sugars as being of markedly lower cariogenicity. One must keep in mind, however, that this conclusion was based on laboratory studies, and many animal tests with the sugar have been run with *ad libitum* feeding. Since rats do not tolerate lactose very well and tend to eat less, and less frequently, on lactose diets than on controlled diets with other sugars, the lower caries activity on lactose diets may in part be an unspecific effect[29]. It does not seem justified to regard lactose as a virtually non-cariogenic food, a conclusion which was drawn from the publication by Storey[30]. Several papers on observations, referred to above, in babies breast-fed over periods of a year or longer, as it is common practice in Central African Countries [sic], have shown that lactose in milk can be highly cariogenic when drunk frequently[30-35]. The reason for the high cariogenicity of milk in this situation is the habit of *ad libitum* feeding. Infants are not only breast-fed upon demand frequently during daytime, but also are allowed to sleep beside their mother with the nipple of a breast in their mouth, suckling even at night as often as they tend to wake up. The caries prevalence in the deciduous dentition of these children is very high. This practice has the same effect as continuous availability of a nursing bottle with sugar-sweetened contents. Fortunately, if the permanent teeth erupt into a much less sugar-swamped oral environment, they usually remain caries-free.

Sugars in Fresh Fruits

There are a number of studies which seem to confirm that the popular saying 'an apple a day keeps the doctor away' may also apply to '. . . keeping the dentist away'[11,36]. However, these findings do not provide direct evidence of low cariogenicity of fruit-borne sugars since individuals who consume relatively high amounts of fresh fruit may differ in a number of other dietary and oral hygiene variables which affect caries activity.

Indeed, findings in several groups of South African farm workers show a high risk associated with frequent fruit eating[37]. The caries experience of 120 farm workers was analysed. The purpose was to determine the effect of a high intake of citrus fruit or of different varieties, in comparison with the diet of the grain-producing (control) group. The mean daily intake of added sugars (excluding that from the specific fruits to be investigated), was the highest for the control group, however, they had the lowest caries experience, DMFT 9.9, significantly different from the citrus group with DMFT 24.8 and the 'mixed variety' fruit group with DMFT 22.7 ($P<0.001$). This suggests that sugars contained in fruits may be even more cariogenic than extrinsic sugars.

Some fruits tend to cause only moderate falls in plaque pH[6,38,39]. Apples, however, besides containing sometimes high concentrations of free acids, by virtue of their sugars content, can also give rise to formation of acid in plaque[6,40-42]. A host of information with a reliable pH-telemetry method has been gathered by Imfeld[6], including direct comparisons of acidity generated by intrinsic sugars from fruits and sucrose. And apple for instance contains 9 to 11 per cent sugars, mostly fructose. There are favourable factors in an apple that are missing in 10 per cent sucrose solution: fresh apples are fibrous and crisp which makes them self-cleansing, a considerable part of the sugars is likely to remain in the bolus up until it is swallowed, and the citric acid in the apple is a good stimulant for neutralising saliva. Nevertheless not only dried dates and raisins with high content of sugars, but also apples and bananas in Imfeld's studies gave rise to dangerously strong acidity. It is interesting to note that the pH turned and remained low not only in plaque, but also in the oral fluid in which the pH was monitored concomitantly. What is surprising is a lack of acceleration of the oral sugar clearance in the case of the apple; the pH in the oral fluid stayed low even longer than in plaque. The conclusion from these studies is that there is no difference in acidogenicity of fruit-borne and dissolved or soluble sugars, although some properties of fruits appear favourable in theory.

The limited studies of caries in rats fed various fruits indicate that apples, bananas, and grapes can give rise to appreciable levels of caries, sometimes as much or more than sucrose itself[43-46]. Moreover, it has been demonstrated that fruit, especially citrus fruits, carry a risk of acid erosion of tooth enamel[47-50]. It would appear that fresh fruits when consumed infrequently in the normal varied diet do not contribute effectively to caries activity, but they possess a cariogenic potential which may become manifest when they are consumed frequently. Regarding dried fruits, plaque pH measurements and animal feeding studies clearly indicate a high cariogenic potential[38,43].

Complex Carbohydrates (Starches)

Most national dietary surveys in highly developed countries result in recommendations to eat more food with complex carbohydrates. The idea behind this is to reduce fat intake; because of the caries risk associated with consumption of sugars, sugars are not recommended as energy-providing substitutes for fats. Whether this is justified need not be discussed further at this stage, but for the sake of fact-finding, it is necessary in this context to examine whether starches may not, in principle, be as hazardous for dental health as sugars.

Starches cannot directly serve as substrates for bacterial fermentation, but hydrolysis to maltose, isomaltose and glucose is no problem in the oral cavity. Both salivary and bacterial hydrolases can accomplish this, and it has been shown that after the chewing of crackers, potato chips and so forth, glucose clearance is prolonged due to the intermediate starch degradation products maltotriose and maltose[51]. Acid formation can start surprisingly quickly after starchy food has got in contact with dental plaque. Pollard et al.[52] have tested the acidogenicity of white bread, cooked spaghetti, cooked long-grain rice and many other starch products with and without added sugar. Paired t-tests of the minimum pH values measured with indwelling electrodes showed that none of the test products was significantly different from 10 per cent sucrose solution. So there is no doubt that starches are acidogenic in the mouth; how cariogenic starch products are, depends on many factors. In cases of impaction of starchy food in retentive fissures and interdental spaces, especially when the starch has been industrially processed, this may give rise to considerable amounts of acid in their cariogenic potential must be considered high. Observations in individuals with hereditary fructose intolerance (HFI) due to an enzyme defect tended to show that complete lack of fructose and sucrose in the human diet resulted in low caries experience[53]. However, these individuals, who tolerate unlimited amounts of starches, are a very limited, special group, and all normal populations eating preponderantly starches eat them in cooked or baked form and besides also eat much food containing sugars as well. Imfeld[6] refers to a large number of animal experiments showing that cooked starch cannot be considered a non-cariogenic dietary component, and Lingström *et al.*[54] have shown with three different pH-measurement systems that acid formation in plaque after chewing soft bread or potato chips is more intense and lasts longer than after intake of sucrose. Therefore it is highly questionable whether a recommendation to use complex carbohydrates in place of sugars would decrease the caries risk in particular since many starch-containing types of food contains secrets and at the sugars as well.

The Role and Functions of Non-fermentable Sweeteners in Relation to Dental Caries

Sugar alcohols or polyols, with the pentitol xylitol and the hexitols sorbitol and mannitol are sweet, but not cariogenic (in the case of xylitol) or much less cariogenic than sugars (in the case of hexitols). Numerous articles on original clinical research, among them the Turku Sugar Studies[55], the' Michigan Xylitol Programme (1986–1995)' [56], the Belize City chewing gum trial[57] and review papers[58,59] have firmly established the caries preventive effect of these sugar substitutes, especially of xylitol. The stimulating effect on salivary glands is unequivocally established, and of xylitol it is well-known that it can be taken up by oral bacteria, but because in the cells it has the form of a toxic xylitol phosphate it cannot be further metabolised. Only a few questions are still open: does xylitol reduce (initial) caries because it stimulates salivary flow, or has it a specific remineralising power of its own? Does xylitol change the plaque flora[60]? There is no doubt that under certain growth conditions xylitol-resistant mutants of mutans streptococci can emerge, but not all strains of these species show this phenomenon[61]. If such a mutation occurs, the cell is unable to synthesise a cellwall transferase system necessary to transport the xylitol molecules inside. At the same time these resistant mutants of mutans streptococci seem to be less virulent which may result in a less cariogenic plaque flora. The uncertainty as to whether xylitol changes the plaque composition favourably may be due to the inconsistency of strains to develop resistant mutants. As a matter of fact, these open questions do not limit the general use of polyols, especially xylitol, because safety and the overall caries preventive effect are firmly established. Recently, two reports have been published indicating that xylitol can, besides the inhibiting effect on dental caries, also prevent acute otitis media in children[62,63].

That all polyols when eaten in amounts of 20–40g or more do have the side effect of causing osmotic diarrhoea, however, in small confectionery such as chewing gum with amounts of 2g or less per piece, very few children have problems. On the positive side the reduction of the number of sucrose contacts when polyol gum is used in place of sucrose gum can substantially reduce the total time of acid attack on teeth, and thereby reduce the caries risk[64].

A special group which will profit from the beneficial effect of a polyol, especially xylitol chewing gum, are elderly people. Besides the saliva stimulation which is necessary in many cases of xerostomia, dentate individuals with recession and high risk of root caries will profit[65].

Modern 'non-caloric' artificial sweeteners such as aspartame or cyclamate are not carbohydrates and therefore do not give rise to cariogenic acid formation in plaque, however, they can only correct the low sweetness of some polyols but not provide the necessary bulk which sucrose or polyols have to deliver in sweets.

Dietary Components Increasing the Risk of Erosive Loss of Hard Tissues

Caries lesions are caused slowly by diffusion of protons of weak bacterial acids into enamel, thus proteinising the phosphate in apatite which then releases calcium; the pore volume in this pre-carious hard tissue increases until finally it is weakened to a degree that the layer above the carious subsurface porosity collapses, and a carious cavity is formed.

In contrast to the diffusion-controlled caries development, erosion is due to strong acids such as citric acid in fruit and acid beverages. Contact of a strong acid with the tooth causes an immediate stormy dissolution of the surface layer, and mechanical friction afterwards (toothbrushing after a breakfast with grapefruit or apple) whisks away whatever mineral substance at the interface, only loosened by the acid, that otherwise might have a slight chance to remineralise.

Regular removal of plaque is essential for prevention of caries and periodontal disease, but it increases the susceptibility of tooth surfaces to erosion. Therefore it is a very important task of dental professionals to instruct patients regarding the correct time for daily oral hygiene practice, and to instruct the most gentle and efficient manner of cleansing. Not only acid in fruit and drinks is erosive, but all individuals addicted to eating raw vegetables and other unprocessed food run a very high risk of the erosion[66]. In contrast to former assumptions, yoghurt and fresh cheese are not erosive due to the high mineral content and absence of aggressive chelating citric acid[67]. Larsen and Nyvad[68] found that otherwise erosive orange juice, pH 4.0, when supplemented with 40 mmol/1 calcium and 30 mmol/1 phosphate was not erosive anymore because the supplements saturated the juice with respect to apatite. Such a drink has already been launched commercially as a 'functional food' intended to counteract osteoporosis—another hint that medical indications are stronger arguments than dental ones.

A good source of original information and references to erosion literature are the proceedings of the workshop on 'Etiology, Mechanisms and Implications of Dental Erosion' published in 1996[69].

In an affluent society with the possibility to choose from a host of exotic and indigenous varieties of fruit it seems unlikely that the modern trend to eat them will be ignored. Considering the positive health effects of fruit and vegetables it would moreover not be feasible to advise against consuming them. The best compromise seems to advise people to avoid eating the same fruit every day; not always grapefruit for breakfast, but also banana or a pear for a change—variation in the choice of diet is the best general health advice possible not only in order to avoid erosion of teeth, but also to avoid the sequelae of environmental pollution, and to make sure one gets all essential nutrients, vitamins and minerals.

Conclusions from Observations on Dental Health Determinants

Although a relationship between sugars and dental caries is accepted by all clinicians and researchers working in the dental field, the degree of emphasis on the importance of this factor in prevention and control of the disease varies. The information we have available today, based on studies into the situation in the 1990s, should stimulate a sober scientific and rational approach to the role of fermentable carbohydrates in dental caries. If one intended to advise in principle against consumption of all cariogenic food, it would be irrational to advise only against consumption of sucrose. The same applies to sugar substitution in food and snacks; regarding this issue Rugg-Gunn[64] wrote a comment on a recent review article on the beneficial effects of sugar substitutes[58]. It starts with this sentence, 'Substitution of non-sugar sweeteners for non-milk extrinsic sugars in the diet is an important means of preventing caries.' While the statement concerning the usefulness of sugar substitutes is correct, the sentence nevertheless implicitly also contains two misleading statements.

Firstly, to suggest replacing extrinsic sugars only would imply that intrinsic sugars such as fruits are non-cariogenic; that is not true—all sugars are potentially cariogenic. Secondly, to replace non-milk extrinsic sugars only would imply that the lactose in milk is non-cariogenic; this also is not the case.

The choice of sugar-free, especially xylitol-containing chewing gum is a welcome preventive possibility. If the reports on the prevention of acute otitis media by xylitol chewing gum are further confirmed, doctors in well-baby clinics, paediatricians and oto-rhino-laryngologists are the professionals to recommend it as a preventive measure with positive general health effects in childhood. Moreover, any dentist should recommend it individually, especially to mothers with children and elderly people with salivary deficiencies. However, if issued as a message as to what a healthy diet should consist of, it is doubtful whether this would be understood as dietary counseling in the traditional sense of the word. It would be more efficient to stimulate the manufacturers of chewing gum to promote products containing xylitol preferentially.

As a general health message from the medical side, the recommendation of the varied diet seems appropriate from the medical as well as the dental point of view, supplemented by the dental recommendations and instructions regarding oral hygiene and fluoride use. Detailed instruction of patients in gentle, systematic cleansing with a soft brush and a minimum of pressure is of paramount importance since there is a definite trend to consume more fruit and more varieties, many of them with erosive potential.

The most important observation emerging from recent epidemiological studies and reviews on epidemiological studies is that populations in industrialised countries are characterised by very low caries experience in the younger generation, in general independent from intake of sugars and other carbohydrates. The main conclusion is that we should question the necessity of dietary counselling from what has become a specifically dental point of view, focusing predominantly on restrictions of sugars in the diet. The current emerging view underscores the need to adopt a more equilibrated, general-health conscious preventive approach. It should recognise the importance of a good diet, but dietary recommendations should be based primarily on medical and general health considerations and arguments. Prevention of dental disease is possible with other, more direct measures and should concentrate on achieving better personal oral hygiene and appropriate use of fluoride. Where fluoridation of drinking water is not feasible, fluoridating domestic salt is an alternative dietary preventive measure.

For the situation in developing countries, preventive measures requiring expensive professionals may be too costly. In order to achieve the best possible cost-benefit ratio, the special problems of each high-risk populations should be studied and analysed[70]. The results of the analysis should be the basis of an appropriate specific approach to the problem in a developing country; it should not only take into account the causes of the high risk (which may well be high sugar consumption), but also the economic and cultural background. It may be useful to keep in mind that the studies in The Netherlands have shown that despite a continuing high sugar consumption the basic 'personal prevention package' of oral hygiene habits—cleaning with a toothbrush and using fluoride toothpaste—seemed to have been sufficient to keep more than 80 per cent of adolescents caries free. In most of the subjects who are not caries free, the number of carious lesions has become very low; the problem of the few with high caries experience is not that they could not profit from personal preventive measures and additional professional help; their problem is that they do not (yet) react to any advice, and do not seek any kind of professional help.

In short, dental health problems do not require any dietary recommendations in addition to, or other than, those required for maintenance of general health.

Periodontal Health

Maintenance of periodontal health is achieved by preventing chronic inflammation of the gingiva, the periodontal connective tissues and the supporting alveolar bone.

Nutritional Factors

One of the oldest observations on nutrition and periodontal health is James Lind's account of scurvy in the first controlled therapeutic trial conducted in 1747 [See Volume I, Chapter 3]; he experimented on sailors suffering from general weakness and putrid periodontal inflammation on board the ship, *Salisbury*. He subjected them to a number of different treatments, but the only effective one was eating oranges and lemons. This observation strongly biased investigators for more than 200 years, due to the striking evidence that periodontal disease seemed to be a systemic disease caused by nutritional deficiencies. Today it seems more likely that Lind saw cases of acute necrotising ulcerative gingivitis and periodontitis of bacterial causation rather than scurvy, or at least in addition to scurvy.

Before Löe and his team published their clinical-experimental work on the bacterial causation of gingivitis in 1965[71] nutritional and other systemic factors were assumed to be virtually exclusively responsible for periodontal disease(s), even when it was becoming clear that vitamin C deficiency could only explain a small segment of the problem.

Non-nutritional Factors

Up until about 1960 nearly everybody believed that periodontitis was a systemic disease. This explains why scientists up until the early 1960s were still looking mainly for systemic disturbances associated with loss of bone in connective tissue. Research was directed towards malnutrition, hormonal disturbances, occlusal trauma, genetic factors, nutritional deficiencies and systemic dysfunctions. American epidemiologists and nutritionists conducted a study on 21,559 subjects in eight areas around the world: Alaska, Ethiopia, Ecuador, Vietnam, Chile, Colombia, Thailand and Lebanon[72]. Surprisingly, this tremendous and important study tends to be largely ignored nowadays. It was carried out by a multidisciplinary research team of nutritionists, biochemists, physicians and dentists. The dental epidemiologists included, among the items to be studied, a number of local factors such as oral hygienic status. Russell in 1963[72] reported on the oral findings. As far as dental caries was concerned, the Russell study confirmed the caries-preventive effect of fluoride in drinking water; furthermore it corroborated the earlier finding that people who did not have more to eat than was sufficient for one or two meals per day had lower numbers of carious teeth than well-nourished people.

Regarding periodontal health the results of the Russell study were, at that time, quite unexpected. The research team found periodontitis strongly dependent on age in all populations studied, the severity increasing with age in all populations examined. However, periodontitis was much more closely associated with another factor: 12 per cent of the variance could be explained by age, 66 per cent by lack of oral hygiene. In contrast the influence of the only nutritional influence detected, deficiency of vitamin A, was negligible: 1 per cent of the total variance.

Although Russell in the discussion section of this paper uttered the expectation that future computer analysis of the data (a facility in 1963 not yet being available for unimportant projects such as dental research) would still reveal nutritional causes of periodontal disease, these were never found and after 1965 the explanation we now know became generally accepted.

Conclusion Regarding Diet and Periodontal Health

Periodontal diseases are caused by local inflammatory irritation due to overgrowth and differentiation of dental plaque, and not by systemic nutritional deficiencies. Therefore, the rational method of prevention is regular cleaning of teeth and not dietary measures.

Mucosal Health

Diet and nutrition can affect the soft tissues by influencing plaque bacteria, and to some extent the immunological response as well as healing and repair. However, in contrast to the retentive morphology of the teeth and periodontal structures, the mucosa self-cleans by desquamation of peripheral epithelial cells. This continuously minimises the antigenic load of bacteria and food residues. Nevertheless, inflammatory reactions to bacterial colonisation and/or infection occur, and soluble food components can cause irritations. Precancerous lesions and oral cancer develop upon inherited predisposition and a variety of environmental agents, notably alcohol in high concentrations and tobacco, but also nutritional/dietary components.

In the case of risk to mucosal health, medical rather than dental advice is appropriate. In addition to this question of competence, there is a practical aspect: the risk to develop pathology originating from the oral mucosa is high in elderly people, and due to the high percentage of edentates among them it is most likely that they see a doctor more often than a dentist.

SOURCE

König, KG. Diet and oral health. 2000. *Int Dent J* 50:162–74. Copyright 2000 by FDI World Dental Press. Reprinted with permission of FDI World Dental Federation.

CHAPTER 4

ENVIRONMENTAL HEALTH

Treat the earth well. It was not given to you by your parents; it was loaned to you by your children.
   —Native American proverb

Water and air, the two essential fluids on which all life depends, have become global garbage cans.
   —Jacques-Yves Cousteau (1910–1997), French undersea explorer

ON DECEMBER 24, 1968, the three astronauts of Apollo 8, William Anders, Jim Lovell, and Frank Borman, commanded more than the first manned spacecraft to orbit the moon. They commanded our attention as one by one they began their televised reading from Genesis, the story of creation from the Bible. The reading from lunar orbit was done with a backdrop of the earth rising behind the moon, thus creating a striking image depicting the isolation and frailty of our planet. It was that stirring and emotional broadcast from Apollo 8 that launched the global initiative known as the Environmental Movement. Enough momentum was generated that the UN put together a Conference on the Human Environment in Stockholm in 1972, the first time representatives of multiple governments met to discuss the state of the global environment.

Environmental sources of human disease have long been investigated and, in some circumstances, identified. For example, sanitarians of the nineteenth century linked poor air and water quality, solid waste, and substandard housing with infectious disease outbreaks and high mortality rates. In the twentieth century, rising concerns about the contamination of food and drugs, smog, contaminated water and fish from industrial runoff, thinning egg shells in birds of prey exposed to dichlorodiphenyltrichloroethane (DDT), radiation from nuclear fallout, and a population explosion all generated some degree of environmental activism among select groups. However, until that Christmas Eve broadcast, little had galvanized world attention on environmental threats to the entire globe.

In this chapter, we consider the development of environmental health as a specific focus within the public health firmament. Although environmental health is often viewed from the prism of its sister field of occupational health, the focus in this chapter is environmental health without occupational health considerations.

AIR POLLUTION

London may have the longest record of its population suffering the effects of air pollution. As early as the thirteenth century, Edward Longshanks (Edward I) prohibited the use of imported coal in London, as it gave off more acrid smoke than did the domestic variety. In 1684, English writer John Evelyn wrote in his diary that smoke in London was so thick that he could not see across the street and could scarcely breathe. The Industrial Revolution made matters even worse as factories belched out smoke at ever increasing rates. For individuals living and working in industrialized areas, smoke and its constituents sometimes yielded deadly effects, especially during weather inversions. During a weather inversion, warm air is overtopped by a layer of cold air that acts like a blanket, holding it in place. If there is no wind, the warm air becomes trapped and accumulates pollutants. Over the course of several days, the pollutant levels can become deadly. Several such incidents occurred during the twentieth century. The first of these to be documented happened in December 1930 when a cold front descended over Belgium. Temperatures were barely above freezing during the day and dropped to below 10°C at night. With no wind for several days, a cold air blanket held the warmer valley air in place and the Meuse Valley, in particular, began to accumulate industrial pollutants. Within three days, 60 people in the area died, and thousands were sickened with respiratory illnesses. Physicians reported an increase in asthma-like attacks. Many individuals had productive coughs that brought up a frothy, slimy expectorant. Many others, especially the elderly, suffered from pallor and cardiac insufficiency. Birds, rats, and cattle died. When the event was over, a commission investigated the incident and determined that the most probable cause of death was the buildup of an irritant poison, perhaps sulfur dioxide or fluorine from industrial chimney smoke.

In 1948, a weather inversion trapped air pollutants in Donora, Pennsylvania, killing 20 and sickening thousands. In *Eleven Blue Men*, Berton Rouché described Ralph W. Koehler's perceptions of the incident. Koehler served the community as a local physician for many years. On October 26, he looked out a window and was struck by the fact that a train going through the community was belching out smoke in typical fashion, but on this day the smoke did not rise. Instead, it rolled to the ground like ink and stayed there. Local residents complained of pain in the abdomen, headache, and nausea. Some began vomiting blood. A later investigation showed that several stack pollutants, such as fluoride, chloride, hydrogen sulphide, cadmium oxide, and sulphur dioxide, were the likely causes of the health disaster.

The worst of the weather inversion air pollution events in the twentieth century, however, may have been the London fog incident of 1952. In December of that year, an unusually cold winter caused an increase in coal burning and car travel, creating intense smog and acid rain conditions. About 4,000 people died of lung disease and heart failure during the immediate weeks after the worst of the four-day fog, and as many as 12,000 may have eventually succumbed due to permanent health damage.

Weather inversions are not the only causes of health problems related to air pollution. Exposure to particulate matter (PM), even if the chemical composition of the particles is nontoxic, is a concern for human health. Although very large particles (larger than 10 microns) can be trapped in the nose and sneezed or blown out, smaller ones (less than 10 microns) can settle in the lungs and bronchi and cause respiratory illness. The very smallest particles (less than 100 nanometers) may even pass through the lungs and affect other organs, causing vascular inflammation and heart attacks.

Exposures to airborne industrial toxins and radiation are also public health issues. Two significant events of the twentieth century stand out: the accidents at Bhopal and Chernobyl. On the night of December 3, 1984, at a Union Carbide plant in Bhopal, India, water entered a holding tank containing 42 tons of methyl isocyanate. The resulting chemical reaction generated both heat and toxic gases that required the release of pressure in order to prevent an explosion. The cloud of gas released immediately exposed more than half a million people to serious toxic effects. Many woke from the screams of family and friends; others awoke because their own eyes, nose, and lungs were burning from the toxins. Massive panic resulted, with entire households fleeing into the streets to join their neighbors. Once in the streets, many were trampled to death. At least 3,000 people died immediately; 5,000 more died within two weeks. Estimates place the number of premature deaths during the following two decades as high as 20,000. Bhopal stands as the worst industrial accident of the twentieth century. The event clarified the need for enforceable international standards for industrial practices that guarantee environmental safety and population health.

The worst nuclear accident in history occurred on April 26, 1986, when the No. 4 reactor at Chernobyl exploded and burned. The explosion sent a radioactive plume into the atmosphere that was 400 times more deadly than the one created by the bombing of Hiroshima. According to the International Atomic Energy Agency and the WHO, as of 2005 the Chernobyl accident was directly responsible for 56 deaths and perhaps indirectly for 4,000 excess cancer deaths among the 600,000 most highly exposed people. High levels of fallout resulted in the evacuation of more than 335,000 people, especially in the "exclusion zone" of Belarus. The radioactive plume also contaminated Russia, Ukraine, all of Europe, and the northeastern part of North America. In Sweden, for example, fallout from the plume was detected on the clothing of workers with radiation monitors. Twenty years later, farmers in Europe continue to monitor radiation in grazing animals because there are still high levels of fallout in some fields. Germany has detected high levels of radiation on playgrounds and attributed those levels to Chernobyl. Italy, Switzerland, and Sweden recommend restricting the consumption of lake fish and wild mushrooms in order to reduce exposure to fallout. The legacy of the worst nuclear accident in history will have environmental and human health impacts for the twenty-first century and beyond.

Our understanding of the health effects of air pollution, including exposure to low levels of pollutants, is still evolving. Despite the fact that air quality regulations have been put into place in some of the developed nations and global regions, significant problems related to air pollution and human health remain. In the United States, for instance, the worst air quality problems are reported for Los Angeles and Pittsburgh, especially for soot (large particulate matter), smog (a mixture of smoke and fog caused by the burning of fossil fuels), and ozone. The air pollution problem for these cities, however, is often dwarfed by that of Athens, Cairo, Hong Kong, Mexico City, Santiago, São Paulo, Seoul, and Tehran. Indeed, the World Bank has identified China as having 16 of the 20 worst polluted cities in the world and the world's highest levels of nitrogen dioxide. China may have begun to respond to being branded a significant air polluter because of world opinion and national pride. As an acknowledgement of the problem and a goodwill gesture, China expended significant effort to clean up the air in Beijing, at least temporarily, for the 2008 Olympic Games.

THE LEGACY OF LEAD

Lead beads were found in an archeological dig in Turkey dating back to 6400 BCE, testimony to the use of the malleable metal for millennia. The Romans used lead pipes to bring potable water to their cities and to secure blocks of limestone together to create grand public buildings. Because it was easy to extract, purify, and mold into objects, lead became a key ingredient for making pots and pans, mugs, coins, and other everyday objects. Lead was also used as a wine preservative and as a key ingredient of pewter items such as mugs, plates, and utensils.

Because of its widespread use, multiple epidemics of lead poisoning among various population groups have been documented over the centuries. For example, the colic of Poitou was documented by François Citois among residents of a wine region of western France in 1639. The Devonshire colic, this time from apple cider rather than wine, was reported by George Baker in 1647 (See Volume I, Chapter 4). Yet despite the knowledge that lead is harmful to human health, its use persisted. Indeed, it was even assumed that because lead was part of the earth's crust, everyone had some lead in their bodies and it might even be required for proper metabolism.

By the twentieth century, lead was widely used in paint pigments, batteries, solder for pipes, and as an antiknock additive for gasoline. It quickly became ubiquitous in interior and exterior paint for housing stocks, in water delivered through plumbing, in neighborhoods downwind from smelter stacks, in the soils surrounding parking lots and highways, and on children's painted toys. Alice Hamilton (see Volume I, Chapter 23) warned of the hazards of lead and called for the total prohibition of its use in interior paint as early as 1913. During the 1930s, Louis Dublin, statistician for the Metropolitan Life Insurance Company, warned of the potential hazards to children from lead. By 1935, Austria, Belgium, Czechoslovakia, Cuba, France, Great Britain, Greece, Poland, Spain, Sweden, Tunisia, and Yugoslavia had banned or restricted leaded interior paints. Despite mounting evidence that lead was a problem to human health, especially the health of children, the lead industry in the United States aggressively promoted its product. It was not until the 1970s that Congress banned the use of leaded interior paint from federally financed or subsidized housing and the U.S. Environmental Protection Agency (EPA) set a standard for airborne lead. The resistance to regulating lead may have harmed several generations of American children and failure to regulate lead in developing nations continues to impact populations, especially children, worldwide.

MERCURY

Quicksilver, or mercury, the flowing metal, has been used for millennia—in paper- and hatmaking, for scientific instruments, and for treating syphilis when it became epidemic in sixteenth-century Europe. The silvery liquid is an attractive substance that almost has a siren that calls for it to be played with. If a thermometer breaks, it is fun to roll the metal, watching it coalesce and fracture into pellets. Unfortunately, this wonderful toy attacks the liver and kidneys, and it may travel to the brain where it causes lack of coordination and other neurological problems. Far more toxic than inorganic mercury, however, are organic mercury compounds. Because these are soluble, they are able to penetrate membranes, enter the bloodstream, bind to red blood cells, and travel to the brain. During the course of a month or so after exposure to inorganic mercury compounds, neurological signs begin to show, especially numbness, slurred speech, and difficulty walking. Higher levels may lead to severe neurological disease, deafness, blindness, and death.

Two large-scale incidents of mercury poisoning happened in the twentieth century, in Iraq and in Minamata, Japan. In Iraq in 1972, bread was made with seed wheat that had been treated with a fungicide of organic mercury; it sickened 6,500 people and killed 459. In Minamata, a town on the coast of the island of Kyushu, Japan, the first clue that there was a devastating problem came when many of the local cats began to yowl continuously and show neurological problems. Some of the cats fell or jumped into the sea and drowned. Pigs, dogs, and crows died, and humans began to show symptoms shortly thereafter. Individuals who had eaten fish or shellfish taken from Minamata Bay had been poisoned because the Chisso Corporation, an industrial chemical company, had discharged inorganic mercury into the bay for many years. In the sediments at the bottom of the bay, inorganic mercury was converted into organic mercury compounds and became concentrated in the fish and shellfish as it moved up the food chain. Those who ate the fish and shellfish were exposed to 100,000 times the levels of organic mercury found in the bay water. Over time, the human toll of methyl mercury poisoning at Minamata was 700 deaths, 9,000 with permanent paralysis and severe brain damage, and about 50,000 additional people with milder but significant neurological symptoms of mercury poisoning.

Organic mercury crosses the placenta and can affect a fetus. For this reason, public service advisories along many waterways warn pregnant women to limit their consumption of fish and shellfish. In 1990, the WHO issued a warning about a regular diet of fish "perhaps" being hazardous for the unborn. Many Western physicians now counsel their pregnant patients to avoid sushi in order to prevent exposure to mercury.

GLOBAL WARMING

The idea that man's noxious and toxic contaminants could be flushed, diluted, or buried forever, concepts that were held over from the Sanitary Movement of the 1800s, were challenged in the twentieth century. Shocking instances of human and animal health effects that resulted from both the deliberate and accidental practices that contaminated the environment made the public take notice. Air and water pollution, accidents such as Bhopal and Chernobyl, pesticide and heavy metal contamination that moved up the food chain, as well as the growth of holes in the ozone layer brought the importance of environmental health to the fore. None of these, however, captured attention and triggered debate as broadly as did global warming.

In 1999, a team of scientists from France, Russia, and the United States drilled ice cores two miles into the Antarctic ice sheet and determined that greenhouse gases (carbon dioxide, methane, nitrous oxide, chlorofluorocarbons, and others) were at their highest levels in 420,000 years. This multinational scientific effort effectively ended the debate begun in the 1970s about whether human-driven events were influencing global climate change.

The general public and many national governments remain unconcerned about what are seemingly alarmist statements about sea levels rising a few inches or slightly warmer summer seasons. The impacts of global warming, however, are not so simple. As climate differs by region of the earth's surface, so do the effects of global warming. Precipitation patterns are likely to shift, and this will effect crop yields. Livestock are likely to suffer from temperature extremes that will affect their growth and fertility. Pasture lands will likely have to be moved due to drought and swamping. Insects are likely to flourish and expand their ranges, carrying diseases that haven't been seen is certain areas before. Groundwater pollution and saltwater intrusion are likely to increase, and supplying potable water to some regions may become problematic. The growing zones for native plants have already shifted, and weather extremes have already produced more violent storms. How humankind copes with these changes has yet to be resolved.

Selected Readings

The first reading by W. P. D. Logan describes the mortality experience during and immediately following the dense four-day fog in London (the Great Smog) in 1952. Those 4,000 deaths in such a short time period shocked the nation and generated the beginnings of an environmental movement in Britain. The Great Smog clearly demonstrated that pollution could no longer be ignored because it could, in fact, strike with almost unbelievable speed. As a direct result of the incident, Parliament passed the Clean Air Act of 1956 to 1) restrict the use of dirty fuels in industry and 2) ban black smoke. Taking heed of the dangers of burning dirty fossil fuels en masse, the environmental movement began to spread into other industrialized nations, sparking additional legislation elsewhere.

Herbert Needleman's 2000 review article is offered as the second reading as it explains the political machinations by industry to prevent the removal of lead in gasoline in the United States. Needleman gives us in-depth descriptions of the personalities involved in the struggle and a view through the lens of one of the participants in the fray. His persistence in educating the public about the dangers of lead made Needleman a target for attacks, especially from industry, but his work has since been credited with significantly reducing the average blood lead levels of American children.

The third reading, Robert Shope's discussion of global climate change and what that may mean for infectious diseases, is thought provoking. Although it is clearly speculative, Shope's work reminds us of the fragility of the public health successes against malaria, cholera, and yellow and dengue fevers achieved during the twentieth century. Shifting global and regional climactic conditions, whether the result of global warming or other natural or man-made conditions, will pose challenges for large segments of the world's population.

BIBLIOGRAPHY

Armstrong B. 1996. Editorial (Melanoma). *Cancer Causes & Control* 7 (2): 195–96.

Black H. 2000. Environmental and public health: Pulling the pieces together. *Environmental Health Perspectives* 108 (11): A512–15.

Carson RL. 1967. *Silent Spring*. Greenwich, CT: Fawcett Publications Inc.

Davis D. 2002. *When Smoke Ran Like Water: Tales of Environmental Deception and the Battle Against Pollution*. New York: Basic Books.

Dinham B and Malik S. 2003. Pesticides and human rights. *Int J Occup Environ Health* 9 (1): 40–49.

Fears TR, Scotto J, and Schneiderman MA. 1976. Skin cancer, melanoma, and sunlight. *Am J Public Health* 66 (5): 461–64.

Folley JH, Borges W, and Yamawaki T. 1952. Incidence of leukemia in survivors of the atomic bomb in Hiroshima and Nagasaki, Japan. *Am J Med* 13 (3): 311–21.

Fujiwara K. 1975. Environmental and food contamination with PCBs in Japan. *Sci Total Environ* 4 (3): 219–47.

Gochfeld M and Goldstein BD. 1999. Lessons in environmental health in the twentieth century. *Annu Rev Publ Health* 20:35–53.

Hollis MD. 1951. Aims and objectives in environmental health. *Am J Public Health* 31 (3): 263–70.

Lave BL and Seskin EP. 1970. Air pollution and human health. *Science*, n. s., 169 (3947): 723–33.

Mazur A. 1987. Putting radon on the public's risk agenda (in Communicating to Communities). Special issue on the technical and ethical aspects of risk communication, *Sci Technol Hum Val* 12 (3/4): 86–93.

McAlpine D and Arakis S. 1958. Minamata disease: An unusual neurological disorder caused by contaminated fish. *Lancet* 2 (7047): 629–31.

Menzies D and Bourbeau J. 1997. Building-related illnesses. *N Engl J Med* 337 (21): 1524–31.

Picciotto IH and B Brunekreef. 2001. Environmental epidemiology: Where we've been and where we're going. Epidemiology 12 (5): 479–81.

Rahu M. 2003. Health effects of the Chernobyl accident: Fears, rumours, and the truth. *Eur Cancer* 39:295–99.

Redlich CA, Sparer J, and Cullen MR. 1997. Sick building syndrome. *Lancet* 349:1013–16.

Robson M and Toscano WA, eds. 2007. *Risk Assessment for Environmental Health*. San Francisco: Jossey-Bass.

Rogan WJ, Gladen BC, and Wilcox AJ. 1985. Potential reproductive and postnatal morbidity from exposure to polychlorinated biphenyls: Epidemiologic considerations. *Environ Health Perspect* 60:233–39.

Roholm K. 1937. The fog disaster in the Meuse Valley, 1930: A fluorine intoxication. *J Indust Hygiene Toxicol* 19:126–27.

Roueché B. 1953. The Fog. In *Eleven Blue Men and Other Narratives of Medical Detection*. New York: Berkeley Medallion Books.

Schwartz J, Slater D, Larson TV, Pierson WE, and Koenig JQ. 1993. Particulate air pollution and hospital emergency room visits for asthma in Seattle. *Am Rev Respir Dis* 147 (4): 826–31.

Thibodeau LA, Reed RB, Bishop YMM, and Kammerman LA. 1980. Air pollution and human health: A review and reanalysis. *Environ Health Perspect* 34 (Feb): 165–83.

Wedeen RP. 1984. *Poison in the Pot: The Legacy of Lead*. Carbondale, IL: Southern Illinois University Press.

Winkelstein W Jr. and deGroot I. 1962. The Erie County air pollution–pulmonary function study. *Am Rev Respir Dis* 86 (6): 902–6.

Mortality in the London Fog Incident, 1952
(1953)

W. P. D. Logan, M.D. Glasg., Ph.D. Lond. Chief Medical
Statistician, General Register Office

The Meuse Valley fog episode in 1930 caused 64 deaths, and the Donora
(Pennsylvania) episode in 1948 caused 20 deaths. In December, 1952, a
four-day fog in London caused about 4,000 deaths. This paper gives a short
account of when and where these deaths occurred, the age-distribution,
and the reported medical causes. No attempt is made here to present detailed meteorological data or to discuss clinical aspects; these and other
features of the incident, including additional details about mortality, will
no doubt be discussed in a report which, it is understood, will be made to
the Minister of Health when investigations have been completed. Two
papers have already been published concerning the effects of the fog on
hospital admissions[1] and on general practice.[2]

The figures given here are from the Registrar-General's weekly returns, with additional data, and indicate that the incident was a catastrophe of the first magnitude in which, for a few days, death-rates attained a
level that has been exceeded only rarely during the past hundred years—
for example, at the height of the cholera epidemic of 1854 and of the influenza epidemic of 1918–19.

Increase in Deaths

Unusually dense fog developed over practically the whole of the Greater
London area early in the morning of Friday, Dec. 5, 1952, and continued
until early in the morning of Tuesday, Dec. 9. In relation to the periods
for which the numbers of deaths registered are published in the weekly
returns, the fog began towards the close of the week ended Saturday,
Dec. 6, and continued into the first half of the week ended Saturday, Dec.
13; and it was the latter week that the majority of the deaths due to the fog
were registered. Table I shows numbers of deaths registered in the Greater
London area (population about 8½ million) from the week ended Nov. 15,
1952, to the week ended Jan. 10, 1953, compared with the annual averages
in corresponding weeks of the five previous years. Deaths registered increased from 2,062 in the week ended Dec. 6 to 4,703 in the week ended
Dec. 13 and 3,138 in the week ended Dec. 20. In the next week (week
ended Dec. 27) the number of registrations fell to 2,234—less than 200

Table I Deaths Registered in Greater London from Week Ended Nov. 15, 1952, to Jan. 10, 1953, Compared with the Annual Average for Corresponding Weeks of the Five Previous Years, 1947–52

Year	Deaths in week ended								
	Nov. 15	Nov. 22	Nov. 29	Dec. 6	Dec. 13	Dec. 20	Dec. 27	Jan. 3	Jan. 10
1952	1,565	1,699	1,902	2,062	4,703	3,138	2,234	2,977	2,634
1947–52 (av.)	1,747	1,708	1,809	1,805	1,852	1,914	1,923	2,303	2,213

more than in the week before the fog incident. It is possible, therefore, that by that time the effect of the fog had more or less come to an end and was not responsible for the subsequent rise in mortality during the weeks ended Jan. 3 and 10. On the other hand, part of the decline in registrations in the week ended Dec. 27 may have been due to the intervention of the Christmas holidays, during which some registrations may have been postponed. It is not possible to be sure, therefore, that all the deaths brought about by the fog had been registered within the two weeks ended Dec. 13 and 20. Assuming that they were, the number of deaths so caused can be estimated to lie between 3,717 (the excess in the weeks ended Dec. 13 and 20, 1952, over the week ended Dec. 6, 1952) and 4,075 (the excess in the weeks ended Dec. 13 and 20, 1952, over the corresponding average for 1947–51). Having regard to the opposing considerations that all of the excess deaths in the weeks ended Dec. 13 and 20 were not necessarily due to fog, and on the other hand that all of the fog deaths had not necessarily been registered within these two weeks, it is reasonable to estimate that in Greater London approximately 4,000 deaths were brought about by the fog incident.

Table II gives numbers of deaths in the weeks ended Dec. 6, 13, and 20 in Greater London, divided into London administrative county and the outer ring, with the latter also subdivided by county areas, and in the hundred and 160 great towns of England and Wales minus Greater London. Although a certain amount of dense fog was reported in other areas it is evident that it was only in Greater London that there was an appreciable increase in mortality in the week ended Dec. 13. In the remainder of the great towns (aggregate population 14 million) the increase amounted to only 164 deaths, compared with an increase of 2,641 in Greater London. Incidentally the fact that the subsequent rise in numbers of registrations in the weeks ended Jan. 3 and 10, already noted for Greater London, was paralleled in the remainder of the great towns supports the suggestion that this later increase in mortality was independent of the fog.

Table II   Deaths Registered in London Administrative County and the Outer Ring (by county areas) and in the 160 Great Towns of England and Wales: Weeks Ended Nov. 29, 1952, to Jan. 10, 1953

Area	Deaths in week ended							Ratio of week ended Dec. 13 to Dec. 6
	Nov. 29	Dec. 6	Dec. 13	Dec. 20	Dec. 27	Jan. 3	Jan. 10	
London A.C.	853	945	2,484	1,523	1,029	1,372	1,216	2·6
Outer ring:	1,049	1,117	2,219	1,615	1,205	1,605	1,418	2·0
Middlesex		499	942	728				1·9
Surrey		293	564	390				1·9
Kent		103	174	104				1·7
Herts		21	45	33				2·1
Essex		201	494	350				2·5
160 great towns	6,042	6,647	9,452	7,701	6,472	7,842	7,617	1·4
Great towns minus Greater London	4,140	4,585	4,749	4,563	4,238	4,865	4,983	1·04

Within the Greater London area the abrupt increase for the week ended Dec. 13 occurred both in the central area (administrative county) and in the outer ring; as the right-hand column of table II shows, the weekly mortality in the central area almost trebled (ratio 2·6) and in the outer ring had doubled (ratio 2·0). The breakdown of the outer ring into towns within the constituent county areas indicates that mortality increased sharply in the Essex section (ratio 2·5) and least in Kent (ratio 1·7). But clearly no large section of the Greater London area escaped. As examples of what happened in some districts, deaths registered in Stepney increased from 29 to 119 (ratio 4·1), and in East Ham from 16 to 62 (ratio 3·9).

Analysis of Deaths

Age-Distribution

Table III compares the age-distribution of deaths registered in the London administrative county in the weeks ended Dec. 6 and 13. Although the

Table III Deaths Registered in London Administrative County, by Age: Weeks Ended Dec. 6 and 13, 1952

—	Age							
	All ages	Under 4 weeks	4 weeks–1 year	1–14	15–44	45–64	65–74	75 and over
Dec. 6	945	16	12	10	61	237	254	355
Dec. 13	2,484	28	26	13	99	652	717	949
Ratio of week ended Dec. 13 to week ended Dec. 6	2·6	1·8	2·2	1·3	1·6	2·8	2·8	2·7

Table IV Percentage Age-Distribution of Deaths Registered in London Administrative County, Weeks Ended Nov. 29, 1952, to Jan. 3, 1953

Age (years)	Week ended					
	Nov. 29	Dec. 6	Dec. 13	Dec. 20	Dec. 27	Jan. 3
Under 1	3	3	2	2	2	3
1–44	–	11	4	2	4	5
45–64	21	193	95	11	31	25
65 and over	53	494	296	27	124	67
All ages	100	100	100	100	100	100
Total number	853	945	2,484	1,523	1,029	1,372

increase in mortality was greater and older than at younger ages it was slightly less at ages 75 and over (ratio 2·7) than ages 45–74 (ratio 2·8). The mortality of newborn infants almost doubled, and that of infants aged 1–12 months more than doubled. Deaths of children rose by a third (from 10 to 13) ended young adults by close on two-thirds (61 to 99). It is clear, therefore, that all ages shared to some extent in the increased mortality, and that it was by no means confined to the very young or very old. Although there was relatively little disturbance of the usual age-distribution of deaths, as is shown in table IV which gives the percentage of deaths at various stages during several successive weeks.

Causes of Deaths

Deaths registered in the London administrative county increased by about 1,500 in the week ended Dec. 13, and about half of the increase was attributed to bronchitis or pneumonia. Deaths from bronchitis increased by over eight times (from 76 to 704) and deaths from pneumonia by almost three times (from 45 to 168) (table V). In the next week—the week ended Dec. 20—deaths from bronchitis totaled 396, still a very high figure, and deaths from pneumonia numbered 125. Other causes of death that increased greatly in the week ended Dec. 13 were respiratory tuberculosis (from 14 to 77), cancer of lung (from 45 to 69), coronary disease (from 118 to 281), myocardial degeneration (from 88 to 244), and "other respiratory diseases" (from 9 to 52). 24 [sic] deaths were certified as due to influenza compared with 2 in the previous week. There was no increase

Table V   Numbers of Deaths Assigned to Various Causes, London Administrative County: Weeks Ended Nov. 29, 1952, to Jan. 3, 1953

Cause of death	Week ended					
	Nov. 29	Dec. 6	Dec. 13	Dec. 20	Dec. 27	Jan. 3
Respiratory tuberculosis	19	14	77	37	21	24
Cancer of lung	27	45	69	32	36	48
Vascular lesions of C.N.S.	98	102	128	119	91	131
Coronary disease	131	118	281	152	109	150
Myocardial degeneration	79	88	244	131	108	136
Influenza	7	2	24	9	6	4
Pneumonia *	28	45	168	125	91	104
Bronchitis	73	76	704	396	184	215
Other respiratory diseases	8	9	52	21	13	10
Motor-vehicle accidents	1	8	4	10	4	5
Suicide	5	10	10	7	5	12
Total (all causes)	853	945	2,484	1,523	1,029	1,372

* Excluding deaths at ages under 4 weeks.

Table VI Deaths from Bronchitis and from Pneumonia by Age, London Administrative County: Weeks Ended Dec. 6, 13, and 20, 1952

Age (years)	Bronchitis			Pneumonia (at ages over 4 weeks)		
	Dec. 6	Dec. 13	Dec. 20	Dec. 6	Dec. 13	Dec. 20
Under 1	2	6	1	5	9	7
1–44	—	11	4	2	4	6
45–64	21	193	95	11	31	16
65 and over	53	494	296	27	124	96
All ages	76	704	396	45	168	125

Table VII Numbers of Deaths Certified by Coroner or Certified after Post-mortem Examination, Greater London: Weeks Ended Dec. 6, 13, and 20, 1952

Week ended	Total deaths	No. certified by coroner	No. certified after Post-mortem examination		
			Coroners'	Others	Total
Dec. 6	2,062	458 (22%)	452	169	621 (30%)
Dec. 13	4,703	962 (20%)	960	267	1,227 (26%)
Dec. 20	3,138	680 (22%)	680	203	883 (28%)

in deaths from motor-vehicle accidents—possibly because fewer vehicles were on the roads—and there was no increase in deaths by suicide.

The age-distribution of deaths from bronchitis and from pneumonia are shown in table VI. As for deaths from all causes combined, the increases were greatest at advanced ages, but young persons by no means escaped. Deaths from bronchitis at ages under 45 rose from 2 in the week ended Dec. 6 to 17 in the next week, and deaths from pneumonia almost doubled (from 7 to 13).

Deaths Certified by Coroners

One of the results of the sudden increase in mortality was to double the work of coroners and coroners' pathologists. Their reports will provide valuable information about the pathological changes found and may throw some light on the mechanism whereby the deaths occurred. As table VII shows, there was a very large increase in the week ended

December 13 in the number of cases certified by coroners and in the number of post-mortem examinations. In relation to the increased numbers of deaths, however, the proportions of coroners' cases and post-mortem examinations were slightly reduced. Cases certified by coroners include only those where referral to a coroner resulted in an inquest or post-mortem examination; the total number of referrals is not known.

Number of Deaths Each Day

One of the most striking features of the incident was the rapidity at which deaths started to increase. Table VIII shows the number of deaths *occurring* each day (not numbers of registrations as in other tables). Even on Dec. 5, the first day of the fog, there was an obvious increase in the number of deaths, and the daily totals mounted rapidly to their highest levels on Dec. 7 and 8, the third and fourth days of the fog. There was some decline on Dec. 9, and a still greater decline in Dec. 10; but even on Dec. 15 the daily total was almost twice as high as before the fog began (see figure). [p. 79, Ed.]

Previous Incidents

The 1952 incident is not the first in which dense fog in London has caused a sudden increase in deaths; as recently as 1948 a continuous but less dense five-day fog was responsible for some 300 deaths in the London administrative county.[3] But so far as can be ascertained from a rapid search through the weekly returns, such events have been very rare, and only three others have been traced in which an association between dense fog and suddenly increased mortality has been clear-cut. In table IX mortality is related to these three incidents and to those in 1948 and 1952. It is evident that the increase in mortality in the 1952 incident was very much greater than on previous occasions.

There is reason to believe that the fog incident in December, 1952, caused deaths in London on a scale possibly never experienced before from this cause. It is to be hoped that such an event will never recur—or be allowed to recur.

Summary

The dense four-day fog in Greater London in December, 1952, was responsible for some 4,000 deaths during the two following weeks.

The increased mortality affected persons of all ages, but particularly those aged 45 and over.

Deaths assigned to bronchitis and pneumonia increased eight times and three times respectively in one week.

Table VIII Deaths in Greater London and Constituent Areas by Date of Occurrence, Dec. 1–15, 1952 (excluding any deaths occurring within these dates but not registered by Dec. 20). Atmospheric Pollution Readings at Kew Observatory, Richmond (South-West London)

Area	Deaths on Dec.														
	1	2	3	4	5	6	7	8	9	10	11	12	13	14	15
Greater London	259	301	321	288	406	581	894	910	792	543	528	484	501	449	425
London A.C.	112	140	143	120	196	294	513	518	430	274	255	236	256	222	213
Outer ring	147	161	178	168	210	287	381	392	362	269	273	248	245	227	212
Atmospheric pollution (mg. per c.m.), max. reading	0.30	0.95	0.30	0.95	2.55	2.65	1.70	1.95	1.45	0.30	0.30	0.45	0.45	0.95	0.30

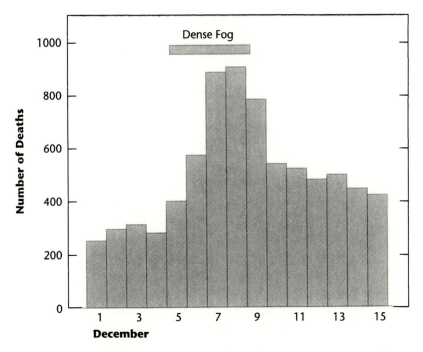

Deaths in Greater London each day from Dec. 1 to 15, 1952.

Table IX Instances of Sudden Increases in Mortality in the London County Area Associated with Dense Fog

Year	Dates of dense fog	Deaths				Ratio*
		Weekly totals				
1873	Dec. 9–11	Dec. 13	Dec. 20	Dec. 27	Jan. 3	1·4
		1,759	2,415	1,540	1,842	
1880	Jan. 26–29	Jan. 31	Feb. 7	Feb. 14	Feb. 21	1·5
		2,200	3,376	2,495	2,016	
1892	Dec. 28–30	Dec. 31	Jan. 7	Jan. 14	Jan. 21	1·4
		1,830	2,509	2,503	2,101	
1948	Nov. 26–Dec. 1	Nov. 27	Dec. 4	Dec. 11	Dec. 18	1·3
		779	1,019	944	891	
1952	Dec. 5–9	Dec. 6	Dec. 13	Dec. 20	Dec. 27	2·6
		945	2,484	1,523	1,029	
* Deaths in week of suddenly increased mortality to deaths in previous week.						

A considerable increase in numbers of deaths occurred even on the first day of the fog.

Four previous London fogs resulting in a sudden increase in deaths have been noted; but the 1952 incident caused by far the largest increase.

SOURCE

Logan WP. 1953. Mortality in the London fog incident, 1952. *Lancet* 1 (7): 336–8. Copyright 1953 by *The Lancet*. Reprinted with permission of Elsevier.

REVIEW
The Removal of Lead from Gasoline: Historical and Personal Reflections
(2000)

Herbert L. Needleman

Tetraethyllead (TEL) was first fabricated for use in gasoline in 1923. Shortly after manufacture began, workers at all three plants began to become floridly psychotic and die. A moratorium on TEL production was put into place, but was lifted in 1926. Between 1926 and 1965, the prevailing consensus was that lead toxicity occurred only at high levels of exposure and that lead in the atmosphere was harmless. Most of the data on lead toxicity issued from a single source, the Kettering Laboratory in Cincinnati. In 1959, the first warnings of adverse health effects of lead at silent doses were raised by Clair Patterson, a geochemist. In hearings before the Senate Committee on Public Works, Senator Edward Muskie raised the question of adverse health effects of airborne lead. As new data accumulated on health effects of lead at lower doses, the movement to remove lead from gasoline gained momentum, and the Environmental Protection Agency examined the question. The removal of lead would take place over the next 25 years, and its accomplishment would require a severe change in the federal stance regarding its hazard. This article details the interaction of various forces, industrial, regulatory, judicial, public health, and public interest, that were engaged in this contest and estimates the value of this step.

Introduction

E.I. DuPont and General Motors formed the Ethyl Gasoline Company in 1922 and began to make commercial tetraethyllead in 1923. Standard Oil began production of [it] in 1924. Shortly after production began, workers in three plants, Dayton, Ohio, Bay Way, New Jersey, and Deep Water, New Jersey, began to die, and many more became floridly psychotic. A moratorium on production was imposed, and the Surgeon General convened a meeting of scientists and industry officials. Shortly after the Surgeon General's committee announced TEL safe for general use in 1926, the Public Health Service recommended that the allowable concentration of tetraethyllead be set at 3 cc per gallon. Ethyl quickly agreed to comply, relieving the government of any pressure to regulate lead in gasoline. For the next 35 years lead toxicity as a health issue virtually disappeared from sight (1).

The struggle to remove lead from gasoline, which began in 1959, would occupy the next three decades. Its removal would require a rearrangement of both the scientific and the public perception of its toxicity and the

181

realization that children's brains were the most sensitive targets. In the process, a fledgling environmental movement would gain strength in contest with the lead industry, while responsible government officials would be forced to jettison their own complacent picture of lead dangers and realign their long held proindustry bias.

Arranging a Lead Consensus

After the Surgeon General's report, a single figure, Robert Kehoe, was cultivated by the industry as the dominant authority on lead. Data on the health effects of lead were sparse, and the only source of funding for research came from industry treasuries. What little research there was issued almost exclusively from Kehoe's group at the Kettering Laboratory in Cincinnati.

C.F. Kettering established the laboratory that bore his name with an initial gift of $130,000 from Ethyl, E.I. DuPont, and General Motors (GM). He had tapped Kehoe, a young toxicologist at the University of Cincinnati, to study the deaths at the Ethyl plant in Dayton and later to direct the laboratory. Kehoe's early studies compared lead concentrations in workers in direct contact with tetraethyllead to men in the same plant with other assignments. He designated this second group "unexposed" controls. When he found lead in the excreta of his unexposed group, he concluded that lead was naturally present in everyone. The presence of it, he argued, could not be taken by itself as an indicator of poisoning. This was a fundamental error, and it was vigorously attacked by David Edsall, Yandell Henderson, and others at the Surgeon General's 1925 meeting, who argued that potentially all workers in the Dayton plant were exposed to TEL fumes. After that meeting, criticism of Kehoe subsided; he had data and few others did. He became a corporate officer at GM and a consultant to DuPont.

Kehoe eventually came to see the merit in his critics' assertions: clearly he had chosen the wrong control group. To answer them, he searched for an unquestionably unexposed group. He visited a remote farming village outside Mexico City, removed from industry or urban pollution. There he sampled food, utensils, and the excreta of the residents. The farmers in this remote area had lead in their excreta. Kehoe concluded, once again, that the lead in these farmers showed that the metal was a "natural" constituent of body chemistry. This observation of natural lead levels in Mexican farmers became the nucleus of Kehoe's position throughout his career. From this he constructed a case that lead in gasoline presented no danger and that the general concern about lead as a health threat was overstated.

Once again Kehoe overlooked the glaring flaw in his conclusions. His Mexican farmers also had increased amounts of lead in their clay dishware. Kehoe's analyses showed this, but he dismissed his own finding. It is difficult to understand how Kehoe, the lead industry, and the public health community could have overlooked such a fundamental state.

Fluctuations in the Tetraethyllead Market

At the end of World War II, automobile production expanded and TEL sales swelled. Then the market began to change. Ethyl's patent expired in 1947, and other chemical companies competed for TEL sales. Oil companies used improved fuel stock that required less TEL to raise octane levels, and jet aircraft, which did not require high-octane fuel, began to replace piston-driven planes (2). In the late 1950s, Ethyl laid off part of its workforce. Facing lowered revenues, the company sought permission from the Public Health Service to raise the amount of lead in gasoline to 4 cc per gallon.

State of Knowledge in the Public Health Service

Ethyl's request was made at a time of growing public concern about the environment. Before World War II, environmental attention has focused on conservation of resources in the service of an industrial economy. Living standards improved after the war ended, and people turned to outdoor recreation. Americans began to regard the environment as an asset with intrinsic value apart from utilitarian purposes. Citizens began to regard the air they breathed and the water they drank (3).

The Public Service had in the past displayed a distinct proindustry bias on lead. Its Medical Director was R.R. Sayers, who had authored the 1925 Bureau of Mines study and had served as the president of the business-oriented American Association of Industrial Physicians. At that time the Environmental Investigations Branch was headed by H.H. Shrenk, who would later become the director of the Industrial Hygiene Foundation at the Mellon Institute.

In 1959 the Lead Liaison Committee was created by the Surgeon General to coordinate research on the health effects from atmospheric lead. Government was represented by the National Air Pollution Control Administration, the Department of Health, Education and Welfare (DHEW), and the California Department of Health. Industry's viewpoint had an abundance of weight. It was represented on the committee by the International Lead Zinc Research Organization, E.I. DuPont, the American Petroleum Institute, the Auto Manufacturers Association, Ethyl Corporation, and the Kettering Laboratory. The Liaison Committee concluded that contemporary levels of lead in the atmosphere presented no hazard. The Committee would occupy a strategic position in regulatory activity that held until the public was given access to minutes of their meetings. Shortly after the proceedings were opened up to public scrutiny the industry's interest in the committee waned, and it was disbanded (4).

The same year the Surgeon General convened a meeting to evaluate Ethyl's request to increase the amount of TEL and fuel. Testimony was taken only from Ethyl Corporation and E.I. DuPont, and the only witness on the health effects of lead was Kehoe (5). The Surgeon General's report acknowledged Kehoe's Mexican study as evidence demonstrating the "contribution of natural sources." While lamenting the sparse data on body burdens of lead, the report concluded that there was no reason not to permit an increase in lead added to gasoline.

A Challenge to the Consensus

In 1965, Kehoe's monopoly on lead science was threatened by a geochemist. Clair Patterson was a research associate in geology at the California Institute of Technology. His measurements of the isotopic ratios of certain minerals convinced him that the long-held consensus of geologists that the age of the earth was 3 billion years old was wildly wrong—by 1.5 billion years. Patterson's studies placed the age of the earth at 4.5 billion years (6). At the time he did this, he swam against a tidal wave of orthodox scientific opinion. His findings were confirmed, his skeptics silenced, and the geology textbooks revised.

Patterson discovered this error because he employed extraordinary measures to avoid contamination while conducting and analyzing his specimens. As a result the isotope ratios were vastly more accurate than those of earlier workers. As he measured the concentration of mineral isotopes, he observed that the lead levels in soil and ice were much higher than would be expected on the basis of natural fluxes. He realized that human activity had severely raised environmental levels of lead.

Most scientists would have treated the contamination of his reagents as a technical annoyance to be overcome and then forgotten. To Patterson it [was] not a nuisance but a clear signal of the contamination by lead of the biosphere. This, he realized, was an unrecognized danger of major proportions to everyone. His conclusions validated the warnings 40 years earlier of Yandell Henderson, David Edsall, and Alice Hamilton that inserting leading to gasoline would contaminate the entire biosphere.

He began to divert a considerable proportion of his extraordinary mind and energy away from the pure science of geochemistry to the study of lead contamination. If Kehoe ignored contamination, Patterson was obsessed by it. He conducted his experiments in an ultraclean chamber entered through an airlock in which the air was filtered, the experimenters gowned and masked, and the reagents and water supply purified of any

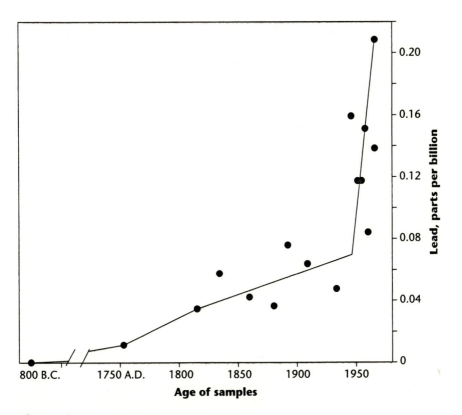

Figure 1 Lead concentrations in Greenland snow cores since 800 BC. From *Morozumi et al.*, 1969. [(39), Ed.]

traces of lead. By these measures he established the true concentrations of lead in his samples.

From the depths of the Pacific Ocean he brought tuna to the surface with extreme care to avoid taint. He studied pre-Iron Age mummies buried in sandy soil and cores of the Greenland ice pack. By slicing the ice cores he was able to precisely date the specimen and show the time course of lead in the atmosphere (see Fig. 1).

The techniques that he developed to obtain clean specimens and taught to scientists around the world would produce for the first time unimpeachable and valuable data on people's contamination of the biosphere by lead and other elements. Patterson and his colleagues showed that technological activity had raised modern human body lead burdens to levels 600 times that of our pretechnologic ancients.

His work began to attract attention outside of the field of geochemistry. In 1965 in response to an invitation by the editor of the *Archives of Environmental Health,* he submitted a long article titled "Contaminated and Natural Lead Environments of Man" based on his findings and speculations

(7). Kehoe was asked to referee the manuscript and decide whether it should be published. Irritated because Patterson did not pay him homage, Kehoe argued for the paper's publication so that Patterson could be offered up for demolition.

> I should let the man, with his obvious faults, speak in such a way as to display these faults . . .

> The inferences as to the natural human body burdens of lead, are I think, remarkably naïve . . . It is an example of how wrong one can be in his biological postulates and conclusions, when he steps into this field, of which he is so woefully ignorant and so lacking in any concept of the depths of his ignorance, that he is not even cautious in drawing sweeping conclusions. This bespeaks the brash young man, or perhaps the not so young [Patterson was 43 at the time] passionate supporter of a cause. In either case hardly the mark off [*sic*] the critical investigator.

> We have been working with the physiological aspects of this problem carefully and step by step for more than thirty years . . . The virtue of the paper is its examination of the manner in which man has altered "the face of the earth" in a variety of ways, and has disturbed the composition of the human internal milieu in doing so. It is strange that Dr. Patterson does not realize that this has happened to the large proportion of mineral components of the earth, and that this is one of the outstanding physiological problems of our time. Can we adapt to these changes, individually and collectively? Are our physiological mechanisms flexible enough to cope with them? It appears, in the case of lead, that they are, and also that we are very nearly able to define the limit beyond which we shall not be able to cope with them. . . . It is disappointing that our work has not been viewed in this manner by Dr. Patterson, but the issue which he has raised, in this article and by word of mouth elsewhere, cannot be "swept under the rug." It must be faced and demolished, and therefore, I welcome its "public appearance." (8)

In this letter Kehoe displayed the second part of this basic argument: humans have achieved a biological adaptation to lead. Patterson's precise point was that human's exposure to lead was new, and that a few thousand years of lead exposure, a Darwinian moment, with nowhere near the time needed to develop adaptive responses.

Patterson's *Archives of Environmental Health* paper fundamentally altered the vocabulary of the debate over the health effects of lead. Kehoe and his partisans had commonly referred to average population values as "normal" levels of lead in blood. Normal also conveys some of the meaning "natural." Patterson understood that because a certain level of lead was commonplace did not mean it was without harm. He argued that normal should be replaced by "typical." Natural should be reserved for those concentrations of lead that existed in the body or environment before contamination by people. Other workers had missed this distinction because their reagents and instruments, the very air they breathed in their laboratories, freighted with lead, swamped their measurements. The so-called "unexposed" subjects in Kehoe's studies in the Dayton plant who did not directly handle TEL breathed it, and the food of Kehoe's "unexposed" Mexican farmers had been cooked in and served from leaded ceramic pots and plates.

The *Archives of Environmental Health* paper released a fusillade of angry responses from the toxicology orthodoxy. They included the editor of the journal in their attacks for publishing it. The furious toxicologists focused on Patterson for his hubris in stepping outside his field to talk about people instead of rocks.

While Patterson seemed to thrive on the controversy, there were other, more serious effects. A group from Ethyl Corporation visited him and tried to (in his words) "buy me out through research support that would yield results favorable to their cause." He responded with a lecture in which he predicted that future scientists would show that Ethyl's activities were poisoning both the environment and people, and their operations would eventually be shut down. Following this meeting, his long-standing contract with the Public Health Service was not renewed, and his substantial contract with the American Petroleum Institute was terminated. Members of the Board of Trustees at California Institute of Technology visited the chairman of his department asking that he be fired (9).

The paper and the attendant controversy crystallized the polar positions embodied by Patterson and Kehoe and exposed the question of lead effects at low or silent doses. Those who adhered to Kehoe believed that lead poisoning occurred only at high doses with obvious signs of severe illness. Patterson clearly spelled out the other position: elevated levels of lead found in all humans were associated with sometimes-silent disturbances in body chemistry. Perhaps, he argued, everyone was to some degree poisoned. Complacency over lead would never be the same.

Publicly vilified and professionally threatened, this contentious, unmovable man, who was content to work as an outsider, would eventually be recognized by the scientific establishment for his extraordinary contributions. He would win the Goldschmidt Medal, the equivalent of the Nobel Prize in geochemistry, be elected to the National Academy of

Sciences, and have a mountain peak in Antarctica and a large asteroid named after him. His friend Saul Bellow would use him as a model, Professor Sam Beech, in *The Dean's December*.[1]

The Muskie Hearings

For any regulation of lead in gasoline to thrive, it would have to originate outside of the Public Health Service (PHS). In 1966, Senator Edward Muskie, Chairman of the Senate Subcommittee on Air and Water Pollution, presided over hearings on the Clean Water Act (10). He gave considerable attention to the status of lead in the air and in gasoline.

The Surgeon General, William Stewart, one of the first to testify, gave testimony that declared the government's concern, perhaps for the first time, about the effects of lead at low doses, particularly in children and pregnant women:

> Existing evidence suggests that certain groups in the population may be particularly susceptible to injury. Children and pregnant women constitute two of the most important of such groups. Some studies have suggested an association between lead exposure and the occurrence of mental retardation among children.

Muskie asked why the PHS was rushing once again to increase lead in fuel without testing for hazard. With unusual frankness, Dr. Richard Prindle of PHS explained the pressure on PHS to raise the TEL limit.

> I think the situation was one of tremendous pressure, frankly, to move forward in what amounts to an economic problem as far as the industry was concerned . . . This was attempted in light of the knowledge.

---

1 In *The Dean's December*, Saul Bellow described Professor Sam Beech, a character easily recognized as Clair Patterson.

> These scientists were diapered babies when they went public with a cause. But Beech somehow inspired respect. There was a special seriousness about him. He was physically, constitutionally serious. His head, for a body of such length, was small. His face was devoid of personal vanity . . . He was indeed an eminent man of science. That was unanimous. He had authoritatively dated the age of the earth, had analyzed the rocks brought back from the moon. Corde was beginning to think that with pure scientists, when they turned their eyes from their own disciplines, there were occasionally storms of convulsive clear consciousness.

Bellow then describes "Beech's theories about the relationship between lead and social disorder, and the chilly reception they received from the orthodoxy.

> Here science which itself was designed for deeper realization, experienced a singular failure. The genius of these evils was their ability to create zones of incomprehension. It was because they were so fully apparent that you couldn't see them.

MUSKIE: If I am out in the woods hunting deer, I don't shoot at a moving leaf but wait until I see something more.

PRINDLE: I think you are probably correct, Senator.

Prindle also cited a recent PHS study of air and blood lead in Los Angeles, Cincinnati, and Philadelphia (the Three Cities Study) as showing increases in blood lead levels:

> We noted a general trend toward an increasing concentration of lead in the blood of various groups of persons as the[y] vary from rural to central urban areas . . .

Once again Kehoe was the industry's principal witness. Two years earlier he had gone on record that there was no health risk from airborne lead and no need for an ambient air lead standard (11). The Ethyl Corporation was jittery; Kehoe's testimony was critical to the fate of their company. ". . . If he had wavered the company would have been faced with disaster," said a member of Ethyl's defense group (2).

Taking a hand in such a high-stakes game in the Senate chamber did not induce a trace of restraint in Kehoe. He began by telling Muskie that he knew so much about the subject that he was forced to abridge his presentation: "I'm afraid we would be here the rest of the week if I were to undertake to do this [tell all that he knew]."

Although science ordinarily recognizes the provisional nature of any research finding, and scientists are expected to display some modesty or tentativeness about the conclusions they draw, Kehoe, with almost every sentence, stepped on this convention. He said that enough was known about TEL toxicity to allow the amount of TEL to be increased without risk:

> The fact is, however, that no other hygienic problem in the field of air pollution has been investigated so intensively, over such a prolonged period of time, and with such definitive results.

An edginess between Kehoe and Muskie quickly became obvious. When Muskie pointed out that the Public Health Service and others disagreed with Kehoe and that many felt that there were unanswered questions and need for more research, Kehoe responded:

> . . . I would simply say that in developing information on this subject, I have had a greater responsibility than any other persons in this country. . . . the evidence at the present time is better than it has been at any time that this is not a present hazard.

Muskie pressed on about finding a substitute for TEL:

... would it be desirable if a substitute for lead in gasoline could be found?

KEHOE: there is no evidence that this has introduced a danger in the field of public health . . . I may say the work of the Kettering Laboratory in this field, that lead is an inevitable element in the surface of the earth, in its vegetation, in its animal life, and that there is no way in which man has ever been able to escape the absorption of lead while living in this planet.

Kehoe went so far as to state that air lead levels in Cincinnati had decreased. When Muskie pointed out what appeared to be a paradox, Kehoe had a novel explanation:

MUSKIE: Over the past three years I assume there has been a tremendous growth in automobiles and in the amount of traffic in Cincinnati, and yet as I understand it, you say that there has been no increase in the concentration of lead in the ambient air?

KEHOE: That is a fact. There has been a change *downward*, since the period of the Second World War . . . we had difficulty in Cincinnati getting the kind of coal that we would like . . . During this period we had to take the coal that could be obtained . . . In 1945 this whole situation was changed and in the period immediately following this the lead content of the atmosphere of Cincinnati went significantly downward.

MUSKIE: What you have just said is that the decrease in the concentration in the atmosphere is due to better control stationary sources of air pollution?

KEHOE: That is right.

MUSKIE: Have you drawn any conclusions as to whether or not the concentration of lead in the atmosphere has gone up, gone down, or remained stationary?

KEHOE: We conclude that there has been no increase.

Kehoe neglected to reveal the whole story, failing to mention two sources of bias in the Cincinnati data. In the early years, different analytic methods were used to measure lead, and more samples were taken from industrial sites, while fewer industrial sites were sampled later. Later, a scientist from Kehoe's own laboratory would publish data showing that lead levels in Cincinnati's air had in fact increased between 1961 and 1968 (12).

MUSKIE: Is it your conclusion that in 1937 to the present time, on the basis of that data, that there has been no increase in the amount

of lead taken in from the atmosphere by traffic policemen, by attendants at service stations or by the average motorist?

KEHOE: There is not the slightest evidence that there has been
a change in this picture during this period of time. Not the
slightest.

Nothing could jostle Kehoe's limitless confidence and optimism.
When Muskie again returned to Kehoe's guarantee that there was no
harm to be expected from atmospheric lead, he received a characteristic response.

MUSKIE: Does medical opinion agree that there are no harmful
effects and results from lead ingestion below the level of lead
poisoning?

KEHOE: I don't think that many people would be as certain as I
am at this point.

MUSKIE: You are certain?

KEHOE: . . . It so happens that I have more experience in this field
than anyone else alive.

One week later Clair Patterson testified. He began by attacking the belief that natural lead cycling and human activity each contributed about
the same amount of lead to the environment. About 10 thousand tons of
lead were naturally recycled each year, he said, while millions of tons
were emitted due to industrial emissions. Large numbers of people are
sickened, he believed, as a result of this unnatural load, and the brain is
the most significant target. Patterson attacked the PHS for relying on
industry-furnished data:

It is not just a mistake for the public health agencies to cooperate
with industries in investigating and deciding whether public health
is endangered—it is a direct abrogation in violation of the duties
and responsibilities of the public health organizations. In the past,
these bodies have acted as though their own activities and those of
the lead industries in health matters were science, and they could be
considered objectively in that sense.

Whether the best interests of public health have been served by
having public health agencies work jointly with representatives of
the lead alkyl industries in evaluating the hazards of lead alkyl to
public health is a question to be asked and answered.

When Muskie asked him if his classification into natural, typical, and
"contaminated" concentrations of lead in food and humans was a logical
approach to follow, Patterson's response was pointed:

"Not if your purpose is to sell lead."

MUSKIE: "Well, I don't think it is the purpose of the Public Service to sell lead."

PATTERSON: "That is why it is difficult to understand why the Public Health Service cooperated with the lead industry in issuing this report which fails to make this distinction."

Muskie was determined to throw Kehoe's industry perspective into contrast with the public health witnesses' position:

> . . . those representing the industry, the American petroleum industry and others, have told us that there is no evidence of increase in the past since sometime in the 1920s that create any cause for concern as to hazards from lead . . . Now what do you say on this and where is their analysis faulty?
>
> PATTERSON: The evidence for an increase in concentration the blood of people in American cities is clear. The difference, as I said, between the concentrations of lead in blood of people living in cities and outside of cities is that between 0.17 and 0.11 parts per million. The difference is not due to food . . . As I say from these known things we can predict that the people in the cities will have higher concentrations of lead in their blood as a consequence of their absorbing the greater amounts of lead and the difference is due to the greater concentration of lead in the air.

He attacked Kehoe's claim that levels that [sic] dropped in Cincinnati:

> . . . there is given on the back side of the page of data from which Dr. Kehoe quoted, another figure which shows the concentrations of lead in that very same city increased. This is data gotten from the National Air Sampling Network which is not the same organization that Dr. Kehoe represents. It shows an opposite trend. The point here is that kinds of data which purport to show that the concentrations of lead in the atmosphere of American cities is decreasing is rather invalid.

Industry had traditionally measured the prevalence of lead toxicity by counting deaths, or at least severe damage to the brain. Muskie raised the question of a larger pool of unrecognized toxic illnesses:

> Is it conceivable that there is something different in the deleterious effects on health from low-level exposure than from more concentrated exposure leading to classical lead poisoning?

PATTERSON: . . . when you expose an organism to a toxic substance it responds in a continuum, to continuously changing levels of exposure to this toxic substance. There is no abrupt change between a response and no response. Classical poisoning is just one extreme of the whole continuum of responses of an organism, human organism, to this toxic metal. There is no reason why this shouldn't be so.

Muskie's aggressive inquiry marked the government's shift away from complacency towards lead. The hearings established a new premise: that lead poisoning was not only a florid disease of workers, it could be an insidious, silent danger. The notion that lead poisoning was an all-or-nothing phenomenon was discredited and replaced by degrees of disease spread gradually across a continuum. Patterson had inserted the concept of the dose-response relationship into the debate. This was the concept that the PHS could no longer casually disregard and it would from then on play a central role in regulation of lead in gasoline.

Silent Lead Poisoning

In the late 1960s, the question of "silent" lead poisoning drew the attention of the civil rights and antipoverty movements, urban advocates, and environmentalists. In an important move, the PHS shifted responsibility for management of childhood lead poisoning to the Centers for Disease Control and in 1974 placed the lead program under Dr. Vernon Houk. The definition for lead poisoning was a level of lead in blood equal or greater than 60 µg per 100 ml of blood. Screening studies of the ostensibly normal children in Chicago, New York, and other cities reported that between 20 and 45% of children considered normal blood lead levels in the range of 40–50 µg/dl. Dr. Jane Lin Fu of the Department of Health, Education, and Welfare, who first raised the question of asymptomatic lead toxicity, reviewed studies (13). Some pediatricians began to think that if 60 µg/dl was toxic, it was dubious that 50 µ/dl was harmless.

In 1970, the Surgeon General called for early identification of children with "undue" lead exposure, the best locution the government could summon. His statement avoided the loaded term "poisoning" but indicated that this was probably more lead than a child should have. It also indirectly suggests that there was a "due" level of lead in blood. For the first time, research funds were allocated from federal sources to study the health impacts of lead on children. The industrial monopoly on scientific data was drawing to an end.

Ethyl's anxiety about sales was exacerbated by the new perspective on lead toxicity. This was not helped by an inning or two of corporate hardball. In 1962 Ethyl was bought by Albemarle Paper Manufacturing, and GM's interest in the [*sic*] Ethyl was liquidated. In 1970 GM announced that it would begin installing catalytic converters in its new models, and as a result, GM stated, it would be necessary to phase out lead in gasoline. To Ethyl's management this was a betrayal: ". . . it struck some people as incongruous—not to use a harsher word—for General Motors to sell half of what was essentially a lead additive firm for many millions and then to advocate annihilation of the lead antiknock business," wrote Ethyl's official biographer (2).

Badly shaken, Ethyl resolved to fight the growing environmental spirit in the United States, stating that it was "fully justified in speaking out for this additive, which had saved billions of dollars for the American economy and helped make possible the modern automobile." To combat lead regulation, it formed a defense team, titling it, with unconscious irony, the "Ethyl Air Conservation Group." The Group was staffed with Ethyl officials and members of the Hunton and Williams law firm. Lawrence Blanchard, a partner in Hunton and Williams and board member of Ethyl, headed the group. Ethyl's biographer captured this step in apocalyptic terms: "Blanchard, in effect, was appointed general in a war . . ."

The Seven Cities Study

In 1968 the PHS commissioned a large epidemiologic study of lead in the atmosphere, directed by Lloyd Tepper of Kettering Laboratory. Once again, questions were raised about the objectivity of the study, because of industry's participation and the fact that inner-city children were excluded from its sample. The planning group at the outset agreed that the results of this study would be withheld from the public until it was completed and reviewed.

Dr. John Goldsmith, Director of Epidemiology in the California Department of Health, and member of the California Air Resources Board (CARB), requested access to the data from Robert Horton, of the Environmental Protection Agency (EPA), to be used in open hearings on airborne lead by the CARB. Horton denied the request, even though some of the data Goldsmith wanted were from California and had been furnished to the EPA by Goldsmith's own group. Then, at the Air Resources Board hearings, Tepper rose to testify on behalf of industry, using his version of the proscribed Seven Cities data to argue against the hazards of airborne lead. Tepper was followed by testimony from Ethyl Corporation, Kettering Laboratories, and Nalco, another TEL producer. All of them used Seven Cities data. Despite this, in 1976 the CARB set a standard for air lead in California of $1.5\,\mu g/m^3$. California's action put increased pressure on EPA to develop a federal standard.

The National Academy of Sciences: Airborne Lead in Perspective

The Clean Air Act of 1970 directed the Environment Protection Agency to name each pollutant known to be dangerous and widespread and then, within 2 years, issue a standard that would define a safe level of exposure. Constructing a lead standard exposed the agency to its first encounter with serious controversy in rule-making. Kenneth Bridbord, an EPA physician and epidemiologist, quickly sent the EPA's administrator a report indicating that millions of Americans were breathing air with lead in excess of what was thought to be an acceptable threshold of $2\,\mu g/m^3$. EPA recoiled from issuing a standard for lead in air. Instead of writing a standard, it deferred to the National Academy of Sciences (NAS), contracting with them to conduct a survey of airborne lead, hoping that NAS would provide both guidance and authority the agency felt unwilling to supply (14).

From the beginning, NAS relied on its informal network of associates and colleagues to select committee members and, as a result, drew criticism from the public health community. Four well-qualified choices, eminent scientists with long experience in lead, were overlooked. Clair Patterson, Harry Schroeder at Dartmouth, who had conducted some of the only transgenerational studies of lead at low dose, and T. J Chow, who had published fundamental studies of atmospheric lead deposition in Greenland ice cores, were excluded. John Goldsmith, head of the California Health Department's Division of Epidemiology, who had published a groundbreaking study of the relationship between air lead levels and blood lead levels in *Science* (15) was omitted from the panel. All of these established scientists were seen by the NAS as alarmists.

The lead industry, in contrast, was handsomely represented on the panel of consultants. Kehoe and Lloyd Tepper came from the Kettering Laboratory. Kamran Habibi and John Perrard were from E.I. DuPont, and Gary Ter Haar came from Ethyl Corporation. Industry scientists were also granted major responsibility for writing sections of the draft. Gordon Stopps of DuPont, who was a member of the oversight committee on Biological Effects of Atmosphere Pollutants, was neither a member of the committee nor an appointed consultant. Nevertheless, he was assigned to write two critical sections of the report: adult epidemiology and lead alkyls. His earlier position on lead was a matter of record: in numerous earlier publications Stopps had stated that TEL was harmless (16).

Harriet Hardy, a widely respected expert in metal toxicity, complained about the imbalance and bias of the panel. T. J. Chow wrote about the propriety of asking industry employees to write chapters on their products. The Academy staff became defensive when questioned about the fairness of the selection process. One staff member told the *Science* magazine reporter covering the NAS selection process that Goldsmith and Schroeder were thought to be potentially disruptive to the work of the Committee (16). The Academy staffer responsible for this project responded to the question of industrial bias: "Rosters of committees and panels consist of people with high competence in specific fields regardless of where they work and the appointment is made with the understanding that the person is thought to serve as an individual and not as a representative of his organization . . ." This same understanding could not, however, extend to Patterson, Goldsmith, or Schroeder.

The NAS report "LEAD: Airborne Lead in Perspective" was a clear failure (17). It spent many pages on discussions of lead in plants and animals, while evading full examination of the specific questions for which it had been commissioned. It virtually ignored the Seven Cities Study, presenting it in one paragraph as a hasty afterthought. The report said that there were no conclusive data to show that atmospheric lead at concentrations below $2\,\mu g/m^3$ contributed to blood lead levels, nor was there any evidence to support toxicity at low levels of lead. The senior review committee of NAS treated the report with unusual harshness and gave failing grades. Because of its vagueness and unwillingness to grapple with lead in the air, the review committee chairman stated that the report "failed miserably to form any sort of a precise conclusion . . . There's no point in being a high-priced data collector."

Despite this caustic review, the ambiguities and bias in the NAS report provided the industry with a new instrument. They trumpeted it, proclaiming that the country's most prestigious scientific body had given TEL a clean bill of health and that any regulation of lead in gasoline was unsound and unnecessary. Once again progress in lead control had been damaged. On the day following the release Ethyl's stock increased by 20%.

EPA's negligence in monitoring the NAS committee was obvious; the agency was new to this controversial area and had internal conflicts about the need to regulate lead. As a result it failed to press the NAS to produce what it paid for: a clear statement about the dangers of lead in the air. Instead EPA took the equivocal language in the NAS report and used it to justify its failure to write the lead standard mandated by Congress.

A Dual Strategy for Regulating Lead in Gasoline

Congress recognized, when it wrote the Clean Air Act, that to control hydrocarbons and carbon monoxide in the exhaust, the catalytic converter was necessary. The catalyst was made of platinum, and platinum is effectively poisoned by lead. EPA now possessed two separate mechanisms through which to control lead in gasoline: protecting the platinum catalyst and protecting human health. Safeguarding the catalyst was easy work; it needed no evidence of adverse health effects. In 1972 EPA issued rules that each gas station have at least one lead-free pump to protect the platinum catalytic converter on new models.

EPA's medical officers continued to struggle for a separate health standard, fearing that if a substitute for platinum was discovered sometime in the future, lead would be returned to fuel. In 1973, EPA, recognizing that 200,000 tons of lead were blowing out of the exhaust of American cars each year, promulgated a regulation facing down lead content in all gasoline. Its target was to reduce lead in gasoline to 0.5 g/gal within 5 years (18).

The White House began its own private review of the issue and relied on the Office of Management and Budget (OMB) for direction (19). Within EPA a small staff of doctors and epidemiologists, handicapped on one hand by the NAS report and pressured on the other by the OMB, found themselves entangled in the struggle with a practiced and well-lawyered lead industry. The EPA administrator once again announced a delay in regulating. It appeared that this would go on indefinitely, when a young lawyer from the National Resources Defense Council, David Schoenbrod, filed suit against the EPA. His claim was upheld by the District Court of Appeals, who found that the administrator had illegally delayed and ordered him to set a standard (18).

The Office of Management and Budget, which had gained increased power under Nixon, conducted its own review and was in a strategic position to halt the process. Other intramural politics were at work. DHEW, which bore ill feelings toward the EPA for taking over some of its roles in health protection, expressed them by discrediting the EPA's health analysis before OMB. Meanwhile, the Arab oil crisis threatened (19).

In this setting, John Sawhill of OMB and John Quarles, deputy administrator of the EPA, met in the Executive Office Building to discuss the impact of lead removal on fuel stocks in the face of the looming oil crisis. The additive industry was skillfully exploiting the growing national anxiety about fuel supplies. EPA estimated the oil penalty from phasing lead out at 30,000 barrels per day. Industry's calculations were different and their public relations arm broadcast them. On December 2, 1973, a full-page ad appeared in the *New York Times* showing an oil barrel bearing an American flag pouring oil down a manhole. Its headline proclaimed that removing lead from gasoline would have the effect of dumping one million barrels of oil a day. Two days later it was published in the *Washington Post* (20).

Sawhill's deputy at OMB, Richard Fairbanks, threatened to veto the regulations, claiming that Melvin Laird, Counsel to President Nixon, said "those regulations would go out over my dead body." This turned out to be a bluff. Laird had no position on lead, and after some compromises by EPA on the timetable, the White House signed on (19).

On December 6, 1973, the final regulations calling for a phased reduction of lead in gasoline to protect health were released. Ethyl Corporation and DuPont sued in court, arguing that removing lead would cost an enormous amount of money and crude oil resources, that no one had been poisoned by lead in air, and that any changes in humans reported at lesser doses of lead were not actual health effects. The court upheld the industry, setting aside the regulations as "arbitrary and capricious." The EPA petitioned for rehearing. The earlier judgment was vacated and the EPA's regulations were upheld (21). Ethyl, PPG Industries, DuPont, NALCO Chemical, and the National Petroleum Refiners Association appealed to the Supreme Court, where they lost.

Setting a Standard

Still, by 1976, the EPA continued to show reluctance to bear down and enforce the regulations. There was no progress in reduction of lead in gasoline. Schoenbrod again went to court, and the EPA was ordered to set an ambient standard and "end the administrative foot dragging."

The statute specified that the first step in setting a standard is to collect and critically summarize the scientific knowledge about the pollutant. These data are assembled and evaluated in what is called a *Criteria Document*. The EPA staffers assigned to write the first draft had a severe tilt toward industry's position. They met with industry representatives, but refused to meet with Schoenbrod (18). Their draft contrasted strongly with other EPA position papers on airborne lead and concluded that an acceptable standard in the atmosphere was 5 $\mu g/m^3$, considerably higher than that found in most American cities.

David Shoenbrod sent me a copy of that draft and asked if I would review it and discuss it at a public meeting of the EPA's Science Advisory Board (SAB). The chemist on my team, Neil Maher, and I examined it and found its survey of the studies of lead's impact on children badly out of date and biased. To us it read as if written by an industry scientist. We wrote a strong critique and presented it at the SAB meeting in Arlington, Virginia. In addition to our testimony, Sergio Piomelli, a pediatric hematologist with considerable experience in treating lead-poisoned children, made a strong case to lower the permissible level of lead in air to 2 $\mu g/m^3$ or less. Two members of the SAB, Samuel Epstein, a professor of environmental health at Case Western Reserve University, and Ruth Levine, Dean of Graduate Studies at the Boston University School of Public Health, also had strong reservations, but the rest of the Board seemed acceptant of the 5 µg/m³ standard.

Almost completely silent during this process were the two academic consultants to EPA, Dr. Julian Chisholm and Dr. Paul Hammond. Chisholm was the dean of childhood lead poisoning. He had spent his career at the Johns Hopkins University Medical School and, more than anyone, had put the diagnosis and management of the disease on a solid footing. Hammond was a veterinarian and had published on the poisoning of cattle and horses near a smelter in Minnesota. On the strength of this he was appointed to chair the 1972 NAS study.

After 2 days of vigorous debate the tide of opinion slowly shifted, and the SAB told the authors of the document to return to the drawing board, discard the first draft, and submit a new revision. The original authors were removed and different writers were assigned. A second draft was completed in 1976. This draft was longer and not as obviously flawed, but it was still far from acceptable.

The SAB recommended that new consultants be appointed to the Criteria Document staff and instructed EPA staff to revise it once again. Piomelli and I were appointed, along with two industry representatives, Emmet Jacobs, a vice president for environmental affairs at DuPont, and Edward McCabe, a pediatrician who was a paid consultant to the International Lead Zinc Research Organization. We met with EPA staff in North Carolina in midsummer heat to hammer out the final version. Representing the EPA were two University of North Carolina faculty members: Lester Grant, a neurobiologist who had done some research on lead, and Paul Mushak, a metals toxicologist who had worked on lead and other pollutants. The six of us spent long sweltering days laying out our positions on the critical issue: the effects of lead at low dose on children. Jacobs and McCabe were at a disadvantage; they had less clinical experience in managing lead-exposed children than Piomelli and I and were not as familiar with the clinical literature. The health effects section was brought up to date to include the latest data.

Late one night after a long day's work, we all had dinner together at the home of an EPA staffer. After dinner and a liberal amount of red wine, I asked Jacobs why DuPont, with its wealth of excellent research chemists, hadn't developed a safer gasoline additive to replace TEL. Jacobs, who had matched my intake, told me that their economists had modeled the future sales of leaded gasoline and projected that the consumption of gasoline would soon level off and perhaps decline. Given such a projection, the company would not invest $100 million in research and development funds.

I learned a valuable lesson that night: the entire debate about scientific studies, about the health risks for children, was merely a shadow play.

The real decision had been made by DuPont's economists. Their plan was clear: don't budge on TEL and seek medical and environmental arguments to support the choice.

The Criteria Document for lead was published in December 1977 and called for a standard of $1.5\,\mu g/m^3$. In some ways it signaled a minor revolution. It stated that lead in air and in dust was a significant source for human exposure and that brain damage occurred in individuals who showed no symptoms (22). Hearings were held on the document that summer. During the hearings, there was a moment of surprise. The two former EPA consultants, Hammond and Chisholm, testified, but now in a different role. They now appeared as witnesses for the lead industry and testified that the analyses in the Criteria Document that they had worked on were faulty. The new Criteria Document was accepted and was then used by the Air Office of EPA to determine a standard. Another step toward the removal of lead from gasoline had been taken.

The Attempt to Put Lead Back into Gasoline

The lead phasedown was by all measures of striking success. With the new standard in place, and the gradual retirement of old cars that ran on leaded fuel, air lead levels began to fall. In 1977 air lead levels in Philadelphia ranged between 1.3 and $1.6\,\mu g/m^3$. In 1980 the concentrations were between 0.3 in $0.4\,\mu g/m^3$. Similar trends were observed in most major cities.

In June of 1980, Lead Industries Association [LIA] petitioned EPA to rescind the regulation, claiming that a study of atmospheric lead in Idaho upon which the regulation relied had contained a serious error. The study in question examined the relationship between air and blood lead levels in the vicinity of a large lead mine and smelter in Kellogg, Idaho (23). The authors, Anthony Yankel and Ian von Lindern, originally estimated that a $1\,\mu g/m^3$ increase in atmospheric lead would increase blood lead by $2\,\mu g/dl$. Yankel later claimed to have found an error in calculations that overestimated the air lead effect. When the case was heard in court, the original calculations were upheld. Yankel, it turned out, no longer worked for the Idaho Health Department. He had taken a job with the lead industry. The judge denied the LIA claim and recommended that the Department of Justice investigate Yankel's behavior (24). The standard had withstood another skirmish.

In 1980 Ronald Reagan, who succinctly expressed his environmental concerns by saying "If you've seen one tree, you've seen them all," was elected to the presidency. By Executive Order, without consulting Congress, he made the OMB the clearinghouse for all government regulations. OMB was given the power to require sweeping analyses of proposed regulations and by doing so delay and halt any that it found objectionable. Reagan appointed Ann[e] Gorsuch to the post of EPA Administrator and assigned his Vice-President, George Bush, a former oil man, to head the Task Force on Regulatory Reform.

Reagan wasted no time. The EPA's budget was cut, and its enforcement section was reorganized out of existence. In 1980, 1,300 cases had been referred for enforcement. One year later, 59 cases were referred. The agency was virtually toothless. Many career EPA staffers in middle management positions were squeezed out or forced to resign. Experienced professionals were replaced by political appointees. The agency was in a confused shambles.

OMB canvassed industries to determine which regulatory programs they felt needed revision. Deregulating lead in gasoline was the first item on the Bush Task Force Agenda. Noting that air lead levels were dropping as older cars were replaced by catalyst-equipped vehicles, DuPont representatives called upon EPA to rescind the lead regulations.

OMB increased the pressure on the EPA to do something about the complaints of the small refiners. Boyden Gray, counsel to Bush and to the Regulatory Task Force, promised that EPA would reexamine the phasedown and consider relief. Richard Wilson, EPA's acting director of enforcement for air, held 32 meetings with refiner representatives to discuss their problems, but none with public health of [sic] public interest officials.

The definition of a *refiner* included those who bought low-lead fuel and mixed it with high-lead-content gasoline. These were refiners without refineries; they made large profits simply by blending fuel stocks. The adjective "small" was also misleading. It referred to those who processed less than 50,000 barrels per day. An EPA staffer defined a "small refiner" as "a short man with pockets full of $1,000 bills" (25).

In December of 1981, Senator Harrison Schmitt arranged a visit of officials of a New Mexico oil refinery, Thriftway, with Administrator Gorsuch. Thriftway executives complained that lowering the amount of lead in gasoline was producing losses of $100,000 a month for them and that they faced eventual bankruptcy. They requested an individual waiver of the regulations on the basis of financial need. Gorsuch told them that if she granted it, she would be forced to give the same dispensation to other refiners. But, she said, a relaxation of the lead phasedown regulations was in the offing, and that it did not make sense to use EPA's limited enforcement powers when the lead regulations were to be changed. The Thriftway people then asked for written assurances that they would not be prosecuted for exceeding the standard. Gorsuch demurred, but told them that they had been assured by the Administrator of the EPA (26). As she left the room, she said to Senator Schmitt's administrative assistant, "I can't tell your client to break the law, but I hope they got the message" (25).

A firestorm ensued over the Administrator's statement that she would not enforce her agency's own regulations, and the episode became the subject of wide publicity capped by a *Doonesbury* cartoon. Congressman Toby Moffett asked the Inspector General to investigate whether any laws had been violated. In February of 1982, EPA bent to OMB and announced the projected relaxation of the regulations that Gray had promised and Gorsuch predicted.

Congressman Moffett, chairman of the Subcommittee on the Environment and EPA, held hearings on the lead phasedown in April 1982. Public health professionals and private physicians, including Vernon Houk, Sergio Piomelli, and myself, turned out to testify on the unsoundness of such an action. The EPA hearings also marked the debut of Dr. Claire Ernhart as the lead industry spokesperson, testifying that the evidence for lead's threat to child health was exaggerated.

The Gorsuch-Thriftway episode had the effect of waking up EPA's demoralized staff. In some ways this became one of EPA's finer moments. EPA's own data indicated that 200,000 children would be poisoned if the rules were relaxed. Despite the purges of their ranks, the deep cuts in their budget, and their damaged morale, EPA's professionals could not countenance inflicting such harm on the nation's children. They took a stand against rescinding the regulations.

Considerable antagonism grew between the large and the small refiners on the need to regulate. Many large fuel companies, including Exxon, Amoco, and Phillips Petroleum, supported the continuance of the phasedown. They pointed out that they had fought against regulation, but, faced with the inevitable, had invested hundreds of million dollars to retrofit their refineries. They were now in compliance and strongly protested granting any competitive advantage to those who had not spent the money to retool.

Congressman Moffett demanded that the president discipline Gorsuch for encouraging refiners to break the law. While the hearings were taking place, Jack Anderson reported that a tanker load of high-lead gasoline purchased from China by a California refiner was on the high seas approaching the West Coast. The lawyer for the refiner who had chartered the ship, and who had served as chairman of Reagan's fundraising committee in California, had visited him in the White House to press for relaxed regulations.

A bipartisan group of 31 congressman joined by 13 senators from both parties petitioned the White House to hold the line on the phasedown. On August 15, 1982, Anne Gorsuch seemed to have experienced a conversion. The *Environmental Health Letter* carried this headline "EPA Reverses Position, Toughens Regulations on Lead in Gasoline."

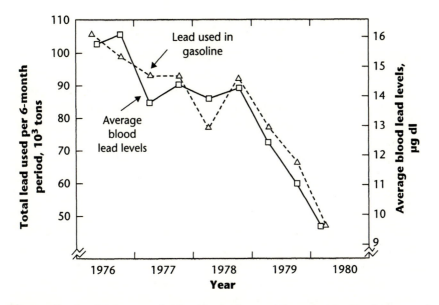

Figure 2 Parallel decreases in blood lead values and the amounts of lead consumed in gasoline between 1976 and 1980. Source: USEPA/Environmental Criteria and Assessment Office (1986).

OMB's move on EPA served to highlight industry's role in influencing health-based regulations and sharpen the focus on the health impacts of airborne lead. In the wake of the administration's embarrassment, the relaxation of the phasedown was quietly buried. The president of the National Petroleum Refiners Association complained bitterly that "EPA is reneging on an implicit promise in the present regulatory scheme." Lawrence Blanchard, vice chairman of Ethyl, and "general" of the company's antiregulatory campaign, who had called EPA "novelists" and "bastards" at an Ethyl stockholders meeting (27), fired another of his smallbore expostulations at the EPA hearings:

> It was misleading at best and fraudulent at worst to talk about symptoms and horrors of lead poisoning. That is just like talking about the horrors of gassing World War I soldiers with chlorine at a hearing as to whether we should chlorinate to purify drinking water (28).

Between 1976 and 1980, the amount of lead consumed in gasoline production dropped by 50% (see Fig. 2). The blood lead level of the average American dropped by 37%. In 1984 EPA's analysts calculated that the benefits of the phasedown exceeded the costs by $700 million.

The Second Criteria Document

In 1982, the EPA was mandated by statute to update and revise its 1977 airborne lead regulations. By this time, a separate Criteria office had been created to read these documents. Lester Grant, a consultant to EPA in the first lead document, was appointed director. A substantial increase in the budget for the lead document was allotted, a panel of external writers was appointed, and a greatly enlarged group of consultants and reviewers was appointed. Important changes had taken place since the publication of the first document. Air lead levels had come down quite sharply, and considerable data had been collected correlating air lead levels, gasoline lead emissions, and blood lead levels. At the time the first Criteria Document was written, there were only hints that lesser levels of lead were toxic to children. In the 5 intervening years, a number of studies had been published showing that children with lower levels of lead had lower IQ scores, language and attentional problems and behavioral disturbances. The work of my group at Harvard was one of these (29), and it was followed by data from England showing similar changes. Claire Ernhart, who had published an early study showing that lead decreased (30), and who now was supported by International Lead Zinc Research Organization, tried to recant her earlier conclusions that low-dose lead was toxic.

The EPA now had a growing health database. The National Academy of Sciences had convened a new committee, which came to much stronger conclusions about the hazards of lead in the atmosphere (31).

To the lead industry this new standard was another crucial battle, and they planned their attack around three salients: (1) The decline in blood lead levels was not due to removing lead from gasoline; the close correlation between gasoline sales and blood lead levels was not causal. (2) While lead at high doses was toxic, there was no solid evidence that at lower doses, humans suffered any effects. The studies of lead in humans were flawed, and the animal work was irrelevant. (3) Not only was lead toxicity overrated, lead was probably an essential trace element.

After thorough review of the literature and the many submissions from external authorities, EPA concluded that the relationship between gasoline production and air lead levels was causal. "The contribution of gasoline lead to total atmospheric emissions has remained high, at 89% . . . Between 1975 and 1984, the lead consumed in gasoline has decreased 73%, while the corresponding composite maximum quarterly average of ambient air lead decreased 71%." See Fig. 3. Industry arguments that this was a spurious relationship were futile.

In the meetings of the EPA Criteria Committees, Ernhart and I represented the two polar positions on health effects in children. We were asked to critique each other's papers before the hearing panel. Ernhart

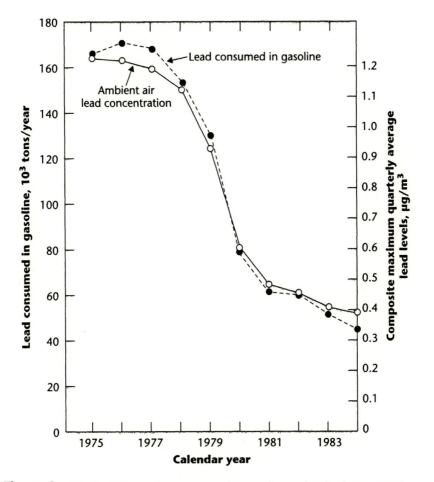

Figure 3 Relation between lead consumed in gasoline and air lead concentrations.
Source: USEPA/Environmental Criteria and Assessment Office (1986).

raised the now traditional criticisms: that I had not controlled for other factors that affect development and that causality worked in the other direction: children with low IQ may ingest more lead. I pointed out the complete covariate control is impossible to achieve, but that many studies controlling for differing factors found a lead effect. This consistency among many studies published at that time was strong evidence that the lead effect was real and not produced by confounders, and this was strongly buttressed by animal studies, which showed similar changes and effectively destroyed the reverse causality hypothesis.

Ernhardt had criticized me for incomplete control, but in her 1974 study she had not controlled for an important factor, socioeconomic status. I pointed this out. She responded that this was because all her subjects were from a single class, welfare parents. I had brought her paper, along with others, with me to the hearing and was able to quote it to her: "they [the parents] ranged from managers, clerical workers, skilled and unskilled workers to service workers and welfare recipients (30).

Lester Grant then appointed a special committee to review both our studies in-depth. The committee consisted of three psychologists, including Sandra Scarr, Lawrence Kupper, a statistician, Paul Mushak, a toxicologist, and Lester Grant. Their draft report asserted that no conclusions could be drawn from either study about the health effects of lead at low dose. I received my copy and counted 11 errors in the committee report, all of which biased against my study. I wired Grant that if he did not correct them, I would insist that he send an errata sheet to everyone who received a copy of the draft. The errors were corrected, but the conclusions were allowed to stand. With financial and statistical support from EPA, I re-analyzed the data to address the special committee's criticisms that had been the source of their assertion of no conclusion. The reanalyses, using EPA's suggestions, showed an even stronger lead effect than I had published earlier. I published this as a letter to *Science* (32). On April 27, 1984, I presented the three analyses to the Clean Air Advisory Committee (CASAC), the highest level of peer review in the EPA.

After CASAC heard my presentation, they declared that my paper was sound and qualified to be included in the Criteria Document and used in the standard setting. Ernhart's paper recanting her earlier findings was also included, but EPA's conclusions differed from her interpretation: ". . . it is notable that an assertion [in Ernhart's paper] between lead and lower Verbal Index scores was nevertheless observed across several of the analyses (at p values ranging from 0.04 to 0.10) and that an association between preschool lead levels and General Cognitive Index scores approached significance at $p < 0.09$." EPA concluded that her study continued to show a lead effect, despite her persistent efforts to discredit it (33).

The sum of data on human health effects dwarfed what had been known in 1977, when the first Criteria Document was issued. The second (1980) NAS report this time was much more declarative about the health effects of lead at low dose.

> The evidence is convincing that exposure to levels of lead commonly encountered in urban environments constitutes a significant hazard of detrimental biological effects in children, especially those less than 3 years old. Some small fraction of the population experiences particularly intense exposures and is at severe risk.

The EPA's Criteria draft in 1986 firmly agreed:

> . . . lead has diverse biological effects in humans and animals . . . the developing organism seems to be more sensitive than the mature individual.

The lead industry drew its last arrow and in doing so exposed their desperation. In the 1970s they had supported a series of investigations attempting to demonstrate that lead was an essential trace element. This was done by growing rodents in lead-free environments on synthetic diets made to contain no lead and comparing them to animals raised on an ordinary lead-containing diet and comparing growth (34). These studies had little credibility. This time they brought two German investigators to EPA to argue their claim for lead's essentiality. This position simply did not withstand investigation by an independent review committee. They criticized the statistical analysis and noted that the method of obtaining blood for analysis was open to contamination and that the animals may have suffered other deprivations. In order to achieve a lead-free diet, the investigators may have deprived the animals of other essential trace elements such as selenium and chromium. They added calcium EDTA to the rat chow. EDTA is an agent long used to treat lead toxicity. This drug also removes other minerals along with lead, resulting in other dietary deficiencies (35).

EPA had traveled a long way since the first *Criteria* draft of 1972. The evidence documenting lead toxicity was now strong enough that the agency, citing the "overwhelming evidence of the threat to humans," proposed to cut lead in gasoline by 91% in 1986 and to achieve a total ban by 1995.

Long accustomed to having their way in regulatory proceedings, the industry was ill-equipped to lose. In a plaintive tone, they blamed the conspiracy of a small group of scientists, environmentalists, and the press. "Ethyl vowed to fight the EPA goals 'in every appropriate manner'" related the *New York Times* (36):

> "We feel wronged at this stage of the game," said Jerome Cole, president of the International Lead Zinc Research Organization. "Five or six scientists, together with the rabid environmentalists, have used the media very skillfully putting over their views, but there's a lot of responsible opinion that doesn't support that." According to Donald R. Lynam, the director of air conservation at Ethyl Corporation:

> "Unfortunately, the atmosphere we're now in prohibits objective scientists from coming forward. And why should they, when they would be crucified by the press, the EPA and the environmentalists."

The payoff for taking lead out of gasoline exceeded the predictions of the most convinced lead advocate. Lead levels in children's and adults' blood continued to drop in direct relationship to the reduction in lead in gasoline. The average American child's blood lead level in 1976 was 13.7µg/dl. In 1988 the Government estimated that 3–4 million American children had blood lead levels greater than 15 μg/dl, the level then assumed to be toxic (37). Six years later, in 1994, it was estimated that 600,000 children had blood lead levels in that range (38). The removal of lead from gasoline spared as many as 3.4 million children from growing up with hazardous concentrations of the toxic metal in their bodies.

Acknowledgements

I am grateful to Julian Chisholm, Jane Lin Fu, Kenneth Bridbord, and Joe Schwarz for unstinting discussions on their roles in lead regulation. Cliff Davidson shared some of his archival data on Clair Patterson with me. I thank John Balaban, Thomas Kane, Paul Mushak, Roberta Needleman, and Ellen Silbergeld for careful review of drafts of this paper.

SOURCE

Needleman HL. 2000. The removal of lead from gasoline: Historical and personal reflections. *Environ Res* 84 Section A: 20–35. Copyright 2000 by *Environmental Research*. Reprinted with permisison of Elsevier.

Global Climate Change and Infectious Diseases
(1991)

Robert Shope

The effects of global climate change on infectious diseases are hypothetical until more is known about the degree of change in temperature and humidity that will occur. Diseases most likely to increase in their distribution and severity have three-factor (agent, vector, and human being) and four-factor (plus vertebrate reservoir host) ecology. *Aedes aegypti* and *Aedes albopictus* mosquitoes may move northward and have more rapid metamorphosis with global warming. These mosquitoes transmit dengue virus, and *Aedes aegypti* transmits yellow fever virus. The faster metamorphosis and a shorter extrinsic incubation of dengue and yellow fever viruses could lead to epidemics in North America. *Vibrio cholera* is harbored persistently in the estuaries of the U.S. Gulf Coast. Over the past 200 years, cholera has become pandemic seven times with spread from Asia to Europe, Africa, and North America. Global warming may lead to changes in water ecology that could enhance similar spread of cholera in North America. Some other infectious diseases such as La-Crosse encephalitis and Lyme disease are caused by agents closely dependent on the integrity of their environment. These diseases may become less prominent with global warming because of anticipated modification of their habitats. Ecological studies will help us to understand more fully the possible consequences of global warming. New and more effective methods for control of vectors will be needed.

The influence of climate in the debate on infectious diseases has been a subject of debate, speculation, and serious study for centuries. Jacob Henle (1) stated in his 1840 treatise *On Miasma and Contagia* "Heat and moisture favor the production and propagation of the infusoria and the molds, as well as the miasmata and contagia, therefore miasmatic-contagious diseases are often endemic in warm moist regions and epidemic in the wet summer months." He included cholera and yellow fever among the miasmatic-contagious diseases, and indeed these two diseases may have a resurgence, as global warming materializes.

For a discussion of global climate change and its possible effect on infectious diseases I shall deal necessarily in hypothetical terms. There is no way of knowing for certain what effect, if any, a rise in temperature and a change in rainfall patterns will have. It is feasible, however, to review the literature and point out where warmer temperatures and increased or decreased rainfall favor transmission of certain pathogenic infections; then the epidemiology of these infections can be dissected to see where the temperature and rainfall are critical to the success of the agent.

It is convenient to adopt the terminology used by Jacques May (2) in his book *The Ecology of Human Disease*. He considers each transmissible disease complex. Those that involve only the causative agent and man are two-factor complexes; those that involve in addition a vector are three-factor complexes; and those that involve yet an intermediate host are four-factor complexes. The ambient temperature will have an influence on each of the factors in the complex. Many of the two-factor complexes are not limited by temperature and therefore are distributed anywhere in the world that the agent is introduced and that is inhabited by people. Examples are poliomyelitis and measles. The distribution, prevalence, and severity of these diseases are not expected to be modified by global climate change. One could argue that mortality rates of measles and poliomyelitis are higher in the tropics than in the temperate zones, and therefore these diseases will become more severe. The increased severity in the tropics is probably related to poorer socioeconomic conditions. To the extent that global warming increases poverty and its associated ills, the two-factor complexes will also be affected. The three- and four-factor complexes by definition include the vector-borne diseases and zoonoses. Only rarely is a given vector-born disease distributed everywhere people live. These diseases are usually limited in their distribution, either by the range of their vector, or by that of a reservoir vertebrate host. The vector and host in turn are limited in range directly or indirectly by temperature and rainfall.

Yellow Fever and Dengue

If I had to guess which vector-borne diseases would pose the greatest threat in case of global warming in North America, I would say that those transmitted by *Aedes aegypti* mosquitoes—yellow fever and dengue. Both diseases are caused by viruses of the family Flaviviridae. There is a single yellow fever serotype and four serotypes of dengue. In the days of sailing ships, *Aedes aegypti* mosquitoes flourished in the water storage vessels on board and were transported each spring north to the Atlantic coastal cities. Dengue in Philadelphia was described in 1780 by Benjamin Rush, and yellow fever epidemics occurred as far north as Boston. This history is important in the context of global warming because the limiting factor in these epidemics was the onset of cold weather. *Aedes aegypti* is killed rapidly at freezing temperatures; 62% of adults died when exposed for 1 hr at 32°F (3), and in a study in Georgia, most larvae died when average weekly ground temperature dropped to 48°F (4).

The northernmost winter survival of *Aedes aegypti* is now about 35° N latitude, or the latitude of Memphis, Tennessee. This distribution is predicted with global warming to move northward and encompass additional large population centers, the numbers depending on how much warming occurs. In addition, the development of mosquito larvae is faster in warm climates than cold ones, and thus with global warming, the mosquito will become a transmitting adult earlier in the season.

The extrinsic incubation period of dengue and yellow fever viruses also is dependent on temperature. Within a wide range of temperature, the warmer the ambient temperature, the shorter the incubation period from the time the mosquito imbibes the infective blood until the mosquito is able to transmit by bite. The implication is that with warmer temperatures in the United States, not only would there be a wider distribution of *Aedes aegypti* and faster mosquito metamorphosis, but also the viruses of dengue and yellow fever would have a shorter extrinsic incubation and thus would cycle more rapidly in the mosquito. A more rapid cycle would increase the speed of epidemic spread.

Persons infected with dengue are entering the United States on a regular basis. In 1987, the diagnosis was confirmed by the Centers for Disease Control in 18 cases by laboratory examination (5). These persons were ill in 10 states and the District of Columbia, and all were presumably infected outside the United States. Three of these were from Florida and Georgia, states with *Aedes aegypti*. Table 1 [Not shown, Ed.] shows the numbers of reported cases of dengue infection over an 11-year period. All four serotypes have been recognized. Importation of dengue cases continues; as recently as 2 months before this conference, we identified dengue type I virus from the blood of a man returning to New Haven, Connecticut, from Thailand. We isolated the same serotype simultaneously from the blood of his traveling companion hospitalized at New York Hospital.

Another vector of dengue virus, the Asian tiger mosquito, *Aedes albopictus*, has recently been introduced to the United States from Asia. This mosquito has established itself in scattered foci as far north as 42° N latitude. With global climate change, predictably this vector will become more prevalent and extend its range even further north, thus compounding the risk of dengue transmission.

One may argue that global climate change will be associated with large areas of drought, thus *Aedes aegypti* will not have sufficient water in which to breed. Paradoxically, this mosquito thrives both in wet and dry climate. In dry areas, people store water in their homes. The mosquito is domestic and breeds readily in cisterns and water storage jars.

How serious are yellow fever and dengue? Yellow fever is a febrile hemorrhagic disease characterized by hepatic and renal failure. Between 20 and 50% of victims with a severe form died, although recovery, when it occurs, is almost always complete. Dengue is usually a nonfatal illness with fever, rash, and protracted malaise. A severe form of dengue with hemorrhagic fever and shock syndrome is described principally in persons suffering a second infection with a different serotype. Most of the hemor-rhagic fever cases are in children, and the case fatality rate is about 5%. An effective vaccine is available for yellow fever, but there is no specific preventive immunization for dengue.

To summarize, we know the following: a) *Aedes aegypti* mosquitoes are prevalent in the southern United States as far north as latitude 35° N. Temperature is a factor limiting northward spread. This species thrives in both wet and dry climates. b) *Aedes albopictus* mosquitoes have recently been introduced into the U.S. And range as far north as latitude 42° N. c) *Aedes aegypti* is an effective vector of yellow fever, and both mosquito species are effective vectors of dengue. The extrinsic incubation period of dengue and yellow fever viruses is shortened by higher ambient tempera-tures, leading to more rapid amplification of epidemic spread. d) All four serotypes of dengue virus have been introduced into the United States in recent years, and introduction is a regular occurrence that can be ex-pected to continue. e) Yellow fever and dengue are serious diseases. There is no vaccine for dengue.

Cholera

Let me turn now to a very different disease, cholera. It is different be-cause it is considered to be a two-factor complex—agent and human being. Cholera behaves ecologically, however, like a three-factor com-plex. There is growing evidence that a reservoir for this disease exists in bays and estuaries and that such a reservoir encompasses the Gulf Coast of the United States (6).

Cholera is characterized by profuse, watery diarrhea leading to loss of body salts and severe dehydration. The disease is rapidly fatal in a high percentage of patients if fluid and salt replacement is not immediately available. The causative agent of epidemic cholera is a bacterium, *Vibrio cholerae* serotype 01, that is motile and grows aerobically at 37°C.

Cholera has been known for centuries in the delta of the Brahmapu-tra and Ganges rivers. Since the beginning of the nineteenth century there have been seven pandemics in which the *Vibrio cholerae* spread rap-idly from endemic foci, usually in Asia, Africa, Europe, and sometimes to North America. Once an epidemic starts, transmission is by fecal-oral spread from carriers recovered from the disease and from asymptomatic, infected persons.

Since 1973, repeated episodes of cholera in persons living in the Gulf Coast focus of Louisiana and Texas, and in persons consuming raw oys-ters from Louisiana, have been recorded. In August 1988, cholera oc-curred in a man in Colorado who ate oysters harvested in a bay off the coast of Louisiana (7). Between August and October of 1988, persons in five other states developed cholera, presumably from oysters harvested in the same area.

Comparison of the cholera toxin gene sequences using a DNA probe (8) confirmed that the strains of *Vibrio cholerae* coming from Louisiana were very similar to each other over a span of several years, and that these isolates differed from those of other parts of the world. Thus the evidence is strong that there is a continuing focus of the agent in Louisiana and that the multiple episodes of disease do not represent repeated introductions.

What does cholera have to do with global climate change? Louisiana has 40% of the coastal wetlands. With a rise in sea level and perhaps diminished river flow rates, the bays and estuaries of Louisiana can be expected to undergo major modifications. The temperature, pH, salinity, and composition of plant and animal life may well change drastically. The focus of *Vibrio cholerae* may thrive or may disappear as a result of these changes; we cannot count on its disappearance, however.

May (2) has plotted the areas of cholera expansion in pandemics of the nineteenth century. These were summer outbreaks and lay between summer isotherms 60° and 80°F in summer isohyets of 2 to 4 inches per month of rain. Little is known about the relation of *Vibrio cholerae* to the ecology of estuaries harboring the agent in the United States. Colwell and associates (9) have made a start. So far, no aquatic animal reservoir has been found, although persistence in shellfish for several weeks has been demonstrated. A better understanding of the ecology would help us predict the effects of global climate change and prepare us to react.

Other Diseases

Dengue, yellow fever, and cholera are not the only diseases that probably will be affected. Predictions of the effects of global warming include relatively severe modifications of some of our forests. As forest habitats decline, so will many of the more fragile species of insect vectors in vertebrate hosts of parasitic, bacterial, and viral infections. We may, for instance, experience a gradual decline in prevalence of LaCrosse encephalitis virus that depends in part on tree-holes of hardwood forests for breeding of its vector, *Aedes triseriatus*, and for maintenance of its vertebrate hosts, squirrels and chipmunks. We may also experience a decline in Lyme disease, caused by *Borrelia burgdorferi*, a spirochete transmitted by the tick, *Ixodes dammini*. Tick populations are dependent in their adult stage on deer for blood meals [although deer population reduction does not always lead to reduce tick populations (10)], and deer populations are dependent at least in part on forests for browsing and cover.

Finally, one must consider the possibility of emergence of new infectious diseases. New diseases have continually appeared, and there is no reason to doubt they will continue. Lyme disease, first recognized in 1975 (11), is now the most prevalent tick-born disease in the United States. The agents of such diseases are not actually new. They have been present in natural wildlife cycles, and it is the ecology that changes, bringing the agent in contact with humans.

The relatively rapid ecologic changes that are now predicted set the stage for a speeding up of the process. As change occurs, creatures extend their distribution and overlap occurs. In the special case of segmented genome viruses, ecological overlap of populations creates an abundant opportunity for reassortment of genes that could increase the virulence of the progeny virus (12). There is no way to anticipate these events, but their potential argues for maintaining a strong biomedical infrastructure and watching closely for new diseases.

Recommendations

What can we do now to prepare for the changes in climate that are expected? I have used examples of infectious diseases that may increase in prevalence or severity. Each of these depends on a reservoir, either a vector, a vertebrate host, or an environmental source, for its maintenance. We know from experience that these diseases have the potential to become epidemic when the ecology changes. We do not know how the ecology will change over the next 50 years, nor do we know enough about the ecological factors essential for the generation of epidemics of each disease.

The first recommendation, therefore, emphasizes the importance of ecological studies. These should be multidisciplinary, involving botany (including forestry), zoology, entomology, microbiology, hydrology, climatology, and epidemiology. The information we need to project what will happen with climate change can best be acquired in the field, studying survival and adaptation, especially at the fringe of the distribution of species of plants, vertebrate animals, and arthropods. Confirmatory laboratory studies will also be needed, especially of arthropod vectors and the interaction of infectious agents with the vector. These laboratory studies will involve survival of the vector and infectious agent under changed temperature and humidity and ability of the agent to multiply or go through its development cycle in the vector under changed conditions. The ecology of water systems that harbor cholera organisms should also be studied. With the information gained, we should be in a better position to project what will happen with specific diseases after global climate change.

The second recommendation relates to arthropod-born disease agents. We need research on the means of control of vectors. The rationale is that whatever climate and ecologic change occurs, we can anticipate an increase in some vector-borne diseases. The only generic defense (other than health education) will be control of vectors.

The study of dengue reported here was sponsored by National Institutes of Health grant AI 01984, U. S. Army grant DMAD 17–87G7005, and the World Health Organization.

SOURCE

Shope R. 1991. Global climate change and infectious diseases. *Environ Health Perspect* 96:171–74. Reprinted with permission *of Environmental Health Perspectives*.

CHAPTER 5

OCCUPATIONAL HEALTH

I learned in the early part of my career that labor must bear the cross for others' sins, must be the vicarious sufferer for the wrongs that others do.
—Mary Harris "Mother" Jones (1837–1930), American labor organizer

When a man tells you that he got rich through hard work, ask him: 'Whose?'
—Don Marquis (1878–1937), American humorist

IN THE EARLY 1950S, THE MEDICAL director of one of the leading British asbestos companies, John Knox, approached a young English epidemiologist, Richard Doll, for help with some statistical analyses on the mortality experienced by workers in Knox's company. Both men were stunned at the extent to which asbestos workers died compared to the general population. Doll was working on a paper reporting their findings when Knox told him to cease because his company did not want the results published. Doll would hear none of it and submitted the paper to the *British Journal of Industrial Medicine* with himself as the sole author. The publication of Doll's paper in 1955 broke the more than decade-long effort by the international asbestos industry to suppress any report linking asbestos exposure with cancer. It also set in motion a series of events that 25 years later led to bankruptcy of that industry, the establishment of governmental occupational health surveillance efforts in the United States, and various legal actions extending beyond the asbestos industry. The establishment of societal norms requiring disclosure of research results also dates back to Doll's paper. More than a half century after it appeared in print, the ripples from Doll's singular act of defiance continued to resonate within public health, most prominently in the occupational health arena.

EARLY TWENTIETH CENTURY OCCUPATIONAL HEALTH ACTIVITIES

The study of occupation as a source of illness and disease predates the development of the modern public health movement. The seventeenth-century Italian physician Bernardo Ramazzini described the hazards observed for workers in 52 occupations in his classic *De Morbis Artificum Diatriba* (Diseases of Workers).

In the nineteenth century, sanitary physicians such as Edward Headlam Green-how in England and Louis-René Villermé in France established occupation as a contributing factor for the development of disease, particularly tuberculosis. During the early part of the twentieth century, concerns about occupation as a contributing factor for various pulmonary conditions resulted in the identification of pneumoconioses, especially coal worker's pneumoconiosis and silicosis. New methods of diagnosing these conditions were developed, including x-rays, which brought to light an elevated mortality risk for silico-tuberculosis.

Silicosis, in particular, was increasing rapidly in the United States due to the growth of heavy industry. Indeed, one of the worst U.S. industrial disasters occurred at Gauley Creek, West Virginia, during the late 1920s. At that time, Union Carbide decided to divert the New River to better harness it for hydroelectric power at a new plant the company was building nearby. The river was to run through a three-mile tunnel drilled through Gauley Mountain. During the construction, the workers mined through large amounts of silica without any form of respiratory protection. An investigation by the U.S. House of Representatives concluded that what happened at Gauley Creek was a disaster created by industry's utter disregard for the workers, most of whom were black and unskilled. Various estimates place the number who died from silicosis from Gauley Creek at about 1,000 of the more than 2,000 workers in the tunnel. Despite what we now know about the dangers of silicosis, the disease remains the most common occupational disease globally.

Concerns about pneumoconiosis–asbestosis arose in the 1920s and 1930s. Frederick Hoffman, an actuary with the Prudential Insurance Company and the founder of the American Society for the Control of Cancer (now the American Cancer Society), called attention to the morbidity and mortality associated with occupational exposure to asbestos. Many asbestos companies feared the liabilities if asbestos exposure also increased the risk of tuberculosis. These fears became particularly acute during the Great Depression, when many workers with silicosis and silico-tuberculosis pressed workers' compensation claims against their employers. The asbestos industry's response was simple: deny and suppress any information that would validate the link. It was, in fact, the industry's concerns about workers' compensation claims during the Great Depression that framed the development of occupational health during the twentieth century.

PNEUMOCONIOSES, X-RAYS, AND ACCEPTABLE LIMITS OF EXPOSURE

Historically, tuberculosis was a major cause of morbidity and mortality among blue-collar men, though the link with occupation was not well understood. Coal mining was one of the basic occupations underpinning the Industrial Revolution in Britain, and miners there developed a form of tuberculosis with its own name—miner's phthisis. Medical researcher Philip D'Arcy Hart gathered information on miner's phthisis in Britain between 1920 and 1940 and demonstrated that the disease was a form of silicosis. Indeed, its incidence was correlated with the silica content of the soil in which the miners worked.

During the interwar period, Coal Worker's Pneumoconiosis (CWP) also emerged as a well-defined entity: the inhalation of coal dust resulted in specific scarring of the lungs. CWP was accepted as a real entity in Britain, but it was resisted as a diagnosis in the United States, possibly because of the economic implications. That is, if the disease were a form of pneumoconiosis, it would have to be a basis for workers' compensation claims. Thus, it took almost three-quarters of a century before CWP was established as a basis for workers' compensation claims in the United States, and it required national legislation in order to cover the disease.

Two developments fostered the identification of CWP as a distinct disease. First, pre-existing knowledge about silicosis allowed physicians to compare the clinical presentation of miners with CWP to an already known entity. Second, the development of x-rays facilitated the diagnosis of pneumoconioses to a degree unfathomable by physicians in the nineteenth century and earlier. X-rays allowed physicians to map areas of pulmonary fibrosis, which facilitated the classification of various lung diseases by characteristic patterns. Several international meetings took place to develop a unified lung disease classification system. The modern system, validated for consistency and external validity, derives from such a meeting in Cincinnati in 1968.

Concurrent with the classification of pulmonary diseases was the development of a new concept: a threshold or limit of exposure below which workers would not develop a known occupational disease. From the late eighteenth century through the first part of the twentieth century, industry boomed in England and in the United States in particular. All manner of new exposures manifested, as did new illnesses among working populations. Thresholds for exposure were published for different compounds from 1900 to 1925; in 1927, the American Chemical Society published exposure limits for 25 gases. Several PHS studies into the effects of occupational exposures were also published during that time and led to the organization of the National Conference of Governmental Industrial Hygienists (NCGIH). This group met initially in 1938 and by 1941 had established the Threshold Limit Values for Chemical Substances Committee. In 1948, the organization began issuing maximum allowable concentrations for various compounds, and in 1956, it introduced the threshold limit value (TLV). In some instances, the development of TLVs occurred with considerable influence from the affected industries, which somewhat undercut the credibility of the TLV approach.

ASBESTOS

At the beginning of the twentieth century, asbestos served as a sobriquet for industrialization. It was used not only in machinery to maximize the usefulness of available energy in steam engines, but also on the brakes that stopped those engines. It was used in building materials, in shipbuilding, and around plumbing and heating pipes. The use of asbestos burgeoned, and the world's largest asbestos manufacturer, Johns-Manville, became a component of the Dow Jones Industrial Average. As critical as the tobacco industry was to the emergence of the consumer-led economy during the past century, so too was the asbestos industry central to global industrialization of the same period.

The occurrence of asbestosis as a consequence of exposure to asbestos fibers ("dust") began to be appreciated in the early part of the twentieth century. Because the silico-tuberculosis link had been defined, the asbestos industry was concerned that there might also be a link between asbestosis and tuberculosis. Working with one of its insurers, the Metropolitan Life Insurance Company, the industry surveyed its workers for signs of asbestosis, silicosis, and silico-tuberculosis. It then contracted with one of the leading tuberculosis facilities in the world, the Saranac Laboratory in upstate New York, to assess whether exposure to asbestos increased the risk of silico-tuberculosis. Using laboratory animals, scientists at Saranac determined that exposure to asbestos did not increase this risk. However, they also found that the animals exposed to asbestos developed an increased number of adenomas, a finding they included in the first draft of their report. Industry's goal was to have an exculpatory document it could use in court in order to contest workers' compensation claims of silico-tuberculosis. The industry attorneys demanded that Saranac remove the reference to adenomas; the section was deleted. Thus began a series of efforts by the asbestos industry to both generate and then suppress scientific data, epidemiologic and otherwise, that related exposure to asbestos with an elevated risk of lung cancer.

In 1955 when Richard Doll found that the mortality for asbestos workers was five times what would be expected for other Britons and succeeded in publishing those results, he lifted the curtain on occupational cancer in general and asbestos-related cancer in particular. Doll stated, "For my own part, I feel that any positive findings with regard to the cause of cancer must be made available to all research workers on the subject . . . it is by free publication that the work can be tested and utilized (or disproved) by others." Doll's publication raised alarm, not only for the increased risks to workers in asbestos plants, but also for the population as a whole. Asbestos use was becoming widespread in both industry and consumer products. Asbestos manufacturers, however, continued to claim that use of their products constituted only minimal risks.

Also during the early 1950s, Irving J. Selikoff, a Paterson, New Jersey, physician, joined with fellow physicians to open a group practice, the Paterson Clinic. One of the groups to whom the clinic marketed itself was the local asbestos union. During the next decade, Selikoff observed a seemingly high number of lung cancer cases among the asbestos workers at the clinic. He gathered the available data on those cases and took it to the ACS National Headquarters in New York City. There he approached E. Cuyler Hammond, an epidemiologist directing the ACS research effort on the etiology of cancer. Hammond compared Selikoff's data with similar data the ACS had collected on men who were not exposed to asbestos. The analysis showed an interaction between cigarette smoking, asbestos, and the development of lung cancer. These results were first reported in 1964 and then refined in a 1968 publication. Selikoff was so shocked by the magnitude of the risks that he began working first with the national asbestos union and then the American Federation of Labor and Congress of Industrial Organizations (AFL-CIO) to persuade the U.S. Congress to pass legislation that would allow workers to petition the federal government for a newly created National Institute for Occupational Safety and Health (NIOSH). The goal was for NIOSH to research a suspected occupational health problem and to provide for regulation to reduce occupational exposures to workers. In 1970, such legislation was passed, and it became a model for other nations, particularly the Scandinavian countries.

The risks associated with exposure to asbestos could no longer be hidden by the industry. When Johns-Manville, the world's leading asbestos manufacturer, declared bankruptcy in 1982, the evidence that the industry had been trying to keep information about the health risks associated with asbestos exposure under wraps became public. As with the tobacco industry (see Chapter 2), the degree to which the industry had succeeded in suppressing scientific data and disclosure of risks exceeded the wildest conjectures of its critics. The industry had systematically suppressed data while asbestos became ensconced in myriad consumer products, including automobile brake pads, acoustic tiles, flooring, and construction materials, as well as in heating system insulation in schools and other public and private buildings. During World War II, unaware of the potentially lethal consequences of exposure to asbestos, the U.S. Navy specified its use in many ships built to fight the war. As a result, lung and other asbestos-associated cancers exploded near the shipyards where the boats were built.

Given the time lag between exposure to asbestos and manifestation of asbestos-associated diseases, health consequences from asbestos exposure will continue in the United States until at least 2025. For workers in developing nations where asbestos is not banned, the effects will be felt well after that.

OTHER OCCUPATIONAL RISKS

Asbestos was not the only source of occupational cancer concern among workers in the twentieth century. Two examples stand out: bischloromethyl ether (BCME) and vinyl chloride. Similar to Selikoff's observations about asbestos exposure, in 1962 a Rohm and Haas physician at a plant in Philadelphia observed three cases of lung cancer among fifty workers in two buildings involved in the manufacture of BCME, an agent commonly used in the manufacture of polymers. None of the workers was older than age 37, and one was a nonsmoker. With some cooperation from the company, a cohort of workers was established and given periodic follow-up to assess whether BCME exposures were associated with an elevated risk of lung cancer. Within a decade, an elevated risk was established, and it was found to be specific for small-cell ("oat cell") lung cancer, which was not associated with cigarette smoking. Workers in other companies with BCME exposure were also found to have an elevated risk of lung cancer. As a result, the companies redesigned their processes to eliminate the exposures.

The same level of enlightened corporate behavior was not in evidence with regard to vinyl chloride. During the 1960s, a relationship between exposure to vinyl chloride and the development of acroosteolysis was observed in more than one company and in workers with differing levels of exposure. Concerned that public disclosure would lead to the rejection of polyvinylchloride plastics by the public, the industry (in both the United States and Europe) sought to suppress all publications about the association, including within the medical literature. At the same time, toxicological studies suggested that vinyl chloride was carcinogenic. Corporate occupational health departments began to observe multiple cases of angiosarcoma of the liver. As this cancer was extremely rare, the existence of more than a single case in a small plant or two heightened concerns. The industry began a course of governmental deception, delaying notifications even as they undertook their own studies in which they found vinyl chloride to be an extraordinary carcinogen, not merely for angiosarcoma of the liver but also for other organ systems. Governments around the globe were confronted with the issue of how best to regulate worker exposures in a modern economy. Should they wait for data indicative of a problem, or should they use toxicological data as an indicator of where problems might exist with present-day exposures? Although many countries, including the United States, addressed the issue by using toxicological data to set threshold limit values to assure worker safety, a definitive answer for whether such an approach is sufficiently protective remains elusive and will require additional analyses for many years to come.

Not all occupational health issues in the twentieth century concerned cancer or respiratory diseases. During the 1960s and 1970s, petrochemicals were a common feedstock for enhancing agricultural output and creating new materials. Mr. McGuire's line "Just one word . . . Plastics." from the 1968 movie *The Graduate* summed up the seemingly limitless potential for petrochemicals at the time. One example of petrochemical expansion is that of dibromochloropropane (DBCP), used as a fumigant to control nematodes in crops in the United States and elsewhere. In September 1977, a significant proportion of factory workers involved in the production of DBCP were observed to be sterile. Subsequent investigations found DBCP to be a gonadotoxin in laboratory animals, and the product was banned in the United States. When lead was determined to be a threat to the developing fetus, the U.S. Occupational Safety and Health Administration (OSHA) imposed upper limits of exposure for pregnant women. Industry responded by requiring women to provide proof of sterility and by demoting pregnant women into lower-paying positions with less lead exposure. These labor practices persisted until the United States Court of Appeals, Seventh Circuit declared them illegal in 1989.

Exposure to radiation was yet another occupational health concern that emerged in the twentieth century. Women painting radium dials on watch faces in the early part of the century developed a variety of adverse health outcomes, ranging from destroyed jawbone to elevated risks for developing various cancers. Radiologists and radiological technicians were found to be at high risk for radiation exposure, especially before technological innovations facilitated reductions in the dose of radiation required for each radiograph taken. Those working on the Manhattan Project and later on nuclear bomb production during the Cold War also had elevated health risks, particularly for cancers. And even in the latter part of the century, studies of workers at the Hanford, Washington, nuclear works, itself a creation of the Manhattan Project, raised concerns about elevated risks for a variety of cancers, even among workers with low dosimeter readings. It seems likely that controversy about the safety of occupational radiation exposures will continue for some time to come.

Most of the exposures discussed in this chapter arose from producing various goods rather than from providing services. However, in the late twentieth century, an interest in occupational health issues in the service industries began to surface. Two conditions of concern were back injuries and carpal tunnel syndrome, the rise in the latter being associated with omnipresent computer technology. Almost every aspect of the worker's ergonomic situation began to be scrutinized by the end of the century, and data gathering to study potential ergonomic problems is only in the beginning stages. All that can truly be said is that as work changes, so will its risks.

Although there were some egregious acts committed by industry to suppress knowledge about dangerous occupational exposures during the course of the twentieth century, much was achieved in the field of occupational health and safety. Some governments, especially those in developed nations, enacted occupational health legislation that limited known dangerous exposures. Some provided a legal means for redress when the regulations were not followed. Unfortunately, most workers throughout the world are not covered by such legislation. The WHO estimates that there are about 2 million occupational deaths per year, with less than 15 percent of workers having access to occupational health services. Such figures exemplify the pervasive global philosophy that the health and safety of workers are subservient to the needs of business and industry.

Selected Readings

The first reading for this chapter is Richard Doll's 1955 paper describing the excess in lung cancer mortality for asbestos workers in Britain. Doll's paper, now a classic, sets the stage for the demise of the asbestos industry and serves as the piece that broke the silence on occupational risks long suppressed by industry in general.

The 1960 paper by J.C. Wagner, C.A. Sleggs, and Paul Marchand appears second. It was the first paper drawing a distinct link between exposure to asbestos fibers, specifically crocidolite, and mesothelioma, a rare tumor of the pleura. The work is abridged in that we have removed the x-ray and histology photos as they are not necessary for understanding the public health importance of the piece. This work appeared at a terrible time for South African industry, which was struggling to keep pace with the international demand for asbestos. Indeed, there were rumors that the industry was considering having Wagner shot. In 1962, Wagner left South Africa for Britain where he continued to work on asbestos-related cancers and received the Charles S. Mott Prize for his research on cancer prevention in 1985.

The last reading for this chapter is by W. G. Figueroa, Robert Raszkowski, and William Weiss. It shows how the editorial climate was changing with regard to printing results from occupational studies. This 1973 paper, published in the *New England Journal of Medicine*, was the first report to directly connect occupational exposure to chloromethyl methyl ether (CME) with lung cancer.

The paper is now considered a landmark in occupational medicine as it aided in CME being classified by the EPA as a human carcinogen.

BIBLIOGRAPHY

Centers for Disease Control. 1999. Achievements in Public Health, 1900–1999: Improvements in workplace safety—United States, 1900–1999. *MMWR* 48 (22): 461–69.

Cochrane AL, Davies I, and Fletcher CM. 1951. "Entente Radiologique" A step towards international agreement on the classification of radiographs in pneumoconiosis. *Brit J Ind Med* 8:244–55.

Cochrane AL, Fletcher CM, Gilson JC, and Hugh-Jones P. 1951. The role of periodic examination in the prevention of coal workers' pneumoconiosis. *Brit J Ind Med* 8:53–61.

Corn JK. 1992. *Response to Occupational Health Hazards: A Historical Perspective.* New York: Nostrand Reinhold.

Davis L, Wellman H, and Punnett L. 2001. Surveillance of work-related carpal tunnel syndrome in Massachusetts, 1992–1997: A report from the Massachusetts Sentinel Event Notification System for Occupational Risks (SENSOR). *Am J Ind Med* 39 (1): 58–71.

Dinham B and Malik S. 2003. Pesticides and human rights. *Int J Occup Env Heal* 9:40–52.

Fry SA. 1998. Studies of US radium dial workers: An epidemiological classic. Radiat Res 150 (Suppl. 5): S21–29.

Glass RI, Lyness RN, Mengle DC, Powell KE and Kahn E. 1979. Sperm count depression in pesticide applicators exposed to dibromochloropropane. *Am J Epidemiol* 109:346–51.

Gochfeld M. 2005. Chronologic history of occupational medicine. *J Occup Environ Med* 47 (2): 96–114.

Hunter D. 1955. *The Diseases of Occupations*, 1st ed. London: English Universities Press.

Lloyd JW. 1975. Angiosarcoma of the liver in vinyl chloride/polyvinyl chloride workers. *J Occup Med* 17 (5): 333–34.

Meiklejohn A. 1951. History of lung diseases of coal miners in Great Britain: Part I, 1800–1875. *Brit J Ind Med* 8:127–37.

Meiklejohn A. 1952. History of lung diseases of coal miners in Great Britain: Part II, 1875–1952. *Brit J Ind Med* 9:208–29.

Meiklejohn A. 1952. History of lung diseases of coal miners in Great Britain: Part III, 1920–1952. *Brit J Ind Med* 9:208–29.

Rosner D and Markowitz G, eds. 1987. *Dying for Work: Workers' Safety and Health in Twentieth-Century America.* Bloomington, IN: Indiana University Press.

Rosner D and Markowitz G. 2006. *Deadly Dust: Silicosis and the On-Going Struggle to Protect Workers' Health.* Ann Arbor, MI: University of Michigan Press.

Selikoff IJ, Churg J, and Hammond EC. 1962. Asbestos exposure and neoplasia. *JAMA* 188 (4): 22–26. Reprinted as a Classic in Oncology. 1984. *CA–Cancer J Clin* 34:48–56.

Selikoff IJ, Hammond EC, and Churg J. 1968. Asbestos exposure, smoking, and neoplasia. *JAMA* 204 (2):106–12.

Wagner JC, Sleggs CA, and Marchand P. 1960. Diffuse pleural mesothelioma and asbestos exposure in the North Western Cape Province. *Brit J Ind Med* 17:260–71.

Weiss W and Nash D. 1997. An epidemic of lung cancer due to chloromethyl ethers: 30 years of observation. *J Occup Environ Med* 39:1003–9.

Mortality from Lung Cancer in Asbestos Workers
(1955)
From the Statistical Research Unit,
Medical Research Council, London

Richard Doll

Sixty-one cases of lung cancer have been recorded in persons with asbestosis (Boemke, 1953; Hueper, 1952) since Lynch and Smith (1935) reported the first case. In view of the infrequency of asbestosis, this large number of cases suggests—but does not prove—that lung cancer is an occupational hazard of asbestos workers. The strongest evidence that it may be a hazard has been produced by Merewether and by Gloyne. Merewether (1949) found that lung cancer was reported at necropsy in 13.2% of cases of asbestosis (31 out of 235) against 6.9% in silicotics (55 out of 796). Neither author gave full details of the sex composition of the group examined, but since women form a higher proportion of asbestos workers than persons employed in occupations liable to give rise to silicosis (coal-miners, stonemasons, pottery workers, foundry men, metal grinders) and since lung cancer is less common among women, the differences in the proportions of cancer cases cannot be accounted for by differences in sex distribution. In fact the proportions which are more properly comparable with the findings in silicotic subjects are the proportions of lung cancer found among men with asbestosis, 17.2% in Merewether's series and 19.6% in Gloyne's.

Animal experiments are inconclusive. A positive result was reported by Nordmann and Sorge (1941) who found that of 10 mice which had been exposed to asbestos dust and survived for 240 days, two developed lung carcinoma. Smith (1952), however, considers that one of the "carcinomas" was, in fact, an example of squamous metaplasia and that the other, an adenocarcinoma, may have developed spontaneously from the common mouse adenoma. A negative result has been reported by Vorwald and Karr (1938). The majority of workers (cited by Hueper, 1952) consider that a causal relationship between asbestosis and lung cancer is either proved or is highly probable and the reality of the relationship was agreed at the recent International Symposium on the Epidemiology of Lung Cancer (Council of the International Organizations of Medical Sciences, 1953). A minority, however, remains skeptical (Cartier, 1952; Warren, 1948), and, according to Heuper (1952), Lanza and Vorwald, so that it was thought desirable to undertake a fresh investigation.

Necropsy Data

Since 1935, records have been collected of all the coroners' necropsies on persons known to have been employed at a large asbestos works.*

---

* Necropsies on asbestos workers are ordered by the coroner when, in his opinion, there may be a question of asbestosis being a contributory cause of death.

Table 1 Causes of Death Diagnosed at Necropsy among Persons
Employed in Asbestos Works (1933–52)

Cause of death	Asbestosis present	Asbestosis absent	All cases
"Heart failure"	34	11	45
Pulmonary tuberculosis	12	9	21
Lung cancer	15	3	18
Other diseases of the respiratory system	10	4	14
Other diseases	4	3	7
All causes	75	30	105

Pathological diagnoses in 105 consecutive cases are summarized in Table 1. Details of the cases in which lung cancer was found are shown in Table 2. During the first half of the period, eight deaths occurred in which lung cancer was found in association with asbestosis, while in the second half of the period there were seven such cases and a further three in which lung cancer was found without asbestos. The number of asbestos workers employed at the works increased steadily from 1914, and a great increase in the number of lung cancer deaths was also recorded among the whole population of England and Wales over the same period. It might, therefore, have been anticipated that a larger number of cases in which the two conditions were associated would have been found in the last 10 years. National regulations for the control of asbestos dust were, however, introduced in 1931 (Asbestos Industry Regulations, 1931) and the precautions taken to prevent dust dissemination in the works had become effective by the end of the following year. All the subjects in whom the two diseases were found together had been employed for at least nine years under the old conditions, and although 11 of the 15 men and women died within 30 years of their first exposure, the association of the two conditions has not yet been found in any person taken into employment during the last 31 years (1923–53). It is, therefore, possible that the reason more cases were not found in the second half of the period is that reduced exposure to dust has already begun to lessen the incidence and severity of asbestosis.

Table 2 Occupational History and Necropsy Data of Asbestos Workers with Primary Lung Cancer

Year of death	Sex and age	Occupation	Period of exposure	Years of exposure	Years of exposure before Jan. 1, 1933	Years from first exposure to death	Years from last exposure to death	Pathological report Asbestosis	Histological type of primary long cancer
1935	M. 62	Weaver	1919–32	13	13	16	3	Present	"Carcinoma"
1935	M. 54	Weaver	1909–32	23	23	26	3	"	Epithelial carcinoma
1936	M. 65	Fiberizer	1913–36	23	19	23	Less than 1	"	Endothelioma of pleura
1938	M. 47	Weaver	1910–12 1920–37	19	14	28	1	"	"Carcinoma"
1939	M. 49	Disintegrater	1910–14 1919–39	24	17	29	Less than 1	"	"Carcinoma"
1940	M. 52	Disintegrater	1911–15 1919–21 1923–39	22	15	29	Less than 1	"	"Carcinoma"
1941	M. 52	Weaver	1913–19 1924–38	20	14	28	3	"	Oat-celled carcinoma
1942	M. 59	Bag carrier	1913–41	28	19	29	1	"	Oat-celled carcinoma

(continued)

Table 2 *(continued)*

Year of death	Sex and age	Occupation	Period of exposure	Years of exposure	Years of exposure before Jan. 1, 1933	Years from first exposure to death	Years from last exposure to death	Pathological report Asbestosis	Pathological report Histological type of primary long cancer
1948	M. 59	Weaver	1912–14 1918–48	32	16	36	Less than 1	"	Anaplastic carcinoma
1948	M. 53	Weaver	1922–35	13	10	26	13	"	"Carcinoma"
1948	M. 48	Spinner	1922–48	26	10	26	Less than 1	"	"Carcinoma"
1948	M. 65	Maintenance man	1919–48	29	13	29	Less than 1	"[1]	Oat-celled carcinoma
1950	F. 51	Spinner	1915–42	27	17	35	8	"	"Carcinoma"
1951	M. 74	Fiberizer	1917–43	26	15	34	8	"	Adenocarcinoma
1951	M.. 60	Weaver	1919–25 1929–50	27	9	32	1	"	"Carcinoma"
1944	M. 36	Weaver	1942–44	2	0	2	Less than 1	Absent	Oat-celled carcinoma
1951	M. 43	Fiberizer	1939–48	9	0	12	3	"	Anaplastic carcinoma
1952	M. 51	Weaver	1941 (3/12) 1945–52	7	0	11	Less than 1	"	"Carcinoma"

[1]Also pulmonary tuberculosis.

Method of Estimation of Risk

Although the necropsy data shown in Tables 1 and 2 suggest (1) that some groups of asbestos workers have suffered an increased risk of lung cancer, and (2) that the risk may now have decreased, it is not possible to be certain of either of these propositions without a more detailed knowledge of the whole mortality experience of the workers. The first proposition has, therefore, been tested by comparing mortality experience by that section of the male employees of the works referred to above, who had worked for at least 20 years in "scheduled areas"*, with the mortality reported for all men in England and Wales; and the second proposition by comparing the incidence of lung cancer among men employed for different periods under the pre-1933 conditions. The investigation was limited to the small group of men who had been employed for at least 20 years, since the labour involved in searching out the individual records of men employed for shorter periods would be disproportionately great and, so far as was known from Table 2, would be comparatively unrewarding.

The date of birth, date of completing 20 years' work in the "scheduled areas," and, where applicable, date of ceasing employment and date and cause of death were obtained, for each man, from the records of the firm's Personnel Officer. Full details were, in most instances, already available for the men who had ceased employment as well as for the greater number who continue to be employed, since some of those who had left were registered as having asbestosis and the attention of the firm had been drawn to the death of others, in view of the possibility of the cause of death being industrial in origin. All the remaining men were successfully traced and the relevant details obtained. This was not difficult since, by limiting the study to men who had been employed in one place for 20 years, few were found to have changed their job or to have moved out of the region.

From the data the numbers of men alive in each five-year age group were counted separately for each of the years from 1922 (the first in which a man was recorded as having had 20 years' service) to 1953. A man who had completed the 20 years before the beginning of the year and who was alive at the end of it was counted, for that year, as one unit; a man who completed the period before the beginning of a year but who died during it, and a man who completed the period during a year and who survived to the end of it, were each counted, for that year, as half a unit; the one man who died in the same year as he completed his 20-year period was counted as a quarter of a unit.

---

* By "scheduled areas" [it] is meant those areas where processes were carried on which were scheduled under the Asbestos Industry Regulations of 1931 as being dusty.

The causes of death were recorded as they were given on the death certificate or, when available, as they were finally determined by necropsy. The causes were classified into five categories (see Table 4), and the numbers in each category were then compared with those which might have been expected to occur by multiplying the numbers of men alive in each five-year age group by the corresponding mortality rates for men in England and Wales over the same period. Because of the small numbers, however, populations were not considered separately for each year, but were added together to form five groups living in the periods 1922–33, 1934–38, 1939–43, 1944–48, and 1949–53, and the mortality rates used for each group were those for the years 1931, 1936, 1941, 1946, and 1951. The rates for 1931 were used for the period 1922–33, rather than those for the mid-years, since disproportionately few men were under observation during the early part of the period. As an example of a method, the mortality rate for all neoplasms other than lung cancer among men in England and Wales aged 55 to 59 in 1951 was 2.778 per 1,000. The numbers of years lived in this age group in the five years 1949–53 were respectively 15 years, 15 years, 17½ years, 19 years, and 19 years. The number of deaths expected in the period was, therefore, estimated to be $(15 + 15 + 17½ + 19 + 19) \times 2.778/1,000 = 0.238$. The total number of deaths expected from each category of diseases was obtained by adding the numbers thus calculated for each age group for each of the five periods.

The great majority of the men lived and, when they died, died in the town in which the works was situated, so that it would have been preferable to have basic calculation of the expected death on the death rates observed in that town rather than on the rates for all England and Wales. These, however, were not known in sufficient detail. Little error in the expected number of deaths from lung cancer is likely to have been introduced on this account since, according to Stocks (1952); the age-adjusted death rate for lung cancer among men in the town concerned was 96% of the rate for England and Wales. Stocks's figure was calculated only for the period 1946–49, but the proportion is unlikely to have varied greatly over the longer period of the investigation. The expected number of deaths from all causes is, however, likely to be somewhat underestimated since the age-adjusted rate from all causes for the town is about 25% higher than the England and Wales rate (*i.e.* the excess was 22% in 1950, 28% in 1951, and 22% in 1952).

Results

The number of men studied was 113; the numbers of man-years in each of the five periods in each age group are shown in Table 3. The total number of deaths from all causes and the number of deaths observed in each

Table 3 Number of Man-years Lived by Men with 20 or More Years of Work in a "Scheduled Area"

Age (years)	Period					All periods
	1922–33	1934–38	1939–43	1944–48	1949–53	
30–	0	0.5	1.5	0	0	2
35–	4.5	2	11	17.5	9	44
40–	9.5	16	33.5	48	55	162
45–	9.5	19.5	50	78.5	84	241.5
50–	6.5	25.5	39.5	85	96.5	253
55–	12	6	30	52	85.5	185.5
60–	15	3	5.25	25.5	36	84.75
65–	1	13.5	3	10	21.5	49
70–	0	2	9	3	3.5	17.5
75–79	0	0	1	1.5	0.5	3
All ages	58	88	183.75	321	391.5	1042.25

of the five disease categories, together with the expected number of deaths, are shown in Table 4. From Table 4 it appears that the men who had been exposed to asbestos dust suffered an increased mortality from lung cancer, other respiratory diseases and cardiovascular diseases, in association with asbestosis, but that their mortality from other diseases with close to that expected.

Four explanations of the findings are possible: (1) that all the men who had died of lung cancer were recorded because of interest in the condition, but that some of the records of other men dying of other diseases or still alive were omitted, with consequent underestimation of the expected number of deaths; (2) that lung cancer was incorrectly and excessively diagnosed among the asbestos workers; (3) that lung cancer was insufficiently diagnosed among the general population of England and Wales; or (4) that the asbestos workers studied suffered an excess mortality from lung cancer.

It certainly cannot be claimed that the records of the Personnel Office were necessarily complete, but they were believed to be complete and no deficiency on this score would account for the total excess of deaths unless it were so gross that more than half the defined population had been omitted. Moreover, the number of deaths due to conditions unrelated to asbestosis was close to the estimated number and this is unlikely to have

Table 4 Causes of Death among Male Asbestos Workers Compared
with Mortality Experience of All Men in England and Wales

| Cause of death | No. of deaths | | Test of significance of difference between observed and expected (value of P) |
	No. observed	Expected on England and Wales rates	
Lung cancer:[1]			
with mention of asbestosis	11	–	<0.000001
without mention of asbestosis	0	0.8	
Other pulmonary diseases (including pulmonary tuberculosis) and cardiovascular diseases:			
with mention of asbestosis	14	–	<0.001
without mention of asbestosis	6	7.6	
Neoplasms other than lung cancer	4	2.3	>0.1
All other diseases[2]	4	4.7	
All causes	39	15.4	<0.000001

[1] Including one case with pulmonary tuberculosis.

[2] Including two cases (benign stricture of oesophagus and septicaemia) in which asbestosis was present but was not thought to have been a contributory cause of death.

happened unless the population had been estimated approximately correctly and the deaths from all causes fully reported.

All the 11 deaths attributed to lung cancer were confirmed by necropsy and histological examination so that the excess number cannot be attributed to incorrect diagnosis among the group of asbestos workers. Some of the excess may well be due to an underestimation of the expected deaths since part of the increase in mortality attributed to lung cancer over the past 30 years is certainly due to improvements in diagnosis and therapy (Doll, 1953). Even, however, if it were postulated that the whole of the recorded increase between 1931 in 1951 was spurious and that the real mortality from the disease throughout was that ascribed to it in 1951, the expected number of deaths is increased to only 1.1 and the observed excess is still grossly significant. For the actual number of lung cancer cases to be so little in excess of the expected as to be reasonably attributable to chance, it would be necessary for the expected cases to be 6.2, that is 5.6 times the number estimated on 1951 rates. In other words, it would be necessary to postulate that in 1951 (and throughout the previous 20 years) there was 5.6 times as much cancer of the lung as was recognized in 1931, which would mean that the condition would have to have been present and capable of detection in over 20% of all men at death. Moreover, even if this were so, it would still not account for the fact that all the cases of lung cancer were found in association with asbestosis.

It is, therefore, concluded that the fourth explanation is the most reasonable one and that the asbestos workers who had worked for 20 or more years in the "scheduled areas" suffered a notably higher risk for lung cancer than the rest of the population.

To test if the risk has altered since the 1931 regulations were introduced, it is not only necessary to make allowance for duration of employment before the end of 1932, but also to allow for the men's ages and for the total durations of their employment in the "scheduled areas," since the men employed in the earlier periods can also have been employed longer and lived to be older. On the other hand, there is no need to consider the changing incidence of lung cancer in the total population of England and Wales since the non-industrial risk has been shown to be small in comparison with the industrial one. The data required for comparing the risks among men employed for under 10 years, for 10 to 14 years, and for 15 years and over in the pre-1933 conditions are shown in Table 5. The ages shown are the ages of deaths of the men who have died and the ages in mid-1953 for the men who are still alive. The expected numbers of men in each pre-1933 employment group found to have asbestosis or asbestosis and lung cancer are estimated by multiplying the numbers in each age, total employment, and pre-1933 employment subgroup by the proportions of men with asbestosis or with asbestosis and lung cancer in the same age and total employment group for all lengths of pre-1933 employment combined. For example, three out of the nine men aged 50 to 54 years who had been employed for 20 to 24 years in the areas in which they might be exposed to asbestos dust were found to have asbestosis and lung cancer. Since three men had worked for under 10 years in the pre-1933 conditions, three had worked for 10 to 14 years, and three had worked for 15 or more years, the expected number of cases in each of the pre-1933 employment groups would have been the same, i.e., $3 \times 3/9$, or 1. In fact, the numbers of cases found were 0, 1, and 2. The total numbers expected in each pre-1933 employment group are obtained by adding the numbers calculated for each of the age and total employment groups within it. The results are as follows:

Table 5 Numbers of Men Employed for Different Periods before 1933 and Numbers Known to Have Asbestosis and Lung Cancer in Association with Asbestosis Divided by Total Duration of Employment in a Scheduled Area and by Age

Total length of employment in "scheduled area" (years)	Age at June 30, 1953, or at death (years)	Length of employment before January 1, 1933									All Lengths of employment before January 1, 1933		
		0–9 years			10–14 years			15+ years					
		No. of men	No. of men with asbestosis	No. of men with cancer of lung	No. of men	No. of men with asbestosis	No. of men with cancer of lung	No. of men	No. of men with asbestosis	No. of men with cancer of lung	No. of men	No. of men with asbestosis	No. of men with cancer of lung
	35–	1	–	–	1	1	–	0	–	–	2	1	–
	40–	4	–	–	1	1	–	0	–	–	5	1	–
	45–	7	1	–	0	0	–	1	1	1	8	2	1
	50–	3	2	–	3	3	1	3	3	2	9	8	3
20–24	55–	5	3	–	2	1	–	0	0	0	7	4	0
	60–	3	1	–	1	1	–	1	1	0	5	3	0
	65–	2	0	–	0	–	–	1	1	1	3	1	1
	70–	0	0	–	0	–	–	1	1	–	1	1	–
	75–9	1	1	–	0	–	–	0	–	–	1	1	–

25–29	40–	3	–	–	0	–	–	0	–	–	3	0	–
	45–	10	2	–	2	1	1	0	–	–	12	3	1
	50–	6	2	1	0	0	0	0	–	–	6	2	1
	55–	6	1	–	8	4	0	1	1	–	15	6	0
	60–	3	–	–	1	1	0	3	3	1	7	4	1
	65–	1	–	–	1	1	1	0	0	0	2	1	1
	70–	0	–	–	0	–	–	1	0	0	1	0	0
	75–	0	–	–	0	–	–	1	1	1	1	1	1
	80–4	0	–	–	0	–	–	1	0	–	1	0	–
30–34	45–	2	–	–	0	–	–	0	–	–	2	0	–
	50–	2	–	–	5	–	–	2	1	–	9	0	–
	55–	1	–	–	1	–	–	3	2	1	5	2	1
	60–	1	–	–	0	–	–	2	1	–	3	1	–
	65–	0	–	–	0	–	–	0	0	–	0	0	–
	70–4	0	–	–	0	–	–	1	1	–	1	1	–
35+	55–	0	–	–	0	–	–	1	–	–	1	0	–
	60–	0	–	–	0	–	–	1	–	–	1	0	–
	65–9	0	–	–	0	–	–	2	–	–	2	0	–

(continued)

Table 5 (continued)

Total length of employment in "scheduled area" (years)	Age at June 30, 1953, or at death (years)	Length of employment before January 1, 1933									All Lengths of employment before January 1, 1933		
		0–9 years			10–14 years			15+ years					
		No. of men	No. of men with asbestosis	No. of men with cancer of lung	No. of men	No. of men with asbestosis	No. of men with cancer of lung	No. of men	No. of men with asbestosis	No. of men with cancer of lung	No. of men	No. of men with asbestosis	No. of men with cancer of lung
	35–	1	–	–	1	1	–	0	–	–	2	1	–
	40–	7	–	–	1	1	–	0	–	–	8	1	–
	45–	19	3	–	2	1	1	1	1	1	22	5	2
	50–	11	4	1	8	3	1	5	3	2	24	10	4
All lengths of employment in any "scheduled area" (20 yrs.+)	55–	12	4	–	11	5	0	5	3	1	28	12	1
	60–	7	1	–	2	2	0	7	5	1	16	8	1
	65–	3	0	–	1	1	1	3	1	1	7	2	2
	70–	0	0	–	0	–	–	3	2	0	3	2	0
	75–	1	1	–	0	–	–	1	1	1	2	2	1
	80–4	0	–	–	0	–	–	1	0	–	1	0	–
	All ages	61	13	1	26	14	3	26	16	7	113	43	11

		Length of employment before January 1, 1933		
		Under 10 years	10–14 years	15 years and over
Total number of men with asbestosis	observed	13	14	16
	expected	21.9	10.3	10.8
Number of men with asbestosis and lung cancer	observed	1	3	7
	expected	5.5	2.4	3.1

The differences between the numbers of men observed and the numbers expected in each employment group, had the incidence of the conditions remained steady throughout, are statistically significant (total asbestosis, $\chi^2=7.52$, n=2, P=0.025; asbestosis and lung cancer, $\chi^2=8.72$, n=2, P=0.01*). They are highly so if the trend, that is, the biologically important reduction in the proportion between observed and expected numbers as the length of pre-1933 employment is reduced, is also taken into consideration. It is clear, therefore, that the incidence both of asbestosis and lung cancer associated with asbestosis have become progressively less as the number of years during which men were exposed to the pre-1933 conditions has decreased.

The extent of the risk of lung cancer over the whole period among the men studied appears to have been of the order of 10 times that experienced by other men. This agrees well with the data reported by Merewether (1949), but it is somewhat greater than that suggested by Gloyne's data (1951). The great reduction in the amount of dust produced in asbestos works during the period has been accompanied by a reduction in the incidence of lung cancer among the workmen so that the risk before 1933 is likely to have been considerably greater—perhaps 20 times the general risk. Whether the specific industrial risk of lung cancer has yet been completely eliminated cannot be determined with certainty; the number of men at risk, who have been exposed to the new conditions only and to have been employed for a sufficient length of time, is at present too small for confidence to be placed in their experience. It is clear, however, that the risk has for some time been greatly reduced. The extent

---

* The expected numbers of lung cancer are small and the probability that the differences could arise by chance has consequently been somewhat, but not seriously, underestimated. If all men with more than 10 years pre-1933 employment are grouped together and Yates' correction made for small numbers, $\chi^2=5.82$, n=1, P=0.02.

of the reduction is particularly striking when it is recalled that between 1933 and 1953 the incidence of the disease among men in the country at large has increased sixfold.

Summary

The cause of death, as determined at necropsy, is reported for 105 persons who had been employed at one asbestos works. Lung cancer was found in 18 instances, 15 times in association with asbestosis. All the subjects in whom both conditions were found had started employment in the industry before 1923 and had worked in the industry at least nine years before the regulations for the control of dust had become effective.

One hundred and thirteen men who had worked for at least 20 years in places where they were liable to be exposed to asbestos dust were followed up and the mortality among them compared with that which would have been expected on the basis of the mortality experience of the whole male population. Thirty-nine deaths occurred in the group whereas 15.4 were expected. The excess was entirely due to excess deaths from lung cancer (11 against 0.8 expected) and from other respiratory and cardiovascular diseases (22 against 7.6 expected). All the cases of lung cancer were confirmed histologically and all were associated with the presence of asbestosis.

From the data it can be concluded that lung cancer was a specific industrial hazard of certain asbestos workers and that the average risk among men employed for 20 or more years has been of the order of 10 times that experienced by the general population. The risk has become progressively less as the duration of employment under the old dusty conditions has decreased.

I would like to offer my thanks to the management of the firm concerned for permission to carry out this work and to the Medical Officer and members of the staff of the works were the men were employed, who carried out the greater part of the work on which this report is based.

SOURCE

Doll, R. 1955. Mortality from lung cancer in asbestos workers. *Brit J Industr Med* 12:81–6. Reprinted with permission of BMJ Publishing Group Ltd.

Diffuse Pleural Mesothelioma and Asbestos Exposure in the North Western Cape Province

(1960, Abridged)

From the Pathology Division, Pneumoconiosis Research Unit of the Council for Scientific and Industrial Research, Johannesburg, West End Hospital, Kimberley, and the Department of Thoracic Surgery, University of the Witwatersrand and Johannesburg General Hospital

J. C. Wagner, C. A. Sleggs, and Paul Marchand

Primary malignant tumours of the pleura are uncommon. Thirty-three cases (22 males, 11 females, ages 31 to 68) of diffuse pleural mesothelioma are described; all but one have a probable exposure to crocidolite asbestos (Cape blue). In a majority this exposure was in the Asbestos Hills which lie to the west of Kimberley in the north west of Cape Province. The tumour is rarely seen elsewhere in South Africa.

Mesothelioma of the pleura is regarded as an uncommon tumour. In the last four years we have seen 33 histologically proven cases; 28 of these had some association with the Cape asbestos field and four cases had been exposed to asbestos in industry.

The tumour is rarely encountered elsewhere in South Africa. During the past five years, with the exception of the present series, no neoplasm of this nature has been diagnosed amongst 10,000 lungs examined at the Pneumoconiosis Bureau in Johannesburg, or in the Technology Department of the South African Institute for Medical Research. Higginson and Oettle (1957) did not observe a single case in a survey of malignant tumours occurring in the Bantu and Cape Coloured population of Johannesburg and the North Eastern Transvaal.

Our first necropsy specimen of pleural mesothelioma was examined at the Pneumoconiosis Research Unit in February, 1956 (Case 1). During the early months of that year, one of us (C.A.S.) in the Northern Cape treated six patients with gross pleural thickening. Pleura biopsies from two of them showed the features of mesothelioma. In the ensuing two years, eight further cases were found from this region and five from elsewhere in the Union. During this period C.A.S. had become perturbed at the number of these unusual tumours occurring amongst his patients, and stimulated an investigation. At this stage there were two reasons to suggest that asbestos may be implicated. First, asbestos was found in the lungs of the first case (Case 1), and secondly, 10 of the cases came from a hospital to which suspected cases of tuberculosis were referred from a large asbestos mining area. This hypothesis could not be supported at once from the original histories obtained from the patients, for they included housewives, domestic servants, cattle herders, farmers, a water bailiff, an insurance agent, and an accountant, none of whom were working on the asbestos mines at the time. We therefore undertook a detailed investigation of their past occupation and place of residence, and the association with asbestos exposure was discovered. The cases are summarized in Table 3. Previous biopsy specimens were examined, and new cases diagnosed, including asbestos miners. In only one case do the relatives deny that the patient either visited the asbestos mines or was exposed to asbestos.

This is a preliminary publication and the problem is being intensively investigated

The Asbestos Area of the North-West Cape

According to Hall (1930) asbestos was discovered by Lichenstein near Prieska during his travels between 1803 and 1806. Since then it has been established that the asbestos deposits extend from 20 miles south of Prieska, northwards through the western part of the magisterial district of Hay, to the eastern portion of the magisterial district of Postmasburg and finally, to the western area of the district of Kuruman (Fig. 1). These deposits occur in the slopes of a range of hills covering an area of approximately 8,000 square miles. Known as the "Asbestos Mountains", these hills extend more or less longitudinally between 22.30° and 23° E. The whole area is semi-arid, sparsely populated, and, apart from mining, cattle ranching is the only important occupation. In the Kuruman area several large tracts of land in or abutting on these mountains have been reserved for the aboriginal inhabitants and here whites may only reside in the immediate vicinity of the mines.

The type of asbestos mined throughout this area is crocidolite, better known as Cape Blue Asbestos. The chemical analysis of the fibre is given in Table 1. Crocidolite is the fibrous form of reibeckite and all stages of transformation from a massive reibeckite rock through lamellar reibeckite to asbestiform crocidolite occur in this region. Magnetite is frequently associated with crocidolite (Vermass, 1952).

Mining of asbestos first began in the Prieska district in 1893 and gradually spread northward. In 1908 production had begun in the Kuruman district. Between 1916 and 1918 a large number of claims were taken up.

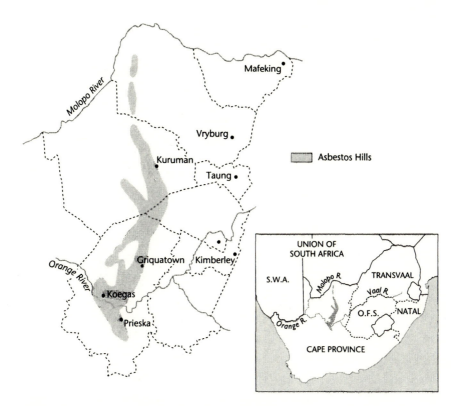

Figure 1   Map of Griqualand West asbestos fields.

This northward trend has continued and in about 1950 mining started at Pomfret near the Bechuanaland border (Table 2).

Initially the ore was quarried in numerous small open cast workings. This was followed gradually by a type of shallow mining; inclined shafting became more common after 1930.

According to Frood (1915), the quarrying was a family affair undertaken by the local inhabitants. The men quarried the rock, which was sorted and then hand cobbed by the women and children. Hand cobbing consists of separating the fibre from the banded ironstone by striking the rock cob with a small hammer. As the market was selective, a rotary sieve was sometimes used to grade the fibre and eliminate the small particles of dust. After grading, it was bagged and weighed. The asbestos was then transported by donkey wagon to the nearest rail-head. Before the establishment of the railway in this area between 1923 and 1930, such a journey could last as long as 10 days. This transport was generally undertaken by white youths (farmers' sons) under contract. The white inhabitants played very little part in actual recovery of the fibre, being nearly always employed in the role of managers or overseers, issuing stores and

Table 1   Chemical Analyses of Crocidolite and Amosite (from Vermaas, 1952)

	Crocidolite	Amosite
SiO_2	51.94	49.47
Al_2O_3	0.20	0.63
Fe_2O_3	18.64	4.15
FeO	19.39	35.63
MgO	1.37	6.57
CaO	0.19	0.52
Na_2O	6.07	0.02
K_2O	0.04	0.20
H_2O-	0.31	0.07
H_2O+	2.58	2.33
TiO_2	—	0.25
MnO	—	0.61
F	—	0.10
Total	100.73	100.46

Table 2   Population of the Magisterial Districts in Which the Asbestos Fields Are Situated (taken from Union Census 1921, and 1951)

District	Population 1921			Population 1951		
	Whites	Non-whites	Total	Whites	Non-whites	Total
Prieska	3,430	4,879	8,309	3,361	10,847	14,208
Kuruman	4,713	16,698	21,411	4,818	23,779	28,597
Hay	4,499	8,814	13,313	2,757	9,631	12,388
Postmasburg	Included in the Hay District			4,887	21,019	25,906

supervising the grading and weighing of the fibres. Farming activities were and are still carried out round the mines.

Since the 1939–1945 war, the demand for crocidolite has enormously increased. The lucrative claims have been bought by registered companies, others have been abandoned. As deeper and richer deposits have been found, vertical shafts are being sunk. However, the mines with large shallow deposits are still using the inclined shaft and tunnel, and quarrying is still used by the few remaining smaller producers. With the building of more mills, hand cobbing has diminished. In 1915 the first crushing mill was established at Koegas in the south. This was followed by a large mill at Kuruman (operated between 1926 and 1931) where it was situated within 300 yards of the main street, close to which cobbing was also done for a few years (1927–1930). This was followed by a mill at Prieska in 1930, which was completely rebuilt in 1957. Griquatown had a small mill in 1928. The practice today is for one mill to serve several mines in the immediate vicinity.

In the early days the manager and labourers lived within a few yards of their place of work, and even today the non-white prefers to live as close as possible, and the children play on the dumps from the mine and mill.

Case Histories

The following case histories illustrate various aspects of the disease and the different types of exposure to asbestos dust.

CASE 1.—B.P., a Bantu male, 36 years of age (born 1920), was a mine labourer, and was the first case diagnosed as a mesothelioma with evidence of asbestosis. He was born in the Kuruman district but it is not known whether he worked in the asbestos mines. He was employed on the Witwatersrand gold-mines underground for two years and in the change rooms for a further 11 years.

A radiograph taken at a mine hospital on August 18, 1955 showed a massive right-sided pleural effusion, and 3,000 ml. of fluid was withdrawn. He was admitted to the Witwatersrand Native Labour Association Hospital on August 24, 1955, and two days later aspiration yielded 1,000 ml. of thick gelatinous pus "which could be pulled out in threads". He was treated with frequent aspirations and installation of varidase but without improvement, and he died on February 15, 1956 (Martiny, 1956).

At autopsy a right thoracic cavity was occupied by a large gelatinous tumour which displaced the mediastinum and compressed the left lung. The tumour had infiltrated the pericardium. The right lung was completely compressed by neoplastic tissue (Fig. 2) but the right bronchial tree did not show any evidence of a primary bronchogenic carcinoma. Histological sections of the plural growth showed a papillary mesothelioma (Fig. 3). There was evidence of asbestosis in both lungs (Fig. 4). [Figures here and throughout the case series not shown, Ed.]

CASE 4.—K.H., a white female of 56 years of age (born 1898), was a social worker, who could only have a short exposure to asbestos as a child and probably a further slight exposure as a young woman. She may have paid several short visits to the mines with her husband at a later period.

She was born in Griquatown where she lived until she was 5 years of age. Her family then moved to Kimberley where from 1916 to 1922 she worked as a clerk in an asbestos warehouse. Her husband owned an asbestos mine from 1933-1940.

She was referred to the West End Hospital, Kimberley, on July 19, 1954, because of dyspnoea and right chest discomfort of acute onset. The chest radiograph showed a loculated pleural effusion at the right base. Straw-coloured fluid was aspirated, which on examination was found to be negative for *M. tuberculosis* but contained mesothelial cells arranged in acini. At thoracoscopy in Johannesburg on August 11, 1954 tumour nodules were seen on the parietal pleura. Histological examination of the biopsy specimen showed a mesothelioma. Deep therapy and radio-active gold instillation in September, 1955 caused initial repression of both the pleural fluid and nodules but did not arrest the progress of the disease. She received a further course of x-ray therapy without improvement and died in January, 1957. The liver was enlarged and nodular before death but no necropsy was done. (Figs. 5, 6, 7, and 8 show the radiological development of the tumour in this case.)

CASE 14.—S.S., a Bantu male, 40 years of age (born 1918), was an asbestos miner. He was born in the Kuruman district and as a child often played on the asbestos dump near an asbestos mine. He subsequently worked with asbestos for several years, being employed at an asbestos mine weighing fibre from 1938-41. In 1942 he worked on a Witwatersrand gold mine but returned to the Kuruman district in 1943 where he worked as a farm labourer until his final illness.

He was admitted to the West End Hospital on March 3, 1959. He had been well until July, 1958 when he became aware of pains in the right side of his chest. In addition he had a slightly productive cough and shortness of breath on exertion. Chest radiograph on March 9, 1959 showed obliteration of the right lung field. Asbestos bodies were found in the sputum. Needle biopsy showed histological features consistent with a mesothelioma.

[Autopsy findings and five additional cases are presented. They have been deleted here to save space. Ed.]

Discussion

In 1924 Robertson denied the existence of primary malignant tumours of the pleura and considered them to be secondary in origin. Since then, on the one hand, Willis (1948, 1953) and Smart and Hinson (1957) have supported Robertson's views, while on the other hand, primary neoplasms of this nature have been described by many authors in recent years. These include Tobiassen (1955) in Sweden, Belloni and Bovo (1957) in Italy, Godwin (1957) in the United States, and McCaughey (1958) in Britain. Evidence in support of the mesothelial origin of these tumours can be found in the tissue culture experiments of Stout and Murray (1942) and Sano, Weiss, and Gault (1950).

The variegated histological pattern of tumours arising from the mesothelium of the pleura was remarked on by Klemperer and Rabin (1931). Such a variation is appreciated when the multipotentiality of the cells lining coelomic cavities are considered. Maximow first demonstrated this feature in 1927. Novak (1931) stated that the mucosa of all parts of the Müllerian canal and the germinal epithelium were derived from these cells. Keasbey (1947) showed that in the embryo, the mesonephros, metanephros, Wolffian body, genital ridge, and all dependent urogenital structures are derived from the mesothelium.

Campbell (1950) considered the presence of both epithelial and mesenchymal elements a major diagnostic feature. In describing the histology of 11 of these tumours McCaughey (1958) demonstrated that either the epithelial or the mesenchymal element might predominate. He classified his cases into the following four groups: Tumours of epithelial character; tumours of mesenchymal type; tumours of mixed type; and tumours of anaplastic type.

Using McCaughey's classification on our series of tumours, the majority are, as in Campbell's series, of the mixed type. Of the remainder, a few showed the papillary tubular structure of the "tumours of epithelial character", and there were several of the anaplastic type. One case had the appearance of a "tumour of mesenchymal type" but even in this case primitive tubular structures were seen.

Apart from the original case all the histological diagnoses were made on biopsy material. Three of these biopsy findings were confirmed at necropsy. In the remainder, we have had to rely on clinical and radiological examination to exclude other primary sites of malignancy.

Following the work of Meyer and Chafee (1939, 1940), the possibility of demonstrating hyaluronic acid in these tumours both chemically and histochemically has been considered as a diagnostic aid. Both these investigations are still in an early stage (Harington, 1959).

Preliminary results of the histochemical experiments show that there is no achromatic substance in both the stroma and glandular structures of the tumours. This metachromasia can be reversed by incubation with testicular hyaluronidase. This material stains strongly with Hale's (1946) colloidal iron method. The periodic acid Schiff technique has given variable reactions. These results are not specific for hyaluronic acid but are strongly suggestive of its presence.

The amount of metachromatic substance in these tumours has varied considerably. This we think is partly due to the fact that until recently we had not appreciated the solubility of hyaluronic acid in aqueous media and the majority of these tumours were fixed in 10% formol-saline. Further, Lison (1953) states that the metachromasia of hyaluronic acid is optimal at a concentration of 1/10,000 and gradually decreases at higher levels. When the high concentrations that Meyer and Chafee (1939, 1940) found in their tumours are considered, this variation in metachromatic properties seems to have been partially explained. In addition, with the great differences in the histology of the various lesions, it would be logical to expect certain tumours with a marked adenoid appearance to secrete more than those with an essentially non-glandular structure.

Three of the five autopsies performed showed evidence of peritoneal metastases. In the other two, intra-thoracic spread was observed, in one case to the other lung and chest wall, and in the second to the mediastinal lymph glands and pericardium. Biopsy evidence of metastases has been attained in two cases, one from the omentum and the other from the subcutaneous tissue of the chest wall; while a third patient developed an implantation nodule in the thoracotomy scar which showed a similar appearance to that of the previous biopsy specimen.

The first recorded case of carcinoma of the lung associated with asbestos was described by Lynch and Smith (1935). By 1955, according to Doll, a total of 61 cases had been reported. Included in these cases was one mesothelioma. Cartier (1952) mentioned two cases of diffuse mesothelioma from a Canadian chrysotile mine. A further three cases were described by van der Schoot (1958). Unfortunately no indication is given in the literature regarding the type of asbestos to which the majority of recorded cases of carcinoma were exposed. However, discussion with management and medical officers of two of the factories, in which the majority of the cases reported in Britain were employed, suggest that most of these workers were handling chrysotile asbestos (Wagner, 1958). The possibility that some of these people may also have been exposed to crocidolite dust cannot be excluded.

Attempts to produce tumours in experimental animals by exposing them to asbestos dust have been made. Vorwald and Karr (1938) were unsuccessful. Lynch, McIver, and Cain (1957) succeeded in producing tumours in mice, but lung neoplasms in his control animals were far too numerous for the results to be considered significant. On the other hand, Schmähl (1958) working in Druckrey's laboratory has been able to produce sarcomas in rats. This has occurred after subcutaneous and intraperitoneal inoculation of both asbestos fibres and dust. He states that "mineral asbestos" was used but does not name the variety.

In our series of mesotheliomata, histological evidence of asbestos has been observed in eight of the 10 cases in which lung parenchyma was included in the specimen examined. No lung tissue was present in the biopsies for the remaining 23 cases. It was only in the four cases that came to necropsy that large sections of the lung tissue were available for examination. In all of these specimens evidence of asbestosis was found.

At first it was thought that the presence of numerous asbestos bodies, fragments of fibre, and dust immediately below the pleural elastic laminae in these specimens, might have been significant in the pathogenesis of the tumours. However, it is more probable that this distribution is a result of the marked atelectasis. Similar features have been observed in atelectatic lungs and asbestos miners in which no mesotheliomas have been observed.

Pleural fibrosis is a common finding in cases of asbestosis and in some cases large pleural plaques measuring up to 1.0 cm in thickness have been seen. These plaques, which were first described by Gloyne (1933), have been observed following exposure to both amosite and crocidolite asbestos dusts. In these cases of benign pleural thickening no evidence of stromal metachromasia has been observed.

In all the histological sections of pleura examined in the cases of these mesotheliomas and in more than 100 cases of asbestosis, no asbestos bodies, fragments of fibres, or dust have been observed beyond the plural elastic laminae.

Three patients from the Kuruman district, with clinical and radiologic features consistent with those of diffuse pleural mesothelioma had markedly abnormal cells in the pleural fluid. These cells showed no specific features to distinguish them from cells originating in secondary malignant pleural deposits nor from the grossly atypical cells sometimes seen in non-malignant pleural effusions. As no biopsy or autopsy examinations were obtained in these cases they have been excluded from the series.

The pathological evidence for associating these tumours with asbestos exposure is not conclusive. As previously stated, only in eight of the 33 cases has evidence of asbestos been demonstrated. Of these, six had a definite mining history and one had been exposed to asbestos while lagging steam pipes. The other case was born in the Kuruman district and nothing else is known of him, until his arrival at a Witwatersrand goldmine at the age of 23. In the remaining 25 cases we can only present circumstantial evidence of exposure to asbestos dust (Table 3). Eighteen of these 25 cases were born in the vicinity of the mines and two arrived in the district as infants. Of these 18 people 11 admit definite childhood exposure to the dust and two others were exposed industrially in later

Table 3 Diffuse Pleural Mesothelioma: Association with Asbestos

(1) Case no.	(2) Year of birth	(3) Age at diagnosis	(4) Race	(5) Sex	(6) Born on asbestos field	(7) Asbestos exposure	(8) Diagnosed on biopsy	(9) Necropsy	(10) Histological evidence of asbestosis	(11) Survival from initial symptoms (in months)
1	1920	36	B	M	+	Other history unknown until came to the Witwatersrand at the age of 23	–	+	+	8
2	±1913	±42	MXD	M	+	Mined asbestos from 1930–33; left area at the age of 27	–	+*	–	29
3	1902	53	B	F	+	Lived whole life in a location near an asbestos mill	+	–	–	11
4	1896	58	W	F	+	Lived on asbestos fields until the age 5; worked in asbestos warehouse 1916–20	+	–	–	30
5	1925	31	B	M	+	Spent all his working life in the vicinity of mines	–	+*	–	11
6	1903	53	W	F	+	Lived all her life in the vicinity of mines	+	–	–	15
7	1920	36	W	M	+	Lived all his life in the city of mine; worked as a miner	+	–	+	24
8	1894	63	MXD	F	+	From the age of 24 lived in a village serving local mines; often visited mines; watched cobbing outside houses	+	–	–	5

9	1905	52	MXD	M	+	Whole life spent near mines, digging wells	+	–	–	5
10	1909	49	W	M	+	Lived at the mine from age 7–17 years; played on dumps and in mine as a boy; returned to assist from age 21–25	+	–	–	13
11	1898	60	MXD	M	+	Whole life spent near mines; miner 1931–33	+	+	+	12
12	1910	48	B	M	+	Lived near mines until the age of 17; miner 1927	+	–	+	Still alive
13	1909	50	W	F	+	Lived near mine until the age of 21; played with fibre as a child	+	–	–	7
14	1918	40	B	M	+	Whole life spent near mines; miner 1938–41; played on dumps as a child	+	+	+	9
15	1916	42	W	F	+	Daughter of Case 22; lived at mine until age 20; went to school near cobbing sheds	+	–	–	Still alive
16	1896	60	W	M	+	Went to school near mines; transporting asbestos 1914–16	+	–	0	42
17	1911	48	MXD	F	+	Lived on major wagon route till age of 15	+	–	–	3
18	1920	38	B	M	+	Whole life in the vicinity of the mines; miner 1945–58	+	+	+	22

(continued)

Table 3 *(continued)*

(1)	(2)	(3)	(4)	(5)	(6)	(7)	(8)	(9)	(10)	(11)
Case no.	Year of birth	Age at diagnosis	Race	Sex	Born on asbestos field	Asbestos exposure	Diagnosed on biopsy	Necropsy	Histological evidence of asbestosis	Survival from initial symptoms (in months)
19	1922	37	MXD	M	+	Family lived at mine; miner 1938–1959	+	–	+	Still alive
20	1906	53	W	F	+	Spent whole life in village on wagon route to Kimberley	+	–	–	8
21	1912	44	W	M	+	Lived in the vicinity of mines until the age of 16; often on dumps as a child	+	–	–	16
22	1889	68	W	M	+	Whole life in the vicinity of the mines; miner 1913–32, and 1945–52	+	–	–	12
23	1895	63	W	F	+	Lived in the vicinity of the mines until the age of 30	+	–	–	8
24	1922	35	W	M	–	Lived in the vicinity of a mill from the ages of 1–7; played on the dumps as a child	+	–	–	48
25	1899	50	W	F	–	Lived in a mining area from the age of 10 to 18 years; after 1918 spent whole life in the same town as Case 24	+	–	–	Still alive

26	1895	49	W	M	−	Mined and transported asbestos from 1929–33 as overseer	+	−	−	13
27	1904	52	W	M	−	Born in North West Cape; transported asbestos from 1920–24	+	−	0	15
28	1899	60	W	M	−	Lived whole life on farm in mining area from the age of 12; transported asbestos 1916–21	+	−	−	Still alive
29	1913	44	W	M	−	Maintaining locomotive boilers 1931–45	+	−	−	7
30	1909	50	W	M	−	Maintaining steam pipes in explosive factories 1930–40	+	−	+	Still alive
31	1913	44	W	M	0	Worked as fitter on railways, maintaining locomotive boilers, dates unknown	+	−	−	6
32	1908	49	W	M	−	Making asbestos blankets for the Air Force 1939–45	+	−	−	7
33	1890	59	W	F	−	No history of exposure to asbestos	+	−	−	8

Keys:

Column 4–Race:	Column 6	Column 9	Column 10
W = White	+ = Born on asbestos fields	+ = Necropsy done	+ = Positive histological evidence of asbestosis
MXD = Mixed (Coloured)	– = Not born on asbestos fields	– = Necropsy not done	– = No lung tissue submitted
B = Bantu	0 = Unknown	* = Only small fragments of parietal pleura submitted at autopsy for histological examination	0 = Small fragments of lung tissue, but no evidence of asbestosis

life. In addition two patients with childhood exposure later worked in the asbestos mines. Three cases arrived in the region at an older age but were employed either on the mines or in transporting asbestos. A further three of these 25 cases have had industrial exposure, and in only one case do the relatives deny any exposure to asbestos dust.

The four industrial cases are significant. Two of the patients were lagging locomotive boilers and one was lagging steam pipes. A man, who was an upholsterer by trade, was employed in making fire-proof clothing from 1939-1945. As far as can be ascertained, these people were never in the Griqualand district. These findings tend to add support to asbestos being the common factor in the development of these tumours, and to counter the suggestion that there may be some other environmental cause in the region of Griqualand West.

If asbestos dust is a factor in the occurrence of these tumours, similar cases might have been expected from the neighbourhood of the Transvaal asbestos mines in the Pietersburg and Lydenburg districts, where crocidolite and amosite asbestos is mines. According to Vermaas (1952), crocidolite and amosite occur in the same seams in the Pietersburg district. As can be seen from Table 1, amosite is similar in composition to crocidolite. In the past four years the lungs of 24 cases of asbestosis from the Lydenburg district have been examined. In this material two cases of adeno-carcinoma have been observed. The one was in a white minor with 19 years' service, who had an adeno-carcinoma arising from a bronchus. The other case was a Bantu miner who had a peripheral tumour. No service record was attainable in this case. Only one case of asbestosis has been received from the Pietersburg area. All of these men were actually employed on the mines at the time of death, the majority having had a relatively short service. Our findings suggest that mesothelioma occurs 20 to 40 years or more after exposure to dust. Until comparatively recently the mining in the Transvaal has been on a small scale, and there were no settlements in the vicinity of the mines.

The lungs of 20 asbestos miners from the Cape Asbestos Field have been examined, in whom no mesothelioma was observed. One autopsy specimen consisting of three fragments of lung showed asbestosis and an adeno-carcinoma. Radiological features of asbestosis have been observed in many miners from this region, without any suggestion of tumour formation. However, pleural involvement has been a common finding in these cases (Hurwitz, 1959). It is possible that there has not been a sufficient length of time after exposure for tumour development in these cases. Further, the factor of individual susceptibility must also be considered.

We wish to record the great assistance that we have received in this investigation from the medical practitioners of the Griqualand West District and the thoracic surgeons and pathologists in Johannesburg, Pretoria, and Durban.

We thank the Secretary of Health for permission to publish this paper.

Addendum

By the end of June 1960, a total of 47 cases of mesothelioma had been identified. In 45 of these a possible association with exposure to crocidolite has been established. In one case a mesothelioma of the peritoneum was present.

SOURCE

Wagner JC, Sleggs CA, and Marchand P. 1960. Diffuse pleural mesothelioma and asbestos exposure in the North Western Cape Province. *Brit J Indust Med* 17:260–271. Copyright 1960 *British Journal of Industrial Medicine.* Reprinted with permission of BMJ Publishing Group Ltd.

Lung Cancer in Chloromethyl Methyl Ether Workers
(1973)

W. G. Figueroa, M.D., Robert Raszkowski, M.D.,
and William Weiss, M.D.

ABSTRACT.—An increased incidence of lung cancer (about eight times) occurred among men exposed to chloromethyl methyl ether at a chemical manufacturing plant. Of 14 men in whom lung cancer developed, histologic confirmation was obtained in 13, and 12 had oat-cell carcinomas. Three of the 14 men had never smoked. These observations suggest that the agent is an occupational hazard.

Although cigarette smoking appears to be the major etiologic factor in bronchogenic carcinoma occurring in the general population, certain occupational groups have an increased risk of acquiring the disease. These include uranium miners, workers in nickel refining, and people exposed to asbestos or chromium. The following observations implicate another industrial hazard that increases the risk of lung cancer.

Estimation of Risk

In a chemical manufacturing plant with approximately 2,000 employees periodic chest x-ray surveys were carried out for years. In 1962 management became aware that an excessive number of workers suspected of having lung cancer were being reported in one area of the plant (Cases 1–3, Table 1), and turned to a chest consultant, who recommended a program to establish the degree of risk by semiannual screening.

The program, begun in December, 1962, was patterned after the method of the Philadelphia Pulmonary Neoplasm Research Project[1] and was run in conjunction with it. Briefly, this consisted of a 70-mm chest photofluorogram and questionnaire regarding age, smoking habits and respiratory symptoms. Each man was interviewed at the first examination by one of us (W. W.).

A group of 125 men were studied over the next five years: 14 were lost at various intervals during the investigation because of job termination. In four (Cases 4–7, Table 1) of the remaining 111 men lung cancer developed during the five-year period of observation. Eighty-eight men were in the age group from 35 to 54, and all four cases of lung cancer occurred in this group, giving a five-year incidence of 4.54 per cent.

Table 1 Lung Cancer in CMME Workers

Case no.	Age (yr)	Smoking history*	Duration of exposure to CMME (yr)	Date of diagnosis	Histo-logic type	Survival (mo)
1	37	None	7	1962	Unknown	Unknown
2	33	1 ppd/20	8	1962	Oat cell	7
3	39	1 ppd/20	8	1962	Oat cell	6
4	47	1 ppd/20	10	1963	Oat cell	18
5	52	1 ppd/20	4	1964	Oat cell	11
6	47	1 ppd/20	3	1964	Oat cell	8
7	43	1 ppd/20	14	1966	Oat cell	4
8	53	2 ppd/20	10	1969	Oat cell	4
9	48	1 ppd/20	5	1970	Oat cell	11
10	50	1 ppd/20	1?†	1970	Squamous	24
11	55	1 ppd/20	12	1970	Oat cell	4
12	43	Pipe only	12	1970	Oat cell	20
13	37	None	14	1971	Oat cell	5
14	44	None	12	1971	Oat cell	10

*Packages/day (ppd) smoked/no. of yr.
†1 mo according to fellow workers.

The best estimate of the expected number of cases must be derived from the youngest age group under investigation in the Pulmonary Neoplasm Research Project. In that study there were 2,804 men 45 to 54 years of age, in 16 (0.57 per cent) of whom proved lung cancer developed in the first five years of observation. Smoking habits were very similar in the plant workers and the men under investigation in the Research Project: the proportions of cigarette smokers were 78 and 74 per cent respectively, and the proportions of current cigarette smokers using one or more packages per day were 24 and 20 per cent respectively. The slightly higher age of the Pulmonary Neoplasm Research Project groups makes the figure of 0.57 per cent an overestimate of the expected number, but if we accept it as the best available figure, a five-year incidence was eight times higher in the plant workers. With the use of the binomial theorem, this difference is statistically highly significant at a probability of 0.0017.

While this small risk study was in progress, plant management made a careful investigation of the work histories in several men whose lung cancers developed while they were working in the area under suspicion, and concluded that the only common denominator was exposure to chloromethyl methyl ether (CMME). Management is as yet unable to provide exact information on the exposure of the employees to CMME.

Further interest that CMME could be a carcinogen was stimulated by Case 14, a 44-year-old man admitted to Germantown Dispensary and Hospital in December, 1971, because of cough and hemoptysis. A detailed occupational history revealed that he was a chemical operator who had been exposed to CMME for 12 years. The patient stated that 13 of his fellow workers had lung cancer, and he suspected that this was his diagnosis. All had worked as chemical operators in the same building of a local chemical plant, where they mixed formalin, methanol and hydrochloric acid into two 3,800-liter kettles to produce CMME. During the process fumes were often visible. To check for losses, the lids on the kettles were raised several times during each shift. The employees considered it a good day if the entire building had to be evacuated only three or four times per eight-hour shift because of noxious fumes.

Characteristics of the Lung-Cancer Cases

A retrospective investigation of the 14 cases was made by examination of hospital records and autopsy results when available and by consultation with family physicians. The pertinent data are summarized in Table 1.

Age at diagnosis ranged from 33 to 55 years. Three men had never smoked, a fact that was confirmed in the interviews of Cases 13 and 14 during the risk study. One man smoked pipes only. The remaining 10 men smoked one package of cigarettes or more per day.

Estimates on duration of exposure to CMME were obtained from Case 14 since company management was unable to provide this information. Because they depend on one man's memory these estimates are only approximate, and the exact chronologic relation between exposure to CMME and diagnosis of the cancer is uncertain. The duration of exposure ranged from three to 14 years in 13 cases. Case 10 had been exposed for only one month according to Case 14, but the company stated that he had had no known exposure.

The histologic type of cancer was determined in 13 men; only a gross autopsy examination was made in Case 1. Oat-cell carcinoma was found in all men except case 10—his tumor was a squamous-cell carcinoma, and it is of interest that there is doubt about his exposure to CMME. All the men with oat-cell carcinoma died within 20 months of diagnosis.

Discussion

Chloromethyl methyl ether (CMME) and bis chloromethyl ether (BCME) are widely used in the chemical industry as intermediates in organic synthesis and in the preparation of ion-exchange resins. Commercial CMME contains 1 to 7 per cent BCME.

Recently, these agents have been found to be highly carcinogenic for mice and rats. [2-5] Indeed, the inhalation of as little as 0.1 ppm of BCME has produced squamous-cell carcinoma of the lungs in rats.[4] A recent report of six cases of lung cancer suspected of being due to occupational exposure to CMME in California[6] is a rare reference to a possible carcinogenic effect of this chemical in man.

The current study revealed certain findings of interest in the men in whom lung cancer developed. They were rather young, most being in the fourth and fifth decades at diagnosis, but the findings were largely due to the fact that the workers at risk were also primarily in this age group. The facts that three of the 14 men had never smoked and that all but one of the 13 histologically confirmed cancers were of oat-cell type are unusual. These peculiarities, together with the greatly increased risk demonstrated in the periodic screening study of the chemical-plant workers, strongly suggest that an industrial hazard is associated with CMME.

We are indebted to Dr. B. J. Miller, Department of Surgery, Germantown Dispensary and Hospital, for referring the index case to us and to Dr. Catherine Boucot Sturgis for advice in preparation of the manuscript.

SOURCE

Figueroa WG, Raszkowski R, and Weiss W. 1973. Lung cancer in chloromethyl methyl ether workers. *New Engl J Med* 288:1096–97. Copyright 1973 by *New England Journal of Medicine*. Reprinted with permission of Massachusetts Medical Society.

CHAPTER 6

WOMEN'S HEALTH

If men got pregnant, there would be safe, reliable methods of birth control. They'd be inexpensive, too.
> —Anna Quindlen (b. 1951), American journalist and author
> The *New York Times*. Living Out Loud, p. 31 (1988)

Violence against women is a worldwide yet still hidden problem. Freedom from the threat of harassment, battering, and sexual assault is a concept that most of us have a hard time imagining because violence is such a deep part of our cultures and our lives.
> —Boston Women's Health Book Collective
> *Our Bodies, Ourselves For The New Century* (1998, p. 158)

THE TWENTIETH CENTURY BEGAN STEEPED IN the Progressive Era, with women in many developed nations marching for the right to vote and the right to control their reproductive health (see Volume I, Chapter 22, Margaret Sanger). Everything changed mid century, however. The right to vote had been recognized in many nations, and oral contraceptives fostered an explosion of sexual freedom and women's pursuit of careers. New demands emerged as views changed, i.e., "equal pay for equal work," breaking the "glass ceiling," and challenges to "de-medicalize" childbirth (recognizing childbirth as a natural process rather than one requiring medical management). Access to safe and legal abortions became a battle cry for some even as the training for physicians to perform the procedure disappeared. Still others focused on eliminating domestic violence.

In developing nations, women continued to struggle with reproductive issues and poverty. Fertility control via imposed contraceptive implants and a one-child policy raised ethical challenges. Globally, violence against women, sex trafficking of women, female genital mutilation, and sexually transmitted diseases remained significant women's health issues. For example, the WHO reported that in the year 2000, in every country without exception, between 10 and 50 percent of women were physically abused by an intimate partner during their lifetime. In 1995 alone, the European Union estimated that half a million women were trafficked into their member nations for the sex trades. Such figures show that despite progress on some fronts, women's health and human rights issues remain dramatically interwoven.

REPRODUCTIVE ISSUES

Efforts to control fertility brought a variety of actors to the stage in the twentieth century. Some had Malthusian concerns and sought a safety valve for what they felt was an impending global population explosion and collapse. Others had a strong belief in eugenics and sought to selectively reduce the number of poor and other undesirables. Feminists seeking control of their bodies clashed with traditionalists and those with strong religious convictions about both birth control and abortion. Pharmaceutical research developed new birth control methods and brought them to market, but some of them yielded unexpected side effects. Furthermore, the need for economic development prompted some rapidly developing nations to take drastic steps to control their populations. Across the globe, fertility control and reproductive issues emerged in several forms: greater availability of barrier contraception, the introduction of oral contraceptives (which attended a variety of social issues), family limitation with increased availability of abortion and sterilization, and the development of postcoital contraception ("morning after" pill).

Barrier Contraceptives

The two most commonly used varieties of barrier contraceptives are the condom and the diaphragm, with the cervical cap and the sponge distantly trailing in popularity. There is some evidence that condoms were used in ancient times, but the idea that they were used specifically for contraception remains controversial. Gabriel Falloppio, a renowned Italian physician and anatomist, first described using condoms to prevent syphilis in the 1500s. It was more than a century later, however, before condoms were accepted as a regular means of birth control. Since that time, condom use has continued to grow. A female condom has even been developed, though it has a limited following.

The cervical cap was developed in the 1830s and the diaphragm in the 1880s. Both devices were improved when the rubber vulcanization process was invented in the late 1800s, making the items more resilient. The cervical cap was particularly popular in Europe in the early half of the twentieth century. It enjoyed some popularity in the United States though it was less popular than the diaphragm. Legal barriers prevented the dissemination of the diaphragm in the United States prior to the 1920s; the only manufacturer was in Europe, and importation into the United States was illegal. Birth control advocate Margaret Sanger bankrolled the founding of a United States diaphragm manufacturer, and she also financed the successful effort to overturn the federal laws prohibiting the transportation of such devices across state lines. By 1940, one-third of married women in the United States were using diaphragms. However, physicians remained reluctant to prescribe them for single women.

In the later part of the twentieth century, specifically as a response to the development of the HIV epidemic, condom use increased worldwide. Condoms became ubiquitous in some societies, even being required by statute for prostitutes to ply their trade legally. In other societies, condoms were viewed as an attempt to limit the right to procreate, as a challenge to masculinity, and as a promotion of promiscuity. As late as 2008, for instance, Pope Benedict XVI reaffirmed the Catholic Church's condemnation of artificial birth control, including the use of condoms by married couples in which one partner was known to have HIV. However, it seems unlikely that the HIV epidemic can be controlled, much less abated, without the use of condoms to prevent transmission of infection. How religious and spiritual authorities reconcile hostility to condoms with the challenges presented by the HIV epidemic remains to be seen.

Oral Contraceptives

Oral contraceptives represent the confluence of two developments: understanding the hormonal events underlying the menstrual cycle and the ability to synthesize steroids, in particular, variants of the sex hormones estrogen and progesterone. Advances in endocrinology during the first part of the twentieth century indicated that if one demarcated the menstrual cycle by menstruation, ovulation occurred mid cycle. Previously, it was thought that ovulation coincided with the period. In the 1920s, the demonstration of the relationship between ovulation and the presence of estrogen and progesterone was critical to establishing how to intervene in the cycle to prevent ovulation. In 1945, an oral contraceptive was proposed in a paper published in an obscure journal. Other scientists noted the ability to control apparent ovulation through manipulation of estrogen and progesterone levels. However, the challenge was the inability to synthesize estrogen and progesterone.

The innovation in the manufacture of the female sex hormones came with the development of a synthetic process using yams from Mexico. The Syntex Corporation was organized in Mexico to exploit this process; it secured a monopoly on the yams and began to produce the needed steroids. Many pharmaceutical companies in the United States used these steroids as the core for a variety of chemicals mimicking estrogen. Using these estrogenomimetic compounds, in 1957 G. D. Searle, in collaboration with Harvard gynecologist John Rock and contraceptive pioneer Gregory Pincus, developed Enovid. While Enovid was released for the treatment of menstrual disorders, it was clearly being used off label for contraceptive purposes. Within a decade it was being used by more than 40 percent of young American women as a means of birth control.

Soon after oral contraceptives (OCs) were introduced in England, reports surfaced of a thrombotic (blood clot) risk associated with their use. Investigations by health authorities and academics confirmed the risk. OC labels were revised to incorporate this additional risk, and further epidemiologic studies were initiated. In this manner, the field of pharmacoepidemiology and drug safety was born. Two further "generations" of OCs were introduced, each with lower amounts of estrogens than the prior one. Additional studies suggested that the thrombotic risk declined with the reduction in estrogen levels, but it was not eliminated. Later research found that OCs were protective against ovarian cancer and uterine cancer. The question remains as to whether the use of OCs increases the risk for breast cancer.

The introduction of OCs brought forth considerable social change. At first, there were many state laws banning the distribution of contraceptives to women who weren't married. During the 1960s, the U.S. Supreme Court reviewed such laws and declared them unconstitutional. The United States was not the only venue for such change. OCs became a popular approach to fertility control in many nations. For example, in 2000, 45 percent of French women aged 18 to 44 were current oral contraceptive users. Whether such use will continue with the identification of further health effects associated with the use of OCs remains to be seen.

One nation that did not jump onto the oral contraceptive bandwagon was Japan, where the pill was illegal until the very end of the twentieth century. Throughout that century, family planning in Japan consisted of abortion and condoms only, as there were concerns that the pill would not only promote promiscuity, but also lead to estrogen pollution of the environment and low sperm counts among Japanese men. With the development of drugs for erectile dysfunction, these concerns were diminished, but not eradicated, and the pill was approved in June 1999. Because of 40 years of bad publicity, Kunio Kitamura, head of Japan's family planning association, said "I didn't think it would take this long . . . The pill has such a bad image that now I will have to educate women about its advantages." At the time of this writing, the pill will still not be available through Japan's national health service.

Family Limitation and Abortion

The UN estimates that about one-fifth of all pregnancies worldwide end in abortion and that 95 percent of all abortions are performed in developing countries. The risk of maternal death from unsafe abortions in the year 2000 was estimated at 1 in 150 in developing nations, and 1 in 150,000 in developed ones—figures that tell of the nature of desperation of many women. Being the target of sexual violence or the tool of an unsafe sex trade makes abortion an unhappy choice for many. For others, it is an economic decision. Indeed, one more mouth to feed may mean the difference between being able to feed, clothe, and possibly educate a family's children and keeping the family mired in poverty. Various reports during the last decade of the twentieth century show the abortion rates highest in Eastern Europe, especially the Russian Federation (68 percent of pregnancies), Romania (63 percent), and Belarus (62 percent). Abortion rates were also over 50 percent in Cuba.

A major consideration in most reviews of global economic disparities and inequities is lack of access to family planning services. But access to such services, including safe and legal abortion, is not the same as forcing abortion on families as a means of fertility control. For example, after mid century when rapid population growth became a rising concern, the People's Republic of China issued "reproductive norms" as a means of controlling fertility. As of 1970, men were expected to wait to marry until they were at least 28 years old (25 in rural areas), and women were to be at least 25 years old (23 in rural areas). Beginning in 1979, households were limited to one child with additional children being subject to significant fines.

In India, the most common form of contraception remains tubal ligation, the female form of sterilization. This method is preferred in India as there is no need to teach large numbers of illiterate women how to use pills or intrauterine devices (IUDs), no cost for condoms or other barrier methods, and no need for follow-up. Unfortunately, the practice of sterilization is often done in an assembly line under unsanitary conditions. Thus, most women will not consent to sterilization until they have already borne half a dozen children. In the 1960s, a transistor radio was offered as an incentive for undergoing a vasectomy, but with the growth of the Indian economy, that approach has been retired.

CERVICAL CANCER SCREENING

Georgios N. Papanicolaou was born in Greece in 1883 and studied medicine in Athens and Munich before immigrating to New York in 1913. In 1914, he began working at the Weill Medical College of Cornell University under the direction of the chairman of the anatomy department, Charles Stockard. One of Papanicolaou's tasks at Cornell was to harvest guinea pig oocytes. In order to determine the best time to collect the eggs, he first needed to first determine the animals' menstrual cycles. Using a nasal speculum, Papanicolaou collected smear samples from the guinea pig vaginas and examined them under the microscope.

Finding that the cells in the smears yielded distinct cytological patterns at different times in the menstrual cycle, he was able to chart the changes each day in order to predict the best time to harvest the eggs.

Papanicolaou and Stockard published these results in the *American Journal of Anatomy* in 1917. Expanding upon his idea of mapping menstrual cycles, Papanicolaou began taking vaginal scrapings from women. He noticed that malignant cells were sometimes visible and hypothesized that because cancer cells rapidly reproduce, their presence in the vaginal smears could provide a means of early cancer detection. In 1920 he published his theory in the journal *Growth*. In 1928 he presented these results openly at the Race Betterment Conference in Battle Creek, Michigan, where the audience of physicians and scientists (invited by John Harvey Kellogg for the purpose of fostering eugenics) considered the idea of looking at dead cells ludicrous. They were sure that only a biopsy and histological exam could detect the disease.

In 1938, Papanicolaou teamed with Herbert F. Traut, a gynecologic pathologist at Cornell, to conduct a clinical study that could evaluate the vaginal smear as a diagnostic tool for uterine cancer. All women admitted to the gynecologic service of the New York Hospital submitted to a vaginal smear, and Papanicolaou took it upon himself to interpret each one. He found that many asymptomatic cancer cases were detected at an earlier stage than was detectable by biopsy. The findings were published in 1943, and the vaginal smear became widely known as the Pap smear. Although it took years for the Pap smear to become routinely administered to asymptomatic women, the effectiveness of the technique could not be denied as the mortality rate from cervical cancer dropped significantly.

VIOLENCE

Violence against women comes in many forms. In patriarchal societies, women are considered property, and the female victims of domestic violence are commonly charged with bringing the violence upon themselves. It is not atypical, for example, for family members, clergy, police, and medical professionals to side with the abuser, blame the victim, and leave her with nowhere to go except back home to more abuse. When women are killed by their abusers in the global North, society often terms these events "crimes of passion." In the global South, these same deaths are called "honor killings." Both terms are useful for defending perpetrators and helping to excuse their actions. Indeed, as honor killings are often considered private family affairs, few countries even keep official statistics on them. Zaynab Nawaz, program assistant for women's human rights at Amnesty International, says, "Females in the family—mothers, mothers-in-law, sisters, and cousins—frequently support the attacks. It's a community mentality." As we entered the twentieth century, the UN estimated that about 5,000 women were killed in honor killings annually, primarily because they in some way sullied the family name. The United Nations International Children's Emergency Fund (UNICEF) estimates that in India about 5,000 brides are killed annually because the families of the grooms consider their dowries insufficient. Most of the perpetrators in these instances go unpunished.

Not all violence against women ends in death, but the mental and physical effects as well as the social consequences for victims can be severe. For example, rape is effective in instilling terror and thus is widely practiced in war zones and refugee camps. In the last decade of the twentieth century alone, rape was revealed as a war tactic in Algeria, Angola, the Russian Federation (Chechnya), Cote d'Ivoire, the Democratic Republic of Congo, East Timor, India (Kashmir), Liberia, Rwanda, Sierra Leone, Sri Lanka, Sudan, northern Uganda, and the former Yugoslavia. In Darfur, innumerable international media reports documented that men wearing military uniforms routinely held women and young girls at knifepoint and publicly raped them to terrify and destroy the social cohesion of the surviving refugees. Aid workers in Darfur reported that women and girls sent out to collect firewood were repeatedly raped by militiamen. The situation became so dire that men in the camps became unwilling to accompany the women and girls on firewood gathering expeditions because they feared for their own lives if they tried to defend the women. On December 14, 2004, the British Broadcasting Company (BBC) reported the words of one rape survivor on its Africa News front page: "They want to destroy everything—by violating us, they want to make our men ashamed and to demoralise [sic] them." Authorities in Darfur, however, deny that rape and out-of-control militias exist. Instead, they claim that the refugees make up such stories for the press.

Public rape and gang rape also occur outside of war zones, especially in public institutions such as prisons and schools, as a means of social control. For example, if sexual violence at school threatens girls' safety, parents may choose to keep their daughters at home, thus diminishing their daughters' future earning power and reducing the likelihood of future social change. As resisting change may be a primary goal for some societies, public rape often goes unpunished. Most rape is private, however, with the perpetrators of the rapes being intimates of the victims, not strangers. Data from various surveys show that 14 to 20 percent of women in Canada, Korea, New Zealand, and the United States experience rape at some time during their lives. Statistics from Peru, Malaysia, the United States, and many other countries indicate that 60 to 80 percent of victims know their rapists. The psychological, as well as physical, scars left by rape can be significant. Furthermore, exposure to HIV/AIDS and other sexually transmitted diseases as well as the risk of pregnancy are frighteningly real. Unfortunately, the shame of being victimized by an intimate may prevent women from seeking medical care quickly enough to minimize these risks.

Human trafficking for forced labor and the sex trades is another form of violence against women and a global health issue. At the beginning of the twentieth century, both the U.S. government and the UN estimated that about 800,000 people were trafficked across international borders each year, and the vast majority were women and girls destined for the sex trades. At least 150,000 of these victims were from South Asia alone, and 50 percent were under the age of 18. A study by the European Union showed that 95 percent of women trafficked for prostitution were violently assaulted; more than 60 percent reported fatigue, neurological symptoms, gastrointestinal problems, back pain, and/or gynecological infections, including HIV/AIDS. A nine-country study of trafficked women found that 89 percent wanted to escape, 63 percent had been raped, 68 percent had post-traumatic stress disorder, and many suffered severe depression as well as suicidal tendencies. Unfortunately, little progress has been made to stem the problems of human trafficking. In 2000, the UN General Assembly issued the *Protocol to Prevent, Suppress, and Punish Trafficking In Persons, Especially Women and Children*, but the impact of that effort was less than hoped. In February 2008, the UN convened the first global forum against human trafficking in Vienna. Antonio Maria Costa, the executive director of the UN Office of Drugs and Crime, stated that trafficking remains "a monster whose shape, size, and ferocity we can only guess."

Women's health is a broad arena, with concerns dependent upon economic status, cultural expectations, and national norms. Women in developed nations may have better access to health care and family planning measures, but they are more likely to be at risk for chronic diseases and the unintended consequences of new therapies. In contrast, women in developing nations continue to struggle with lack of access to both health care and family planning measures. Globally, women of all cultures and economic statuses struggle against violence. The domestic violence literature alone abounds with descriptions of physical injury, depression, suicide, gynecological problems or infections, and pregnancy with complications (vaginal bleeding, premature labor, low birth weight, miscarriage, and stillbirth). The repercussions of rape and trafficking include all of the above plus the risk of sexually transmitted diseases, including HIV/AIDS.

Selected Readings

The first reading, by George N. Papanicolaou and Herbert F. Traut, is abstracted from their monograph *Diagnosis of Uterine Cancer by the Vaginal Smear*, published by The Commonwealth Fund in 1943. This slim volume brings together the scientific quest for understanding the menstrual cycle (which eventually led to the development of oral contraceptives) and the breakthrough in cytology that led to the development of a successful screening tool for cervical cancer. It is abridged here, removing the technical aspects of the laboratory techniques and the photos of the many cytology slides included in the original work. We believe our abridged version pays honor to the findings and the public health impact of the work. Today, women expect a Pap test or smear as part of routine gynecologic care, including women in developing countries. Indeed, since its introduction, Pap smear screening has been successful in reducing mortality from invasive cervical cancer by 70 to 90 percent. Limitations to the success of the Pap screening test include false negative results from inadequate samples and inaccurately read smears by poorly trained technicians. Pap smear screening programs are also reliant on health care systems that provide for clinical follow-up when a patient is identified as having abnormal results.

The second reading, by Louise Tryer, provides an excellent review of the introduction and social consequences of OCs. Some of these consequences were expected, such as the reduction in unwanted pregnancies as well as the moral, legal, and religious challenges that emerged. Other consequences, however, were not anticipated, especially the health concerns that arose from the original formulations. Tyrer puts it all together for the reader, showing the massive impact that the pill has had on not only women's physical health, but also on society as a whole.

Finally, L. Heise, M. Ellsberg, and M. Gottmoeller provide a global perspective on gender-based violence in the third reading. Beginning with the statement that violence against women is a human rights violation, they build the case that women suffer physically, emotionally, and economically from violence. They also explore the cultural roots of violence and show that violence leaves its impact on multiple generations. This work calls for change in the way health providers approach gender-based violence, but the challenge, unfortunately, remains a global issue.

BIBLIOGRAPHY

Agnihotri AK, Agnihotri M, Jeebun N, and Purwar B. 2006. Domestic violence against women—an international concern. *Torture* 16 (1): 30–40.

Anderson AD and Kring GG. 1958. The value of the Papanicolaou smear in the diagnosis of carcinoma of the uterine cervix and of the uterine fundus. *Wis Med J* 57 (7): 257–60.

Benangiano G and Schei B. 2004. A FIGO initiative for the 21st century: Eliminate all forms of violence against women worldwide. *Int J Gynecol Obstet* 86 (2): 328–34.

Bogen E. 1935. The cause of breast cancer. *Am J Public Health* 25 (3): 245–50.

Casper MJ and Clarke AE. 1998. Making the Pap smear into the 'right tool' for the bob: Cervical cancer screening in the USA, circa 1940–95. *Social Studies of Science* 28 (2): 255–90.

Centers for Disease Control and Prevention. 1999. Achievements in Public Health, 1900–1999: Family planning. *MMWR* 48 (47): 1073–80.

Clark JH. 2006. A critique of women's health initiative studies (2002–2006). *Nuclear Receptor Signaling* 4:e023.

Clarke AE and Casper MJ. 1996. From simple technology to complex arena: Classification of Pap smears, 1917–90. In: Biomedical technologies: Reconfiguring nature and culture. *Med Anthropol Q* 10 (4): 601–23.

Collaborative group for the study of stroke in young women. 1973. Oral contraception and increased risk of cerebral ischemia or thrombosis. *N Engl J Med* 288 (17): 871–78.

Collaborative group for the study of stroke in young women. 1975. Oral contraceptives and stroke in young women. *JAMA* 231 (7): 718–22.

Colton FB. 1992. Steroids and "the pill": Early steroid research at Searle. *Steroids* 7 (12): 30.

Davis JP, Osterholm MT, Helms CM, Vergeront JM, Wintermeyer LA, Forfang J, Judy LA, Rondeau J, Schell WL, and the Investigation Team. 1982. Tri-state toxic-shock syndrome study. II. Clinical and laboratory findings. *J Infect Dis* 145 (4): 441–48.

Dawson DA, Meny DJ, and Ridley JC. 1980. Fertility control in the United States before the contraceptive revolution. *Fam Plann Perspect* 12 (2): 76–86.

Djerassi C. 1992. Steroid research at Syntex: "the Pill" and corticone. *Steroids* 57 (12): 41.

Fremont-Smith M and Graham RM. 1952. Screening for cervical cancer in internist's office by routine vaginal smears. *J Am Med Assoc* 150 (6): 587–90.

Garcia CR, Pincus G, and Rock J. 1958. Effects of three 19-nor steroids on human ovulation and menstruation. *Am J Obstet Gynecol* 75 (1): 82–97.

Germain A. A new agenda for girls' and women's health and rights. Available at http://www.iwhc.org/resources/anewagenda.cfm.

Grimes DA, Mishell DR, Shoupe D, and Lacarra M. 1988. Early abortion with a single dose of the antiprogestin RU-486. *Am J Obstet Gynecol* 158 (6, Part 1): 307–12.

Herbst AL and Scully RE. 1970. Adenocarcinoma of the vagina in adolescence: A report of 7 cases including 6 clear-cell carcinomas (so-called mesonephromas). *Cancer* 25 (4): 745–57.

Herbst AL, Ulfelder H, and Poskanzer DC. 1971. Adenocarcinoma of the vagina: Association of maternal stilbestrol therapy with tumor appearance in young women. *N Engl J Med* 284 (15): 878–81.

Herbst AL, Ulfelder H, Poskanzer DC, and Longo LD. 1999. Adenocarcinoma of the vagina: Association of maternal stilbestrol therapy with tumor appearance in young women. 1971. *Am J Obstet Gynecol* 181 (6): 1574–75.

Herrero R. 1996. Epidemiology of cervical cancer. In: National Institutes of Health Consensus Conference on Cervical Cancer. *J Natl Cancer Inst* 22 (1): 1–6.

Hillis SD and Wasserheit JN. 1996. Screening for clamydia—A key to the prevention of pelvic inflammatory disease. *N Engl J Med* 334 (21): 1399–401.

Kaunitz AM. 1999. Oral contraception health benefits: Perception versus reality. *Contraception* 59 (Suppl. 1): 29S–33S.

Krantz G. 2002. Violence against women: A global public health issue! (Editorial). *J Epidemiol Community Health* 56 (4): 242–43.

Lanes SF and Rothman KJ. 1990. Tampon absorbency, composition, and oxygen content and risk of toxic shock syndrome. *J Clin Epidemiol* 43 (12): 1379–85.

La Vecchia C, Franceschi S, Decarli A, Fasoli M, Gentile A, and Tognoni G. 1984. "Pap" smear and the risk of cervical neoplasia: Quantitative estimates from a case-control study. *Lancet* 2 (8406): 779–82.

Lindsay S. 1949. The Papanicolaou-Traut method of cancer diagnosis: Its use as a routine pathologic laboratory procedure. *California Medicine* 70 (5): 413–16.

Marks LV. 2001. *Sexual Chemistry: A History of the Contraceptive Pill.* New Haven, CT: Yale University Press.

National Institutes of Health. 2005. NIH Consensus and State-of-the-Science Statements: Management of Menopause-Related Symptoms. *J Natl Cancer Inst Monogr* 22 (1). Available online at http://consensus.nih.gov/2005/2005MenopausalSymptomsSOS025main.htm.

Nelson HD, Haney E, Humphrey L, Miller J, Nedrow A, Nicolaidis C, Vesco K, Walker M, Bougatsos C, and Nygren P. 2005. *Management of Menopause-Related Symptoms. Evidence Report/Technology Assessment No. 120 (AHRQ 05-E016-2).* Rockville, MD: Agency for Healthcare Research and Quality.

Nelson HD, Humphrey LL, Nygren P, Teutsch SM, and Allan JD. 2002. Postmenopausal hormone replacement therapy: scientific review. *JAMA* 288 (7): 872–81. Comment in Grodstein. 2003. Letter. *JAMA* 289 (1): 44–45; author reply 45.

Norris JW. 1989. Oral contraceptives and stroke. *Stroke* 20 (4): 559–61.

Osterholm MT, Davis JP, Gibson RW, Mandel JS, Wintermeyer LA, Helms CM, Forfang JC, Rondeau J, and Vergeront JM. 1982. Tri-state toxic-state syndrome study. I. Epidemiologic findings. *J Infect Dis* 145 (4): 431–40.

Osterholm MT, Mandel JS, Davis JP, and Gibson RW. 1985. The impact of bias in the Tri-State Toxic-Shock Syndrome Study. *Arch Intern Med* 145 (4): 763–64.

Papanicolaou GN and Stockard CR. 1917. The existence of a typical oestrous cycle in the guinea pig; with a study of its histological and physiological changes. *American Journal of Anatomy* 22:225–83.

Perse T. 1985. The birth control movement in England and the United States: The first 100 years. *JAMA* 40 (4): 119–22.

Peterson HB and Lee NC. 1989. The health effects of oral contraceptives: Misperceptions, controversies, and continuing good news. *Clin Obstet Gynecol* 32 (2): 339–55.

Peterson HB and Lee NC. 1990. Long-term health risks and benefits of oral contraceptive use. *Obstet Gynecol Clin North Am* 17 (4): 775–88.

Rennie JWR. 1953. The early diagnosis and treatment of breast tumours. *Can Med Assoc J* 8 (2): 127–30.

Rosenberg L, Hennekens CH, Rosner B, Belanger C, Rothman KJ, and Speizer FE. 1980. Oral contraceptive use in relation to nonfatal myocardial infarction. *Am J Epidemiol* 111 (1): 59–66.

Scholes D, Stergachis A, Heidrich FE, Andrilla H, Holmes KK, and Stamm WE. 1996. Prevention of pelvic inflammatory disease by screening for cervical chlamydial infection. *N Engl J Med* 334 (21): 1362–66.

Shapiro S. 1997. Periodic screening for breast cancer: The HIP Randomized Controlled Trial. *J Natl Cancer Inst Monogr* 1997 (22): 27–30.

Sharp GB and Cole P. 1991. Identification of risk factors for diethylstilbestrol-associated clear cell adenocarcinoma of the vagina: similarities to endometrial cancer. *Am J Epidemiol* 134 (11): 1316–24.

Spencer SM. 1966. The birth control revolution. *Saturday Evening Post,* January 15, 1966.

U.S. Department of Health and Human Services, Office on Women's Health. 2002. *A Century of Women's Health 1900–2000.* http://www.womenshealth.gov/archive/owh/pub/century/century.pdf (accessed May 12, 2007).

U.S. House of Representatives. 2006. Hearing before the Subcommittee on Criminal Justice, Drug Policy, and Human Resources of the House Committee on Oversight and Government

Reform. *Women And Cancer: Where Are We In Prevention, Early Detection and Treatment Of Gynecologic Cancers? Serial 109–128.* 109th Cong., September 7, 2005. http://www.access .gpo.gov/congress/house/house07ch109.html (accessed June 10, 2007).

Vessey MP and Doll R. 1968. Investigation of relation between use of oral contraceptives and thromboembolic disease. *Brit Med J* 2 (5599): 199–205.

Vessey MP, Villard-Mackintosh L, McPherson K, and Yeates D. 1989. Mortality among oral contraceptive users: 20 year follow up of women in a cohort study. *BMJ* 299 (6714): 1487–91. Comment in *BMJ* 300 (6720): 330–31.

World Health Organization. 2008. *Eliminating Female Genital Mutilation: An Interagency Statement by UNAIDS, UNDP, UNECA, UNESCO, UNFPA, UNHCHR, UNHCR, UNICEF, UNIFEM, and WHO.* Geneva: WHO Press. www.un.org/womenwatch/daw/csw/csw52/statements_ missions/Interagency_Statement_on_Eliminating_FGM.pdf (accessed June 15, 2007).

World Health Organization. 2005. *Multi-country Study on Women's Health and Domestic Violence Against Women: Summary Report of Initial Results on Prevalence, Health Outcomes and Women's Responses.* Geneva: WHO Press.

Writing Group for the Women's Health Initiative. 2007. Risks and benefits of estrogen plus progestin in healthy postmenopausal women: principle results from the Women's Health Initiative Randomized Controlled Trial. *JAMA* 288 (3): 321–33.

Young B. 1963. Some aspects of mammography. *Proc R Soc Med* 56 (9): 772–75.

Diagnosis of Uterine Cancer by the Vaginal Smear
(1943, Abridged)

George N. Papanicolaou, M.D., Ph.D.
Department of Anatomy, Cornell University Medical College
And
Herbert F. Traut, M.D.
Department of Obstetrics and Gynecology, Cornell University
Medical College and the New York Hospital

Foreword

Although the great importance of cancer of the uterus is generally recognized and the need for techniques whereby its early diagnosis is possible is fully appreciated, progress has been slow and after many decades of the observation of malignant growths we are still hampered by the lack of adequate methods for revealing the presence of cancer in its incipient state. Cancer in its later and more advanced forms was known and described as early as the beginning of the Christian era. Paul of Aegina (*circa* 600 a.d.) probably qualifies as the first expert in the diagnosis and treatment of the disease, particularly cancer of the uterus and breast; however, it was not until well into the era of the microscope that Virchow gave us a cellular definition of the disease. A relatively short period of time has elapsed between the application of the microscope to the diagnosis of the disease in tissues and the next phase upon which we are now entering, namely, that of its recognition in individual cells or small groups of cells quite apart from the site of origin. We are just learning the intimate changes within the cells which are produced by malignant disease, and are thus attaining the ability to recognize them when they are cast off or become separated from the original growth, as in ascitic fluid, in metastases, in pleural fluid, and in vaginal secretions. Progress in this direction has been such that it seems quite possible that in time the cancer cell may be routinely recognized in gastric fluid and fecal and urinary excretions. Virchow taught that the only absolute means of knowing whether a tissue was malignant was by demonstrating its invasion of surrounding structures. It has been learned more recently that there are pre-invasive phases in the life cycle of malignant neoplasms and that these can be recognized by minute changes in the cells themselves. Some of these changes are irregularity in the shape of the cells and of their nuclei, anisocytosis or anisonucleosis, hyperchomatism, atypical structure, and atypical arrangement of the chromatin elements and of the nucleoli, abnormal mitosis, fragmentation of the nuclei, and many others.

Knowledge of the atypical architecture caused by malignancy in the individual cell has made possible the diagnosis of the pre-invasive state of cancer but, more than that, it has made cancer recognizable in locations apart from its origin, because detached cells carry with them the stigmata of the disease.

> G.N.P.
> > H.F.T.
>
> *January, 1943*

CHAPTER I
Diagnosis of Uterine Cancer by Means of Vaginal Smears

Introduction

In the struggle to control cancer, knowledge of the many phases of the disease process as well as the ability to recognize it in its early stages has been so inadequate that the development of any new method of approach to the problem is of importance. This is particularly true of malignant disease of the uterus. Although methods for treating uterine cancer have undoubtedly been improved so that a greater number of women in whom the disease is recognized can be cured, the total death rate ascribed to the disease in the United States has undergone scant diminution during the past twenty-five years. This unsatisfactory status, it is generally recognized, is due to the difficulties which surround early diagnosis and hence to the infrequent opportunities to treat the disease in its most susceptible stage.

The biopsy method which is the mainstay of the present routine for the demonstration of the disease is, after all, an operative procedure, requiring proper facilities and a technique which is somewhat time-consuming and expensive, and hence it cannot be applied upon the scale necessary to reveal the early lesions in women of the cancer-bearing age. Treatment of uterine cancer has therefore been limited almost entirely to the well-developed or late stages of the disease and the final results are somewhat disappointing. It is clear that any contribution to a knowledge of the disease which will permit the diagnosis and treatment of the very early lesions excites interest and comment. The need and the importance of a simple and inexpensive method of examining large numbers of prospective cancer bearers are obvious. The purpose of this study is to describe a method which is new in its application to the field of cancer diagnosis. The method has been in continuous use in the Women's Clinic of the

New York Hospital–Cornell Medical College Association for the past three years. An analysis of diagnostic results is also presented here.

For many years Papanicolaou (6) has studied the cellular content of the vaginal smear, both in the laboratory animal and in the human, in an effort to establish the morphological and pathological variations and their significance. The work relating to rodents (14) is well known and has been of great importance in advancing knowledge of endocrine physiology. In an attempt to apply the vaginal smear technique to the sex hormone problems of women (10) it was found that the picture was complicated by many pathological conditions. It thus became obvious that the variations due to these factors must be sorted out and identified as well as those related to the normal physiological processes. An association was therefore made between the present authors to carry out this purpose.

In the course of his studies, Papanicolaou discovered some years ago that cancer cells could be recognized in the human vaginal smear (4). The relationship of the malignant cells to the various types of uterine cancer and the demonstration of the vaginal smear as a reliable means for diagnosing early as well as firmly established lesions are new contributions which have a theoretical as well as a practical importance.

This volume presents a study of the abnormal cells characteristic of uterine carcinoma. It is hoped that ability to recognize and differentiate these cells in the vaginal smear will lead to the application of this method of diagnosis to many women, thus making possible the early recognition and effective treatment of the disease. It is also hoped that study of the early lesions, discovered by means of the vaginal smear, will lead to further knowledge and a better understanding of the primary chapters in the life history of the disease process.

Cancer of the uterus arises from a considerable number of different cell types. Within broad limits, the resulting growth follows a characteristic sequence depending upon its cellular inheritance. However, with the partial exception of adenoma malignum which originates in the gland-bearing mucosa of the endocervix and in the endometrium, all types of carcinoma of the uterus (including the very early stages of the disease) have a common characteristic, namely, they are exfoliative growths. By this is meant that they are constantly shedding superficially placed cells. These liberated cells float singly or in groups into the secretions of the uterus, the cervix, or the vagina, mix with normal cells, and are eventually passed into the vagina where they tend to accumulate.

This exfoliative characteristic makes it possible to observe in preparations of the vaginal secretion cells representing all the epithelial tissues, normal or pathological, which line the uterus or vagina at the time of investigation. In contrast, the curettage and biopsy techniques bring to the microscope only those cells actually reached by instrumentation which at best is a sampling procedure. Therefore, it cannot be considered completely thorough and is particularly ineffectual in the early stages of the disease when the lesion is small. Moreover, the preparation of the vaginal smear is so simple that the procedure can be widely applied and as often as necessary, without the restrictions of monetary and time costs imposed by curettage or biopsy.

The technique for preparing the vaginal smear will be dealt with in the section which follows. However, it must be emphasized that two criteria must be fulfilled before the vaginal smear method of diagnosis can be successful or reliable. In the first place, it is not recommended as a means of ultimate diagnosis. It should be used as a preliminary or sorting procedure and should be confirmed as a matter of routine by biopsy and tissue diagnosis. The reasons for this stipulation will become clear to all those who use the method, as they will not infrequently encounter smear preparations which contain so many abnormal cell forms that, while most suspicious of cancer, they are not able to make an absolute diagnosis. In other words, there are many criteria of probable malignancy in the smear preparations in addition to those which may be characterized as absolutely pathognomonic. In the second place, evaluation of individual cells or those arranged in small groups is a much more difficult task, requiring greater knowledge of cytology, than the recognition of cancer in tissue preparations where orientation of the abnormal cells to one another and to the basement membrane is of great assistance in making a diagnosis. In many ways the use of the vaginal smear preparation for the recognition of malignant cells is analogous to the use of blood-smear preparations in the diagnosis of diseases of the blood and blood-forming organs. Patient and repeated search of multiple preparations by well-trained microscopists is essential to success.

[The remainder of Chapter 1 describes the preparation and staining of vaginal smears. Chapters II through VII discuss the differentiation of cell types and are not reproduced here, Ed.]

CHAPTER VIII
Discussion of the Use of the Vaginal Smear as a Diagnostic Procedure

A very large number of vaginal smears, probably between seven and ten thousand, were prepared from the vaginas of 3,014 adult women, most of whom were in the cancer-bearing age of life. In this group of patients, 179 were found to have cancer which was primary in the uterus. Four women were found to have cancer of the ovary which had metastasized to various parts of the lower genital tract, producing lesions which shed cells that could be detected in the vaginal smears. Three others had cancer of the bladder or urethra producing cells that appeared in the vaginal spreads, all of which could be recognized as malignant in character, although the source was not always discernible. Finally, there were seven instances of carcinoma of the vulva, all but one of which were productive of cells that were found and recognized in the vaginal smears (Plate H, 19-21) [Not shown, Ed.]. Thus there were 193 instances of carcinoma involving the uterus and some part of the lower genital tract. The malignant processes which were primary in the uterus were the only ones occurring in sufficient numbers to provide a basis for forming any adequate concept of the value of the vaginal smear as a method of diagnosing the presence of the carcinomatous process.

Carcinoma of the Cervix

There were 127 cases of carcinoma of the cervix. Of these, 107 were squamous carcinomas. Six were of the adenoma malignum variety, while twelve were frank adenocarcinomas and two were adenoacanthomas. Of the whole group, seven were found to be very early intradermal types of squamous carcinoma, and all of these were productive of abundant cellular desquamation so that their presence could be easily detected, although nearly all of them were invisible upon close inspection of the cervix.

In the total group, twenty-four had been treated with radiation therapy and many of these showed a greatly reduced tendency to shed cells as well as being characterized by the production of atypical cells showing radiation effect (Plate F, 31-35) [Not shown, Ed.]. Of this group of postradiational lesions there were only two which did not shed cells. We have not included a considerable number of cases with healed lesions as the result of radiation treatment, because these uniformly showed no shedding of malignant cells, which is what might be expected. It would seem therefore that the vaginal smear method is of use not only in the diagnosis of carcinoma of the cervix, but also in following the results of therapy. There is a close relationship between the shedding of the malignant cells and the process of degeneration and of final healing.

In the entire group of 127 patients with demonstrable lesions of the cervix, failure to detect the malignant cells in the vaginal smears occurred four times. Analysis of these four cases yields the following information: one patient had an unhealed cervix which had been amputated previously at another institution and repeated smears failed to reveal the presence of any surviving carcinoma; a second patient had an early adenoma malignum which failed completely to make its presence known by exfoliating cells; the third patient had an adenoma malignum of greater proportions which had been treated with intracanalicular radium and which also remained undiscovered; the fourth patient had a Grade II squamous cell carcinoma which, though not completely healed after treatment with radium, could not be detected. The incidence of negative smears for the series as a whole is therefore 3.2 per cent. If the postradiational cases are excluded, the incidence of negative findings is 1.6 per cent.

This experience would seem to indicate that the vaginal smear method in the hands of careful workers forms a reliable accessory method for the study of carcinoma of the cervix of the uterus. It would seem that with the exception of the adenoma malignum, the method offers a distinct advance in the field of diagnosis.

Carcinoma of the Fundus

There was a total of fifty-three patients in this series who had primary carcinoma of the fundus. Forty-one were well-defined papillary and undifferentiated lesions. One patient had a mesodermal type of carcinosarcoma which shed its cells copiously (Plate H, 17-18) [Not shown, Ed.]. There were five instances of adenoacanthoma and six of the well-differentiated adenoma malignum variety. Of the entire group of fifty-three patients, eight were found to have very early superficial and circumscribed lesions. There were five instances of postradiational carcinoma, two of which failed to show any surface cells surviving when the uterus was opened for inspection.

Failure to diagnose carcinoma in the entire series occurred seven times. Analysis of these instances yields the following data: two cases were postradiational and had no surface cells surviving, four were adenoma malignum, and one was an adenocarcinoma associated with pyometra and an occluded cervix. Excluding the postradiational cases which could hardly have been expected to yield positive smears under the circumstances, the percentage of failure is found to be 9.3. This percentage is much higher than in the case of the carcinomas of the cervix, but, as will be seen, it is due, for the most part, to the relatively high incidence of adenoma malignum, which as has been pointed out, is slow to shed. However, the conclusion is inescapable that the vaginal smear method is not as accurate for the diagnosis of carcinoma of the fundus as it is for that of carcinoma of the cervix.

It should be pointed out, however, in evaluating the method, that the routine use of the vaginal smear in the care of gynecological patients was the only means which brought the presence of unsuspected adenocarcinoma to the attention of the clinicians in nine instances in this series. In other words, failure to diagnose carcinoma on seven occasions in which it was demonstrated by curettage is offset by nine instances in which the presence of the tumors was primarily revealed through the examination of vaginal smears. As these patients were under forty-five years of age and gave no symptoms leading to an indication for curettage, the value of the vaginal smear is enhanced as a diagnostic procedure. On two occasions the vaginal smears revealed adenocarcinoma correctly when repeated curettage failed to do so because of the inaccessible location of the lesion. Furthermore, it should be pointed out that the detection of adenocarcinoma cells arising from the fundus is much more difficult from the cytological point of view than in the other forms of uterine cancer. As the study has progressed, a marked increase in proficiency was evidenced. It may be, therefore, that with added experience this handicap can be further reduced.

Other Forms of Carcinoma

For the sake of completeness, our experience in encountering other forms of cancer of the lower genital tract has been mentioned. These lesions resulted from metastases or direct extension to the uterus, the cervix, or the vagina and vulva. It is quite remarkable that these processes should also produce cells which can be recognized as malignant in nature. They form a complicating factor, however, and stress the importance of careful clinical observation of the patient, and the need for alert and discriminating observation on the part of the microscopist. It is noteworthy that most of these lesions presented cells of such a bizarre form that we had difficulty in accounting for them until the patient had been most carefully studied. The cells from the transitional epithelium of the urinary tract, for instance, are very clearly defined and quite typical in nature (Plate C, 27) [Not shown, Ed.]. In similar manner the metastatic lesions from carcinoma of the ovary produced cells which could not be accounted for as coming from the uterus or vagina (Plate H, 2-5) [Not shown, Ed.]. The vulva can usually be counted upon to produce such large and atypical cells as to call one's attention at once to some unusual lesions (Plate H, 19-210 [Not shown, Ed.].

In four cases, one of carcinoma of the cervix, one of adenocarcinoma of the endometrium, one of adenoma malignum, and one of adenocarcinoma of the cervix, the patients were having treatments with estrogenic hormone during the period of the study. As a result of this treatment, the leucocytes decreased considerably in number and the erythrocytes became less numerous. The small basal cells were largely replaced by superficial squamous cells, many of the acidophilic type. The malignant tumor cells of the cervix and of the endometrium, however, persisted at all times and could be much more easily recognized and identified. In the case illustrated in Plate K, 3-4 [Not shown, Ed.], eight milligrams of stilbestrol had been administered from June 9, 1941, when the first smear was taken, to June 14, 1941, the date of the second smear. Although the number of treated cases was relatively small, the results have conclusively demonstrated that such a method of treatment may facilitate the recognition of malignant cells in the vaginal smear.

SOURCE

Papanicolaou GN and Traut HF. 1943. *Diagnosis of Uterine Cancer by the Vaginal Smear.* New York: The Commonwealth Fund. Reprinted in 1945, 1957, and 1949. The abridged 1949 version with updated bibliography is reprinted here by permission of the Commonwealth Fund.

Introduction of the Pill and Its Impact
(1999)

Louise Tyrer

Introduction of the birth control pill in the United States in 1960 marked the end of a relatively short period of time (<10 years) to intentionally produce an oral contraceptive, and the beginning of a relatively long period of controversy surrounding the use of the pill. Availability of the pill had an impact on various aspects of social life, including women's health, fertility trends, laws and policies, religion, interpersonal relationships and family roles, feminist issues, and gender relations, as well as sexual practices among both adults and adolescents. The pill proved to be highly effective from the outset. Although safety issues developed with the earlier formulations, continued evolution of pill hormones and doses has resulted in a greatly improved and safe oral contraceptive. A broad range of noncontraceptive health benefits also is associated with the pill. These health effects are significant, as they include protection against potentially fatal diseases, including ovarian and endometrial cancers, as well as against other conditions that are associated with substantial morbidity and potential hospitalization and associated costs. The popularity of the pill has remained high, with rates of use in the past 30 years in the United States ranging from one-quarter to almost one-third of women using contraception. Almost 40 years after its introduction, the pill's contraceptive efficacy is proven, its improved safety has been established, and the focus has shifted from supposed health risks to documented and real health benefits. *CONTRACEPTION 1999;59:11S–16S © 1999 Elsevier Science Inc. All rights reserved.*

KEY WORDS—oral contraceptives, introduction of the pill, noncontraceptive health effects, history of oral contraceptives

Introduction

Introduction of the birth control pill in the United States marked both an end and a beginning. First, it marked the end of a relatively short period of time (<10 years) to intentionally produce an oral contraceptive. It also marked the beginning of a relatively long period of controversy surrounding the use of the pill. The controversy comprised various social influences including legal, religious, and feminist issues, as well as health concerns. Almost 40 years later, it is useful to examine the relative role of social factors in pill use today, as well as the shift in focus from health risks to health benefits.

Stages in Approval of the Pill

Stages leading to the approval of the pill are summarized in Figure 1. Around the same time that combinations of progestin and estrogen were

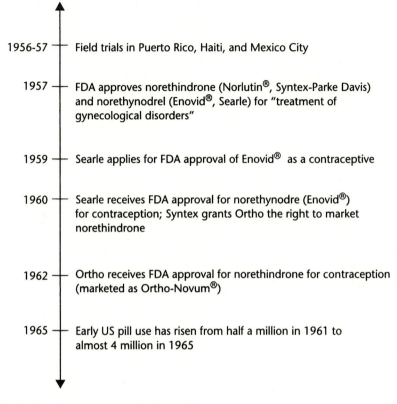

1956-57 — Field trials in Puerto Rico, Haiti, and Mexico City

1957 — FDA approves norethindrone (Norlutin®, Syntex-Parke Davis) and norethynodrel (Enovid®, Searle) for "treatment of gynecological disorders"

1959 — Searle applies for FDA approval of Enovid® as a contraceptive

1960 — Searle receives FDA approval for norethynodre (Enovid®) for contraception; Syntex grants Ortho the right to market norethindrone

1962 — Ortho receives FDA approval for norethindrone for contraception (marketed as Ortho-Novum®)

1965 — Early US pill use has risen from half a million in 1961 to almost 4 million in 1965

Figure 1 Stages in approval of the pill.[1]

being field-tested for contraception in a sufficient sample of women who consented to enroll in the study, in Puerto Rico, Haiti, and Mexico City, the Food and Drug Administration (FDA) approved two such drugs in the United States.[1] Parke-Davis (Morris Plains, NJ) applied for FDA approval of the Syntex (Palo Alto, CA) product, norethindrone (Norlutin®), for which it had obtained marketing rights from Syntex.[1] Similarly, Searle (Chicago, IL) applied to the FDA for approval of its progestin, norethynodrel (Enovid®)[1]. In 1957 both drugs received FDA approval, but were specifically limited to the treatment of gynecologic disorders.[1]

Everyone in the pharmaceutical industry knew that these drugs could be used for contraceptive purposes, but most were reluctant to consider applying for FDA approval for that indication for several reasons. For contraceptive purposes, a healthy woman would be required to take a drug every day for 21 days, a concept most industry experts felt women would have difficulty accepting. Such use would cost about $10 each month, which was expensive at that time.[1] There were concerns about religious disapproval in the population, and top executives of some companies that opted not to pursue the pill were themselves Roman Catholic (e.g., Parke-Davis's chairman and Merck's chief executive).[1] Manufacturers also worried about potential side effects, including the long-term effect of suppressing ovulation. Furthermore, the prohibition against disseminating birth control information in some states (e.g., Connecticut, Massachusetts) presented legal problems.

Ultimately, Searle was the first to risk marketing a birth control pill when it applied in 1959 for an FDA indication for contraception for Enovid, in the same formulation currently being used for menstrual disorders.[1] On May 11, 1960, the FDA approved the first drug for contraception, Searle's norethynodrel formulation (Enovid).[1] Meanwhile, Syntex, which still held the patent on norethindrone, signed a contract with the Ortho Division of Johnson & Johnson (Arlington, TX) to market it as a contraceptive.[1] Ortho planned to immediately submit an application to the FDA; however, Parke-Davis was unwilling to release some preclinical data it had collected. Therefore, Ortho repeated several studies that resulted in FDA approval of the Syntex formulation containing the progestin norethindrone, in 1962.[1] Ortho marketed the second contraceptive pill to reach the market as Ortho-Novum®.[1]

Questions about whether women and society would accept a contraceptive pill were soon answered. Whether or not ideological objections to the pill existed, its use did not seem to have been hindered. It became clear that women were desperately looking for a convenient, effective means by which they could control their fertility. In 1961, an estimated 408,000 women in the United States were using the pill. In 1962 the number was 1,187,000, which climbed to 2.3 million in 1963, and to 3.8 million in 1965.[1] By 1967, the number of women using the pill worldwide was estimated to be >12.5 million.[1] Use of the pill continues to grow; however, misperceptions about potential negative effects persist.

Although FDA approval of the pill led to its use by increasing numbers of women, many concerns still faced health professionals as well as women using the pill. These concerns posed the following questions to users of the pill, their clinicians, and the larger society: Was it safe? Was it legal? Did it conflict with one's religious beliefs? Was it going to adversely affect gender relations, morals, or society in general? Was it going to encourage irresponsible sexual behavior? (For example, what would the effect be of separating sexual activity from procreation?) Would it be affordable or available to all women? Would it advance the interests of women, or were potentially negative aspects of the pill a hindrance? Some of these questions remain today.

Health Issues Concerning the Pill

One of the major concerns associated with the early pill, which contained relatively high doses of hormones, was related to potential adverse health effects. As observed in the field trials, immediate side effects were associated with pill use in some women. Some of the more commonly reported effects included headache, nausea, and dizziness.[1] However, within a few years of FDA approval, serious cardiovascular effects were observed in a small proportion of users, including stroke, venous thromboembolism, and myocardial infarction. In addition, there continued to be concerns related to the long-term effects of taking the pill. People wondered whether the long-term suppression of ovulation would present problems when women later decided to discontinue the pill to become pregnant. Also, long-term consumption of hormones raised questions about potential cancer risk. In light of these concerns, critics wondered if oral contraceptives had been tested extensively enough before their approval. Furthermore, later criticisms were made concerning the primary population in which the pills were tested, that is, women not in the United States.

Development of Serious Threats to Health

As early as 1962, reports of serious adverse effects associated with the first pills were accumulating, notably 132 reports of thromboembolism, which included 11 deaths.[1] Indeed, early epidemiologic studies of oral contraceptives containing high doses of estrogen (>50μg) reported increased risks of several cardiovascular events, including venous thromboembolism, stroke, and myocardial infarction.[2,3] Later studies controlling for confounding variables would identify the role of certain preexisting health conditions such as hypertension, and particularly the risks to smokers, as factors that increased the incidence of cardiovascular events among women who used the pill.[2,3] Today, these data enable healthcare providers to screen women for any of these risk factors before prescribing the pill.

Role of Steroid Amount

The relation of amount of steroid to serious adverse effects of the pill was a major focus of pharmaceutical companies. By 1965, Searle had introduced a revised version of Enovid (Enovid-E) that contained 100μg estrogen and 2.5mg progestin, compared with 150μg estrogen and 9.85mg progestin in the original formulation.[4] By 1970, Wyeth (Philadelphia, PA) had introduced a pill with 50μg estrogen and 0.5mg progestin (Ovral®).[4] These formulation changes and dose reductions continued with the introduction of a progestin-only pill in 1973 and combination pills containing as little as 20μg estrogen in 1974. In the early 1980s, biphasic and triphasic pills were introduced, which varied the levels of estrogen and progestin delivered over the course of a cycle.[4]

Other Issues Concerning the Pill

Legal Issues

Although enforcement of laws concerning contraception may not have been a practical concern, it is noteworthy that some laws were still on the books concerning dissemination of birth control information around the time that oral contraception became available in the United States. In the late 1950s, after Enovid and Norlutin were approved for treatment of disorders, 17 states had laws limiting the sale, distribution, or advertising of contraceptives.[1] Connecticut law made it a crime to use contraceptives. In fact, the last law to be repealed was the Massachusetts law making it a felony to exhibit, sell, prescribe, provide, or give out information about contraceptives. It was not repealed until 1972.[1]

The United States legal environment may have become more favorable toward women using the pill; however, this is not necessarily the case throughout the world. In Japan, another industrial democratic society like the United States, the pill is still not approved for contraception; condom use is high, and there is a high rate of elective abortion.[1,5]

Religious Issues Concerning the Pill

A major factor involved in the controversy surrounding the introduction of the pill was its violation of certain religious prohibitions against contraception, particularly those of the Roman Catholic Church. Although forms of barrier contraception existed, they were either less used (due to lack of effectiveness) or quietly used. Their availability was not publicized in the same way as that of the new oral contraceptives.

Use of the pill presented dilemmas among certain religious groups and individuals. Because consumption of the pill on a daily basis was required for contraception, in the eyes of the Catholic Church women would be committing sin on a daily basis. Unlike barrier methods, used only at the time of intercourse, or sterilization, which was an action undertaken only once, taking the pill made the sin of contraception more of a dilemma for both women and their partners. Furthermore, physicians with certain strong religious beliefs had to choose between their medical responsibility to their patients and their personally held responsibility to their church. Despite church prohibition, 53% of American Catholics polled in 1967 were using the pill or another method rather than the church-approved rhythm method, and 80% of those <35 years of age said that they would like the church to approve use of the pill.[1]

Psychological Issues

Availability of an effective, reversible contraceptive that women could use independent of the sexual act presented a variety of psychosocial issues. For example, a woman could use the pill without relying on her partner to use a condom or having to prepare herself with a diaphragm, foam, or other coitally related method. Thus, pill use led to greater control over her fertility. In addition, by being able to limit the number and determine the timing of pregnancies, women were now in a position to better pursue their personal life goals, including education, employment, and professional endeavors. The equal rights movement for women that occurred in the 1960s and 1970s has been tied to many other events around the same time, but significantly relates to the availability of the pill.

Although concern about married women's use of the pill was high, potential adolescent use of the pill was clearly viewed as a problem. There were concerns that teenage sexual activity would increase. However, a 1972 survey revealed that more than three-fourths of sexually active women had used contraceptives only sometimes or never.[1] Despite availability of the pill for >10 years, a reluctance to use contraception existed among young women. Cultural factors, including appearing "ready" for sex rather than spontaneously performing "an act of the moment," seem to have played a greater role in teenage behavior than the presence of the pill. This factor continues today to influence adolescent attitudes toward contraception.

If women no longer had to rely on their partners for contraception, some tensions would likely be created if partner approval of method choice or overall contraceptive use had previously been required. Theoretically, a woman could determine the purposes of her fertility without her partner's input. Because this capability could then allow her to make other life choices, including work, the potential arose for a significant impact of the nature of relations between wives and husbands, women and men.

Economic Issues

About the same time the pill was approved, its cost was estimated at approximately $10 each month.[1] This amount was considered expensive 40 years ago, and was probably affordable only for the middle or upper economic classes. However, by 1964 the United States government had established a pilot project with Federal support of birth control for the poor.[1] In 1970, President Nixon announced a new national goal of family planning services for everyone who wanted but could not afford them.[1] Shortly after the pill became available in the United States, England's National Health Service (NHS) was subsidizing the cost of the pill; women paid two shillings (US $0.28) for a month's supply of pills and the British government paid the difference (about $2.08).[1]

More recently, in 1994 Federal and state funding for contraceptive services and supplies totaled $715 million.[6] Federal funding comes from a mix of sources including Title X of the Public Health Service Act; Titles V, XIX, and XX of the Social Security Act (also known as the maternal and child health block grant); Medicaid; and the social services block grant.[6] In addition, states also provide funding. Of all United States women who use reversible forms of contraception, one-quarter (24%) obtain family planning services from either a publicly funded clinic or a Medicaid provider.[7] It has been estimated that if these services were not available, 1.3 million additional unplanned pregnancies would occur annually in the United States.[7] Thus, the government's role in the provision of economic support for family planning has had a major impact on women's lives through the avoidance of unintended pregnancy. Although all government family planning programs currently make oral contraceptives available to their clients, reimbursement from private insurers for contraception in general, and the pill specifically, remains highly variable. This holds true for government employees as well. The Lowey Amendment, requiring that Federal Employees Health Benefits (FEHB) plans provide contraception coverage, was passed by Congress as part of the 1999 national budget. All FEHB health plans are now required to cover five reversible forms of contraception (pill, diaphragm, IUD, implant, and injectable). (Plans with religious affiliations can exempt themselves from this requirement on religious grounds and individual providers can refuse on moral grounds to provide contraceptives.) Previously, only 19% of plans covered all five of these methods, and 10% did not cover any method.[8]

Feminist Issues

Although it is safe to say that the pill was the brainchild of two early "feminists," Margaret Sanger [See Volume I, Chapter 22, Ed.] and Katharine McCormick, over time their motivation for promoting development of a contraceptive pill has been questioned. In various correspondences, their hopes for such a pill alternately rested on a desire for women to be able to control their fertility and therefore their lives, and a desire to reduce the fertility of certain types of women (namely, impoverished and so-called "dysgenic types").[1] This latter motive fueled criticism among feminists who viewed the pill as a discriminatory population-control mechanism, in addition to being a "harmful" method in light of its early but rare adverse effects. Another aspect of feminist criticism focused on what was considered an exploitative approach to testing the pill. The fact that early tests were carried out on non-American women in Puerto Rico,

Haiti, and Mexico was questioned. Although the high level of use of the pill stands as a testament to its acceptance and popularity, certain feminist attacks on the pill have focused on its potential harm to women's health (primarily based on studies of the early, high-dose formulations); the fact that it cannot be used by men and, therefore, situates the entire responsibility for contraception with women; and its lack of protection against sexually transmitted diseases.

Safety of Oral Contraceptives

Misperceptions Related to Pill Use

Many early concerns about the pill stemmed from the lack of long-term experience with its use. Although the pill had been tested in thousands of women before it entered the market, it had not been used in these women for many years or, ideally, one generation. Thus many concerns and misperceptions abounded. Because pill use consisted of daily administration of hormones, both users and physicians alike believed that some kind of periodic "break" from the pill was necessary. Early pill users wondered if they would jeopardize future fertility by suppressing current fertility with the pill. Furthermore, there was concern that the "excess" hormones present in women's bodies could somehow adversely affect the next generation of daughters eventually born to them. This concern arose because of the experience with diethylstilbestrol, which did have an adverse effect on the reproductive tracts of some of the offspring of women receiving this experimental therapy to treat threatened abortion. Probably the overriding misperception was that the pill would lead to breast cancer.[9]

Evolution of Pill Dose and Safety

In the 40-year history of the pill, both the content and dose of its steroid components have changed significantly. A study of changes in pill content from 1964 to 1988 documented a steady decline in mean estrogen and progestin doses in all types of formulations, which was accompanied by changes in the types of steroids used as well.[10] Although estrogen doses >50 µg comprised the majority of prescriptions between 1964 and 1971, they were steadily taken over by formulations with 50 µg into the early 1980s. From around 1983 to present, the majority of pill prescriptions have been for formulations <50 µg estrogen. Scientists now conclude that, "The data demonstrate that oral contraceptive formulations in wide use today differ in hormone content and side effects from those of the past, when most of the major studies addressing the risks associated with oral contraceptive use were completed."[10]

A review of the epidemiology of oral contraceptives and cardiovascular disease among current users of today's pills is unwarranted.[3] In addition to changes made in pill content and dose, the other important factor in the improved safety profiles relates to the identification of women with risk factors, such as smoking, high blood pressure, history of cardiovascular disease, and diabetes with vascular disease.[3] Better selection of users coupled with safer formulations have made the "risks" associated with pill use far less than those associated with full-term pregnancy.[3]

Identification of Pill Health Benefits

The story of pill would not be complete without a discussion of the noncontraceptive health benefits that have been associated with the use of the pill.[11]

Conclusions

Introduction of the pill into American society almost 40 years ago stands out as an epochal event in human history. It has had an impact on various aspects of social life, including women's careers, health, fertility trends, laws and policies, religion, interpersonal relationships and family roles, feminist issues, and gender relations, as well as sexual practices among both adults and adolescents. In short, it has forced society to reexamine many long-standing beliefs that seemed to come together at the point of women's control over their fertility. Although introduction of the pill resulted in controversy in many areas of social life, early rates of use in the United States exceeded 20% of currently married white women aged 18–39 years,[12,13] and, in the past 30 years, have ranged from one-quarter to almost one-third of women using any method of contraception.[12-14] By the end of the reproductive years, >80% of United States women have used the pill for an average of about 5 years.[15]

From the outset, the pill proved to be highly effective. Although rare safety issues developed with the earlier formulations, continued evolution of pill content and hormone dose has resulted in a greatly improved and safer oral contraceptive. Clinical refinements in the identification of risk factors, such as smoking and certain preexisting medical conditions (cardiovascular disease, hypertension), have permitted better patient selection. Currently, most healthy nonsmokers can take the pill until menopause, at which time they should be encouraged to switch to hormone replacement therapy for additional benefits. In addition to contraceptive efficacy, a broad range of noncontraceptive health benefits is associated with the pill. These health effects are significant, as they include protection from potentially fatal diseases as well as other conditions that are associated with substantial morbidity.

Although it is useful to understand the impact the pill has had on society, it is also important to view its impact within the more specific context of its benefits for the individual woman who uses it, both from the perspective of contraceptive effectiveness and from that of supplemental health benefits. It is here where one can fully appreciate the significant contribution the pill has made in so many areas of modern life.

SOURCE

Tryer L. 1999. Introduction of the pill and its impact. *Contraception* 59:11S–16S. Copyright 1999 *Contraception*. Reprinted with permission of Elsevier.

A Global Overview of Gender-based Violence
(2002)
Program for Appropriate Technology in Health (PATH), Washington, DC, USA

L. Heise, M. Ellsberg, M. Gottmoeller

Abstract

This paper provides an overview of the extent and nature of gender-based violence and its health consequences, particularly on sexual and reproductive health. © 2002 International Federation of Gynecology and Obstetrics. Published by Elsevier Science Ireland Ltd. All rights reserved.

KEYWORDS:—Violence; Women; Gender; Health

Violence against women is the most pervasive yet least recognized human rights violations in the world. It also is a profound health problem, sapping women's energy, compromising their physical health, and eroding their self-esteem. In addition to causing injury, violence increases women's long-term risk of a number of other health problems, including chronic pain, physical disability, drug and alcohol abuse and depression. Women with a history of physical or sexual abuse are also at increased risk for unintended pregnancy, sexually transmitted infections (STIs), and adverse pregnancy outcomes.

Despite its high costs, almost every society in the world has social institutions that legitimize, obscure and deny abuse. The same acts that would be punished if directed at an employer, a neighbor, or an acquaintance often go unchallenged when men direct them at women, especially within the family.

For over two decades women's advocacy groups around the world have been working to draw more attention to the physical, psychological, and sexual abuse of women and to stress the need for action. They have provided abused women with shelter, lobbied for legal reforms, and challenged the widespread attitudes and beliefs that support violent behavior against women [1].

Increasingly, these efforts are having results. Today, international institutions are speaking out against gender-based violence. Surveys and studies are collecting more information about the prevalence and nature of the abuse. More organizations, service providers, and policymakers are recognizing that violence against women has serious adverse consequences for women's health and for society.

1. Extent and Nature of the Problem

Gender-based violence includes a host of harmful behaviors that are directed at women and girls because of their sex, including wife abuse, sexual assault, dowry-related murder, marital rape, selective malnourishment of female children, forced prostitution, female genital mutilation, and sexual abuse of female children. Specifically, violence against women includes any act of verbal or physical force, coercion or life-threatening deprivation, directed at an individual woman or girl that causes physical or psychological harm, humiliation or arbitrary deprivation of liberty and that perpetuates female subordination [2].

2. Intimate Partner Violence

The most pervasive form of gender violence is abuse of women by intimate male partners. A recent review of 50 population-based studies carried out in 36 countries indicates that between 10 and 60% of women who have ever been married or partnered have experienced at least one incident of physical violence from a current or former intimate partner [2]. Although women can also be violent and abuse exists in some same-sex relationships, the vast majority of partner abuse is perpetrated by men against their female partners.

Representative sample surveys indicate that physical violence in intimate relationships is almost always accompanied by psychological abuse and, in one-third to over one-half of cases, by sexual abuse [3–5]. Most women who suffer any physical aggression generally experience multiple acts over time. However, measuring 'acts'of violence does not describe the atmosphere of terror that often permeates abusive relationships. For example, in Canada's 1993 national violence survey one-third of women who were abused physically in a relationship said they had feared for their lives at some time [6]. Women often say that the psychological abuse and degradation are even more difficult to endure than the physical abuse itself.

3. Sexual Coercion and Abuse

Sexual coercion and abuse also emerge as defining features of the female experience for many women and girls. Forced sexual contact can take place at any time in a woman's life and includes a range of behaviors, from forcible rape to non-physical forms of pressure to compel girls and women to engage in sex against their will. The touchstone of coercion is that a woman lacks choice and faces severe physical or social consequences if she resists sexual advances.

Studies indicate that the majority of nonconsensual sex takes place among individuals known to each other—spouses, family members, courtship partners, or acquaintances [7, 8]. Ironically, much nonconsensual sex takes place within consensual unions. For example, in a 15-country qualitative study of women's HIV risk, women related profoundly troubling experiences of forced sex within marriage. Respondents frequently mentioned being physically forced to have sex and/or to engage in types of sexual activity that they found degrading and humiliating [9].

Regrettably, much sexual coercion takes place against children or adolescents in both industrial and developing countries. Between one-third and two-thirds of known sexual assault victims are age 15 or younger, according to information from justice systems statistics and rape crisis centers in Chile, Peru, Malaysia, Mexico, Panama, Papua New Guinea and the United States [10].

Sexual exploitation of children is widespread in virtually all societies. Child sexual abuse refers to any sexual act that occurs between an adult or immediate family member and a child, or any nonconsensual sexual contact between a child and a peer. Laws generally considered the issue of consent to be irrelevant in cases of sexual contact by an adult with a child, defined variously as someone under 13, 14, 15, or 16 years of age.

Because of the taboo nature of the topic, it is difficult to collect reliable figures on the prevalence of sexual abuse in childhood. Nonetheless, the few representative sample surveys provide cause for concern. A recent review of 17 studies worldwide indicate [sic] that anywhere from 11 to 32% of women report behavior constituting sexual abuse in childhood. Although both girls and boys can be victims of sexual abuse, most studies report that the prevalence of abuse among girls is at least 1.5 to 3 times that among boys [11]. Abuse among boys may be underreported compared with abuse among girls, however.

Studies consistently show that, regardless of the sex of the victim, the vast majority of perpetrators are male and are known to the victim [12–14]. Many perpetrators were themselves sexually abused in childhood, although most boys who are sexually abused do not grow up to abuse others [15].

Although for some children effects of sexual abuse are severe and long-term, not all will experience consequences that persist into later life [16, 17]. Sexual abuse is most likely to cause long-term harm when it extends over a long period, is by a father or father figure, involves penetration, or uses force or violence [16, 18, 19].

4. Explaining Gender-based Violence

While violence against women is widespread, it is not universal. Anthropologists have documented small-scale societies—such as the Wape of Papua New Guinea—where domestic violence is virtually absent [20, 21]. This reality stands as testament to the fact that social relations can be organized in such a way to minimize abuse.

Why is violence more widespread in some places than in others? Increasingly, researchers are using an 'ecological framework' to understand the interplay of personal, situational, and socio-cultural factors that combine to cause abuse [22]. In this model, violence against women results from the interaction of factors for different levels of the social environment.

The model can best be visualized as four concentric circles. The innermost circle represents the biological and personal history that each individual brings to his or her behavior in relationships. The second circle represents the immediate context in which abuse takes place: frequently the family or other intimate or acquaintance relationship. The third circle represents the institutions and social structures, both formal and informal, in which relationships are embedded in neighborhoods, the workplace, social networks, and peer groups. The fourth, outermost circle is the economic and social environment, including cultural norms.

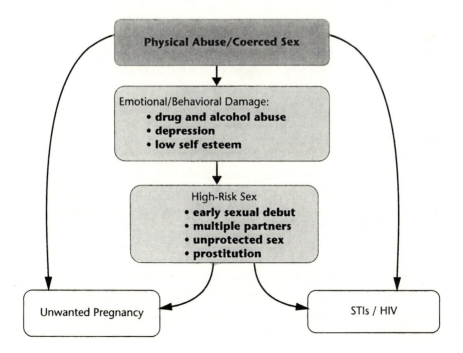

A wide range of studies agree on several factors at each of these levels that increase the likelihood that a man will abuse his partner:

(1) At the individual level these include being abused as a child or witnessing marital violence in the home [23], having an absent or rejecting father [24], and frequent use of alcohol [25].

(2) At the level of the family and relationship, cross-cultural studies cited male control of wealth and decision-making within the family [21] and marital conflict as strong predictors of abuse [23].

(3) At the community level women's isolation and lack of social support, together with male peer groups that condone and legitimize men's violence, predict higher rates of violence [26, 27].

(4) At the societal level studies around the world have found that violence against women is most common where gender roles are rigidly defined and enforced and where the concept of masculinity is linked to toughness, male honor, or dominance [22]. Other cultural norms associated with abuse include tolerance of physical punishment of women and children, acceptance of violence as a means to settle interpersonal disputes, and the perception that men have 'ownership' of women [21, 22].

By combining individual-level risk factors with findings of cross-cultural studies, the ecological model contributes to understanding why some societies and some individuals are more violent than others and why women, especially wives, are so consistently the victims of abuse.

Other factors combine to protect some women. For example, when women have authority and power outside the family, rates of abuse in intimate partnerships are lower [21]. Likewise, prompt intervention by family members and friends appears to reduce the likelihood of domestic violence. By contrast, where the family is considered 'private' and outside public scrutiny, rates of wife abuse are higher [21].

Justifications for violence frequently evolve from gender norms—that is, social norms about the proper roles and responsibilities of men and women. Many cultures hold that men have the right to control their wives' behavior and that women who challenge their right—even by asking for household money or by expressing the needs of the children—may be punished. In countries as different as Bangladesh, Cambodia, India, Mexico, Nigeria, Pakistan, Papua New Guinea, Nicaragua, Tanzania, and Zimbabwe, studies find that violence is frequently viewed as a physical chastisement—the husband's right to 'correct' an erring wife [2]. As one husband said in a focus-group discussion in Tamil Nadu, India, 'If it is a great mistake, then the husband is justified in beating his wife. Why not? A cow will not be obedient without beatings'[28].

Worldwide, studies identify a consistent list of events that are said to 'trigger' violence. These include: not obeying her husband, talking back, not having food ready on time, failing to care adequately for the children or home, questioning him about money or girlfriends, going somewhere without his permission, refusing him sex, or expressing suspicions of infidelity. All of these represent transgression of dominant gender norms.

5. The Impact of Violence on Women's Reproductive Health

A growing number of studies document the ways in which coercion and violence undermine women's sexual and reproductive autonomy and jeopardize their physical and mental health (see Table 1). Although violence can have direct health consequences, it also increases women's risk of future ill health. Physical violence and sexual abuse could put women at risk of infection and unwanted pregnancies *directly*, if women are forced to have sex, for example, or fear using contraception or condoms because of their partners' potentially violent reaction. A history of sexual abuse in childhood also can lead to unwanted pregnancies and STDs *indirectly* by increasing sexual risk-taking in adolescence and adulthood. Therefore, like tobacco or alcohol use, victimization can best be conceptualized as a risk factor for a variety of diseases and conditions [2].

5.1 Reduced Sexual Autonomy Leads to Unwanted Pregnancies and STIs/HIV

In many parts of the world marriage is interpreted as granting men the right to unconditional sexual access to their wives and the power to enforce this access through force if necessary. Women who lack sexual autonomy often are powerless to refuse unwanted sex or to use contraception and thus are at risk of unwanted pregnancies.

As a 40-year-old woman in Uttar Pradesh said, 'What can I do to protect myself from these unwanted pregnancies unless he agrees to do something? Once when I gathered the courage and told him I wanted to avoid sex with him, he said what else have I married you for? He beats me for the smallest reasons and has sex whenever he wants' [29].

Many women are afraid to raise the issue of contraception for fear that their partners might respond violently [30–36]. In some cultures husbands may react negatively because they think that protection against pregnancy would encourage their wives to be unfaithful. Where having many children is a sign of male virility, a wife's desire to use family planning may be interpreted as an affront to her husband's masculinity [30].

Table 1 Health Outcome of Violence against Women

Partner abuse, sexual assault, child sexual abuse	
Fatal outcomes	
	Homicide
	Suicide
	Maternal mortality
	AIDS-related
Nonfatal outcomes	
Physical health	Injury
	Functional impairment
	Physical symptoms
	Poor subjective health
	Permanent disability
	Severe obesity
Chronic conditions	Chronic pain syndromes
	Irritable bowel syndrome
	Gastrointestinal disorders
	Somatic complaints
	Fibromyalgia
Mental health	Post-traumatic stress
	Depression
	Anxiety
	Phobias/panic disorder
	Eating disorders
	Sexual dysfunction
	Low self-esteem
	Substance abuse
Negative health behaviors	Smoking
	Alcohol and drug abuse
	Sexual risk-taking
	Physical inactivity
	Overeating
Reproductive health	Unwanted pregnancy
	STIs/HIV
	Gynecological disorders
	Unsafe abortion
	Pregnancy complications
	Miscarriage/low birth weight
	Public inflammatory disease

For women living with men who are violent, the fear of the negative reaction is often enough to cut off discussion of contraception. As one woman said of her husband, 'Whenever he hears people discussing family planning over the radio, he fumes and shouts . . . If he can threaten a wireless, what would he do to me if I open the topic?' [33].

Violence influences the risk of HIV and other STIs directly when it interferes with women's ability to negotiate condom use. For many women, asking for condoms can be even more difficult than discussing other contraceptives because condoms are often associated with promiscuity, infidelity, and prostitution.

Raising the issue of condom use within marriage or other primary partnerships is especially difficult [37]. As a 46-year respondent in Brazil said, "If I ask my husband to use a condom now, he is going to ask 'why?' He is going to think I am fooling around or that I am accusing him of fooling around, two things that shouldn't be happening" [38].

Sexual victimization in childhood appears to place young women at increased risk of pregnancy during their teenage years. In the early 1990s studies began to find a consistent association between sexual abuse in childhood and adolescent pregnancy [39–41]. The studies also found a clear and consistent link between early sexual victimization and a variety of risk-taking behaviors, including early sexual debut, drug and alcohol use, more sexual partners, and less contraceptive use.

Childhood abuse has also been linked to unintended pregnancies among adult women. A study of 1,200 women in the US found women who reported being psychologically, sexually and/or physically abused, or whose mother was beaten by a partner, had higher rates of unintended first pregnancies than women who did not experience abuse. The likelihood of an unintended first pregnancy increased with both the number of different types of abuse women experienced, and its frequency [42].

In a 1999 speech, Peter Piot, the Executive Director of UNAIDS, noted that violence against women has many links to HIV/AIDS. 'Violence against women is not just because of the AIDS epidemic,' he noted, 'it can also be a consequence of it.' Sexual abuse in childhood appears to increase the incidence of STIs among adults, largely through its effect on high-risk sexual behavior ([43–50]) [*sic*]. Several studies have linked a history of sexual abuse to higher risk of selling sex for money or drugs [39, 50–53]. Abuse in childhood also increases the risk of HIV/AIDS through its effect on drug use. Sexually abused or assaulted women often turn to drugs as a coping mechanism, in addition to such unhealthy behaviors as having unprotected sex and trading sex for money or drugs [54–61].

In some places, fear of men's reaction has also hindered efforts to encourage voluntary HIV/AIDS counseling and testing among women [62].

This has implications both for controlling sexual transmission of the virus and for efforts to reduce mother to child transmission.

5.2. Violence Increases Risks for Other Gynecological Problems

Sexual and physical violence appears to increase women's risk for many common gynecological disorders, some of which can be debilitating. An example is chronic pelvic pain (CPP), which in many countries accounts for as many as 10% of all gynecological visits and one-quarter of all hysterectomies [63–65].

Although CPP is commonly caused by adhesions, endometriosis, or infections, about half the cases of CPP did not have any identifiable pathology. A variety of studies have found that women suffering from CPP are consistently more likely to have a history of childhood sexual abuse [64], sexual assault [63, 66–69], or physical and sexual abuse by their partners [70, 71].

Past trauma may lead to CPP via unidentified injuries, by stress, or by somatization—the expression of psychological distress through physical symptoms [63]. Also, sexual abuse in childhood has been linked to increased sexual risk-taking, and thus to STIs, which can lead to CPP, often due to pelvic inflammatory disease.

Other gynecological disorders associated with sexual violence including regular vaginal bleeding [72], vaginal discharge, painful menstruation [68, 73], pelvic inflammatory disease [74], and sexual dysfunction (difficulty in orgasms, lack of desire and conflicts over frequency of sex) [71, 73, 74]. Sexual assault also increases risk for premenstrual distress, a condition that affects 8 to 10% of menstruating women and causes physical, mood, and behavioral symptoms [75]. The number of gynecological symptoms appears to be related to the severity of abuse suffered, whether there was both physical and sexual assault, whether the victims knew the offender, and whether there were multiple offenders [76, 77].

5.3. Violence Leads to Adverse Pregnancy Outcomes

Around the world, as many as one woman in every four is physically or sexually abused during pregnancy, usually by her partner [78–87]. Estimates vary widely, however. Within the US, for example, estimates of abuse during pregnancy range from 3 to 11% among adult women and up to 38% among teenage mothers [80]. Some of this variation is likely due to differences in how the questions were asked, how often, and by whom [81, 88].

Violence before and during pregnancy can have serious health consequences for women and their children. Pregnant women who have experienced violence are more likely to delay seeking prenatal care [80, 89–94] and to gain insufficient weight [80, 95]. They are also more likely to have a history of STIs [96], unwanted or mistimed pregnancies [81, 94, 97], vaginal and cervical infections [80, 90, 91], kidney infections [97], and bleeding in pregnancy [80, 90].

Violence may also have a serious impact on pregnancy outcomes. Violence has been linked with increased risk of miscarriages and abortions [83, 98], premature labor [97], and fetal distress [97]. Several studies also have focused on the relationship between violence in pregnancy and low birth weight, a leading contributor to infant deaths in the developing world [80, 90, 93, 94, 97–103]. Although the findings are inconclusive several studies suggest that violence during pregnancy contributes substantially to low birth weight, at least in some settings. In one study at the regional hospital in Leon, Nicaragua, for example, researchers found that after controlling for other risk factors, violence against pregnant women was associated with a threefold increase in the incidence of low birth weight [94].

How violence puts pregnancies at above-average risk is unclear, but several explanations have been suggested [82, 88]. Blunt abdominal trauma can lead to fetal death or low birth weight by provoking preterm delivery. Extreme stress and anxiety provoked by violence may also lead to preterm delivery or fetal growth retardation by increasing stress hormone levels or immunological changes. Finally, violence may affect pregnancy outcome indirectly by increasing women's likelihood of engaging in such harmful health behaviors as smoking and alcohol and drug abuse, all of which been linked to low birth weight

6. The Role of Reproductive Health Professionals

Health professionals can do much to help their clients who are victims of gender-based violence. Yet providers often missed opportunities to help by being unaware, indifferent or judgmental. With training and support from health care systems, providers can do more to respond to the physical, emotional and security needs of abused women and girls. First, health care providers can learn how to ask women about violence in ways that their clients find helpful. They can give women empathy and support. They can provide medical treatment, offer counseling, document injuries and refer their clients to legal assistance and support services.

Reproductive health professionals have a particular responsibility to help because:

- Abuse has a major—although little recognized—impact on women's reproductive health and sexual well-being;

- Providers cannot do their jobs well unless they understand how violence and powerlessness affect women's reproductive health and decision-making ability;
- Reproductive health care providers are strategically placed to help identify victims of violence and connect them with other community support services.

Providers can reassure women that violence is unacceptable and that no woman deserves to be beaten, sexually abused, or made to suffer emotionally. If one client said, 'Compassion is going to open up the door. And when we feel safe and are able to trust, that makes a lot of difference' [104].

SOURCE

Heise L, Ellsberg M, and Gotmoeller M. 2002. A global overview of gender-based violence. Int J Gynecol Obstet 78 (Suppl. 1): S5–S14. Copyright 2002 by *International Journal of Gynecology and Obstetrics*. Reprinted by permission of Elsevier.

CHAPTER 7

MATERNAL CHILD HEALTH

Half a million women die each year around the world in pregnancy. It's not biology that kills them so much as neglect.
　—Nicholas D. Kristof (b. 1959), American journalist

There is very little genuine perception that mature people come from small beginnings, that they've had a perilous passage every moment of the way.
　—Pauline Stitt (1909–1996), Director of Maternal Child Health and
　　Crippled Children Services, U.S. Children's Bureau (1949–1955)

Prophet Mohammed didn't circumcise his four daughters.
　—Sheikh Ali Gomma (Gomaa), Grand Mufti of Egypt
　　Spoken at the International Conference on Female Genital Mutilation
　　Al-Azhar University, Cairo on November 22, 2006

AT THE DAWN OF THE TWENTIETH CENTURY, global statistics for maternal–child health were grim and remained so at century's end. In 2000, the United Nations estimated more than 1,500 women died daily from complications of pregnancy and childbirth—more than half a million maternal deaths annually. Additionally, about 10,000 babies born each day didn't take even one breath. Of those born alive, 10,000 more died daily, never living even one month. The WHO reports that at the beginning of the twenty-first century, newborns (one month of age or less) died from different causes than did infants (less than one year). Globally, one-third of newborn deaths were attributable to prematurity and congenital anomalies, one-third to asphyxia, and the remaining third to infectious diseases (especially diarrhea and tetanus). After the one-month mark, infant deaths were most likely to be from acute respiratory infections, diarrhea, measles, and malaria. Save the Children publishes a "Mother's Index" ranking the best and worst countries for becoming a mother and raising a child. The top three, or best, places in the world to become a mother in 2000 were all Scandinavian countries (Sweden, Norway, and Iceland). The bottom three were Yemen, Chad, and Niger, where only one-third of births were attended by trained personnel. Despite some gains in maternal–child health during the twentieth century, significant public health challenges remain for reducing maternal mortality and improving child survival.

MATERNAL AND INFANT MORTALITY

In 1751, Sweden measured maternal mortality for the first time and determined that 900 women died of childbirth complications for every 100,000 births. This abominable statistic led Swedish authorities to push for improved physician and midwife training. In 1900, the U.S. maternal mortality rate was about 850 deaths per 100,000 live births, rivaling the Swedish rate from 150 years earlier. By that time, however, Sweden had already cut their rate to 250 deaths per 100,000 live births.

Wet nurses had gone out of favor during the nineteenth century. By the beginning of the twentieth, many women were no longer breastfeeding their infants, relying instead on both poor quality cows' milk and newly developed infant formula preparations. Having an alternative source of infant nutrition was important for women who had to work, as well as for women of means who, given the option, preferred not having to breastfeed. Marketing campaigns made Liebig's Food the infant formula preparation of choice in London; Mellin's Food became popular in the United States; and Nestle's Milk Food led infant formula sales in Europe. Unfortunately, all of these alternatives to breast milk put infants at risk. Milk from poorly nourished cows kept in unclean conditions, as well as powdered milk formulas that were reconstituted with water from unsafe public water supplies kept infant mortality rates high. Indeed, statistics from 1900 London show that infant mortality was higher among the affluent, those who could afford infant formula, than among the poor, who could not.

In an attempt to save some infants from contaminated feeding practices, New Jersey pediatrician Henry Leber Coit developed a system of certifying clean milk. In 1903, New York City pediatricians W.L. Park and L. Emmet Holt supported efforts toward opening clean milk stations; hundreds opened across the nation. Commercial baby foods were introduced in 1928, with Daniel Gerber leading the way with strained peas. Prepared formulas improved and were successfully marketed around the world. By mid century, breastfeeding-only rates in both the United States and the United Kingdom hovered at around 20 percent. Rising social, economic, and marketing trends were making it harder for mothers to choose and succeed at breastfeeding. In response, seven women from Illinois founded La Leche League in 1956. That organization's mission was to improve rates of breastfeeding by supporting, encouraging, and generally providing information about the practice to women. By 1981, La Leche League had grown to international status, even becoming a consulting agency for UNICEF.

As birthrates declined in developed nations around mid century, formula manufacturers began targeting women in developing nations. Because of sanitation problems, infant mortality rates spiked in the developing nations that accepted infant formula. Response by reformers was swift. In 1977, a boycott of Nestle products was organized, and activists called for that corporation to cease marketing infant formula in developing nations. The Infant Formula Action Coalition (INFACT), the International Baby Food Action Network (IBFAN), Save the Children, the WHO, UNICEF, and the World Health Assembly (WHA), as well as the U.S. Senate, the U.K. Advertising Standards Authority, and the European Parliament, called for Nestle to cease marketing efforts for infant formula in developing nations. Near century's end, the WHO issued breastfeeding guidelines that simply stated that, with few exceptions, infants should be breastfed until six months old.

During the course of the twentieth century, reformers focused on much more than infant feeding practices to improve infant survival. In 1909, Lillian D. Wald, founder of the Henry Street Settlement in New York City, and Florence Kelley, her friend from the National Consumers League, petitioned President Theodore Roosevelt to establish a Children's Bureau. It took several years and a change of administration before Congress passed Public Law 62–116 in 1912, making the United States the first nation with a government agency focused solely on children. President William H. Taft appointed Julia C. Lathrop as chief of the Children's Bureau, the first woman to lead a U.S. federal agency. The agency, however, was unpopular with both business and conservatives as it regulated child labor.

In 1921, Congress passed the Maternal and Infancy (Sheppard-Towner) Act, providing federal matching funds for state maternal–child health education programs. The program was vigorously opposed by two groups: 1) the AMA, whose members believed it allowed untrained birth attendants to attend maternity cases and created a bridge toward socialized medicine, and 2) suffragist Alice Paul and her followers in the National Women's Party, who believed the act labeled all women as mothers. Despite the success of the act in reducing both the maternal and infant mortality rates, Congress yielded to lobbying pressure and failed to renew it in 1929.

Investigations into the components of maternal mortality by J. Whitridge Williams at Johns Hopkins University and Louis I. Dublin at the Metropolitan Life Insurance Company showed the clear benefit of improving maternal–child health through access to care during the peripartum period. Their findings encouraged the creation of best practice guidelines for hospital deliveries and forged significant efforts to provide both prenatal and hospital care for all deliveries. During the latter half of the century, new technologies, such as antibiotics, safer methods of blood transfusion, new screening tests for sexually transmitted and other diseases, treatments for hypertension, improved maternal nutrition, and access to fertility control (safe and legal birth control, as well as abortion) also helped reduce maternal and infant mortality rates, primarily in developed countries. These advances were not always welcome, however. Some women felt motherhood was becoming "medicalized" rather than remaining a natural process, and others viewed access to birth control and abortion as immoral. Despite the push back, the successful reduction in maternal and infant mortality rates by these innovations could not be denied.

By the end of the twentieth century, most developed nations reduced maternal mortality below 4 deaths per 100,000 live births and infant mortality to below 10 deaths per 1,000 live births. Unfortunately, as the twenty-first century unfolded, many of the advances in reducing maternal–infant mortality remained out of the reach of those living in the lesser developed countries where to become a mother, be born alive, or remain alive for even one year remained a significant challenge.

Congenital Anomalies

Congenital anomalies are defined by the WHO as "conditions present at birth, whether detected at the time of birth of not." They can be lethal (causing stillbirth or certain death), severe (lethal or causing significant handicap unless there is medical intervention), or mild (may require medical intervention but doesn't impact life expectancy). The etiology of some anomalies is genetic (inherited) in origin. This happens when one or both parents carry a trait for an anomaly, or it may occur because normal genetic code is passed incorrectly to the embryo at the time of conception. When the presence of only one gene is needed for the expression of an anomaly, it is considered dominant, as exemplified by polydactyly (extra fingers or toes). When both parents must carry the gene for a congenital anomaly for it to occur, it is recessive. Examples of recessive anomalies are sickle cell anemia, Tay-Sachs disease, cystic fibrosis, and phenylketonuria (PKU). The third type of genetic anomaly happens at the time of conception when too many, too few, or broken chromosomes are passed to the embryo. Two major risk factors for this type of anomaly have been identified: consanguineous pregnancies and advanced maternal age.

Consanguineous pregnancies result in increased rates of mental retardation, malformations such as cleft lip or cleft palate, and congenital blindness. When blood relatives mate, the risk of offspring with genetic errors is amplified. Thus, most Americans, Europeans, and many Africans generally disapprove of consanguineous marriages, even banning the practice in some places. Yet in large parts of the world, in a swath across North Africa through Pakistan and India, and in some parts of China, consanguineous marriages are arranged to deal with issues of dowry and family status or to preserve tribal alliances and family wealth. Arranged consanguineous marriages foster both strong family loyalties and common enemies, often resulting in "blood feuds." Traditional societies, in particular, continue the practice of consanguineous marriages, thus fostering tribal or clan loyalties. For instance, estimates for the last decade of the twentieth century placed the proportion of marriages between first cousins in Iraq at 50 to 60 percent, including that of Saddam Hussein and his first wife, Sajida. In Sudan, in parts of Egypt, among Traveller's in Northern Ireland, and among Gypsies in the United States, the rates were even higher, with 60 to 70 percent of marriages taking place between first or second cousins.

Down syndrome, first described in 1866 by physician John Langdon Down, is the most common genetic anomaly, occurring about once in every 800 live births unless selective abortion is practiced. Down observed that some of the residents of the Royal Earlswood Asylum of Idiots in Surrey, England, resembled each other so much they appeared to come from the same family, though they clearly did not. He also stated that the largest proportion of mental defectives in the asylum were "congenital idiots," looking like "typical Mongols," regardless of their ethnic background. Down found that most of the "Mongoloid" individuals in the asylum were trainable and noted that they had shortened life expectancies. During the 1960s, Mongolia, as a new member of the WHO, requested that the term be banned, suggesting instead that the condition be called Down's or Down syndrome. The change was rapidly adopted.

The etiology of Down syndrome was identified in 1959 by French pediatrician and geneticist Jerome Lejeune. Intrigued by the 1956 discovery of the 23 pairs of human chromosomes and considering the possibility that Down syndrome might be genetic in origin, Lejeune took a skin biopsy from one of his affected patients and discovered an extra copy (called a trisomy) of chromosome 21. He thusly verified that Down syndrome begins at conception, when the twenty-first pair of chromosomes in either the mother or the father does not fully separate and the genetic information passed to the embryo is in error. A major risk factor for Down syndrome is maternal age over 35 years. In the second half of the twentieth century and into the twenty-first, it became increasingly common for women to postpone marriage or childbearing to pursue their education or careers or to remarry and begin second families. These older mothers carry an increased risk of bearing infants with Down syndrome. However, as genetic screening became available, many women became comfortable with postponing motherhood, even using technologies to improve their chances of getting pregnant because they had the option of legal, selective termination of their pregnancies.

Beyond genetic causes, about 15 percent of congenital anomalies are environmental in origin, from exposures to infectious diseases (TORCH infections, i.e., toxoplasmosis, rubella, cytomegalovirus, herpes simplex, and others), radiation, teratogenic drugs (such as thalidomide or phenytoin), alcohol, smoking, or environmental pollutants (such as polychlorinated biphenyls or polycyclic aromatic hydrocarbons). The link to infectious agents was widely resisted by the scientific community at the beginning of the twentieth century. In 1941, a rubella outbreak flared in Australia. Soon thereafter, Sydney pediatric ophthalmologist Norman McAlister Gregg began seeing infants born with cataracts. Since the cataracts had to form *in utero*, Gregg considered the exposures the mothers had in common and found that all had been infected with rubella during their pregnancies. He reported a 50 percent risk of being born with congenital defects if the mother was infected with rubella in the first trimester of pregnancy; some risk remained if the infection occurred in the second trimester. Prior to Gregg's report, the medical community believed that the placental barrier protected the fetus from infectious exposures. Other investigators reported similar findings, however, and the search was on for a cure. The rubella virus was identified in 1962. Despite the fact that a rubella vaccine was developed and licensed for use in the United States in 1969, the CDC estimates that 100,000 infants are born with congenital rubella syndrome annually throughout the world.

About 60 percent of congenital anomalies have an unknown etiology or are likely caused by a complex combination of genetic and environmental factors. Complex congenital anomalies happen when an embryo carries a genetic predisposition for an anomaly but the gene is only turned on when one or more environmental factors are present. For example, the neural tube defect spina bifida is complex in origin and is mostly preventable through folic acid supplementation of the mother's diet in the period around conception. Globally, the WHO estimates that more than 300,000 newborns worldwide are affected by spina bifida, but the rates are coming down where folic acid supplementation or dietary fortification of foodstuffs with folic acid has been implemented (see Chapter 1).

In developed nations, preventing congenital anomalies has been aided by new techniques for genetic screening, genetic counseling, vaccine programs, vitamin supplementation, and fortification of foods, as well as by educational programs about avoiding smoking and drinking alcohol. Warnings on teratogenic drugs and knowledge about dangerous occupational and environmental exposures have also helped reduce congenital anomalies. Newborns in the developed world are routinely screened for metabolic disorders and hearing loss, conditions that can be medically managed to help affected individuals maximize their quality of life. Yet in large portions of the world, little progress has been made on preventing congenital anomalies, maximizing infant survival, and improving the quality of life for mothers and their children. Despite the fact that the UN lists both maternal and child health as priorities, progress in this area has far to go.

Female Genital Mutilation

Female genital mutilation (FGM; variously called female genital cutting or female circumcision) has only recently been internationally recognized as a violation of human rights. The practice remains a significant factor in adverse health outcomes for both women and girls. According to various UN sources, between two and three million women, mostly African girls under the age of 15, are subjected to FMG each year, putting them at risk not only from the procedure, but also from its long-term effects, especially at the time of childbirth. FGM is deeply embedded in local cultures, and there is significant social pressure to continue the practice. Although the practice is not codified by any religion, some clerics support the practice's continuance, and others have taken a strong stand against it.

There are four categories of FGM. Type 1: the clitoris and/or prepuce are partially or totally removed (clitoridectomy); Type 2: the clitoris and labia minora are partially or totally removed (excision); Type 3: the vaginal opening is narrowed with a covering created by cutting and moving the labia minora and/or the labia majora (infibulation); and Type 4: all other pricking, piercing, incising, scraping, and cauterizing of the female genitalia for nonmedical purposes. The practice has been described in detail by Ayaan Hirsi Ali. Raised in a strict Muslim family in Somalia, Ali writes that despite her father's insistence that his daughters remain "uncut," her grandmother arranged for all three of his children to be circumcised, both male and female, in his absence. Ali describes her experience at the age of five, being held down by women and hearing the snip of the scissors as a strange man cut out her inner labia and clitoris. Screaming through the pain, she remembers a blunt needle sewing up her outer labia and the strange man cutting the thread with his teeth. Afterward, she reports that her legs were tied together in order to create a strong scar. She found that it hurt terribly to urinate and shortly after she began to wet the bed. Although she healed in about a week, Ali reports that her sister developed fever, had nightmares, lost a significant amount of weight, and suffered from a personality change from which she never recovered. Yet Ali understands that her grandmother was doing what she understood was necessary in order for her grandchildren to eventually be acceptable as husbands and wives in Somali society.

Between 100 and 140 million women are estimated to be living with the adverse consequences of FGM despite its being outlawed by some countries, as well as active programs by the UN and UNICEF to stop the practice. The potential immediate adverse health effects from the practice include hemorrhage, infection, and death from the procedure. Long-term effects include physical and psychological scarring, urinary and menstrual flow retention, painful intercourse, and severe tearing and other complications during childbirth. To address the problem, Egypt's First Lady, Suzanne Mubarak, opened an Expert Conference in Cairo in 2003. Statements by Mohammed Sayed Tantawy, the Sheik of Al Azhar and Egypt's' highest Islamic authority, and Bishop Moussa, a representative for H.H. Pope Shenouda III, Patriarch of the Coptic Church, reported to the conference that FGM has no basis in either Islam or Christianity. As a result, the "Cairo Declaration for the Elimination of Female Genital Mutilation" was written at the conclusion of the conference, and it encouraged all governments to pass legislation to eliminate FGM. A few days later, the Maputo Summit of the African Union approved the "Protocol to the African Charter on Human and Peoples' Rights on the Rights of Women in Africa," which reinforced passing national laws to prevent FGM. In 2006, ten of the world's top Islamic scholars met in Cairo at the International Conference on Female Genital Mutilation. The scholars pronounced the custom to be a crime against humanity, one that can no longer be practiced by Muslims. The clerics then ordered that the word be spread. As FGM predates the advent of Islam, it may take more than declarations to eliminate the practice.

WOMEN AND CHILDREN AS SPECIAL POPULATIONS

Maternal–child health was a difficult area in which to achieve public health progress during the twentieth century. Obstetrics and gynecology emerged as a medical specialty, which helped to develop best practices for safer pregnancy and childbirth for women in the developed world, where trained birth attendants were generally available. Pediatrics also emerged as a force for treating children and preventing disease over the twentieth century, but it could be argued that reformers had far more impact than did those trying to cure disease. Reformers agitated for child labor laws and took on corporations marketing infant formula to vulnerable populations. Reformers also created organizations to advance breastfeeding and fight birth defects. Science cracked the genetic code, identifying risk factors for many congenital anomalies. It also created vaccines to save infants from blindness and death. Developed nations dedicated resources to creating a safety net that allowed mothers and their infants a better chance at a healthy life. However, mothers and infants in the developing world have not been so lucky.

SELECTED READINGS

Reading 1, by William H. Davis (1912), provides some of the first available data on infant mortality stratified by feeding practice (breast vs. bottle). Davis was born in Holyoke, Massachusetts, in 1871, graduated from Harvard Medical School in 1887, and practiced medicine in Boston from 1900–1916. He served as the vital statistician for the Boston Department of Health from 1908 to 1916, at which time he accepted appointment as chief statistician for the U.S. Bureau of the Census. Davis represented the United States at the International Conference in Paris where the International List of Causes of Death (ICD classification system) was revised in 1920 and 1929. His mantra for U.S. Vital Statistics was "Every State in the Registration Area by 1930." The paper reproduced here was read before a meeting of the Massachusetts Association of Boards of Health in 1912 and later published in the *American Journal of Public Health*. In it, Davis makes a point that if all infants were appropriately breastfed, infant mortality would improve regardless of nativity.

The second reading, by Godfrey P. Oakley, Jr., Myron J. Adams, and Charlotte M. Dickinson (1996), calls for the fortification of foods with folic acid. Oakley, director of the Division of Birth Defects and Developmental Disabilities at the CDC, was a forceful advocate of folic acid for the prevention of neural tube defects (spina bifida and anencephaly). Not satisfied with simply providing prenatal vitamins to women, Oakley agitated for and succeeded in getting the FDA to approve the fortification of grains with folic acid in 1996.

The third reading is from the *WHO Chronicle* (1986) and describes the practice and health consequences of female genital circumcision. At the time the piece was written, the WHO stance was that the practice required cultural understanding rather than criticism and that any change would have to be from the ground up rather than from the top down. The WHO changed its stance in a relatively short period of time and moved to condemn the practice as a violation of the human rights of girls and women. Indeed, by the turn of the century, the WHO had changed its terminology from "female circumcision" to "female genital mutilation," reflecting its change in policy.

BIBLIOGRAPHY

Ahlburg D. 1998. Intergenerational transmission of health (in Intergenerational Relations). Papers and Proceedings of the Hundred and Tenth Annual Meeting of the American Economic Association. *The American Economic Review* 88 (2): 265–70.

Alarcon AG. 1949. Rubella as a cause of congenital malformations. *Am J Dis Child* 78 (6): 914–16.

Ali, AH. 2007. *Infidel*. New York: Free Press.

Apgar V. 1953. A proposal for a new method of evaluation of the newborn infant. *Anesth & Anal* 32 (4): 260–67.

Apgar V, and James LS. 1962. Further observations on the newborn scoring system. *Am J Dis Child* 104: 419–28.

Apgar V. 1966. The newborn (Apgar) scoring system: Reflections and advice. *Pediatr Clin North Am* 13 (3): 645–50.

Armstrong MD and Tyler FH. 1955. Studies on phenylketonuria. I. Restricted phenylalanine intake in phenylketonuria. *J Clin Investigation* 34 (4): 565–80. Reprinted in *Nutr Rev* 1983;41 (1): 15–18.

Auld PA, Rudolph AJ, Avery ME, Cherry RB, Drorbaugh JE, Kay JL, and Smith CA. 1961. Responsiveness and resuscitation of the newborn: The use of the Apgar score. *Am J Dis Child* 101:713–24.

Bleyer A. 1932. Indications that mongoloid imbecility is a gametic mutation of degressive type. *Am J Dis Child* 47:342–48.

Bronstein, IP and Brown AW. 1934. Hypothyroidism and cretinism in childhood: III. Mental Development. *Am J Orthopsychiat* 4:413.

Brown AW, Bronstein IP, and Kraines R. 1939. Hypothyroidism and cretinism in childhood. VI. Influence of thyroid therapy on mental growth. *Am J Dis Child* 57:517–23. Reprinted in *Nutr Rev* 1984;42 (1): 20–22.

Czeizel AE, Intödy Z, and Modell B. 1996. What proportion of congenital abnormalities can be prevented? *Brit Med J* 306:499–503.

Dam H, Dyggve H, Larsen H, and Plum P. 1952. The relation of vitamin K deficiency to hemorrhagic disease of the newborn. *Adv Pediatr* 5:129–53.

Dublin LI. 1923. The mortality of early infancy. *Am J Hygiene* 3:211–23.

Dublin LI. 1939. A problem of maternity—a survey and forecast. *Am J Public Health* 29:1205–14.

Dublin LI and Corbin H. 1930. A preliminary report of the Maternity Center Association of New York. *Am J Obst Gynecol* 20:877–81.

Eichholzer M, Tönz O, and Zimmermann R. 2006. Folic acid: A public-health challenge. Review. *Lancet* 367 (9528): 1352–61.

Fildes V. 1992. Breastfeeding in London, 1905–1919. *J Biosoc Sci* 24:53–75.

Fildes V, Marks L, and Marland H, eds. 1992. *Women and Children First: International Maternal and Infant Welfare, 1970–1945*. London: Routledge.

Filippi V, Ronsmans C, Campbell OMR, Graham WJ, Mills A, Borghi K, Koblinsky M, and Osrin D. 2006. Maternal health in poor countries: The broader context and a call for action. *Lancet* 368 (9546): 1535–41.

Gregg, N McA. 1941. Congenital cataract following German measles in the mother. *Trans Opthal Soc Aust* 3:35–46.

Laurence KM, James N, Miller MH, Tennant GB, and Campbell H. 1981. Double-blind randomised controlled trial of folate treatment before conception to prevent recurrence of neural-tube defects. *Br Med J* (Clin Res Ed) 282 (6275): 1509–11.

Levy J. 1919. Reduction of infant mortality by economic adjustment and by health education. *Am J Public Health* 9 (9): 676–81.

McCarthy J and Maine D. 1992. A framework for analyzing the determinants of maternal mortality. *Studies in Family Planning* 23 (1): 23–33.

Mellin GW and Katzenstein M. 1962. The saga of thalidomide: Neuropathy to embryopathy, with case reports of congenital anomalies. *N Engl J Med* 267 (23): 1184–93.

Mosley WH and Chen LC. 1984. An analytical framework for the study of child survival in developing countries (in Introduction and Conceptual Framework). *Population and Development Review* 10 (Suppl. Child Survival: Strategies for Research): 25–45.

MRC Vitamin Study Research Group. 1991. Prevention of neural tube defects: Results of the Medical Research Council Vitamin Study. *Lancet* 338 (8760): 131–37.

Rubin RA and Balow B. 1979. Measures of infant development and socioeconomic status as predictors of later intelligence and school achievement. *Developmental Psychology* 15 (2): 225–27.

Smithells RW, Sheppard S, and Schorah CJ. 1976. Vitamin deficiencies and neural tube defects. *Arch Dis Child* 51 (12): 944–50.

Stevenson RE, Allen WP, Pai GS, Best R, Seaver LH, Dean J, and Thompson S. 2000. Decline in prevalence of neural tube defects in a high-risk region of the United States. *Pediatrics* 106 (4): 677–83.

Stromland K and Miller MT. 1993. Thalidomide embryopathy: Revisited 27 years later. *Acta Ophthalmologica* 71 (2): 238–45.

Udani PM. 1979. Nutritional problems in developing countries. *Paediatrician* 8 (Suppl. 1):48–63.

Williams, JW. 1912. Medical education and the midwife problem in the United States. *J Am Med Assoc* 58:1–76.

World Health Organization. 2008. *Eliminating Female Genital Mutilation: An Interagency Statement—OHCHR, UNAIDS, UNDP, UNECA, UNESCO, UNFPA, UNHCHR, UNHCR, UNICEF, UNIFEM, WHO.* Geneva: WHO Press. www.un.org/womenwatch/daw/csw/csw52/statements _missions/Interagency_Statement_on_Eliminating_FGM.pdf. (accessed June 15, 2009).

Prevention of Infant Mortality by Breast Feeding
(1912)

By William H. Davis, M.D.,
Vital Statistician of Boston Board of Health

Much has been said from time to time in favor of breast feeding of infants; and statements have been made that 80 or 85 per cent of infant
deaths occur among bottle-fed babies.

But such statements have lacked force because it has not been apparent
how many mothers nurse their babies and how many bring them up on
the bottle.

If 80 per cent of infant deaths occur among bottle-fed babies, and if it
should be found that 80 per cent of all babies are bottle fed, then there
would be no case at all against bottle feeding.

In order to find out the percentage of babies that are bottle fed, the
Boston Board of Health recently sent about 900 letters to mothers who
had births recorded within the past year. Care was taken to select proportionate numbers of babies of various age periods, namely, two weeks to
one month, one to three months, three to six months, six to nine months
in nine to twelve months, and to select proportionate numbers of babies
from the various wards and from the various mother nativities—the
number of births in 1910 in the various wards of various mother nativities being taken as the basis for these proportions. Aside from obtaining
the proportionate numbers of babies in the way just indicated, care was
taken not to select these babies in any way but to take them at random
from the birth returns furnished by the Registry Department. The circular sent to each mother was as follows:

> *"Dear Madam:*–To assist the Board of Health in its campaign to save
> the babies of Boston, will you please answer the following questions
> regarding your child and return this slip at once in the enclosed
> envelope.
>
> "Is this child breast fed? (Answer yes or no.)
>
> "How long was it breast fed?
>
> "Is this child bottle fed? (Answer yes or no.)

Read before the Massachusetts Association of Board of Health, January 25, 1912.

"How long has it been bottle fed?

"If bottle fed, what food has been used?"

Replies were received promptly from over half of the mothers addressed, and an additional 200 replies were obtained through the Board of Health nurses, who went to the homes for the information.

Table I gives the results of this investigation—the number of replies received for babies of various ages and mother nativities and the percentages of breast and bottle fed babies.

The number of replies was 736, of which 533, or 72.4 per cent, were breast fed and 203, or 27.6 percent, were bottle fed. But the information thus obtained is only for living children. To determine what proportion of all babies are bottle or breast fed, it is necessary to add a proportionate number of the deaths of 1911. These necessary additions are given in Table II. Adding the figures in each square of Table II to the figures in the corresponding square of Table I, totals may be obtained which show the relative proportions of breast and bottle fed babies in Boston. The corrected percentages shown in Table II were thus obtained. At various places in the table there appear higher percentages of breast feeding for the older babies than for the younger. This, of course, is an error due to too few replies and would be rectified if answers from all the mothers of 1911 could be tabulated. But the evidence furnished by the 736 replies is very striking and may be used for present calculations.

Italy leads, with 83 per cent breast fed; Russia and Poland, with 79 per cent breast fed; Ireland and the United States follow, with 73 per cent and 59 per cent, respectively; while Canada makes the poorest showing, with only 51 per cent breast fed. The replies from mothers born in England, Scotland and Wales, Germany and Scandinavia, were too few to warrant any estimate for the babies of these mother nativities.

Table III gives for 1911 the total mortality of infants by age, my mother nativity and by feeding (for infants over two weeks of age).

Table IV gives for 1911 the total mortality of infants by month, by age and by feeding (for infants over two weeks of age).

Notice in Table IV that there is only a slight increase of deaths among breast-fed babies during the summer months. July, August and September, with 39 and 40 such deaths each month, are lower than February, March and April with 49, 41 and 38 deaths, respectively. The number of deaths among bottle-fed babies, however, jumps up tremendously in July, August and September.

Table III shows that only 26 per cent of infant deaths between the ages of two weeks and one year occur among breast-fed babies. And of infants over two weeks old, born of native mothers, only 16 percent of the deaths occur among breast-fed children; while of babies over two

Table I Living Babies—Breast or Bottle Fed

Mother nativity	2 weeks to 1 year	2 weeks to 1 year		2 weeks to 1 month		1 to 3 months		3 to 6 months		6 to 9 months		9 to 12 months		Percentage breast fed
		Breast	Bottle	Breast	Bottle	Breast	Bottle	Breast	Bottle	Breast	Bottle	Breast	Bottle	
United States	272	174	98	44	8	33	23	42	19	24	29	31	19	64
Ireland	120	93	27	17	1	24	6	23	8	16	5	13	7	77
England, Scotland, and Wales	20	15	5	1	–	3	1	4	1	3	2	4	1	–
Germany	2	1	1	–	–	–	–	1	1	–	–	–	–	–
Canada	69	38	31	5	1	8	7	8	9	8	8	9	6	55
Scandinavia	10	8	2	1	–	1	1	2	–	3	1	1	–	–
Italy	123	106	17	24	2	23	4	23	2	18	2	18	7	86
Russia and Poland	120	98	22	20	2	21	7	21	6	17	6	19	1	82
Totals	736	533	203	112	14	113	49	124	46	89	53	95	41	72
Percentages		72	28	89	11	70	30	73	27	63	37	70	30	

weeks of Italian mothers, 53 per cent of the deaths occur among breast-fed children.

Bottle-fed babies between the ages of one and three months show the highest mortality, especially those babies having mothers born in the United States.

Interesting and instructive as the foregoing figures and rates may be, ten times more interesting and instructive are the estimates which can be obtained from the tables. Many such estimates are tabulated in Table V.

If 74 per cent of infant deaths above the age of two weeks are among bottle-fed babies and only 32 per cent of babies over two weeks are bottle fed, then the bottle-fed infant over two weeks old is six times as likely to die as the breast-fed infant.

Again, if all the infants above the age of two weeks have been breast fed, or equally well fed (for it is by no means proven that bottle feeding may not be so safeguarded that the mortality will be no greater than among breast-fed babies), there would have been only 1,253 infant deaths last year, while if all had been bottle-fed there would have been 4,352 such deaths.

The actual number is infant deaths last year was 2,245, which gives a rate of 127 per thousand births.

Breast feeding of all babies would have saved nearly a thousand lives last year, and the death rate of 1,000 births would have been 71 instead of 127.

There would have been 470 less deaths among the children of native mothers; 161 less deaths among the children of Irish mothers: 97 less deaths among the children of Canadian mothers; 87 less deaths among the children of Italian mothers; and 85 less deaths among the children having mothers born in Russia and Poland.

A large part of the saving of infant life is to be expected in the great reduction of deaths from diarrhea and enteritis. Of 621 deaths from diarrhea enteritis last year between the ages of two weeks and one year, 87 were breast fed and 534 bottle fed; i.e., 86 per cent were bottle fed. If all babies had been breast fed the estimated number of these deaths would have been 493 less than actually occurred.

These figures are so startling that I feel that this investigation ought to be continued till 5,000 or 10,000 replies have been received from others, so that no opportunity be given to criticise [sic] the figures on the score of paucity of data.

These estimated rates measure the possible reduction in infant mortality if all babies could be breast fed, and they also show in what nationalities most of the improvement is to be expected.

Such a saving of infant life is not a mere fancy. The reduction of infant mortality rate from 127 to 71 is entirely within the range of possibilities.

Table II Death Additions to Table I Necessary to Obtain Corrected Percentages of Breast- and Bottle-Fed Babies

Mother nativity	2 weeks to 1 year		2 weeks to 1 month		1 to 3 months		3 to 6 months		6 to 9 months		9 to 12 months	
	Breast	Bottle	Breast	Bottle	Breast	Bottle	Breast	Bottle	Breast	Bottle	Breast	Bottle
United States	5	27	1	3	1	9	1	7	1	4	1	4
Ireland	3	9	–	1	1	2	1	2	–	2	1	2
England, Scotland and Wales	1	1	–	–	–	–	1	1	–	–	–	–
Canada	2	7	–	1	1	2	1	2	–	2	–	–
Scandinavia	–	1	–	–	–	1	–	–	–	–	–	–
Italy	6	6	1	1	1	1	1	1	2	2	1	1
Russia and Poland	3	5	1	–	1	1	–	2	1	1	–	1
Totals	20	56	3	6	5	16	5	15	4	11	3	8

Corrected Percentages for the Various Age Periods

Percentage	2 weeks to 1 year		2 weeks to 1 month		1 to 3 months		3 to 6 months		6 to 9 months		9 to 12 months	
	Breast	Bottle	Breast	Bottle	Breast	Bottle	Breast	Bottle	Breast	Bottle	Breast	Bottle
	68	32	85	15	64	36	68	32	59	41	67	33

Corrected Percentages of Breast-Fed Infants of Various Mother Nativities

Children of mothers born in the United States,	59
" " " " " " Ireland,	73
" " " " " " Canada,	51
" " " " " " Italy,	83
" " " " " " Russia and Poland,	79

Table III 1911 Mortality of Infants by Age, by Mother Nativity and by Feeding (for infants over two weeks of age)

| Mother nativity | Total deaths under 1 year | Total deaths | | | | | | | | | | | | Per cent of deaths 2 weeks to 1 year breast fed |
| | | 2 weeks to 1 year | | 2 weeks to 1 month | | 1 to 3 months | | 3 to 6 months | | 6 to 9 months | | 9 to 12 months | | |
		Breast	Bottle	Breast	Bottle	Breast	Bottle	Breast	Bottle	Breast	Bottle	Breast	Bottle	
United States	927	106	544	26	58	20	172	31	144	15	93	14	77	16
Ireland	345	48	179	7	20	16	47	8	53	8	29	9	30	21
England, Scotland and Wales	61	13	25	1	2	4	6	5	10	1	4	2	3	34
Germany	12	3	6	1	–	–	2	–	1	1	–	1	3	33
Canada	232	32	128	5	10	7	40	7	33	7	35	6	10	20
Scandinavia	30	5	15	–	3	2	4	3	4	–	3	–	1	25
Italy	292	124	112	13	13	26	21	21	27	37	32	27	19	53

Russia and Poland	37	20	8	23	13	29	11	21	17	8	11	101	60	230
Other countries	29	10	4	18	6	10	5	12	6	1	–	51	21	87
Unknown	4	5	–	3	–	3	1	13	–	1	–	25	1	29
Totals	26	178	71	240	88	314	92	338	98	116	64	1,186	413	2,245
Percentages		71	29	73	27	77	23	78	22	64	36	74	26	

Note: There were four deaths over two weeks where method of feeding was not known.

Table IV 1911 Mortality of Infants by Month, by Age and by Feeding (for infants over two weeks of age)

Month	Total deaths under 1 year	2 weeks to 1 year		2 weeks to 1 month		1 to 3 months		3 to 6 months		6 to 9 months		9 to 12 months	
		Breast	Bottle	Breast	Bottle	Breast	Bottle	Breast	Bottle	Breast	Bottle	Breast	Bottle
January	162	34	64	7	6	10	21	8	20	5	9	4	8
February	175	49	65	8	5	13	17	7	16	13	13	8	14
March	196	41	101	10	8	11	35	7	22	9	27	4	9
April	191	38	102	8	10	9	28	10	23	7	22	4	19
May	181	34	85	7	15	4	22	11	20	5	13	7	15
June	129	21	61	4	8	6	19	3	10	6	14	2	10
July	280	39	184	3	10	8	46	10	46	10	49	8	33
August	260	40	181	5	14	6	40	12	64	8	38	9	25
September	224	40	137	2	16	7	39	10	39	10	23	11	20
October	172	26	86	1	5	9	27	6	28	3	13	7	13
November	138	24	62	3	9	9	24	3	12	5	10	4	7
December	137	27	58	6	10	6	20	5	14	7	9	3	5
Totals	2,245	413	1,186	64	116	98	338	92	314	88	240	71	178

Table V Actual Death-rates and Estimated Death-rates If All Children Had Been Breast Fed

| | Mother nativity | | | | | |
	United States	Ireland	Canada	Italy	Russia and Poland	Totals for Boston
Births, 1910	6,226	2,816	1,747	2,703	2,479	17,668
Deaths under one year, 1911	927	345	232	292	230	2,245
Rate per 1,000 births (using the 1910 births)	149	123	133	108	93	127
Percentage of children between two weeks to one year, breast fed (estimated),	59	73	51	83	79	68
Deaths, 1911, of children between two weeks and one year	653	227	160	236	162	1,603
Percentage of deaths between two weeks and one year, breast fed	16	21	20	53	37	26
Estimated total infant deaths, 1911, if all above age of two weeks, had been breast fed	457	184	135	205	145	1,253
Lives saved if all above age of two weeks had been breast fed	470	161	97	87	85	992
Estimated death-rate if all above two weeks have been breast fed	73	65	77	76	58	71
Estimated reduction in death-rate if all above two weeks have been breast fed	76	58	56	32	35	56

New Zealand in 1909 had a rate of 62 and South Australia for the same year had a rate of 61.

Discussion

DR. CHAPIN. It is a great pleasure to have a paper like this presented here showing such interesting facts in such a clear and impressive way. We have had data of this kind from Berlin, London and other places, but to have them from a place right here will better carry conviction to the public. We all realize, I think, from these figures, as we have to some extent before, the great advantage of breast feeding. How to secure more breast feeding has been the great problem. In conversation with nurses in Providence it has developed that it is their opinion that a good deal of bottle feeding is due to the fact that the mothers do not know how to conserve the breast milk. We have, in order to assist mothers in this respect, prepared an circular explaining the best way of securing a good secretion of breast milk and maintaining it, and that's circular has been used very largely by the nurses in instructing the mothers. But it is certainly a great help to us to have home figures with which to back up arguments.

SOURCE

Davis WH.1912. Prevention of Infant Mortality by Breast Feeding. *Am J Public Health* 2 (2): 67–71.

More Folic Acid for Everyone, Now[1]
(1996)

Godfrey P. Oakley, Jr., Myron J. Adams and Charlotte M. Dickinson

Division of Birth Defects and Developmental Disabilities, National Center for Environmental Health, Centers for Disease Control and Prevention, Atlanta, GA 30341-3724

ABSTRACT—Research during the last 5 years has made it clear that people who do not take folic acid supplements are at increased risk for functional folate deficiency, which has been proven to cause spina bifida and anencephaly and also has been associated with an increased risk for occlusive cardiovascular disease. The overriding folate policy issue is how to increase dramatically the folate consumption of 75% of the population who are not now consuming 0.4 mg of folic acid in a supplement. The most expeditious way to increase consumption is through fortification of the food staple. Public health programs are also needed to educate people about the vital importance of increased consumption of folic acid vitamin supplements and of foods rich in natural folates. It is *urgent* that fortification of cereal-grain products be implemented now. The level proposed by FDA would accomplish some prevention, but much more prevention would occur if the fortification were 2.5 times that level. Fortification at the higher level would prevent about 1,000 spina bifida and anencephaly birth defects each year and perhaps as many as 50,000 premature deaths each year from coronary disease. Available data have not demonstrated that increasing consumption of folic acid by 0.1 to 0.25 mg of folic acid a day is harmful. If a policy needs to be established on the assumption that people who take vitamin supplements could be harmed, a good policy option is available: require that all folic acid vitamin supplements also contain 0.4 mg of vitamin B-12. J. Nutr. 126: 751S–755S, 1996.

INDEXING KEY WORDS:

- folic acid
- spina bifida prevention

---

1 Presented at The Ceres Forum™ program "Making Health Claims Work, Fortifying Policy with Science—The Case of Folate" held at Georgetown University in Washington, DC, on June 14, 1995. The program was cosponsored by The Ceres Forum™ and the American Institute of Nutrition. Guest editor for the supplement publication was Gerald E. Gaull, Georgetown University, Washington, DC.

- neural tube defects
- homocyst(e)ine
- food fortification

The amount of folate that needs to be consumed for human health has been greatly underestimated. In 1973 in the United States, the allowable folic acid (pteroyl-monoglutamic acid) level in over-the-counter vitamin supplements was quadrupled from 0.1 to 0.4 mg (Food and Drug Administration 1973). This action provided a natural experimental setting in which to observe the benefits of increased consumption of folic acid. In addition to the naturally occurring folates in their usual diets, ~25% of the American population for two decades has been consuming 0.4 mg of folic acid as a vitamin supplement pill or in those breakfast cereals containing 0.4 mg of folic acid per serving. Those who take supplements consume considerably more active folate than those not taking supplements. The benefits for those who consume folic acid supplements include preventing spina bifida and other neural tube defects and the possibility of preventing cardiovascular disease (Boushey et al. 1995, Centers for Disease Control and Prevention 1992). The increased consumption of folic acid has not been associated with the reporting of adverse effects. The major public policy issue related to folate consumption now is how to provide the necessary amount to the large segment of the population that is not using supplements.

Extra Folic Acid Proven to Prevent Spina Bifida and Anencephaly

Results of two randomized controlled trials have shown that when women consume folic acid supplements, in addition to the naturally occurring folates, a large proportion of the cases of spina bifida and anencephaly is prevented (Czeizel and Dudas 1992, MRC Vitamin Study Research Group 1991). These and other data provided the basis for a recommendation by the U.S. Public Health Service in September 1992 that all women who could become pregnant should consume 0.4 mg of folic acid daily to prevent spina bifida and other neural tube defects (Centers for Disease Control and Prevention 1992). This recommendation is targeted at all women capable of becoming pregnant because many pregnancies are unplanned, and adequate folate must be present early in pregnancy when the fetal nervous system is developing—a time before most women are aware they are pregnant. The Public Health Service (PHS) recommendations suggest increasing folate consumption via three routes: foods rich in naturally occurring folates, vitamin supplements, and fortification of a food staple.

Thousands of Cases of Folic Acid-Preventable Spina Bifida Continue to Occur

Spina bifida and anencephaly are serious and common birth defects. Fortunately, the majority (50–70% in the United States) of cases of spina bifida and anencephaly are folic acid-preventable (Centers for Disease Control and Prevention 1992). Spina bifida is the most common cause of infantile paralysis today, yet an effective program to prevent these birth defects has not been implemented. This lack of effective programs is a personal tragedy for the six to nine women each day whose pregnancies are affected by folic acid-preventable spina bifida and anencephaly. Each year, there are more infants who have contracted these mostly preventable birth defects then there are infants who contract pediatric AIDS. It is urgent that we implement policies and programs that will prevent all cases of folic acid-preventable spina bifida and anencephaly.

Proposed Regulations to Fortify Enriched Cereal Grains with Sufficient Folic Acid

Preventing spina bifida and anencephaly requires increasing consumption of folic acid by 0.4 mg a day for the 75% of women of reproductive age not currently consuming a supplement. The fortification of cereal grains with sufficient folic acid would be an inexpensive and relatively easy method of achieving this goal. The Food and Drug Administration (FDA) concurs and has proposed that cereal grains be fortified at a level of 140 µg of folic acid per 100 g of grain, a level of fortification that would provide the average woman of reproductive age with an additional 0.1 mg of folic acid each day (Food and Drug Administration 1993). Adding 0.1 mg to the average diet falls far short of the PHS recommendation of 0.4 mg daily to prevent spina bifida and anencephaly. The Centers for Disease Control (CDC) Folic Acid Working Group recommended fortification at 2.5 times this level (350 µg per 100 g) to provide prevention to a more substantial number of women. The primary reason that the FDA proposed fortification at the lower level was the concern that older Americans who use folic acid supplements might be harmed by consuming too much folic acid if they were to consume extra folic acid in fortified grain products.

Paradigm Shifts Required

Two paradigm shifts are needed to have sufficient folic acid added to grains. It is necessary to assume the following: 1) it is safe to increase folic acid fortification to ensure that most of the population will consume 0.4 mg of folic acid daily, even though such fortification will mean that some people—a small proportion of those who consume folic acid-containing supplement pills—will consume more than 1.0 mg per day of total folate, a level that is the upper safety threshold that the FDA used to arrive at its recommended fortification level and 2) a substantial part of the population consumes insufficient folic acid. There are powerful data to support these paradigm shifts.

Folic Acid Is Safe

The first paradigm shift needed is to assume that it is safe to consume more than 1.0 mg/d of total folate. Public policy in the area of folate nutrition has been dominated by safety concerns, specifically, the concern that folic acid may correct the anemia associated with vitamin B-12 deficiency and thereby possibly delay the diagnosis and treatment of this deficiency, increasing the risk of permanent neurological damage. Vitamin B-12 deficiency is manifested clinically by anemia, neurological signs and symptoms, or both and is most commonly caused by the loss of intrinsic factor (an endogenous protein that facilitates the obstruction of dietary vitamin B-12 in the gastrointestinal tract). With aging, an increasing proportion of people lose the ability to make intrinsic factor.

There is good evidence that folic acid can correct the anemia of vitamin B-12 deficiency in some people for varying periods of time (Savage and Lindenbaum 1995). The increased consumption of folic acid that occurred after FDA's regulatory change in the early 1970s provided the opportunity for widespread consumption of a milligram or more of folic acid. For example, people could take a vitamin supplement and eat two servings of a breakfast cereal fortified with 100% of the U.S. Recommended Daily Allowance (RDA) and thus consume 1.2 mg/d of extra folic acid in addition to the natural folates in their diets. In a randomized controlled trial of folic acid supplementation, Ubink et al. (1993) reported that men who consumed 2.0 mg/d of folic acid in addition to the folates in their usual diets, had mean plasma concentrations of 39 nmol/L. This level is somewhere to the 47 nmol/L mean reported in the upper decile for survivors in the Framingham study (Selhub et al. 1993), leading to the conclusion that many of these people are also consuming 2.0 mg or greater each day. Thus, thousands of older Americans may have consumed an extra 1.0 mg or more of folic acid for many years and many of these people may also have developed clinical vitamin B-12 deficiency.

Since 1973, there have been no published studies or case reports documenting that folic acid consumption resulted in correcting the anemia and delaying the diagnosis of vitamin B-12 deficiency. Recently published reports on this deficiency suggest that the current major clinical issue is when to treat an asymptomatic individual who has a plasma B-12 level in the lower quartile (Lindenbaum et al. 1994). If the increased consumption of folic acid among the elderly were causing delays in the diagnosis of B-12 deficiency, one might expect more people to be diagnosed and treated for more serious neurological complications of B-12 deficiency. The lack of reports of increases in these cases suggest [sic] the delay in diagnosis must be an uncommon event, if it occurs at all. Perhaps the frequent measurement of serum B-12 today, made possible by the availability of serum B-12 tests and third-party payment for these tests (e.g., Medicare), has led to the timely diagnosis and treatment of the vast majority of people with vitamin B-12 deficiency. Dickinson (1995) in a new review of the literature in this field, also argues that recently the lack of anemia has not delayed the treatment of vitamin B-12 deficiency. He further states that "folic acid even in the full therapeutic dose (e.g., 4 or 5 mg/d) will neither cause nor accelerate neurological deterioration in pernicious anemia." (Dickinson 1995)

An upper threshold level should be described in terms of folic acid, not total folate, consumption because almost all studies of folic acid supplements or treatment have not measured the folates in foods. Accurately determining consumption of foods and the folate content of them is difficult. Further, the amount of free folate from foods will be small compared with 0.4 mg of folic acid daily. Using a safety threshold of 1.0 mg or greater of folic acid seems justified. The widespread exposure to folic acid levels >2.0 mg and higher over the last 20 years and the lack of reported morbidity suggest that the threshold could be raised much higher. Evidence that folic acid prevents spina bifida and anencephaly and may prevent occlusive vascular disease provides new incentive for raising the threshold level of folic acid.

Vitamin B-12 and Supplements: Solution to Concern about Delay of Diagnosis of B-12 Deficiency

If policy is made assuming that there is the potential for harm >1.0 milligram of total folate, there is an option that eliminates this concern. The people at risk are those consuming folic acid supplements. The daily oral consumption of 0.4 mg of vitamin B-12 is a proven way to treat people with vitamin B-12 deficiency caused by pernicious anemia or by other causes (Hathcock and Troendle 1991). Vitamin supplements contain 0.4 mg folic acid and also 0.4 mg of vitamin B-12 would provide health benefits associated with folic acid and prevent B-12 deficiency, eliminating the concern of the delay in the diagnosis of this deficiency (Savage and Lindenbaum 1995). It would also mean that ~20% of the elderly who take supplements would never develop B-12 deficiency (Lindenbaum 1994). This policy options needs consideration.

New Definition of Folate Deficiency Needed

The second paradigm shift is to assume that a substantial part of the population consumes insufficient amounts of folic acid. The most powerful evidence that the population consumes too little folate is that extra folic acid at nutritional levels (0.4 mg/d) prevents many cases of spina bifida. Kirke et al. (1993) published dose-response data from a cohort of Irish women that makes it clear that most women who have infants with spina bifida have red blood cell (RBC) concentrations >150 ng/ml, the usual low normal baseline. This low baseline level was developed to protect people from folate deficiency anemia. It is no longer appropriate to term as low only those RBC concentrations that are <150 ng/ml. The low concentrations should be set by determining what constitutes the lower 5th percentile for RBC or plasma folate for women who consume their usual diet and also consume an extra 0.4 mg of folic acid per day. Thus, policy would be set to ensure that folate consumption is sufficient for developing fetuses. This redefinition would mean that the low normal baseline for RBC folate would be much higher than the current 150 ng/ml.

Functional Folate Deficiency Is Widespread among Adults

In 1987, Kang et al. (1987) demonstrated a striking relationship between levels of plasma folate and plasma total homocyst(e)ine and adults. Below mean values in his samples, there was an increasing level of homocyst(e) ine as the plasma folate went down. Above the mean, homocyst(e)ine remained at a steady low level. Lewis et al. (1992) reported a similar relationship and suggested that a plasma folate level of ~15 nmol/L was needed to ensure adequate tissue folate. He pointed out that the National Health and Nutrition Examination Survey (NHANES) II low cut off level of 7 nmol/L should have been ~14 nmol/L. Therefore, the generally accepted low normal threshold level that is based on adult red blood cell levels is too low and must be raised if there is to be folate homeostasis by most people. More recent studies by Jacob et al. (1994) and by O'Keefe et al. (1995) support the need to increase our estimates of the amount of folate needed for good health and to raise substantially what should be considered as the low plasma and RBC concentrations of folate.

Selhub et al. (1993) reported the relationship between homocyst(e)ine and plasma folate levels but with an important twist. Their data show that 50% of the 65 to 93-year-old survivors of the Framingham study had homocyst(e)ine levels above the low baseline that was associated with plasma folates >15 nmol/l. Thus, 50% had elevated homocyst(e)ine and insufficient plasma folate levels. Data from Sweden also suggest that 40%

of adults have elevated homocyst(e)ine levels because of insufficient consumption of folates (Brattstrom 1994).

It is reasonable to conclude that functional folate deficiency is prevalent; therefore, it is no longer reasonable to consider appropriate the current RDA consumption levels of folate nor the current low normal threshold levels for RBC and plasma folate concentrations. Recommendations for levels of total folate consumption should be adjusted upward. And RDA near 1.0 mg/d for folic acid should be considered on the basis of the current evidence. The low normal threshold should be reevaluated, and levels near 15 nmol/l, as suggested by Lewis, should be considered (Lewis et al. 1992).

Homocyst(e)ine a Risk Factor for Cardiovascular Disease

A substantial portion of the elderly population has high levels of plasma homocyst(e)ine because they do not consume sufficient amounts of folates (Selhub et al. 1993). This finding is of critical clinical importance because plasma homocyst(e)ine concentrations are emerging as a risk factor for cardiovascular disease among adults. Homocyst(e)ine levels can be reduced by long-term, daily consumption of multivitamins containing 0.4 mg folic acid (Lindenbaum et al. 1994). Although folic acid has not been proven, through randomized controlled trials, to prevent cardiovascular disease, the meta-analysis of Boushey et al. (1994) summarizes the findings of 27 existing studies and concludes that there is strong evidence of a causal relationship. They suggest that 10% of all mortality from coronary artery disease, ~50,000 deaths/y, could be prevented by increasing the daily consumption of folic acid by fortification at the 0.35 mg/100 g grain (Boushey et al. 1995). Substantial mortality prevention for cerebral vascular disease and peripheral arterial disease is also likely. Thus, increased consumption of folic acid is known to prevent many cases of spina bifida and may improve the lives of tens of thousands of adults each year by preventing occlusive cardiovascular disease.

Fortify Cereal Grains Now with 0.35 mg of Folic Acid/100 g Grain

Now is the time to prevent all of the cases of folic acid-preventable spina bifida and anencephaly. Fortifying as 0.35 mg/100 g grain, 2.5 times the average FDA proposal, would add ~0.25 mg to the average diet. The CDC Folic Acid Working Group proposed that this be the fortification level. If the safety threshold is raised to 2.0 mg of folic acid, then fortification could occur at 0.70 mg/100 g grain, a level that would ensure that many more women would consume the 0.4 mg of folic acid recommended by the PHS, and more cases of spina bifida would be prevented. Preventing spina bifida and anencephaly are reasons enough for fortification. Additionally, there is growing evidence, suggesting that fortification at the 0.35 mg/100 g grain may prevent substantial mortality, morbidity and disability resulting from occlusive cardiovascular diseases. If there is resistance to assuming that fortifying at these levels is safe, an additional policy option of adding 0.4 mg of vitamin B-12 to folic acid-containing vitamin supplements could also be implemented.

Research during the last 5 years had made it clear that people who do not take folic acid supplements are at increased risk for functional folate deficiency, which in turn has been proven to cause spina bifida and anencephaly and which also has been associated with an increased risk for occlusive cardiovascular disease. The overriding folate policy issue is how to increase dramatically the folate consumption of 75% of the population who are not now consuming 0.4 mg of folic acid in a supplement. The most expeditious way to increase consumption would be for fortification of a food staple. Public health programs are also needed to educate people about the vital importance of increased consumption of folic acid vitamin supplements and increased consumption of foods rich in natural folates. It is *urgent* that fortification of cereal grains be implemented now. The level proposed by the FDA would accomplish some prevention. Much more prevention would occur if the fortification were 2.5 times the level that was proposed by the FDA. Fortification at the higher level would prevent ~1000 spina bifida and anencephaly birth defects each year and perhaps as many as 50,000 premature deaths each year from coronary disease. Available data have not demonstrated that increasing consumption of folic acid by 0.1–0.25 mg of folic acid a day is harmful. In addition, if a policy needs to be established on the assumption that people who take vitamin supplements could be harmed, a good policy option is available: required that all folic acid vitamin supplements also contain 0.4 mg of vitamin B-12.

SOURCE

Oakley GP, Adams MJ, and Dickinson CM. 1996. More folic acid for everyone, now. *J Nutr* 126:751S–755S. Copyright 1996 *Journal of Nutrition*. Reprinted with permission American Society for Nutrition.

A Traditional Practice that Threatens Health—
Female Circumcision
(1986)

In recent years the merit of the traditional practice of female circumcision has begun to be questioned, and in some cases publicly condemned, by those who have traditionally been most ready to condone it—the women and men to whom it is part of everyday life, and who have hitherto looked on it as a passport to social acceptance. This is one of the most hopeful signs to WHO, whose official position against this dangerous practice has been coupled with an insistence that change should come not from outside campaigners but from the countries where female circumcision is still entrenched.

The traditional practices of a society are closely linked with the living conditions of the people and with their beliefs and priorities. In societies where women's needs have been subordinated to those of men, traditional practices often serve to reinforce their disadvantage, with direct and indirect effects on their health.

Traditionally, the reproductive role of women is surrounded by myths and taboos that underpin practices pertaining to menstruation, pregnancy and childbirth. Some of these practices are health-promoting but many are dangerous, even life-threatening. Precocious childbearing—pregnancy and delivery in adolescent girls who are not themselves fully mature—is one of the most lethal. Closely spaced pregnancies are similarly fraught with danger for mother and child, as is grand multiparity. The constellation of beliefs surrounding delivery in many societies—e.g., that the process itself is ceremonially impure and polluting and must be conducted in a dark secluded place, that a prolonged or difficult labour is punishment for marital infidelity and curable only by the woman's confession of her misdeed—introduces further pain and risk into an already risky process (there are an estimated half million maternal deaths in the world every year, most of them avoidable).

Another constellation of beliefs and practices is summed up in the term "son-preference." This involves a preference for male children and, often although not necessarily, a neglect of and discrimination against female children, who are less highly valued for both ideological and straightforward economic reasons. The discriminatory practices affect many areas—duration of breast-feeding, intrafamilial allocation of food, immunization against childhood diseases, quantity and quality of care during illness, type and length of education. Separately and cumulatively, these underinvestments in the girl take a toll on her health and often even her life. In countries where son-preference is coupled with extreme neglect of females during infancy and childhood, the inherent biological advantage of the female—reflected in a lower mortality rate than that of the male—is nullified to such an extent that female mortality in these age groups not merely equals male mortality but exceeds it.[1] Every year this neglect results in excess deaths that must be reckoned in the hundreds of thousands if not in the millions. As for the girl who survives she is married off—usually underfed and uneducated—at an early age to begin bearing children whose own chances for survival and a healthy life are severely diminished by these maternal disadvantages.

Female Circumcision

One traditional practice that has attracted much attention in the last decade is female circumcision. Although not the most lethal of the practices affecting women's health, its adverse effects are undeniable. Seventy million women are estimated to be circumcised, with several thousand new operations performed each day. It is a custom that is still widespread only in Africa north of the equator, though mild forms of female circumcision are reported from some countries in Asia, too. However, history reveals that female circumcision of some kind has been practiced at one time or another on every continent. In Britain during the last century clitoridectomy was thought by some to be a remedy for all manner of "ills," from epilepsy and hysteria to nymphomania and masturbation. Even today, removal of the clitoral prepuce is occasionally performed in the USA to counter failure of a woman to attain orgasm.

At the World Health Assembly in 1976, Dr. Halfdan Mahler, Director-General of WHO, stated that there was a need to combat superstition and practices detrimental to the health of women and children, and he drew particular attention to female circumcision. Since then, concerted efforts have been made to generate awareness of the adverse health effects of the practice.

In 1979 a Seminar on Traditional Practices that Affect the Health of Women and Children, organized mainly by the Regional Office of the Eastern Mediterranean, was held in Khartoum, Sudan. The Khartoum seminar was one of the first interregional and international attempts to exchange information on female circumcision and other traditional practices, to study their implications, and to make specific recommendations of the approach to be taken by the health services.[2]

What the Practice Entails

There are three main types of female circumcision.

1. *Circumcision proper*, known in Muslim countries as *sunna* (which means "traditional"), is the mildest but also the rarest form. It involves the removal only of the clitoral prepuce.

2. *Excision* involves the amputation of the whole of the clitoris and all or part of the labia minora.

3. *Infibulation*, also known as *Pharaonic circumcision*, involves the amputation of the clitoris, the whole of the labia minora, and at least the anterior two-thirds and often the whole of the medial part of the labia majora. The two sides of the vulva are then stitched together with silk, catgut or thorns, and a tiny sliver of wood or a reed is inserted to preserve an opening for urine and menstrual blood. The girl's legs are usually bound together from ankle to knee until the wound has healed, which may take anything [*sic*] up to 40 days.

Initial circumcision is carried out before a girl reaches puberty, the age range being anywhere from one week to 14 years. The operation is generally the responsibility of the traditional midwife who rarely uses even a local anaesthetic. She is assisted by a number of women to hold the child down, and these frequently include the child's own relatives. Sometimes amulets are worn or magico-religious ceremonies performed to ward off a child's anxieties at the prospect of "cutting."

In societies where Pharaonic circumcision is practiced, women are commonly re-infibulated after each delivery, after divorce, and on the death of their husband.

Health Consequences

Most of the adverse health consequences are associated with Pharaonic circumcision (see box). Haemorrhage and shock from the acute pain are immediate dangers of the operation, and, because it is usually performed in unhygienic circumstances, the risks of infection and tetanus are considerable. Retention of urine is common. Sometimes the opening left is too small to allow the free passage of menstrual blood—a condition that can have particularly ironic and tragic consequences. Cases have been reported in which infibulated unmarried girls have developed swollen bellies owing to obstruction of the menstrual flow. Together with the absence of menstruation, this state has convinced their families that they were pregnant—a social disgrace which in some cultures can be wiped out only by murder.

Adverse Effects of Pharaonic Circumcision (infibulation) on Physical Health
IMMEDIATE
Shock due to pain and/or haemorrhage
Infection of the wounds
Urine retention
Damage to urethra or anus
GYNAECOLOGICAL AND GENITOURINARY
Haematocolpos
Keloid formation
Implantation dermoid cysts, including abscesses
Chronic pelvic inflammation
Calculus formation
Dyspareunia
Infertility
Urinary tract infection
Difficulty of micturition
OBSTETRIC
Perineal lacerations
Consequences of anterior episiotomy, e.g.:
blood loss
injury to bladder, urethra or rectum
late uterine prolapse
puerperal sepsis
Delay in labour and its consequences, e.g.:
vesicovaginal and rectovaginal fistulae
fetal loss
fetal brain damage

Implantation dermoid cysts are a very common complication; these often grow to the size of a grapefruit. Keloid scars, which commonly form on the vulval wound, have been known to become so enlarged that they obstruct walking, though in most cases keloids do not constitute a real problem except during labour.

Infections of the vagina, urinary tract and pelvis occur frequently. Pelvic infection can result in sterility. Between 20% and 25% of infertility in Sudan has been attributed to Pharaonic circumcision.

Not surprisingly, a woman who has been infibulated suffers great difficulty and pain during sexual intercourse, which can be excruciating if a neuroma has formed at the point of section of the dorsal nerve of the clitoris. Consummation of marriage often necessitates the opening up of the scar by the husband using his fingers, a razor or a knife. Very little research has been done on the sexual experience of circumcised women, a subject surrounded by taboos and personal inhibition in most societies. However, the operation is known to destroy much or all of the vulval nerve and pressure endings, and seems likely to delay arousal and impair orgasm. During childbirth infibulation causes a variety of serious problems including prolonged labour and obstructed delivery, with increased risk of fetal brain damage and fetal loss. Even with anterioepisiotomy the perineum is often lacerated. Sometimes obstruction leads to the formation of vesicovaginal or rectovaginal fistula. A woman who becomes incontinent as a result is generally repudiated by her husband and shunned by society.

Why Is Female Circumcision Practised?

Though some observers believe female circumcision was originally a means of suppressing female sexuality and attempting to ensure chaste or monogamous behaviour, others believe that it was started long ago among herders as a protection against rape for the young girls who took the animals out to pasture. In fact its origins have proved impossible to trace. Not surprisingly, a variety of reasons are advanced by its adherents for continuing to support the practice today. As the word "sunna" suggests, some Muslim people believe it is religiously ordained. However, there is no support for female circumcision in the Koran, nor is it practiced in Saudi Arabia, the cradle of Islam. Other adherents believe that intact female genitalia are "unclean"; that an uncircumcised woman is likely to be promiscuous; even that the operation improves the life chances of a woman's offspring. Some say it is a ritual initiation into womanhood.

None of the reasons given bears close scrutiny. They are, in fact, rationalizations for a practice that has woven itself into the fabric of some societies so completely that "reasons" are no longer particularly relevant, since invalidating them does not stop the practice.

Significantly, female circumcision is usually associated with poverty, illiteracy and low status of women—with communities in which people face hunger, ill-health, overwork, lack of clean water. In such settings an uncircumcised woman is stigmatized and not sought in marriage, which helps explain the paradox that the victims of the practice are also its strongest proponents. They can scarcely afford not to be. In the best of circumstances people are reluctant to question tradition or take an independent line lest they lose social approval. In poverty-stricken communities struggling to survive, social acceptance and support may mean the difference between life and death.

However, the signs are that education and a widening range of choices for women are slowly but surely undermining the practice. And men, too, from societies that customarily circumcise the women are beginning to express their own ambivalence or outright dislike of the custom.

Campaigning against Female Circumcision

Wherever it has come to the attention of people who do not practice it, female circumcision has elicited reactions of horror and very often condemnation. While this has helped break the silence surrounding the subject, experience shows that such a reaction generally blinds outsiders to the complexities of the issue, and can even exacerbate the problem.

Wherever a colonial administration of the past or a government of today has tried to ban it outright, it has simply been practiced with greater secrecy, and those suffering health complications have been inhibited from seeking professional help. Such an approach ignores the fact that those practicing female circumcision believe in it, and that deeply entrenched attitudes of and towards circumcised women cannot be changed overnight. It ignores the need to *replace* the practice and not merely repress it: girls and women need to find other forms and types of social status, approval, and respectability. It ignores, too, the fact that the operation is a principal source of income to traditional birth attendants and even midwives, who cannot afford to relinquish it unless an alternative living is available.

Roman Catholic missionaries in Ethiopia in the sixteenth century tried to stop the practice among their converts, but when men refused to marry the girls a reversal of the policy had to be demanded urgently from Rome. Today abolitionists who attempt to move fast similarly come up against the brick wall of a conservative society feeling itself threatened, or, if the campaigners are outsiders, against suspicion that they are meddling in cultural affairs that are none of their business. Many of these lessons have been learned, and the present approach is through national or local organizations, using as far as possible the skills and experience of those whose work is among villagers normally, such as teachers, social workers and health personnel.

Often the extremely sensitive subject of female circumcision is approached as part of a health, nutrition or education programme for women, and campaigners are encouraged to listen to and respect the community's own perceptions of the custom. With an understanding of its social, economic and cultural value, they are better able to establish a real dialogue that will open the way to change.

Though it is now generally accepted that the initiative for abolition of female circumcision must be taken by women themselves from the societies that practice it, it is also recognized that such national and local initiatives can be greatly helped by outside support. For the past eight years WHO has played a role that has included technical and financial support for national surveys, for the relevant training of health workers, and for grassroots initiatives. For example, WHO has supported the Working

---

An African Man Speaks Out

"Many popular songs and sayings state that woman gives birth to prophets, savants, great warriors and rich men, but that a woman may never herself be a prophet, a savant, a warrior or a rich person. In these societies a woman can never act or state her opinions freely, and the work she does, although a tremendous burden, is never paid for. She is guaranteed no property rights whatsoever, either in her home or in the community, neither by law nor custom. Her social status is always inferior to the man's.

"The origins of this discrimination go right back to the dawn of African history. In most of our societies the birth of a girl has been regarded as a misfortune, whereas that of a boy has been welcomed with great joy. All the rites marking the stages of life emphasize the difference between the sexes. Girls are brought up strictly to play their allocated role in life, that of wife and mother. This inferiority has always seemed so natural that women have been relegated to a closed world on the fringe of their country's history, which has consistently belonged to the man. . . .

"Accused of fickleness, instability, physical and psychological weakness and narrow-mindedness, [the African woman] has been continually violated and mortified by practices such as circumcision, infibulation and force-feeding, supposedly justified, in an essentially 'phallocratic' society, by the need to restrain her 'natural inclination' to be unfaithful. . . .

"Traditions die hard, it is true. But when they prevent an individual from reaching full development or are even life-threatening, to let them continue would amount to masochism or a collective death-wish."

—From: Diallo, B. The dream of domination. *World Health,* April 1985, pp. 26–27.

Group on Female Circumcision that was formed in 1977 by members of 20 nongovernmental organizations (NGOs), with an African woman as its coordinator.[3]

In August 1982 WHO made a formal statement of its position to the United Nations Commission on Human Rights.[4] This statement endorsed the recommendations of the Khartoum seminar, namely:

- that governments should adopt clear national policies to abolish the practice, and to inform and educate the public about its harmfulness;

- that programmes to combat it should recognize its association with extremely adverse social and economic conditions, and should respond sensitively to women's needs and problems;

- that the involvement of women's organizations at the local level should be encouraged, since it is with them that awareness and commitment to change must begin.

In the same statement the Organization expressed its unequivocal opposition to any medicalization of the operation, advising that under no circumstances should it ever be performed by health professionals or in health establishments. Together with UNICEF, WHO also stated its readiness to support national efforts against female circumcision and continue collaborating on research and the dissemination of information.

In 1983, during the Thirty-sixth World Health Assembly, WHO together with the NGO Working Group convened an informal meeting on the subject with African delegates to the Health Assembly.

In 1984, WHO headquarters, together with its Regional Offices for Africa and for the Eastern Mediterranean, joined UNICEF and the United Nations Fund for Population Activities (UNFPA) in helping to finance a seminar in Dakar organized by the NGO Working Group and sponsored by the Government of Senegal. The Dakar seminar gave further impetus to the establishment of national committees in all the countries where female circumcision is practised. It set up an Inter Africa Committee to act as a bridge between the groups working among the people and the outside supporters of their work.[5]

The subject of female circumcision, along with other harmful practices, was subsequently discussed during the Regional Workshop on Women, Health and Development jointly sponsored by WHO, UNFPA and UNICEF in November 1984 in Damascus, Syrian Arab Republic. At this workshop, participants from countries where female circumcision is practised reported on the activities that had been initiated following the Dakar seminar. Women's groups and nongovernmental women's organizations had proved to be more effective than community workers or health personnel in persuading women to abandon the practice. Parallel efforts to convert the men helped to ensure a positive impact of the campaign among women.

Though the pace of change is slow and adherence to the practice of female circumcision still very strong in some societies, abolitionists believe they are on the right path and that, given adequate resources, commitment and time, the phenomenon will disappear from the countries where it is still practised as surely as it has done from other countries in the past. As was said earlier in this article, there are other traditional practices affecting the health of women and children that are more widespread and even more damaging than female circumcision. One set of practices concerns pregnancy and delivery, of which a particularly striking reflection is found in neonatal tetanus, which kills more than half a million infants a year in the developing world. Through its Expanded Programme on Immunization, through its efforts to promote and support the training of traditional birth attendants, and through health education, WHO is hoping to see this problem reduced to negligible proportions by the year 2000. Son-preference and the neglect of female children, which may well cause even more deaths every year, is a much more complex problem. However, there are countries where the abnormal sex ratio of infant and childhood mortality has been reversed over the space of little more than one generation. This has happened where female literacy has expanded and where women have entered the labour market as skilled workers or professionals—

thereby demonstrating to parents that investing in a girl's health makes economic sense. Obviously, WHO's role in relation to literacy is not central, but the Organization has a duty to document the discriminatory practices responsible for countless excess deaths and enable its Member States to chart the effects of these practices. Many differences in feeding and health care, only now coming to light, would have been revealed much sooner if health and vital statistics had everywhere been collected separately by sex. To rationalize the collection of the needed information, WHO is continuing to develop what are called "gender-specific indicators" for the use of countries. The widespread use of these indicators by governments and organizations—as urged by the Nairobi conference marking the end of the United Nations Decade for Women[6]—would be a giant step in the right direction.

SOURCE

A traditional practice that threatens health–female circumcision. 1986. *WHO Chronicle* 40 (1): 31–36. Reprinted with permission of WHO Press.

PART II

Diseases, Therapies, and Prevention

Chief objective: To determine whether a . . . poliomyelitis vaccine would afford protection against naturally occurring paralytic poliomyelitis in selected groups of children . . . and if protection is provided, the degree of such protection.

> —Evaluation of the 1954 Field Trial of Poliomyelitis Vaccine: Final Report, 1957

CHAPTER 8

TUBERCULOSIS

The Lord shall smite thee with consumption, and with fever, and with inflammation, and with extreme burning, and with sword, and with blasting, and with mildew; and they shall pursue thee until thou perish.
　　—Deuteronomy 28:22

... My mother was a saint. And I think of her, two boys dying of tuberculosis, nursing four others in order that she could take care of my older brother for three years in Arizona, and seeing each of them die, and when they died, it was like one of her own.
　　—Richard M. Nixon (1913–1994), president of the United States
　　Spoken at his White House farewell, 1974

War is expensive, and World War II was no exception—in both lives and money. Although victorious at war's end, Great Britain was broke. By 1948, Britain no longer controlled India, its fount of wealth, and the nation contemplated how to best fund its national health care system, the National Health Service (NHS). A major consideration was how to deal with tuberculosis (TB). The discovery of streptomycin in 1943 by Selman Abraham Waksman at Rutgers University promised the first antibiotic cure for the killer disease. Unfortunately, the new drug carried with it a hefty price tag. If the drug was efficacious, it would have great value and reduce overall costs for the NHS. If it was not, then precious funds would be wasted.

The British MRC turned to Professor A. Bradford Hill for an answer: Hill's response, generally recognized as the first modern randomized clinical trial, demonstrated the efficacy of streptomycin for treating TB. The NHS accepted the trial as statistically sound and determined that investing in the drug would be worth the cost. Public health officials appeared ready to deliver on the 1920s prediction of Louis Dublin, statistician for the Metropolitan Life Insurance Company in New York, that TB would be eliminated from the United States by the 1980s. But Dublin's prediction did not come to pass. Although TB began to wane in the 1900s as a result of Waksman's antibiotic, it came back with a vengeance, this time in drug-resistant

341

forms. The opportunity to eradicate TB was sadly lost because the disease re-emerged in a more deadly form.

EARLY EFFORTS

During the first two decades of the twentieth century, TB continued its reign as the "Captain of Death," a name given to it by John Bunyan, a seventeenth-century English writer and preacher. TB not only killed, but also did so in the prime of a person's economic life, often leaving families destitute. The occupational dimension of TB has been covered elsewhere in this volume (see Chapter 5), and the British, in particular, continued to explore the link between occupation and disease. Treatment, however, increasingly focused on developing facilities specifically designed to attend to tubercular patients while isolating them from the rest of the population. Sanatoria emerged in the late nineteenth century on the premise that clean air and a relaxed environment would allow the patient's immune system to battle the disease. The first sanatorium was established in Gorbersdorf, Germany, by Hermann Brehmer in 1854. However, it was another two decades before the concept began to spread throughout Europe, particularly in Switzerland and Finland, as well as Japan.

The United States also saw sanatoria multiply, particularly in the "fresh air" areas of upstate New York and west of the Rocky Mountains. The first such institution was the Adirondack Cottage Sanitarium, founded in 1882 by Edward Trudeau in Saranac Lake, New York. As the numbers of sanatoria mushroomed, TB mortality continued its decline and Bunyan's captain of death began to be more feared in the past tense than in the present one. In 1917, renowned British physician Sir William Osler observed in *The Lancet*, 'In his [Bunyan's] day it may have been true of consumption; it is so no longer . . .'

The decline in TB mortality did not change the importance of TB as a major societal force. French physician Louis-René Villermé described the concept of disease as a social force in the early 1800s; TB clearly fit the mold. By 1900, French TB control efforts focused on the working class, almost to the detriment of all other contributory factors. In Japan, too, TB (kekkaku) was viewed at the beginning of the century as having an occupational or social class basis for its occurrence. By the early 1920s, care for TB patients in England (principally in sanatoria) consumed almost as many resources as did maternal and child health efforts.

The study of the epidemiology of TB began during the first quarter of the century as well. Although occupation had been identified as a major risk factor, particularly for silicotuberculosis, other factors were also found to be important determinants of disease occurrence, including age, race, and geographical location (urban versus rural). Charles Mantoux developed and demonstrated the usefulness of a screening test for exposure to the tubercle bacillus (known as the Mantoux or protein purified derivative [PPD] test). However, the Mantoux test showed only that an individual was exposed; it could not determine whether he or she was actually infected. Until the prevalence of exposure in the population declined, the test would have limited utility.

The development of x-ray technology helped to identify persons who were infected, but even then, tracing the source of the infection often challenged public health officials. For example, Wade Hampton Frost, chair of the first department of epidemiology in the United States at Johns Hopkins University, demonstrated in a classic cohort analysis that TB infections in older adults did not reflect new infections *per se* but reactivation of old ones. Thus, public health efforts at tracing the source of the disease would be futile.

During the 1930s, tuberculosis mortality continued to fall, even as laid-off American workers with TB took their former employers to court with allegations of occupational torts. However, with the rise of fascism in Europe and the Far East and the accompanying global rearming, the economic challenges of the Great Depression began to fade. Societal concerns changed. Were potential recruits for military service infected with TB? Did TB threaten the ability of the population to produce the arms needed for victory?

After World War I, the U.S. PHS was directed to develop a Bureau of Tuberculosis. This group was to develop and implement a strategy for the control of TB in the United States. By the time of the United States's entry into World War II, the bureau had begun recruiting a cadre of scientists who could assess the effectiveness of its activities. One such person was Jacob Yerushalmy, a biostatistician who questioned the soundness of physicians' diagnoses of active TB. Yerushalmy asked the question, "Of those who really have tuberculosis, how many are correctly diagnosed as such? Of those who really don't have tuberculosis, how many are correctly diagnosed as such?" He described these proportions as "sensitivity" and "specificity"; these measures are now typically used to describe screening programs.

TUBERCULOSIS CONTROL

The global chemical industry developed sulfa drugs during the 1930s, and they were the first pharmaceuticals to hold a bacterial infection in check. However, it was not until the discovery of streptomycin in Waksman's laboratory in 1943 that the demise of TB became more than just a dream for public health officials. Unfortunately, like most of the antibiotics of its era, it was expensive to manufacture and, therefore, to purchase. The United States, coming out of World

War II with its economy intact, could afford streptomycin and all variety of the other antibiotics of the era, such as penicillin and chloramphenicol. Great Britain was not similarly situated. It needed to discern whether the scarce health care funds should go to purchase streptomycin or be allocated for other, more efficacious purposes. Bradford Hill's MRC streptomycin trial not only demonstrated the efficaciousness of streptomycin but also established Hill's randomized trial study design as the definitive way to assess the efficacy of a treatment—and it has been used for more than six decades.

With the use of streptomycin and isoniazid (its antituberculosis properties were discovered in 1951), mortality from TB, as well as prevalence and incidence, declined in the developed world. Among the first to receive streptomycin in Britain after the MRC trial findings were published was George Orwell. Unfortunately, he suffered from its side effects and had to stop taking the drug. Later that year (1948), he died from TB, though not before donating his streptomycin to the wives of two physicians with the disease. They both recovered.

These developments with antibiotics occurred as use of a TB vaccine began in earnest. The Bacillus Calmette-Guérin (BCG), an attenuated live bovine tubercular bacillus, was developed by Albert Calmette, a French bacteriologist, and his assistant, Camille Guerin, in 1909. The team continued to develop the agent as a basis for a vaccine, and the first human administration took place in 1921. Further research, including that by George Comstock, demonstrated that the vaccine has some efficacy, though it is not 100 percent. The vaccine is more effective in children than in adults, and there are geographical differences with respect to the vaccine's efficacy. Hence, the BCG vaccine is widely used but not everywhere, such as in the United States and the Netherlands. The rationale for this decision by public health officials is that the vaccine seroconverts an individual from being PPD negative to PPD positive. If it were to be used in the United States, for example, where the number of tubercular cases declined to very low levels, it would become impossible to determine who was exposed to the tubercle bacillus and should receive prophylactic treatment. Under Scandinavian leadership with financial support from the WHO, BCG is used for mass vaccination programs to protect children from tubercle meningitis and the general population from TB. However, where infections rates are low, BCG presents problems for TB control.

By the 1970s, the prevalence of active TB cases in Western and Central Europe and the United States had declined so steeply that it appeared the disease would soon disappear from all developed countries. Although resistance to both streptomycin and isoniazid had been reported, other antibiotics with antitubercular activity had been developed. To minimize the impact of resistance, triple therapy was developed—a cocktail of antibiotics to defeat the captain of death.

However, with TB in decline, the political will to support programs focused on its elimination was lacking. Funds for TB control, particularly (but not exclusively) in the United States, became difficult to obtain.

FAILURE OF CONTROL EFFORTS

With TB in decline, politicians and even some in the public health arena argued that tax dollars should be spent in other areas that would produce a greater impact on population health. Pharmaceutical companies dropped their efforts to develop new antibiotics to treat TB as public health funding priorities shifted. Although the disease seemed on the brink of eradication in the developing world, the premature shifting of public health efforts away from TB control allowed the disease to re-emerge, this time in new forms more resistant to treatment.

In economics, the term for inaction is "opportunity cost." In medicine and public health, the concept is known as "lives lost." So in the early 1980s, when a new disease appeared that decimated a patient's immune system, TB took its opportunity. First called "gay cancer," then AIDS, and finally HIV infection when its viral origin was confirmed (see Chapter 12), HIV severely compromised the ability of those infected to hold a tubercular infection in check. People infected with HIV not only were at an elevated risk of developing the tubercle bacillus, but they also served as new foci for the spread of the disease. TB challenged the developed world first and then, as the HIV epidemic spread, the rest of it. African nations, which had seen the effects of malaria, smallpox, and HIV at rates not seen elsewhere, now needed to increase efforts for TB control as well.

Other geopolitical and economic forces present during the 1980s and 1990s would intervene in the developed world to force vigilance against TB. Immigration created a new challenge. Many immigrants to the United States, especially those from Mexico and Asia who entered illegally, refused to enroll in treatment programs as they feared deportation if they were identified by the government. A similar situation developed in Great Britain with migration from the Indian subcontinent, in France with migration from North Africa, and in Germany with migration from Turkey. With governments shifting their priorities away from TB control and denying the looming HIV epidemic, a perfect storm had developed for TB to flourish.

An additional challenge for public health officials emerged during the last two decades of the twentieth century: drug-resistant strains of TB. Earlier in the century, when the tubercle bacillus became resistant to streptomycin, other antitubercular agents were developed (isoniazid, rifampin, and ethambutol). However, when TB found its way into an immunosuppressed host, such as one infected with HIV, standard TB treatment cocktails were no longer effective. In fact, the cocktail treatment selected *for* the growth of multidrug-resistant (MDR) strains. It is the MDR TB cases that present the greatest challenge for TB control programs today. One of the foci for TB emerging during the last two decades of the twentieth century was prisons. Although the phenomenon was described in the United States and may be reflective of the HIV epidemic among IV drug users (who are frequently imprisoned in the United States), it has been observed globally. For example, the former Soviet Union controlled TB in prisons by administration of antibiotics. However, when the Soviet Union dissolved, these programs lacked funding, and TB returned to an endemic state among prisoners. With the addition of MDR TB to the prison population, the opportunity cost of not eliminating TB during the 1970s begins to assume its full dimensions.

Selected Readings

The first selected reading focuses on streptomycin, the first efficacious therapy for the treatment of TB. Although the efficacy of the new antibiotic was conclusively demonstrated by the Medical Research Council Streptomycin Trial, the paper by William H. Feldman and H. Corwin Hinshaw describing a new antibiotic was typical for its era, the Golden Age of Antibiotics (1945–1960). Feldman and Hinshaw noted the potential for streptomycin, described its observed toxicity and clinical use, and suggested that the drug addressed a critical unmet medical need. Unknown to both clinicians was the tubercle bacillus's impending resistance to streptomycin. Within a decade, streptomycin would yield to newer antibiotics to treat TB, such as isoniazid, which would power the global antituberculosis campaign.

The second reading is a description by one of the doyens of TB, George Comstock, of the organization and early implementation of the post-World War II global campaign against TB. The WHO played a key role in the organization of this campaign, as did a host of other national and international agencies, including the Danish Red Cross and UNICEF. Of course, the challenges of working with such a diverse set of agencies, each representing the culture in which it developed, were considerable. Comstock notes these challenges, as well as the truly global reach of the TB control campaign. He also reports on the extensive use of BCG vaccination as one means of reducing the number of infected persons from which the bacillus could be spread. Although Comstock was one of the architects of the United States's policy in which BCG vaccination was not used, he makes clear the different circumstances presented in the global campaign, particularly the endemic nature of the disease. The success of the campaign can be gauged by the data in Table 3. Perhaps the international cooperation shown in this campaign presaged that needed (and provided) in the global smallpox eradication effort.

In the third selected paper, Arata Kochi describes both the global state of TB at the end of the twentieth century and the efforts underway to control the disease. The challenges presented by TB are reviewed, particularly the challenge of TB in those infected with HIV. When reading this selection, one should remember it was written before the development of highly active antiretroviral (HAART) therapy. The challenges in TB control presented by HIV infection in the twenty-first century are considerably different from those faced by Kochi. Unknown to Kochi was the extent to which the global community would be willing to underwrite the efforts needed for TB control. At the time, the first Persian Gulf War had just ended, and the extent to which funds would be available for such efforts as TB control had not been established. Unfortunately, the opportunity to control TB in the 1960s and 1970s had been lost, and the larger effort needed in the age of AIDS was only one of the consequences.

BIBLIOGRAPHY

Abdel Aziz M, Wright A, Laszlo A, De Muynck A, Portaels F, Van Deun A, Wells C, Nunn P, Blanc L, and Raviglione M, for the WHO/International Union Against Tuberculosis And Lung Disease Global Project on Anti-tuberculosis Drug Resistance Surveillance. 2006. Epidemiology of antituberculosis drug resistance (the Global Project on Anti-tuberculosis Drug Resistance Surveillance): An updated analysis. *Lancet* 368:2142–54.

Anderson P and Doherty TM. 2005. The success and failure of BCG—implications for a novel tuberculosis vaccine. *Nat Rev Microbiol* 3:656–62.

Barnes DS. 1995. *The Making of a Social Disease: Tuberculosis in Nineteenth-Century France.* Berkeley, CA: University of California Press.

Bass JB, Jr. 1985. Lieutenant of the men of death. *Chest* 88:483–84.

Bastian H. 2006. Down and almost out in Scotland: George Orwell, tuberculosis and getting streptomycin in 1948. *JRSM* 99:95–98.

Bonah C. 2005. The 'experimental stable' of the BCG vaccine: Safety, efficacy, proof, and standards, 1921–1933. *Stud Hist Phil Biol and Biomed Sci* 36:696–721.

Brewer TF and Heymann SJ. 2004. To control and beyond: Moving toward eliminating the global tuberculosis threat. *J Epidemiol Community Health* 58:822–25.

Brimnes N. 2008. BCG vaccination and WHO's global strategy for tuberculosis control 1948–1983. *Soc Sci Med* 67:863–73.

Centers for Disease Control. 1999. Achievements in Public Health, 1900–1999: Control of infectious diseases. *MMWR* 48 (29): 621–29.

Comstock GW. 1994. Tuberculosis: Is the past once again prologue? *Am J Public Health* 84:1729–31.

Comstock GW, Woolpert SF, and Livesay VT. 1976. Tuberculosis studies in Muscogee County, Georgia. Twenty-year evaluation of a community trial of BCG vaccination. *Public Health Rep* 91 (3): 276–80.

Corbett EL, Watt CJ, Walker N, Maher D, Williams BG, Raviglione MC, and Dye C. 2003. The growing burden of tuberculosis: Global trends and interactions with the HIV epidemic. *Arch Intern Med* 163 (9): 1009–21.

Crofton J. 2006. The MRC randomized trial of streptomycin and its legacy: A view from the clinical front line. *JRSM* 99:531–34.

Diamond J. 1997. *Guns, Germs, and Steel: The Fates of Human Societies.* New York: W.W. Norton & Company.

Dickey LB. 1950. The BCG controversy. *Dis Chest* 18:502–7.

Doll R. 1998. Controlled trials: The 1948 watershed. *BMJ* 317:1217–20.

Dye C, Garnett GP, Sleeman K, and Williams BG. 1998. Prospects for worldwide tuberculosis control under the WHO DOTS strategy. *Lancet* 352:1886–91.

Dye C, Scheele S, Dolin P, Pathania V, and Raviglione. 1999. Consensus statement. Global burden of tuberculosis: estimated incidence, prevalence, and mortality by country. WHO Global Surveillance and Monitoring Project. *JAMA* 292:677–86.

Enarson DA. 2004. Children and the global tuberculosis situation. *Paediatric Resp Rev* 5 (Suppl. A): S143–45.

Ernst JD, Trevejo-Nuñez G, and Banaiee N. 2007. Genomics and the evolution, pathogenesis, and diagnosis of tuberculosis. *J Clin Invest* 117:1738–45.

Fine PEM. 1995. Variations in protection by BCG: Implications of and for heterologous immunity. *Lancet* 346:1339–45.

Frieden TR, Fujiwara PI, Washko RM, and Hamburg MA. 1995. Tuberculosis in New York City—Turning the tide. *N Engl J Med* 333 (4): 229–33.

Frieden TR, Lerner BH, and Rutherford BR. 2000. Lessons from the 1800s: Tuberculosis control in the new millennium. *Lancet* 355:1085–92.

Frieden TR, Sterling TR, Munsiff SS, Watt CJ, and Dye C. 2003. Tuberculosis (Review). *Lancet* 362:887–99.

Frost WH. 1937. How much control of tuberculosis? *Am J Public Health Nations Health* 27 (8): 759–66.

Gómez I, Prat, J, and Mendonça de Sousa SMF. 2003. Prehistoric tuberculosis in America: Adding comments to a literature review. *Mem Inst Oswaldo Cruz* (Rio de Janeiro) 98 (Suppl. 1): 151–59.

Gómez-Reino JJ, Carmona L, and Descalzo MA. 2007. Risk of tuberculosis in patients treated with tumor necrosis factor antagonists due to incomplete prevention of reactivation of latent infection. *Arthritis Rheum* 57 (5): 756–61.

Hill Sir AB. 1990. Suspended judgment: Memories of the British Streptomycin Trial in tuberculosis. *Controlled Clin Trials* 11:77–79.

Laserson KF and Wells CD. 2007. Reaching the targets for tuberculosis control: The impact of HIV. *Bull WHO* 85:377–86.

Lee T. 1942. The history of tuberculosis in China. *Chin Med J* 61:272–79.

Lönnroth K and Raviglione M. 2008. Global epidemiology of tuberculosis: Prospects for control. *Semin Respir Crit Care Med* 29:481–91.

MacNeil JR, Lobato MN, and Moore M. 2005. An unanswered health disparity: Tuberculosis among correctional inmates, 1993–2003. *Am J Public Health* 95:1800–1805.

Mahler H. 1966. The tuberculosis programme in the developing countries. *Bull Int Un Tuberc* 37:77–82.

Marshall G, Blacklock JW, Cameron C, et al. [Medical Research Council]. 1948. Streptomycin treatment of pulmonary tuberculosis. *BMJ* 2:769–82.

Mitchison DA. 2005. The diagnosis and therapy of tuberculosis during the past 100 years. *Am J Respir Crit Care Med* 171:699–706.

National Tuberculosis Center. 1996. *Brief History of Tuberculosis*. Newark, NJ: New Jersey Medical School. http://www.umdnj.edu/~ntbcweb/history.htm (accessed June 10, 2009).

Nunn PP, Elliott AM, and McAdam KPWJ. 1994. Impact of human immunodeficiency virus on tuberculosis in developing countries. *Thorax* 49:511–18.

Ogden J, Rangan S, Uplekar M, Porter J, Brugha R, Zwi A, and Nyheim D. 1999. Shifting the paradigm in tuberculosis control: Illustrations from India. *Int J Tuberc Lung Dis* 3 (10): 855–61.

Pearce-Duvet JMC. 2006. The origin of human pathogens: Evaluating the role of agriculture and domestic animals in the evolution of human disease. *Bio Rev* 81:369–82.

Raviglione MC, Dye C, Schmidt S, and Kochi A. 1997. Assessment of worldwide tuberculosis control. WHO Global Surveillance and Monitoring Project. *Lancet* 350 (9078): 624–29.

Raviglione MC and Pio A. 2002. Evolution of WHO policies for tuberculosis control, 1948–2001 (Review). *Lancet* 359:775–80.

Robitzek EH, Selikoff IJ, Mamlok E, and Tendlau A. 1953. Isoniazid and its isopropyl derivative in the therapy of tuberculosis in humans: Comparative therapeutic and toxicologic properties. *Dis Chest* 23 (1): 1–15.

Sharma SK and Liu JJ. 2006. Progress of DOTS in global tuberculosis control. *Lancet* 367:951–52.

Shilova MV and Dye C. 2001. The resurgence of tuberculosis in Russia. *Phil Trans R Soc B* 356:1069–75.

Small PM. 1999. Tuberculosis in the 21st century: DOTS and SPOTS. *Int J Tuberc Lung Dis* 3 (11): 949–55.

Stuckler D, Basu S, McKee M, and King L. 2008. Mass incarceration can explain population increases in TB and multidrug-resistant TB in European and central Asian countries. *PNAS* 105 (36): 13280–85.

Tsogt G, Levy M, Sudre P, Norval PY, and Spinaci S. 1999. DOTS pilot project in Mongolia, 1995. *Int J Tuberc Lung Dis* 3 (10): 886–90.

Villarino ME, Geiter LJ, and Simone PM. 1992. The multidrug-resistant tuberculosis challenge to public health efforts to control tuberculosis. *Pub Health Rep* 107 (6): 616–25.

World Health Organization. 1995. Global tuberculosis programme and global programme on vaccines: Statement of BCG revaccination for the prevention of tuberculosis. *Weekly Epidemiological Record* 70:229–31.

World Health Organization. 2006. *Guidelines for the Programmatic Management of Drug-Resistant Tuberculosis: WHO/HTM/TB/2006.361*. Geneva: WHO. http://whqlibdoc.who .int/publications/2006/9241546956_eng.pdf (accessed July 10, 2007).

World Health Organization. 2006. *Tuberculosis and Air Travel: Guidelines for Prevention and Control: WHO/HTM/TB/2006.363*. Geneva: WHO.

Yerushalmy J. 1947. Statistical problems in assessing methods of medical diagnosis, with special reference to X-ray techniques. *Pub Health Rep* 62:1432–49.

Yoshioka A. 2002. Streptomycin in postwar Britain: A cultural history of a miracle drug. *Clin Med* 66:203–27.

Zetterstrom R. 2007. Selman A. Waksman (1899–1973) Nobel Prize in 1952 for the discovery of streptomycin, the first antibiotic effective against tuberculosis. *Acta Pediatrica* 96:317–19.

Streptomycin: A Valuable Anti-Tuberculosis Agent
(1948)

By William H. Feldman, D.V.M., M.Sc., D.Sc.
Division of Experimental Medicine, Mayo Foundation
And
H. Corwin Hinshaw, M.D., Ph.D., D.Sc.
Division of Medicine, Mayo Clinic, Rochester, Minnesota

To find a specific therapeutic substance that will arrest or impede the progress of tuberculosis and permit the intrinsic factors of healing to operate successfully has been the goal of countless investigators since the beginning of the modern era of chemotherapy. Certainly the need for a specific drug treatment to assist in combating human tuberculosis has been and continues to be a compelling one.

During the past decade many infectious diseases have proved to be highly vulnerable to therapeutic attack by a variety of chemotherapeutic agents. Tuberculosis, however, has until recently resisted specific drug treatment successfully. In the quest for an effective substance in the treatment of tuberculosis little, if any, real basis for encouragement was evident until the advent of the sulphonamide compounds.[1] The observations that sulphanilamide had exerted a slight but definite deterrent action on the pathogenesis of tuberculosis in guinea-pigs prompted additional work with a large number of other sulphonamides in experimental tuberculosis. The results indicated that none of these drugs met the requirements of a therapeutic weapon sufficiently to justify their use in clinical tuberculosis.

Eventually drugs remotely related to sulphanilamide but chemically definitely dissimilar in certain important aspects were found to be greatly superior to any of the sulphonamide compounds in combating experimental tuberculosis. These latter drugs—known commonly as sulphone compounds—were derivatives of 4,4'-diaminodiphenyl sulphone. Among the better-known sulphone drugs that have figured in the recent revival of chemotherapy of tuberculosis are "promin" (known as "promanide in Britain), "diasone," and "promizole."

Historical Résumé

Since the ability of certain of the sulphone compounds to suppress tuberculosis almost completely in the highly susceptible guinea-pig was so unprecedented, and since the significance of this phase of the recent development of tuberculo-chemotherapy to the present status of the drug treatment of leprosy is seldom recounted, a brief résumé of the development of the more recent antibacterial attack on tuberculosis seems appropriate.

As mentioned previously, the observations concerning the effects of sulphanilamide on the progress of tuberculosis in guinea-pigs suggested that the sulphonamide drugs and related compounds were worthy of further exploration. In October, 1940, Feldman, Hinshaw, and Moses reported the first experimental study of the use of promin in experimental tuberculosis induced by human tubercle bacilli.[2] The results when confirmed provided sound evidence that the drugs had exerted marked deterrent effects on the progress of a potentially lethal infection. With the recognition of this fact tuberculosis could properly be removed from the list of infections previously considered resistant to the suppressive action of chemotherapeutic agents.

After this initial observation with promin the effectiveness of several other sulphone compounds as anti-tuberculosis agents was demonstrated (Feldman, 1946b). This phase of the work served to establish firmly the ability of a number of complex synthetic organic compounds to exert a measurable therapeutic effect on infections induced experimentally by human tubercle bacilli.

Parenthetically it is of interest to note that the work with the sulphone compounds, especially promin, in experimental tuberculous infections stimulated an important development in the chemotherapeutic attack on leprosy. Several reports now available indicate definitely that promin and subsequently promizole and diasone have ushered in an important new era in the specific drug treatment of this disease. An objective appraisal of the results up to the present time indicates that this newer therapy in leprosy is definitely encouraging (Faget *et al.*, 1946).

The advent of specific therapy with antibiotics which followed the development of penicillin again focused attention on the possibility of successful chemotherapy of tuberculosis with antibiotic substances. This was not a new approach to the problem of specific drug therapy in tuberculosis by the use of antagonistic substances of bacterial origin. As a matter of fact a report on this form of therapy had been published by Cantani in 1885. A review of the many subsequent reports of different investigators who have explored this approach to the treatment of tuberculosis discloses many antibiotic agents capable of antagonistic action against tubercle bacilli (Feldman, 1946a, 1946b, 1946c; Hart, 1946; Waksman, 1947). However, observations on the range of activity of the substances studied were, with few exceptions, limited to *in-vitro* tests. A notable exception is streptomycin, which, in addition to demonstrating its antagonism to tubercle bacilli in the test-tube, has demonstrated its effectiveness against tuberculous infections (Feldman and Hinshaw, 1944; Feldman, Hinshaw, and Mann, 1945; Youmans and McCarter, 1945). As the search continues, the possibility exists of eventually obtaining not one but perhaps several additional antibiotic agents that will be equal if not superior in potency to streptomycin.

As a result of the information that has accumulated since the first report on the use of sulphanilamide in experimental tuberculosis was published, a chemotherapy of tuberculosis of practical significance has been evolved. At last, after countless disappointments, the practical therapeutics of tuberculous infections has been advanced by a drug of considerable specificity and usefulness. By the use of streptomycin it is now possible for the first time to arrest by specific chemotherapy the progress of several different clinical types of potentially fatal tuberculosis.

Streptomycin in Experimental Tuberculosis

THERAPEUTIC EFFICACY.—The effect of streptomycin on the course of experimental tuberculosis in guinea-pigs and in mice is striking. Under prescribed conditions the potency of this antibiotic is sufficient to alter to a marked degree the usual pathogenesis of infections established by fully virulent tubercle bacilli of the human and of the bovine types. It is of much significance that guinea-pigs inoculated subcutaneously with an effective dose of tubercle bacilli will respond to treatment usually in a dramatic manner. Compared with untreated controls, such animals have an extended longevity, and the residual signs of infection either are not demonstrable grossly or microscopically or, if present, are usually inactive lesions characterized by fibrosis, calcification, or other signs of quiescence. In the experimentally infected animals the tempo of the therapeutic effects is relatively rapid. Evidence of deterrent action may be observed after three weeks' treatment.

The specificity of streptomycin for tubercle bacilli and its ability to alter the course of otherwise irreversibly fatal infections are convincing as shown by experiments wherein guinea-pigs are inoculated intravenously with large doses (1 mg.) of virulent tubercle bacilli. Tuberculosis established by this procedure usually becomes a rapidly fulminating process within a short time. However, if treatment with streptomycin is started within three to four days after the animals have been inoculated the treated animals will live many months longer than those not treated (Feldman, Karlson, and Hinshaw, 1947). The same therapeutic restraints can also be observed in white mice inoculated intravenously with virulent tubercle bacilli and treated with streptomycin (Youmans and McCarter, 1945).

Considering the exceedingly formidable character of the widely disseminated infection that follows the introduction of tubercle bacilli direct [*sic*] into the venous circulation, one cannot avoid the conclusion that streptomycin is an anti-tuberculosis agent of considerable potentiality (Feldman, Karlson, and Hinshaw, 1947). It is suggested that in the future new substances antagonistic to tubercle bacilli be subjected to trial in tuberculous infections induced intravenously. Such a procedure should provide valuable data for comparison with the effectiveness of streptomycin.

DOSAGE.—The therapeutic range of streptomycin in the treatment of tuberculous guinea-pigs appears to vary within rather wide limits. In our experience a daily dose of 4 to 6 mg. administered subcutaneously is therapeutically effective for animals weighing 500 to 800 g. Much larger doses do not seem to be more effective. We have found daily doses of 2 mg. inadequate. However, in many infected animals this smaller dose does exert a definite deterrent influence, but the results are, generally speaking, inferior to those produced by doses of greater magnitude. In the treatment of tuberculous mice with streptomycin a daily dose of 3 mg. divided into four injections has proved effective (Youmans and McCarter, 1945).

FREQUENCY OF MEDICATION.—In our earlier studies on streptomycin in experimental tuberculosis we administered the daily dose of the drug in four equally divided injections six hours apart. Later, as a result of experimental observations (Feldman, Hinshaw, and Karlson, 1947), we found that the frequent administration of streptomycin was not essential to a satisfactory therapeutic effect. It was observed that daily doses of 6 mg. divided into two equal injections twelve hours apart were adequate. Furthermore, we observed that animals treated every alternate week appeared to receive essentially the same therapeutic benefit as those on a daily schedule of treatment.

We now prefer to administer the drug every twelve hours. However, it is our impression that streptomycin can be given to tuberculous guinea-pigs, with satisfactory results, once daily or perhaps once every second or third day. There is no evidence indicating that its therapeutic effectiveness in experimental tuberculosis is dependent on frequent administration of the drug. Certainly it is not necessary to administer streptomycin every two to three hours to obtain the desired effects.

TOXICITY FOR ANIMALS.—Although the administration of streptomycin to tuberculous human beings usually provokes certain objective signs of toxicity of varying severity, this drug is well tolerated by guinea-pigs and by mice in doses within the therapeutic level. Guinea-pigs treated daily for five to six months have shown a normal increase of weight and size and have at the end of the experiment the appearance of normal healthy animals. What the maximal tolerated dose for guinea-pigs may be is uncertain. So far as we know, doses of streptomycin even in excess of the therapeutic effective dose do not induce demonstrable damage in the liver or kidneys of guinea-pigs or mice.

In some animals, particularly monkeys and dogs, signs of toxicity have been reported (Molitor *et al.*, 1946). In these animals toxicity was indicated by transient anaemia, mild to severe proteinuria, and casts and blood cells in the urine. Dogs receiving streptomycin have been noted to manifest signs of vestibular dysfunction. Disturbance of metabolism of fat in the liver and kidneys of monkeys and dogs has been reported (Molitor, 1947).

Summary of Evidence in Support of Clinical Trials

In reviewing the evidence to justify the use of streptomycin in the treatment of tuberculous patients several facts of considerable significance may be recounted:

(1) The experimental animal used was the highly susceptible guinea-pig, which has a minimum of intrinsic resistance to infection by virulent mammalian tubercle bacilli. (2) The beginning of treatment was delayed usually from two to seven weeks after the animals had been inoculated with tubercle bacilli. Thus the conditions of the experiments were severe. Furthermore, the conditions were those of therapy and not of prophylaxis. (3) Treatment extended the lives of the infected animals indefinitely. (4) In many treated animals there was a reversal of a previously positive to a negative reaction to tuberculin. (5) As a consequence of treatment the usual course of the disease was dramatically modified even though the animals had been infected by intravenous inoculation. (6) There was a marked tendency for infected tissues to mobilize factors of repair and resistance, and as a result lesions resolved, fibrosed, hyalinized, or calcified. In a word, under the influence of treatment with streptomycin the tuberculous lesions in an infected animal were converted from an advancing destructive process to one of regression and arrest.

The evidence obtained from the experimental studies amply justifies the conclusion that streptomycin is a highly potent antagonistic agent against tuberculous infections in animals.

The favourable therapeutic index of streptomycin in tuberculous guinea-pigs and the further fact that the drug was well tolerated by these animals provided acceptable reasons for extending the investigation to tuberculous patients.

RESIDUAL INFECTIVITY AFTER TREATMENT.—It is our impression that in tuberculous guinea-pigs streptomycin in most instances exerts its beneficial effects by suppressing the normal growth-progression of the tubercle bacilli rather than by acting in a bactericidal capacity. We have, however, observed infected guinea-pigs, treated for a prolonged period with streptomycin, in which no residual infection could be demonstrated in the spleen by *in-vivo* tests. In addition the same animals failed to react to tuberculin, although at the beginning of treatment sensitivity to tuberculin had been noted (Feldman, Hinshaw, and Mann, 1945).

Although the question is difficult to decide with finality, it seems likely that at least in some infected animals most if not all of the infective bacteria are eventually eliminated as a direct or an indirect consequence of treatment. However, in our experience this is not true in the majority of instances. Even after treatment for many months and in the absence of recognizable alteration of tissue the presence of fully virulent tubercle bacilli can be demonstrated in the guinea-pigs by suitable procedures. For this reason it must be concluded that the major effect of streptomycin on tubercle bacilli is that of a bacteriostatic agent.[3] It appears that the concentrations of streptomycin which are attained in the blood and tissues of animals and man are too low to have a direct bactericidal effect.

Streptomycin in Clinical Tuberculosis

The bacillus of tuberculosis produces a number of different diseases in human beings. With this fact recognized, it should not be anticipated that any one form of treatment should be equally applicable to all these diseases. However, these several diseases are all caused by the same microorganism, *Mycobacterium tuberculosis*, and if the organism is so situated as to be exposed to the antagonistic action of streptomycin the suppressive action of the drug should have a certain degree of effectiveness. Studies have shown that streptomycin is not distributed through all tissues of the body in equal concentration (Baggenstoss, Feldman, and Hinshaw, 1947). Furthermore, the mechanical defects which are produced in different structures by the destructive action of tuberculosis will create special clinical and surgical problems which cannot be met completely with any antibacterial agent, regardless of its efficacy (Hinshaw, 1947a).

Miliary and Meningeal Tuberculosis

Generalized haematogenous tuberculosis of human beings most closely resembles the form of tuberculosis which is produced in guinea-pigs and mice experimentally. Such haematogenous forms of tuberculosis as miliary tuberculosis and tuberculous meningitis have in the past been totally refractory to all therapeutic efforts and have had a mortality rate approaching 100%. Until the advent of streptomycin there was no method of treatment which produced even temporary suppression of these diseases or amelioration of the distressing symptoms caused by them.

It is now well established that streptomycin treatment may be effective in bringing about a clinical remission in a considerable percentage of cases of miliary tuberculosis and of tuberculous meningitis (Hinshaw, Feldman, and Pfuetze, 1946; Council on Pharmacy and Chemistry, 1947). It remains to be seen how often these remissions may be prolonged and extended to the point at which one is justified in regarding the disease as cured. We have observed remissions which have lasted for more than two years, and we have patients now under observation who apparently remain well and who eventually can be pronounced essentially cured if this favourable progress continues. When miliary tuberculosis and tuberculous meningitis have been diagnosed at an early stage of the disease and have been treated promptly and adequately, more than 50% of these patients may enjoy a complete remission of all of the infection. Unfortunately, some of these patients will suffer from recurrence of the disease process. In those instances in which the recurrent disease is due to a streptomycin-resistant strain of tubercle bacilli no hope of recovery from the second attack should be entertained. It will probably be at least five years before it can be known to what degree streptomycin treatment will reduce the formerly almost universal mortality rate from these diseases. In the meantime, we would emphasize the importance of starting treatment with streptomycin at the earliest possible moment after the diagnosis of miliary tuberculosis or of tuberculous meningitis has been made.

Pulmonary Tuberculosis

This constitutes the cause of more than 90% of all the deaths from tuberculous infection. The wide variability of tuberculous lesions produced in the lungs and the frequency with which spontaneous recovery from pulmonary tuberculosis is realized make the evaluation of any remedy in this form of disease most difficult (Hinshaw and Feldman, 1944).

Several hundred patients with varying forms of pulmonary tuberculosis have received treatment with streptomycin during the past three years in various American hospitals, and certain conclusions are now tenable (Council on Pharmacy and Chemistry, 1947; Hinshaw, 1947b). All physicians who have employed streptomycin extensively in the treatment of pulmonary tuberculosis have agreed that patients with progressive disease whose symptoms have been marked often enjoy relatively prompt improvement of symptoms, with reduction in the amount of expectoration. There are also a decrease of fever and an improvement of the systemic manifestations of pulmonary tuberculosis. Previously progressive disease becomes at least temporarily quiescent under the influence of streptomycin therapy, and this suppression of the acute disease process is quite uniform during the first few weeks of treatment.

The clinical trend after the first few weeks of treatment depends on whether or not the tubercle bacilli are resistant to the effects of streptomycin and whether or not the destructive nature of the disease is such as to prevent its arrest and the disappearance of bacilli during this period of effective action. Some patients continue to improve for many weeks or months, whether or not streptomycin treatment is continued. The physician is occasionally disappointed to observe a reactivation of the disease within a short time after streptomycin treatment has been discontinued. This tendency to reactivation of previously progressive tuberculosis constitutes strong evidence in favour of the thesis that the drug in vivo is a truly effective suppressive agent. There is increasing evidence that streptomycin combined with collapse therapy and other forms of treatment may be effective when either one alone would probably fail.

Tuberculous Laryngitis and Endobronchitis

TUBERCULOUS LARYNGITIS.—Streptomycin has also been found to be useful in some of the most distressing complications of pulmonary tuberculosis which had previously been refractory to nearly all therapeutic efforts. Tuberculous laryngitis has responded to streptomycin treatment (Figi and Hinshaw, 1946) in a very large percentage of cases, and it is now widely believed that use of the drug is clearly indicated in the more severe and acute phases of this tuberculous disease, even when such treatment is likely to achieve only palliative results. Other ulcerating lesions about the oropharynx and tongue respond to streptomycin in a similar manner. In our experience the most spectacular results with streptomycin treatment of lesions in the larynx have been in those patients with maximal laryngeal involvement and with acute forms of pulmonary tuberculosis without extensive cavitation, and in those patients who have tuberculous laryngitis with minimal evidence of pulmonary tuberculosis.

ENDOBRONCHIAL TUBERCULOSIS.—Active ulcerating lesions of the tracheo-bronchial tree, which are being observed with increasing frequency in the United States, have also responded in a uniform manner to streptomycin treatment (Hinshaw, Feldman, and Pfuetze, 1946 ; Council on Pharmacy and Chemistry, 1947). The serious potentialities of this type of tuberculosis would justify streptomycin treatment under many circumstances. The end-result of tracheo-bronchial tuberculosis is often a bronchial stricture as a result of peribronchial fibrosis. It is immediately obvious that bronchial strictures of this type cannot be precluded and will not yield to any type of antibacterial treatment, and if the degree of obstruction is considerable, pulmonary resection is likely to be required if the stricture is so situated as to make such operation feasible.

Tuberculous Sinuses, Lymph Nodes, Bones, and Joints

Tuberculosis of lymph nodes, of bones and joints, and other types of tuberculosis that produce draining cutaneous sinuses have been treated with streptomycin in a sufficient number of cases to indicate that clinical results are satisfactory in a very high percentage of cases (Hinshaw, Feldman, and Pfuetze, 1946; Council on Pharmacy and Chemistry, 1947; Hinshaw, 1947b). Within a few days to a few weeks after starting treatment the drainage of pus ceases and a scab forms over the sinus, and within a few more weeks, when this scab is dislodged, the sinus appears to be healed. If the sinus tract leads to some large accumulation of pus, such as a cold abscess or an empyema cavity, healing is much less likely to occur, and if it does occur there is much greater danger of a recurrence of drainage of pus. It begins to seem probable that large accumulations of tuberculous pus should be drained by wide-open incision as soon as possible after streptomycin treatment has been instituted. This is in contrast to previously accepted surgical practices. It is probable that tuberculous suppuration may be treated in much the same way as suppurative diseases due to pyogenic bacteria have been treated in the past, provided streptomycin treatment is combined with such surgical intervention.

Cutaneous tuberculosis has not been studied sufficiently to warrant the formation of conclusions, except in the case of scrofulodermia which is associated with tuberculous draining sinuses (O'Leary *et al.*, 1947). This has been discussed in the preceding paragraph. A few patients with lupus vulgaris have been treated, and have appeared to respond sufficiently well to indicate the need for further studies.

Tuberculosis of bones and joints involves a series of problems almost as complicated as those afforded by pulmonary tuberculosis. It is immediately evident that no antibacterial drug can promote the regeneration of destroyed structures, and a comparison with chronic osteomyelitis appears logical. Experience gained thus far has indicated that the principal uses of streptomycin for treatment of tuberculosis of bones and joints are to prevent progression of the disease and to afford protection during and after surgical procedures on the tuberculous joints. In early forms of tuberculosis of joints involving the synovial membrane alone, streptomycin treatment in itself may be adequate to arrest the tuberculous process and hence to avoid subsequent destructive changes, crippling deformities, and the need for surgical treatment.

Tuberculous Enteritis and Peritonitis

Tuberculous enteritis is another most distressing complication of pulmonary tuberculosis. It now seems that streptomycin treatment of this disease yields a gratifying degree of symptomatic relief very promptly in a large percentage of patients. It remains to be determined how permanent these effects may be, but, even if the results prove to be merely palliative, treatment is well worth while, and in some other instance may be the crucial factor in permitting the eventual recovery of the patient.

Tuberculous peritonitis has appeared to respond to streptomycin treatment in the small number of cases in which this treatment has been applied thus far. Judgment of therapeutic results in this disease is more difficult than in other forms of tuberculosis because of the fact that the diagnosis has usually been arrived at as a result of surgical exploration and because of the fact that surgical exploration in itself is thought frequently to exert a beneficial effect on tuberculous peritonitis.

Use of Streptomycin before and after Surgical Procedures

The prophylactic use of streptomycin in conjunction with radical types of thoracic surgical treatment is being put to test in a number of institutions in the United States (Council on Pharmacy and Chemistry, 1947; Glover, Clagett, and Hinshaw, 1947). It has already been determined that streptomycin is of little value in the treatment of advanced and chronic tuberculous empyema (Hinshaw, Feldman, and Pfuetze, 1946). Whether better results will be achieved by surgical treatment of tuberculosis empyema in combination with streptomycin remains to be ascertained. There is reason to hope that streptomycin treatment may prevent the development of tuberculous empyema; our surgical colleagues have not witnessed tuberculous empyema following intrathoracic operations for tuberculosis when operation was performed in combination with streptomycin treatment, except in a few instances in which operation was carried out after the tubercle bacilli had become resistant to the effects of streptomycin.

CLINICAL TOXICITY.—Streptomycin is a drug of moderate toxicity when compared with such drugs as the sulphonamide compounds, but it is definitely more toxic than penicillin. The toxicity of streptomycin is negligible when the drug is used for brief periods in the treatment of non-tuberculous infections. However, when tuberculosis is treated with streptomycin it probably is necessary to utilize the drug for many weeks, and this results in neurotoxic manifestations which are described later. Our colleague Dr. Karl Pfuetze (Medical Director, Mineral Springs Sanatorium, Cannon Falls, Minnesota) has been interested especially in toxicity of streptomycin and the efficacy of the drug when given in small doses. His studies, which have now been in progress for at least two years, have shown clearly that streptomycin is effective in doses as small as 1 g. a day, and perhaps the dose may be still further reduced in many clinical circumstances. When the total daily dose is 1 g., fewer than 50% of patients experience any toxic manifestations whatsoever, and only a few of these complain to any considerable degree. Even these usually recover when treatment is discontinued (Pfuetze, personal communication).

Dosage

The minimal effective dose of streptomycin has not been determined for the various clinical types of disease, but we would suggest that in tuberculosis the average daily dose be approximately 1 g. for a patient of average weight. McDermott (personal communication) has suggested a dose of 20 mg. per kilogram of body weight, which appears to be a reasonable and effective dose and one which will yield minimal toxic results. In previous communications we have recommended that streptomycin be injected at frequent intervals so as to maintain a constantly elevated blood level of the drug. However, as a result of experiments carried out on guinea-pigs (Feldman, Hinshaw, and Karlson, 1947), mentioned above, we have modified this conclusion, and in recent months we have been treating patients by giving the daily dose in a single injection or by dividing the total dose into two injections administered at intervals of twelve hours. The results seem to be equally satisfactory, and this has greatly simplified the clinical use of streptomycin. It remains to be determined whether these infrequent injections and lower doses will be adequate to produce and maintain remissions in such malignant forms of tuberculosis as tuberculous meningitis and miliary tuberculosis.

In previous publications we recommended that in treatment of tuberculous meningitis streptomycin be administered intrathecally as well as intramuscularly (Hinshaw, Feldman, and Pfuetze, 1946). Studies have not been completed to ascertain whether intrathecal injection alone or intramuscular injection alone may possibly suffice. In view of the severe reactions which have occasionally followed the intrathecal administration of streptomycin in doses of 100 to 200 mg., which we recommended previously, we have recently reduced the amount of streptomycin injected intrathecally to 25 to 50 mg. a day. It seems probable that such intrathecal injections every alternate day may suffice.

In the treatment of lesions of the larynx and tracheobronchial tree streptomycin administered by either aerosol or atomizer has often been employed in addition to intramuscular treatment. Recent observations make it seem possible that intramuscular administration of streptomycin alone is adequate for the treatment of these forms of the disease. In the treatment of tuberculous enteritis intramuscular administration of streptomycin is recommended, and it is doubtful if any advantage is gained by the addition of orally administered streptomycin. However, this phase of streptomycin therapy is worthy of further investigation.

Therapeutic Limitations of Streptomycin

Streptomycin, like all other substances of value in chemotherapy, has certain definite shortcomings or limitations.

Antibacterial Potency

Compared with other antagonistic agents effective against tubercle bacilli the antibacterial efficacy of streptomycin against tubercle bacilli is amazingly high. Yet, as was mentioned previously, the major influence of streptomycin on tubercle bacilli in tuberculous infections appears to be that of suppression of the normal pathogenic activities of the organisms. Sterilization of the infective process, even when observed, cannot be attributed to the direct antibacterial action of streptomycin alone. In many instances in clinical tuberculosis during the treatment with streptomycin a marked diminution and eventual disappearance of tubercle bacilli in sputum or other discharges may occur. However, the final elimination of tubercle bacilli from the infected tissues may be dependent only indirectly on the specific action of streptomycin. Most human beings are intrinsically capable of mobilizing mechanisms of resistance and repair which are effective in disposing of tubercle bacilli or inhibiting their aggressive action.

While it would be desirable in the treatment of tuberculosis to have a chemotherapeutic substance of such potency and safety that all tubercle bacilli could be eliminated from the infected host immediately or soon after the administration of a single dose of the drug, the probable results would still be inadequate. In other words, we should distinguish the specific antagonistic effect of the therapeutic substance on the bacterial parasites from the anatomical and purely mechanical factors that were created as a result of the infection. It is illogical to assume that a chemotherapeutic substance, no matter how potent and effective its antibacterial properties may be, can cause in some incredible manner the immediate and complete restoration of tissues that have been irreversibly damaged or destroyed as a consequence of the pathogenicity of the infective agents.

Toxicity[4]

Toxicity must also be considered as another of the limitations of streptomycin as a specific agent in tuberculosis. Like all other agents used in chemotherapy, streptomycin has certain toxic potentialities. However, compared with most other chemotherapeutic agents streptomycin has a reasonable margin of safety when the treatment of severe types of tuberculous diseases is considered. The most important toxic manifestation associated with streptomycin therapy in clinical tuberculosis is the unusual neurological reaction giving rise to dysfunction of the vestibular apparatus. Rarely, auditory function is impaired when large doses are given for prolonged periods or when impaired renal function interferes with the excretion of the drug. Other toxic reactions that have been noted include erythematous rash, fever. eosinophilia, and abnormal urinary sediments.

The toxic reaction to streptomycin referable to the eighth cranial nerve or its end-organs which results in a reduction of the vestibular function is the most serious and was one of the first evidences of toxicity described (Hinshaw and Feldman, 1945; Brown and Hinshaw, 1946; Fowler and Seligman, 1947). The incidence of occurrence of this untoward effect is rather high. At least 90% of patients receiving a daily dose of 2 g. of streptomycin for more than one month will exhibit symptoms of vestibular dysfunction. If the dose is reduced to 1 g. a day fewer than 30% of patients will experience any subjective symptoms or exhibit any objective signs of vestibular dysfunction. Fortunately in most cases the symptoms largely disappear within sixty to ninety days or longer after treatment has been stopped. The most severe symptoms of decreased vestibular function occur in patients receiving doses of 3 g. or more of streptomycin daily. Restoration of vestibular function or compensation phenomena occur more rapidly and more completely in children and young adults than in persons beyond the age of 50 (Hinshaw, Feldman, and Pfuetze, 1946).

While the possible toxic effects of streptomycin should be recognized and carefully considered, extensive clinical trials indicate that in cases of tuberculosis in which the prognosis is unfavourable or uncertain the possible toxic effects of streptomycin do not constitute a valid contraindication to its use (Hinshaw, 1947b). In cases of tuberculosis in which the prognosis is favourable under conventional forms of treatment streptomycin therapy should be used only in exceptional circumstances, if at all.

Streptomycin Resistance

One of the most serious obstacles to the achievement of maximal therapeutic benefits from streptomycin in clinical tuberculosis is the problem of streptomycin-resistant tubercle bacilli. Although the problem of drug-resistant microorganisms is not entirely understood there is evidence that this phenomenon represents a selective process dependent on the capacity of bacteria to undergo spontaneous variation or mutation (Demerec, quoted by Selbie, 1946).

In clinical tuberculosis, while the largest proportion of the bacterial population is sensitive to streptomycin before treatment is started, a few variants are present that are drug resistant in varying degrees (Pyle, 1947). During treatment with a sufficiently potent antibacterial substance such as streptomycin the more sensitive bacterial cells are gradually inhibited and eventually eliminated, while the more resistant cells continue to be propagated. Eventually, if treatment is long continued, there frequently occurs a gradual replacement of the population of tubercle bacilli from one that was predominantly sensitive to streptomycin when treatment began to one that is predominantly streptomycin-resistant. The degree of resistance may be several thousandfold greater than is true of tubercle bacilli sensitive to streptomycin.

In clinical tuberculosis the exact significance of the appearance of varying percentages of streptomycin-resistant tubercle bacilli is somewhat uncertain at the present time. Evidence obtained by animal experimentation shows definitely that infections induced in guinea-pigs by apparently pure cultures of highly streptomycin-resistant strains of tubercle bacilli are not amenable to the therapeutic action of streptomycin (Feldman, Karlson, and Hinshaw—unpublished data; Youmans and Williston, 1946). However, clinically the occurrence after weeks of therapy of some tubercle bacilli highly resistant to streptomycin does not necessarily indicate that the preponderant bacterial population is resistant, and must not be accepted as an indication that treatment may be of no benefit if the need for treatment continues to exist. The fact that patients may continue to improve spontaneously after administration of streptomycin has been discontinued and eventually may become bacteriologically negative (by guinea-pig tests) for tubercle bacilli indicates that treatment may not be required for extended periods.

The time required for the appearance of streptomycin-resistant tubercle bacilli after the beginning of treatment with this substance is variable. Ordinarily, however, the drug-resistant bacteria cannot be demonstrated in appreciable numbers until treatment has been in effect sixty to ninety days. While it is desirable to obtain cultures for the purpose of bacteriological assays for the determination of streptomycin sensitivity[5] at regular intervals after treatment has been started, there is no adequate practical quantitative method of determining when resistant organisms have gained ascendancy. All available tests are only qualitative, and merely indicate that at least a few resistant bacilli are present. This must not be accepted as convincing proof that the end-point of practical treatment has been reached.

Whether or not the administration of streptomycin should be continued after the bacterial population has become predominantly drug-resistant is at the present time a controversial question. It is our opinion, however, that when the vast majority of bacterial cells are no longer susceptible to the antibacterial action of streptomycin further administration of the drug is unwarranted and may even be deleterious. If at a later time streptomycin-sensitive tubercle bacilli again predominate, and other indications are favourable, treatment with streptomycin may be resumed.

How best to meet the problem of streptomycin-resistant tubercle bacilli is at present one of the most important of the many unsolved problems that confront the experimentalist and the clinician. A logical approach would seem to be to use as the therapeutic regimen a combination of two or more drugs each having a high antagonistic efficacy for tubercle bacilli. Streptomycin utilized simultaneously with some other (as yet unknown) antibiotic might prove effective. Streptomycin combined with sulphone compounds or with other synthetic anti-tuberculosis drugs offers possibilities that are now being explored.

Final Comment

During recent years studies in the antibacterial attack on tuberculosis have yielded results sufficient to change to a considerable degree many of the previously held therapeutic concepts of tuberculosis. Most important, it has been adequately demonstrated that this disease is no longer beyond the range of specific drug therapy. Instead, the vulnerability of tuberculous infections to a chemotherapeutic attack has been established experimentally and clinically. While to date the completely ideal anti-tuberculosis drug has not been reported it seems probable that substances equal or superior in effectiveness to known agents may be found. These possibilities warrant expenditure of great effort, and this search may become one of the most important and exciting adventures in medical research.

In the meantime streptomycin seems likely to become generally accepted as a useful drug in certain types of clinical tuberculosis. It must, however, be used intelligently, with full recognition of its shortcomings and limitations. It should frequently be used in combination with other effective methods of treatment, rather than as a substitute for such proved therapeutic procedures as care in a sanatorium, collapse therapy, and surgery.

SOURCE

Feldman WH and Hinshaw HC. 1948. Streptomycin: A valuable anti-tuberculosis agent. *Brit Med J* 4541:87–92. Copyright 1948 by *British Medical Journal*. Reprinted with permission of BMJ Publishing Group Ltd.

The International Tuberculosis Campaign: A Pioneering Venture in Mass Vaccination and Research
(1994)

George W. Comstock

From the Department of Epidemiology, School of Hygiene and Public Health, Johns Hopkins University, Baltimore, Maryland

If an American pediatrician's conversation with Dr. Johannes Holm, a Danish phthisiologist and future director of the International Tuberculosis Campaign, had not been interrupted, the campaign would probably not have become a monumental precedent for world health activities. The International Tuberculosis Campaign was conducted under the auspices of the United Nations International Children's Emergency Fund and three Scandinavian voluntary organizations. In a program that started in the war-torn areas of Europe, nearly 30 million persons underwent tuberculin testing, and almost 14 million were given BCG (bacille Calmette-Guérin) vaccine. In addition, a postgraduate school for physicians was initiated, new laboratories were established and old ones were improved, hundreds of young doctors and nurses were introduced to international public health, and, perhaps most important, research and service were successfully integrated. The success of the campaign led to its becoming the first major disease control and research activity of the World Health Organization.

A Chance Encounter

Historical events sometimes depend on seemingly inconsequential happenings. In a mythical story the absence of a nail in the shoe of the general's horse caused the steed to stumble, starting a chain of events that kept the general from leading his troops to victory. Similarly, a chance telephone conversation determined the nature of one of the first mass projects of disease control conducted by an international health organization. In an unpublished document Dr. Johannes Holm described the circumstances, both formal and "behind the scenes," that led to the formation of the International Tuberculosis Campaign and the major role played by three Scandinavian voluntary health organizations [1].

On 5 December 1947 Holm received a telephone call from Dr. Henry F. Helmholz, a pediatrician at the Mayo Clinic in Rochester, Minnesota, who was in Paris as an adviser to the United Nations International Children's Emergency Fund (UNICEF). The possibility that UNICEF might become involved in campaigns of BCG (bacille Calmette-Guérin) vaccination against tuberculosis had been raised, and Helmholz, who like most Americans knew almost nothing about BCG vaccine, had been referred to Holm for information. At that time, Holm was chief of the Tuberculosis Division in the State Serum Institute in Copenhagen. As an internationally recognized expert on tuberculosis and chairman of the World Health Organization (WHO) Expert Committee on Tuberculosis, not only was he unusually well qualified to instruct Helmholz about BCG vaccinations but he also was familiar with the vaccination campaigns that had already been started in war-torn areas.

Early Relief Efforts by the Danish Red Cross

In the initial relief efforts by the Danish Red Cross following World War II, control of tuberculosis had not been included as a specific program. However, by early 1946 it was apparent to the Danish Relief Mission in Poland that tuberculosis was a major problem and that local facilities were completely inadequate to cope with this disease [2]. They appealed for help.

While this request was being considered, several comprehensive demonstrations of tuberculosis control were under way in Yugoslavia. Here, it was soon discovered that the usual methods of tuberculosis control were not feasible. Early in the postwar recovery period, administration was still disorganized, lack of spare parts and reliable electric power made chest radiography impossible, and facilities for appropriate health education were not available. As a result it was thought that mass vaccination against tuberculosis with BCG vaccine would provide the most good for the greatest number of individuals and that a vaccination campaign would be particularly useful in preventing miliary tuberculosis and tuberculous meningitis in children.

On 21 January 1947 the Polish government agreed to have the Danish Red Cross conduct a mass BCG vaccination campaign. The first tuberculosis workers from Denmark arrived in Warsaw in early April 1947. Although a small building for a clinic had been provided for them, there were no living quarters, and for a time as many as 10 persons slept in a single room of this building [3, 4]. Eventually, a small house was provided that alleviated the crowding somewhat. To make matters worse their luggage was delayed for 3 weeks because of icy roads. When work finally began in May 1947, another effort was made to utilize chest radiography, but again lack of spare parts and reliable electric power defeated this attempt. However, the major thrust of the campaign was a success. In spite of all hardships, almost 208,000 children and young persons underwent tuberculin testing, and nearly 47,000 with negative tuberculin tests received BCG vaccine during the first 6 months of the campaign [3]. With the subsequent extension of the cooperative agreement, several hundred

Polish physicians, nurses, and senior medical students were trained; this training resulted in a dramatic increase in the pace of tuberculosis vaccinations [5].

The Chance Encounter, Again

To return to the telephone conversation on 5 December 1947, Holm told Helmholz about the mass BCG vaccination projects of the Danish Red Cross and learned that UNICEF was to consider assistance to similar projects in Europe at a meeting on 15 December 1947. After one-half hour of conversation, the telephone connection was inadvertently broken. Holm at once called H. H. Koch, director of the Department for International Socio-political Cooperation in the Danish Ministry of Social Affairs, to apprise him of the UNICEF proposal. Koch not only urged Holm to attend the meeting but also offered to pay his expenses. When Helmholz called back Holm told him that instead of giving explanations about tuberculin testing and BCG vaccination by telephone this would be better done in person when he attended the meeting. Helmholz agreed and promised to procure an invitation for Holm.

Danish Relief Proposals Accepted by UNICEF

After 1 week had gone by without any word from Helmholz, Holm called him to ascertain the situation. He was told that Dr. Ludwic Rajchman, chairman of the Executive Board of UNICEF, had stated that Holm's presence was both undesired and absolutely unnecessary because Dr. Thorvald Madsen, formerly with the Danish State Serum Institute, would be at the meeting. As Holm put it in his memoir, "This placed me, of course, in a difficult situation" [1]. Nevertheless, he made arrangements for Helmholz to meet him at the airport in Paris the next day, the Saturday before the scheduled UNICEF meeting on Monday. On Sunday morning Holm was called in his hotel room by Rajchman and Madsen who were in the lobby. Because Holm was still having breakfast in his room, it was agreed that all three would meet at noon. At the appointed hour Rajchman and Madsen invited Holm to have lunch at a restaurant on le boulevard Saint-Germain. He was treated courteously, almost as an old friend. It was clear that his hosts wished to learn about the BCG vaccination projects of the Danish Red Cross, especially the administrative and technical problems. Holm answered all questions freely and in detail but was unable to discover what plans UNICEF had originally had for vaccination programs, either at this meeting or even much later when all three men had become friends and colleagues. It came as a great surprise, therefore, when Rajchman suddenly asked over the after-dinner coffee, "What would you do if you had one or two million dollars to use for tuberculosis control in the war-devastated countries of Europe?" [1].

Without hesitation Holm said that he would give the money to the Danish Red Cross to support and extend its BCG vaccination programs, to develop adequate tuberculosis laboratories in the devastated countries, and to create an international institute to train physicians, nurses, and laboratory technicians from all countries in antituberculosis work. Detailed plans and budgets for these activities had already been made, and the Danish Ministry of Social Affairs was about to ask the United Nations if funds raised in Denmark by the United Nations Appeal for Children could be used for these purposes. After Holm explained what he would do with the money, the conversation became more lively and was "stimulated by several drinks." First, it focused on how the UNICEF funds should be administered and the role of WHO in such projects. UNICEF required that all medical and public health programs conducted under its aegis be approved by its Subcommittee on Medical Projects, which was to have an executive board of three members. Two members had been selected: Professor Robert Debré from France and Rajchman from Poland. The third member was to be named by the Danish government. Holm assumed that Madsen would be this member. A possible objection was raised to the allocation of funds to the Danish Red Cross for a BCG vaccination program. BCG or Calmette's vaccine, as it was commonly known, was a French vaccine. As such France might well wish that its mass administration be supervised by a French organization. Finally, Holm was asked if he might consider accepting a post with UNICEF or WHO to direct tuberculosis activities. His answer was an absolute "no." He had a permanent post in Denmark that allowed him to do the kinds of practical work and research on tuberculosis that he enjoyed. He did not wish to give up his position. However, as technical adviser to the Danish Red Cross, Holm was prepared to assist in any UNICEF-supported activities that might be agreed upon.

At the meeting on Monday, Rajchman announced that he had invited Holm to tell UNICEF what the Danish Red Cross was doing in several European countries and what it was already planning to do in the future. Following this presentation Holm had to answer many technical and organizational questions. At the end of the morning, it was clear that he had been effective in presenting the accomplishments of the Danish Red Cross and the implied advantages of expanding an ongoing program instead of starting a competing effort. In closing the meeting Rajchman stated that he would ask the Subcommittee on Medical Projects to propose financial assistance for the extension of tuberculosis activities of the Danish Red Cross to all European countries in which UNICEF had feeding programs for children.

For a while things moved with remarkable speed. By Tuesday, the day after the meeting, Rajchman had received an informal offer from the Danish government that promised its cooperation with the proposed joint BCG programs. In addition, Rajchman wrote a letter to Holm on Tuesday asking him to direct the planned BCG vaccination campaigns. On Wednesday, at the office in Paris, a draft proposal for support had been prepared by UNICEF. Its preamble reflected admiration for the Danish efforts. "The remarkable initiative taken by the Danish Red Cross in its anti-tuberculosis work on the European continent, and particularly the unprecedented effort in making available the BCG vaccination on the scale never before attempted, represents a lasting contribution for the welfare of European childhood and adolescence and will contribute to a very large degree in speeding up the recovery of the war-devasted [sic] countries. Clearly, therefore, this effort must be recognized as falling fully within the programmes and policies assigned to the International Children's Emergency Fund by the Assembly of the United Nations" [6]. Included in the proposal was an anticipated donation of 2 million kroner by the Danish government. The hope "that suitable arrangement will be made to enable Dr. Johannes Holm to direct ICEF BCG work elsewhere" also was expressed in the proposal. On Thursday Rajchman wrote to Dr. Brock Chisholm, executive director of the WHO Interim Commission, primarily regarding two recommendations from Monday's meeting of the UNICEF Board [7]. Both recommendations dealt with coordinating the efforts of UNICEF and WHO to combat tuberculosis. Rajchman noted that frequent meetings should be held among the following key people in the two organizations: Holm, chairman of the WHO Expert Committee on Tuberculosis; Dr. J. B. MacDougall, the tuberculosis expert from the WHO Secretariat; Dr. B. Borçiç, WHO's liaison officer to UNICEF; and Debré, chairman of UNICEF's Subcommittee on Medical Projects. In this letter Rajchman again mentioned his recommendation that UNICEF appoint Holm as director of the planned BCG vaccination campaigns and that this was known to Holm. Clearly, Holm must have had a change of heart since his absolute refusal only 4 days earlier.

Danish Reactions

Meanwhile, back in Copenhagen, Holm's report of the formal and informal meetings in Paris "created surprise but also great interest in the Ministry of Social Affairs" [1]. Consummation of the proposed UNICEF–Danish Red Cross collaborative tuberculosis work would meet several different but complementary goals. Denmark was justly proud of its assistance to feeding programs and tuberculosis activities in Europe and wished to maintain the international prestige it had earned by these humanitarian efforts [8].

At this time, however, there were serious problems. The United Nations Appeal for Children was being conducted worldwide to support the activities of UNICEF, but Denmark had been reluctant to participate in the program. Monetary regulations forbade the conversion of the appeal's funds into foreign currency. The other alternative, using the revenue to purchase local food, seemed unlikely to be acceptable. Supplying food for European relief efforts had already strained the Danish economy. Furthermore, it had affected the balance of trade adversely, since food comprised a considerable part of Danish exports. As a result it seemed possible that assistance to feeding programs would have to cease within a few months. Taking part in the United Nations Appeal for Children would lead to further economic difficulties and possible domestic repercussions; refusing to take part would damage Denmark's humanitarian reputation.

As a solution to this dilemma, the proposed joint tuberculosis effort could hardly have been better. The United Nations Appeal for Children could proceed. Contributions and the funds promised by the Danish government could be spent in Denmark for items that would not affect the balance of trade, namely, salaries of Danish personnel assigned to the project, support for the already established International Tuberculosis College in Copenhagen, and tuberculin, BCG vaccine, and other medical supplies. The State Serum Institute was already internationally recognized; supplying tuberculin and BCG vaccine to the international enterprise would call the world's attention to the excellence of these products. Although the feeding programs might have to stop, Denmark would still be a leader in a unique international relief effort. On Saturday, December 20, 1947, only 5 days after the meeting in Paris, the Minister of Social Affairs sent a note to the Minister of Foreign Affairs outlining Denmark's relief activities, its current problems, and its support of the UNICEF proposal. Further, the minister requested that this message be transmitted to the secretary-general of the United Nations.

Holm Accepts Directorship with Important Provisos

Negotiations picked up again after the Christmas holidays. On Sunday, January 4, 1948, Holm confirmed earlier suspicions by sending Rajchman a telegram in which he accepted appointment as chief of the tuberculosis campaign. On 6 January 1948, Madsen, who represented the UNICEF office in Paris, met in Copenhagen with representatives of the Ministry of Social Affairs, the Danish Red Cross, and the State Serum Institute's Tuberculosis Division.

Before Madsen's arrival Minister Koch had a conference with Holm. It appeared that Rajchman had insisted that Holm be the director of the joint program. His reasoning, according to Holm [I], was based on fear that WHO would object to the involvement of UNICEF in a medical project and his belief that Holm as chairman of the WHO Expert Committee on Tuberculosis would make UNICEF's participation more acceptable. Responding to this, and apparently without mentioning his Sunday telegram to Rajchman, Holm said he was willing to accept the new post if he could continue to be chief of the Tuberculosis Division in the State Serum Institute. This condition was accepted. When Madsen arrived he merely confirmed that the draft proposal of 17 December 1947 was now official. Following a brief meeting Koch asked the Danish representatives to consider who should be appointed to the UNICEF Subcommittee on Medical Projects. Holm nominated Madsen, but this nomination was not acceptable because Madsen was now a UNICEF employee and could not properly represent Danish interests. Holm was then nominated and appointed to the subcommittee.

The next day Holm confirmed his telegraphed acceptance to Rajchman by writing him a letter but adding certain conditions. The first proviso was that UNICEF accept the Danish government's plans for spending Danish currency, a condition that Madsen had already confirmed as acceptable. There were three personal stipulations: the headquarters must be located in Copenhagen; at least one-half of the UNICEF money for tuberculosis and venereal disease must be allocated to tuberculosis; and Holm must be the chief for all antituberculosis activities financed by UNICEF. The rationale for the last condition was that Holm considered BCG vaccination to be only one part of tuberculosis control; he particularly wished to have funds to train doctors in antituberculosis work and to establish diagnostic tuberculosis laboratories.

Guiding Principles

The first meeting of the UNICEF Subcommittee on Medical Projects met in Paris on 19 January 1948. It was attended by Debré, Rajchman, and Holm, the three executive board members; Borçiç, the secretary; and MacDougall (chief of the WHO Tuberculosis Unit), an official observer. Madsen, chief of the UNICEF Mission to Italy, and Alfred E. Davidson, chief of UNICEF's European office, also were present at the meeting. In addition to reviewing the events of the past month and the role of the Danish Red Cross in current vaccination programs in Poland, Hungary, and Germany, Holm mentioned the proposed Scandinavian Coordination Committee with representatives from the Danish Red Cross, Norwegian Relief Europe, and the Swedish Red Cross. Joint Enterprise was selected as an official name for the tuberculosis projects. Finally, the subcommittee recommended that the UNICEF Executive Board allocate 3 million dollars to the Joint Enterprise in addition to the 2 million kroner pledged by Denmark.

As often happens, important policy decisions were outlined in a bistro over drinks. Holm quoted Rajchman's basic attitude toward international health activities: "If you have made it clear to yourself what you stand for and what you want to achieve, and you have available an acceptable technology, it is not very difficult through a well-planned strategy to obtain the desired results" [1]. Rajchman believed that it was not sufficient that a technology be "generally acceptable"; it also must be endorsed by a group of internationally recognized experts. Because of the numerous variations in tuberculin testing and BCG vaccination procedures, there would be many problems in applying simple and standard techniques in countries with widely different attitudes and conditions. Establishment of the most effective methods would require that a research unit be an integral component of the mass vaccination campaign. It was decided that the unit should be located in Copenhagen in reasonable proximity to the headquarters and should be directed by an internationally recognized research worker.

Another new principle that the Joint Enterprise would introduce into international health activity was the formation of teams of doctors, nurses, and other personnel to be assigned to individual countries from headquarters. Their roles would be to conduct and direct mass vaccination campaigns and to train national personnel to gradually take their places. The Joint Enterprise would not use tuberculosis specialists as chiefs of national missions or on the teams but would "select, educate, and train young people to become good leaders" [1]. As Rajchman said, "We need specialists, but in health care projects, it is much more important to have leaders, and it is easier to make leaders become specialists, than to make specialists become leaders. . . ." [1].

Esprit de corps was considered essential. It was thought that this spirit was best developed by the director, who was to make sure that all personnel knew what the organization stood for and what the realities of assignments were likely to be and that all personnel were trusted completely and implicitly unless they demonstrated that they were untrustworthy. Every effort was to be made to avoid restrictive and suffocating bureaucracy. Achievement of this avoidance would entail considerable financial freedom of action accompanied by financial responsibility. The director of the Joint Enterprise would answer only to the Subcommittee on Medical Projects, not to the Executive Boards of UNICEF or the United Nations. The subcommittee would approve budgets and review periodic financial reports but would not require approval of individual expenditures. Most important, UNICEF's contributions would not go to the Danish government or to the Danish Red Cross but would be deposited in a Danish bank account from which only the director of the Joint Enterprise could withdraw funds. Although the Minister of Social Affairs expressed surprise at such financial freedom, he agreed to the same principles in the use of Danish funds and assigned competent personnel to the Joint Enterprise to assist the director in financial matters, such as preparing budgets and reports of expenditures.

Final Approvals

Two more hurdles for UNICEF remained—approvals by its Programme Committee and its Executive Board. Both groups met in early March 1948 at the temporary headquarters of the United Nations in Lake Success, New York. The Programme Committee readily endorsed the plans for the Joint Enterprise but caught the Subcommittee on Medical Projects by surprise with the suggestion that the Joint Enterprise should not confine its activities to Europe. Objections were raised by the Scandinavian representatives who believed it was most unlikely that their nations could or would be able to support such a major addition. After considerable discussion the Programme Committee recommended that 4 million dollars be allocated to the Joint Enterprise: 2 million dollars together with the Scandinavian contributions to support the European programs and 2 million dollars to be spent on vaccination activities in Africa, Asia, and Latin America with no additional funds from Denmark, Norway, or Sweden.

The next day an informal meeting was held with the UNICEF personnel who would be involved in various administrative and financial matters associated with the Joint Enterprise. Considerable discussion was devoted to how best to maintain an effective liaison among UNICEF, WHO, the Scandinavian Coordination Committee, and the Joint Enterprise. The lead vaccination teams within Europe would be directed and staffed by trained Scandinavian personnel whose salaries would be paid from national funds. If these personnel were later employed outside Europe, they would be paid by UNICEF. Insofar as possible, payment of European expenditures would be divided equally between the UNICEF dollar account and the Scandinavian krone account. This part of the agreement was not written into the formal document prepared by Davidson; it was settled as a gentleman's agreement by a simple handshake between Holm and Maurice Pate, executive director of UNICEF.

Although the Scandinavian representatives to the United Nations had all approved the Joint Enterprise while Rajchman and Holm were in New York, the three voluntary organizations comprising the Scandinavian Coordination Committee had to be persuaded. Not surprisingly, the president of the Danish Red Cross was not happy with the practical arrangements arrived at in New York. Although he was pleased at the international recognition given to the pioneering tuberculosis control efforts of his organization, it was not easy to accept the loss of control implicit in the separate bank account and the gentleman's agreement. Nevertheless, after a "strong exchange of views" and "thorough discussion," the Scandinavian Coordination Committee unanimously approved the UNICEF proposal. At Holm's request Norway and Sweden each agreed to appoint a tuberculosis specialist as an assistant director of the Joint Enterprise.

Many practical details were settled at the meeting in New York. Among them was the decision that all personnel, regardless of the nation from which they were recruited, would spend 1 week at the headquarters in Copenhagen for indoctrination and training. Uniforms were considered essential to identify personnel as members of an international organization. Red Cross uniforms were not acceptable to the Norwegians because the Red Cross was only one of several agencies in Norwegian Relief for Europe. Therefore, it was agreed that the UNICEF uniform would be adopted. A special symbol for uniforms, vehicles, and supplies was to be created from three elements—the UNICEF symbol, the Red Cross, and the double-barred cross of Lorraine (which was the international symbol of the antituberculosis movement). Finally, 1 July 1948 was fixed as the date when the Joint Enterprise would officially take over and expand the tuberculosis work started by the Danish Red Cross.

A Research Unit Is Established

One facet of the tuberculosis campaign was still lacking. The International Tuberculosis College had started its training of epidemiologists, clinicians, and laboratory personnel in Copenhagen in late 1947, and the Joint Enterprise was about to begin its field operations; however, the associated research unit was still in the discussion stage. In February 1948 the WHO Expert Committee on Tuberculosis held its second meeting in Geneva. Holm was the chairman. Two other members, Dr. P. D'Arcy Hart from England and Dr. Herman Hilleboe from the United States, were present. The fourth member, who was from the USSR, was again absent. In addition to welcoming the opportunity to act as advisers to the Joint Enterprise, the committee dealt with two major topics: the formation of a subcommittee on tuberculin and BCG vaccine that would advise the Joint Enterprise on these topics and the proposal of a WHO research unit that would operate in conjunction with the field activities. Although the three members endorsed the idea of a research unit, the topic was tabled in the face of strong opposition from the WHO Secretariat, whose representative stated that research was absolutely outside the possible activities of that organization [1].

In June 1948 UNICEF's Subcommittee on Medical Projects met with WHO's Subcommittee on Tuberculin and BCG. When Rajchman arrived at the meeting, Holm told him of the opposition to the research unit. In what Holm called a "typical fit of rage," Rajchman declared that the Executive Board of WHO and the Executive Board of UNICEF should make the decision on the research unit rather than the WHO Secretariat. He was certain that a meeting on the research unit could be arranged in connection with the forthcoming meeting of the World Health Assembly in July 1948 and that the decision would be favorable. Holm was advised to continue with plans for a research unit but to keep quiet about it for the time being.

One of the experts on the Subcommittee on Tuberculin and BCG was Dr. Carroll Palmer, chief of the Research Unit in the relatively new Division of Tuberculosis Control of the United States Public Health Service. Palmer had accepted this position when it was offered to him by Hilleboe largely because of his belief in the mutual advantages of combining service and research activities. Holm knew Palmer well; he had spent 6 months in Bethesda, Maryland, with Hilleboe's Division of Tuberculosis Control. Palmer had heard of the proposed research unit from Hilleboe and told Holm that the surgeon general of the United States Public Health Service had agreed that he could loan his services part-time to the Joint Enterprise. Although Palmer was favorably impressed with the unique research opportunities, he was always a deliberate man and asked to be allowed to visit Copenhagen and some of the field units before making a decision. Such a visit was tentatively arranged, pending the decision on WHO's involvement in research.

Holm spent the next few weeks in Geneva as a member of the Danish delegation of the first World Health Assembly. This meeting gave him a chance to discuss the problems and opportunities associated with the Joint Enterprise and the proposed WHO research unit with persons who were likely to be elected to the WHO Executive Board. Shortly after closure of the assembly, several members of the new board met with the UNICEF Executive Board and its Subcommittee on Medical Projects. Although the proposed WHO tuberculosis research office was discussed, it was decided that a detailed presentation would first be made to the Joint Health Policy Committee. This committee had just been formed to review and approve all health projects of UNICEF before their initiation and replaced the informal group suggested by the UNICEF Board at their December meeting.

Encouraged by this generally favorable attitude, Palmer returned to Europe in September to visit the research facilities in Copenhagen and field units in Czechoslovakia and Greece. He presented his plans for research to the Subcommittee on Medical Research on 18 October 1948 and to the Joint Health Policy Committee the following day. On the basis of their reports, the WHO Executive Board approved the establishment of a WHO Tuberculosis Research Office in Copenhagen; Palmer was appointed director, and the office's budget was $100,000. The office opened officially in February 1949.

Public and Financial Support

Public support for the Joint Enterprise was also essential. To foster this support a public relations unit was established. The first task of this unit was to select a more appealing and informative name than Joint Enterprise. After several cumbersome suggestions were discarded, the name *International Tuberculosis Campaign* was decided on for publicity purposes. Because it was concise and informative, the International Tuberculosis Campaign gradually replaced Joint Enterprise, even in some official documents.

In spite of the gentleman's agreement regarding the allocation of funds, other administrative aspects of the Joint Enterprise were far from simple. Purchases of $5,000 or more had to be approved by a contract committee at the European headquarters of UNICEF, and if these purchases were to be made in dollars, the New York headquarters of UNICEF had to approve them as well. This approval was to ensure that dollars would not be spent if UNICEF could make soft currency available. Obtaining approval for most major program activities was less complex; approval for these activities usually required only favorable action by UNICEF's Subcommittee on Medical Projects and the Joint Health Policy Committee. Substantive decisions regarding tuberculin testing and BCG vaccination were to be cleared by the WHO Subcommittee on Tuberculin and BCG, while tuberculins, BCG vaccines, and the laboratories producing them were approved by the WHO Expert Committee on Biological Standardization [2].

Financial support was also complicated. There appear to have been three "bank accounts." Two accounts were supplied in large part by funds raised in the annual United Nations Appeals for Children. In the three Scandinavian countries, the funds allocated to the Joint Enterprise were deposited in its kroner account, which was supplemented by the Danish government's contributions. In the other countries appeal funds went to UNICEF, which sent its donation from the Joint Enterprise to the dollar account. The third bank account was the financial support allocated by WHO to its Tuberculosis Research Office and was not under the control of the Joint Enterprise.

All of this financial support for the Joint Enterprise was contingent upon a favorable view of its work among the collaborating agencies. Officially, the work of the Joint Enterprise was reviewed at periodic meetings with designated representatives from the collaborating agencies. Thorough reports of activities were presented, and the comments and advice of the agencies were taken into account in subsequent plans. Liaison was built into the system: the director and the two assistant directors of the Joint

Enterprise represented the Scandinavian participants; the Danish government and UNICEF each had representatives assigned to the Joint Enterprise headquarters; Holm was a member of pertinent UNICEF and WHO committees; and the WHO Tuberculosis Research Office, although officially separate, was specifically charged with preparing detailed reports of tuberculin testing and BCG vaccination in each assisted country as well as with conducting research that would lead to more effective testing and vaccination practices. A close working relationship was fostered by placing most of the statistical staff of the Joint Enterprise under Palmer's direction in the WHO Tuberculosis Research Office [1].

Field Activities

In theory the field work of the International Tuberculosis Campaign was simple. The initial step following requests for assistance was acceptance by the individual governments of a standard agreement with the Danish Red Cross, which acted as an agent for UNICEF and the other Scandinavian countries [9]. In return for the provision of medical supplies, transport, and trained teams to demonstrate how to conduct mass vaccinations, the national governments agreed to pay their appropriate shares of campaign expenses, including salaries of local personnel. They were to see that "the Joint Enterprise is conducted equitably and without discrimination because of race, creed, nationality status or political belief' [9]. Personnel, assets, and supplies of the Joint Enterprise were to be free of all taxes, fees, and import duties. In case of a disagreement regarding compliance, the Programme Committee of UNICEF was to decide what action to take.

After acquainting public health and other authorities with the campaign, personnel made both national and regional efforts to inform the general public about the purposes and nature of the program through newspapers, films, leaflets, and, most successfully, sound trucks operating in the vicinity of the testing sites. It was quickly discovered that a successful campaign depended on providing information to physicians, civic authorities, various key organizations and persons, and the general public [2, 10].

Only persons who had not been infected with tubercle bacilli, i.e., those with a negative reaction to the tuberculin test, were to be vaccinated. By the time the International Tuberculosis Campaign started, preliminary investigations by the Red Cross had shown that only a single tuberculin test was needed. As a general rule this prevaccination test was the Moro patch test for children 11 years of age or younger, and the Mantoux test for older persons; in Mantoux testing personnel most often used the dose of 10 tuberculin units of purified protein derivative to tell which individuals should be vaccinated. By keeping test procedures as uniform as possible, international and regional comparisons would be facilitated.

As the field work started, simple principles became complicated practices. The Moro patch test, which had been so successful for prevaccination testing of young children in Europe, was often unsatisfactory in warmer climates. On sweating skin the patches often dropped off before their scheduled removal at 24 hours, thus leading to false-negative reactions, and sweat-induced sudaminal lesions could be interpreted as positive reactions to the test. Concerns about severe reactions to the Mantoux test caused personnel to deviate from the single dose of 10 tuberculin units; this deviation most often resulted in an additional preliminary test with a dose of 1 or 3 tuberculin units. In Malta the Norwegian team tested older children and adults by the adrenalin-Pirquet scratch test, the tuberculin test preferred in Norway [11]. These unavoidable variations caused the statistical unit considerable difficulty.

BCG vaccine for the Joint Enterprise came from five laboratories that had been approved by the WHO Expert Committee on Biological Standardization. These laboratories were located in Denmark, Sweden, Paris, India, and Mexico. At that time BCG vaccine was available only as a live vaccine dispensed in a liquid medium. It was believed to have a useful life of only a few weeks and had to be protected against light and heat. As a result supplying the field units with fresh vaccine on a regular basis required precise scheduling. Special iced shipping containers were developed that could maintain a temperature of 4°C for 20 hours. Because of the distances involved, air transport was usually needed. At the start of the Joint Enterprise, a small plane owned by the Danish Red Cross was adequate, but as the number of countries involved at a given time rapidly increased during 1949 to a maximum of 15 at year's end, it could no longer meet the demands. In January 1949 a fully equipped DC-3 cargo plane was loaned to the Joint Enterprise by the United States Air Force, which also maintained the aircraft, until March 1950. At that time commercial air facilities had become sufficiently reliable for the weekly shipments and for reicing the vaccine containers on long flights [12].

Service Accomplishments of the Campaign

The scope of the International Tuberculosis Campaign is difficult to describe with certainty because of the variety of definitions that have been used. Although its official start was to be 1 July 1948, some national agreements were signed earlier and some official statistics included work started as early as January 1948. The final day for field operations was 30 June 1951. After that date, "aid to BCG programmes is to be developed as an integral part of WHO's overall tuberculosis service and is to be integrated with the total tuberculosis programme in each area" [2]. WHO was to be responsible for recruiting personnel and for technical matters, UNICEF was responsible for procuring equipment and supplies, and the individual governments were responsible for program operations [13]. Campaign headquarters remained in operation until the end of 1951; it stayed open apparently to assist in the continuation phase by arranging for delivery of equipment and supplies to enable several national governments to complete their vaccination campaigns using teams trained by the Joint Enterprise [14].

A total of 22 countries and the Palestinian refugee camps participated in the International Tuberculosis Campaign. The only published data that are available on all these areas during the campaign's officially prescribed duration are summarized in table 1 [2, 11]. These figures were compiled from the monthly activity reports submitted by all field units. Close to 30 million persons underwent the initial tuberculin tests, and nearly 14 million were vaccinated; an average of 27,103 initial tuberculin tests were performed and 12,671 vaccinations were administered every day for 3 years.

Detailed reports of the campaign were published for only 15 countries and the Palestinian refugee camps [11]. These reports were prepared from individual records of persons who had undergone at least the initial prevaccination tuberculin test. The data in table 2 include the considerable amount of work done in Europe by the Danish and Swedish Red Cross teams during the first 6 months of 1948 as well as that required to complete the mass campaigns in several countries after the official closing date of 30 June 1951. In addition, there are some discrepancies between monthly summaries and individual records that are probably unavoidable considering the large number of field units that often operated under primitive conditions and extremes of weather.

In the European countries the proportions of persons who underwent the prevaccination tuberculin tests—who were therefore present and eligible for vaccination if the tests were negative—were remarkably high considering the complexity of the program in those days. In the early months two preliminary tuberculin tests were considered necessary in many areas, especially for persons older than 12 years of age. Personnel thought a test with a moderately strong dose of tuberculin (5–10 tuberculin units) was needed to avoid the severe reactions that were feared if persons with positive tuberculin tests were vaccinated. To eliminate persons who might have unpleasant reactions to that moderate dose of tuberculin, workers often administered an initial weaker dose, which meant that three visits 3–4 days apart were required to complete the testing.

Other impediments were that specific parental consent had to be obtained for both tuberculin testing and BCG vaccination in Austria and that a parent had to be present during both procedures in Malta. In Syria the religious schools did not favor vaccination, while in Lebanon the

Table 1 The Number of Persons Who Underwent Tuberculin Testing and Who Received BCG Vaccine during the International Tuberculosis Campaign by Country

Country	Period of campaign (month/year)	No. tested	No. vaccinated
Poland	7/48 to 12/49	4,729,033	2,284,829
Finland	7/48 to 6/49	750,000*	362,000*
Czechoslovakia	7/48 to 7/49	3,407,318	2,084,271
Yugoslavia	8/48 to 12/50	3,010,238	1,554,862
Hungary	10/48 to 3/49	1,952,024	771,853
Greece	10/48 to 12/50	1,464,627	1,009,804
India	2/49 to 6/51	4,068,515	1,351,546
Sri Lanka	3/49 to 6/51	306,707	122,764
Morocco	4/49 to 4/51	2,207,507	1,009,589
Austria	5/49 to 7/50	654,293	452,374
Pakistan	8/49 to 6/51	949,987	284,500
Palestine†	9/49 to 12/49	211,323	148,137
Lebanon	10/49 to 3/50	43,463	28,311
Tunisia	10/49 to 4/51	601,502	265,683
Italy	11/49 to 4/50	12,550	6,576
Israel	11/49 to 11/50	365,298	208,851
Algeria	11/49 to 6/51	1,670,665	675,664
Egypt	12/49 to 6/51	2,104,311	661,128
Malta	3/50 to 6/50	54,968	38,770
Syria	3/50 to 8/50	265,285	115,582
Tangier	5/50 to 6/50	21,089	7,493
Mexico	5/50 to 10/50	179,975	83,880
Ecuador	7/50 to 6/51	646,702	346,242
Total	7/48 to 6/51	29,677,380	13,874,709

* Estimated numbers during the period of support by the International Tuberculosis Campaign.

† Refugees from Palestine.

Table 2 Percentage of Persons Who Initially Underwent Tuberculin Testing and Who Returned for Final Results of Tuberculin Testing by Region and Country

Region, country	No. who underwent initial test	% with final test results
Europe		
Austria	693,122	96.6
Czechoslovakia	3,328,810	94.6
Greece	1,609,877	91.1
Malta	55,227	89.0
Poland	4,703,561	93.5
Yugoslavia	3,131,981	90.8
North Africa		
Algeria	2,458,310	70.6
Morocco	2,207,507	78.8
Tangier	21,089	83.4
Tunisia	603,982	77.2
Middle East		
Egypt	4,077,421	63.7
Israel	332,641	89.8
Lebanon	41,744	85.0
Palestine*	208,374	84.3
Syria	265,285	65.3
Latin America		
Ecuador	646,702	85.8
* Refugees from Palestine.		

French schools and physicians were not kindly disposed to the International Tuberculosis Campaign, although they did not object to BCG vaccination [11].

The numbers and percentages of persons with negative tuberculin tests are shown in table 3. The percentages show the proportions of the total number of persons who were eligible for vaccination; their complements,

Table 3 Percentage of Persons with Negative Tuberculin Tests among Those Who Returned for Final Test Results and Percentage of Persons with Negative Tuberculin Tests Who Were Vaccinated by Region and Country

Region, country	Persons with negative tuberculin reactions		
	No.	% with final test results	% vaccinated
Europe			
Austria	526,648	78.6	90.2
Czechoslovakia	2,129,765	67.6	99.5
Greece	1,131,365	77.1	98.8
Malta	39,065	79.5	99.4
Poland	2,276,121	51.7	99.5
Yugoslavia	1,735,540	61.0	98.5
North Africa			
Algeria	1,037,565	59.8*	96.9*
Morocco	1,017,558	58.5*	96.9*
Tangier	8,593	48.9	92.8
Tunisia	286,937	47.5	92.2
Middle East			
Egypt	1,249,774	48.1	98.2
Israel	205,815	68.4	99.1
Lebanon	30,581	73.3	91.1
Palestine†	149,890	71.9	99.4
Syria	113,557	42.8	99.5
Latin America			
Ecuador	334,994	62.2*	99.7*

* Excludes a small proportion of persons who were vaccinated without undergoing preliminary tuberculin testing.

† Refugees from Palestine.

the percentages of persons with positive reactions, give only a rough indication of the extent of tuberculous infection in the various countries because the tested populations are not representative samples. Among the persons eligible for vaccination in all countries, >90% were vaccinated; in 10 of the 16 countries, >98% of eligible persons were vaccinated.

Detailed reports were not prepared for seven countries. Finland did not submit activity reports. Its mass vaccination campaign was already well under way in 1948; it used WHO approved tuberculin testing and BCG vaccination procedures. The only help that Finland required, in addition to the BCG vaccine provided by Sweden, was some additional supplies and transport. Hungary said it needed no trained teams because the Danish Red Cross had been working there since June 1947. However, because it was believed that procedures were not meeting the standards of the International Tuberculosis Campaign, assistance was finally stopped. Only limited demonstrations were possible in Italy because of medical opposition and the desire of the High Commissariat for Hygiene and Public Health for a study rather than a campaign.

In Mexico tuberculin testing and BCG vaccination got off to a good start, were stopped, were started again, and were stopped once more, apparently because of rumors of deaths due to BCG vaccine. After a promise to start once more was not kept, the campaign teams were withdrawn [15]. The rumors may have originated in Puerto Rico. At that time Palmer's research unit from the United States Public Health Service was conducting a controlled trial of BCG vaccine on that Caribbean island; it was modeled after the campaign programs as closely as possible [16]. In spite of strong medical endorsement, the trial was seriously handicapped by unfounded charges from supporters of the opposition political party that BCG vaccine was causing fatalities. In India, Pakistan, and Sri Lanka, only large-scale demonstration programs were conducted, thus leaving mass vaccination up to the national governments at later dates.

After mid-1951 the work started by the International Tuberculosis Campaign was continued and expanded under joint WHO/UNICEF auspices. By the end of 1956, 34 more countries and territories had been assisted in their vaccination campaigns. An additional 160 million people had undergone tuberculin tests, and 60 million of them had been vaccinated [17].

The Research Program

The impressive numbers of persons served by the International Tuberculosis Campaign should not be allowed to overshadow its unique and arguably its most important component, research as an integral part of a service program. The remarkable research opportunities inherent in mass vaccination campaigns had been foreseen by Rajchman, Holm, Debré, and Hilleboe. At their invitation Palmer presented his "Prospectus of Research in Mass BCG Vaccination" [18] to UNICEF and WHO in October and November 1948, respectively.

This prospectus had three general goals: "research on the details of techniques, procedures, and results of tuberculin testing and immunization; basic epidemiological research on tuberculosis infection and disease; and evaluations of the BCG program in the prevention of tuberculosis morbidity and mortality." He gave some specific examples. One of the most pressing problems was how best to select persons for vaccination, namely, how to determine what tuberculin tests and definitions of positive reactions most clearly separated previously infected persons who did not need to be vaccinated from uninfected persons for whom protection was desired.

Because controlled trials of vaccine efficacy did not seem feasible (although Palmer did argue for them), indirect assessments were proposed. One assessment was to study the changes in mortality and morbidity associated with tuberculosis in the wake of the mass vaccination campaigns and to compare tuberculosis rates among vaccinated and unvaccinated persons. A more immediately available assessment was to investigate the degree of postvaccinal allergy (tuberculin sensitivity) that was produced, since it was generally believed that allergy and efficacy were closely related. A corollary to this belief was that revaccination was indicated if tuberculin sensitivity waned, although information on the effects of revaccination was almost completely lacking.

Other suggested research projects included studies on familial characteristics of tuberculin sensitivity, comparisons of chest radiographic findings and tuberculin reactions, and surveys of population samples with histoplasmin skin tests to see if *Histoplasma capsulatum* or a related organism might be causing the tuberculosis-like disease that was then being observed in the United States.

With a sense of urgency akin to that of an archeologist whose dig on an ancient campground is about to be overlain by a superhighway, Palmer stressed the importance of studying tuberculin reactions before BCG vaccination created "artificial" tuberculin sensitivity. He was particularly interested in using the frequency of positive tuberculin reactions among young children to estimate recent levels of exposures to individuals with infectious tuberculosis. He also recognized the importance of what we now call historical cohort studies by urging that campaign records for at least several large communities be "stored separately in a safe place, perhaps in the archives of WHO."

Research Results

The WHO Tuberculosis Research Office was remarkably productive. The office collected 123 reports from 1949 through 1960. Thirty of these reports were published during the existence of the International Tuberculosis Campaign, of which four were annual reports and four were detailed reports of the mass vaccination campaigns in Czechoslovakia, Poland, Syria, and Israel [19]. The remainder, even this early in the development of research projects, reported findings of considerable value for the ongoing mass vaccination campaigns as well as for future work on tuberculosis control.

Among the immediate objectives were "the development of practical methods for the assaying of BCG vaccines, the determination of the effects of a wide variety of factors on BCG, the comparison of vaccines produced in different laboratories, and the correlation of laboratory assays of BCG with results obtained in vaccinated human populations" [20]. Since it was standard policy to screen children who were 11 years of age or younger with the Moro patch test, in 1949 the results of the Moro patch test and those of the Mantoux test for 6,963 Palestinian refugee children aged 0 to 12 years were carefully compared [21]. Fortunately, there was a high degree of agreement ($K = 75.2\%$) between the tests. If the Mantoux test had been accepted as the standard screening test, only 3.4% of the total population would have been wrongly excluded from vaccination by the Moro patch test and 2.3% would have been erroneously vaccinated.

From the earliest days of BCG vaccination, there had been concern that persons with unrecognized tuberculosis might be vaccinated and that later manifestations of tuberculosis might be attributed to a reversion of the BCG vaccine to its original virulent state. This concern was a major reason for hesitancy in accepting the 10-tuberculin-unit test as the only prevaccination screening test. By showing that all 245 patients in a Danish sanatorium who had bacteriologically confirmed tuberculosis strongly reacted to this test dose, the Tuberculosis Research Office strengthened the arguments for discontinuing the use of a second, stronger screening dose [22].

Because of the problems of providing fresh, refrigerated BCG vaccine to the field units, it was important to determine the effects of duration and temperature of storage [20]. When the vaccine was kept at 2°C–4°C, no effect on postvaccinal tuberculin sensitivity was noted with storage times up to 29 days. Surprisingly, this result was also found when the vaccine was stored at 20°C. Even if it was stored for a few days at 37°C, there was little effect on postvaccinal allergy to tuberculin.

In BCG vaccine lots from different laboratories, and even in different lots from the same laboratory, the number of BCG organisms per dose of vaccine varied considerably. Did this variation affect the potency of the vaccine as measured by the production of postvaccinal allergy to tuberculin? In looking at a wide range of dosages, it was found that there was very little postvaccinal effect until the concentration of organisms dropped below one-eighth of the standard number [23].

More important for future research was the recognition that the mean reaction size and its SD were better descriptors of the effects of different doses than was the proportion of persons with positive reactions. Even in these early reports, attention was shifting to descriptions of distributions, an approach that was later to identify the importance of causes of tuberculin sensitivity other than the tubercle bacillus [24].

In assessing BCG vaccination in the field, reliance was placed on the degree of tuberculin sensitivity conferred upon vaccinated persons [25]. To minimize variations due to differences in testers and readers, only specially trained research teams measured postvaccinal tuberculin sensitivity. All children in the selected schools were tested without previous knowledge of prior vaccination to eliminate the observer bias that might occur if only vaccinated children were examined. Emphasis was placed on accurate measurements without regard to definitions of positive reactions. Preliminary results showed that the distributions of postvaccinal reaction sizes were unimodal in every country but that mean reaction sizes differed considerably. Part of the variation was related to the source of BCG vaccine. However, even among individuals given the Danish vaccine, postvaccinal reaction sizes were largest in Denmark, somewhat smaller in Greece and Syria, and much smaller in Egypt.

Subsequent studies after the end of the campaign showed that sunlight was primarily responsible for these variations. Sunlight affected tuberculin only after many hours of exposure [26]. However, BCG vaccine was very sensitive to sunlight. Brief exposures to direct sunshine or moderate exposures to indirect sunshine caused a marked reduction in the number of viable organisms and in the sizes of postvaccinal tuberculin reactions [27]. Exposure of vaccination sites on the skin to sunlight had no effect [28].

Even some basic research was completed and published before the close of the campaign. Two reports [29, 30] dealt with the elusive matter of genetic influences on tuberculosis. By analyzing tuberculin reactions of twins of the same sex and other sibling groups who were examined during a mass vaccination campaign in rural Denmark, it was found that approximately one-half of the variation in postvaccinal tuberculin sensitivity was related to the family and the other one-half was related to the individual.

A concept that was to revolutionize thinking about the cause of tuberculin sensitivity received great support from the campaign. By careful measurement of the transverse diameter of reactions resulting from standardized tuberculin testing, the distributions of reaction sizes of many geographically diverse populations of schoolchildren could be compared [31]. In Denmark and Mexico the distributions were bimodal. One mode was 0 and the other mode was almost 20mm, similar to the mode of reaction sizes among patients with tuberculosis [22]. In Egypt there were also two modes, but the lower mode was 3–4mm; in India the only mode was 0, with a gradually diminishing proportion of reactions in progressively larger sizes. Edwards and Palmer [31] argued that only some nontuberculous cause of tuberculin sensitivity that varied geographically in frequency could explain such contrasting distributions.

The International Tuberculosis Campaign was a major contributor to the now-accepted concept that nontuberculous mycobacteria cause tuberculin reactions that are almost always smaller than those caused by infections with *Mycobacterium tuberculosis*. The International Tuberculosis Campaign and the Tuberculosis Research Office had very little concern for Palmer's third research goal, the evaluation of vaccination programs in preventing morbidity and mortality associated with tuberculosis. Only Finland established a register of persons who were tested and vaccinated in the campaign [1], but an analysis of these individuals with respect to their mortality and incidence of tuberculosis was not conducted until the period 1957–1974 [32]. Mortality was lowest among vaccinated individuals, highest among the nonparticipants, and intermediate among persons with positive tuberculin reactions. However, without controls no conclusions could be drawn regarding the effectiveness of vaccination. Repeated calls for controlled studies had evoked no response in the countries assisted by the International Tuberculosis Campaign, with the sole exception of India. Even there the controlled trial of BCG vaccination was conducted under the auspices of the Tuberculosis Research Office's Field Research Station in Madanapalle, and no support was provided by the International Tuberculosis Campaign [33].

Nevertheless, the International Tuberculosis Campaign and those who led it won notable victories for humanity. Most tangible of these victories were the research findings from investigations of problems faced in conducting mass vaccinations in widely disparate areas and cultures. It is unlikely that so many fundamental facets of BCG vaccination would have been elucidated if the researchers had been isolated in academic institutions and had not been stimulated by their close associations with the field workers. Would the differing geographic patterns of tuberculin sensitivity have been found without the standardized procedures of the mass campaigns? To answer that question one need look only at the mass of data compiled and analyzed by the Tuberculosis Research Office and the relatively little information produced in countries that embarked on programs of BCG vaccination on their own. It was the information generated by the International Tuberculosis Campaign and continued by the WHO-assisted programs that firmly established nonspecific tuberculin sensitivity and the probability that it was caused by nontuberculous mycobacteria, thereby providing answers to many problems of tuberculosis epidemiology and control.

Administrative Lessons

Administratively, the campaign was a pioneer in the health education technique of "each one teach one." In this instance "one" was a vaccination team. The initial instructors were teams from headquarters who trained national teams by working with them under actual field conditions. The teams so trained went on in many instances to train additional teams. In this way stimuli from a few individuals produced the numbers of skilled workers needed to bring BCG vaccination to an entire nation within a relatively short time. Lessons for research administration were also learned. Many service programs produce information that could answer practical and basic research questions. Unfortunately, a number of factors combine to minimize the use of service derived data. One factor is the belief that research is not a proper use of service funds. The founders of the Joint Enterprise wisely recognized that research was essential to maximize the delivery of its services. Another factor is that service personnel often record only the information that they perceive to be useful for a particular person. This problem was largely solved by initially indoctrinating new teams at headquarters and by having statistical personnel visit the teams periodically to check on the completeness of recording and to encourage them in these efforts. Even though incomplete recording became a minor problem, a large number of personnel administered tests and vaccinations and read the results of these procedures. Because of the resulting observer variation, large numbers were required for statistically significant results. For some purposes, such as the frequency of persons with positive tuberculin reactions by age, sex, and geography, the requisite large numbers were available. For other purposes, where precise measurements had to be obtained under conditions in which bias was avoided, the Tuberculosis Research Office developed special research teams and procedures. However, what differentiated their research from most of that done in academia was the development of research questions in close working relationship with the field staff and the knowledge of what the field workers needed to know to make their work more productive.

Summary

A single summary statement of the success of the International Tuberculosis Campaign is not possible. We will never know how many cases of tuberculosis were prevented by the millions of BCG vaccinations. However, a tremendous amount of information was gained informally through the experiences of the field teams and formally by the Tuberculosis Research Office. Assistance was given to tuberculosis laboratories in 13 countries. Useful precedents were set: the use of headquarters teams to train other individuals in their own surroundings, integration of research into a mass campaign, and the introduction of research as a legitimate function of UNICEF and WHO. Through the International Tuberculosis Campaign, the Scandinavian countries, especially Denmark, established a well-deserved reputation for philanthropy. Finally, while we cannot properly assess the efforts of hundreds of individual team members in providing a public health service, often under most difficult conditions, the examples they set for humanitarian service may well have been the most important legacy of the International Tuberculosis Campaign.

Acknowledgments

This paper is largely based on an informal manuscript by Dr. Johannes Holm, the director of the International Tuberculosis Campaign. If Dr. Holm were still living, he should have been the senior author. Insights into work in the field and at headquarters were provided by Dr. Lydia B. Edwards and Mr. Finn C. Nielsen. Dr. Edwards participated in the field activities and became one of the major contributors to research stimulated by and based on the findings reported by the campaign teams. Mr. Nielsen was one of the top administrators at campaign headquarters. He made available letters and other documents relating to the establishment of the campaign. Dr. K. S. Stein provided a description of the early activities in Poland. Mr. Tyge Krogh kindly furnished the English summary of his thesis entitled, "Humanity and Politics." With respect to the origin, goals, and conduct of the International Tuberculosis Campaign, the author has done his best merely to distill the essence of Dr. Holm's memoir and the mass of accompanying documentation. The opinions regarding the successes and failures of the campaign's service and research activities are those of the author. The author is grateful to Kathleen E. Niswander for preparing numerous sequential copies of the manuscript.

SOURCE

Comstock G. 1994. The international tuberculosis campaign: A pioneering venture in mass vaccination and research. *Clin Infect Dis* 19:528–40. Copyright 1994 *Clinical Infectious Diseases*. Reprinted with permission of University of Chicago Press.

The Global Tuberculosis Situation and the New Control Strategy of the World Health Organization
(1991)

Arata Kochi, Chief Medical Officer, Tuberculosis Unit, Division of Communicable Diseases, World Health Organization, *CH–1211 Geneva 27, Switzerland.*

The World Health Organization Tuberculosis Unit undertook a special study [1] in 1989/90 to determine the nature and magnitude of the global tuberculosis problem by reviewing the official statistics and the available data from both published and unpublished studies, including the article by Murray *et al.* [2]. The findings of this study are summarized in Table 1.

Infection

About 1,700 million people, or one third of the world's population are, or have been, infected with *Mycobacterium tuberculosis*. The overall proportion of infected people is similar in the industrialized and developing nations. However, 80% of infected individuals in industrialized countries are aged 50 years or more while 75% of those in developing countries are less than 50 years old. This is the result of differences in the past and current levels of transmission of the infection and in the population structures in these two areas.

Disease

It is estimated that, in 1990, there were 8 million new cases of tuberculosis in developing and industrialized countries: 7.6 million (95%) in the former and 400,000 (5%) in the latter. The largest numbers were in the WHO's Western Pacific region (2.6 million), the South-East Asian Region (2.5 million) and the African region (1.4 million). The highest incidence was in the African Region (272 cases per 100,000).

Death

It is estimated that tuberculosis caused 2.9 million deaths in 1990, making this disease the largest cause of death from a single pathogen in the world. While the largest number of deaths occurred in the South-East Asian Region (940,000), the Western Pacific Region (890,000 and the African

Table 1 The Global Toll of Tuberculosis

Region	People infected (millions)	New cases	Deaths
Africa	171	1,400,000	660,000
Americas*	117	560,000	220,000
Eastern Mediterranean	52	594,000	160,000
South-East Asia	426	2,480,000	940,000
Western Pacific†	574	2,560,000	890,000
Europe and other industrialized countries§	382	410,000	40,000
Total	1,722	8,004,000	2,910,000

*Excluding USA and Canada.

† Excluding Japan, Australia and New Zealand.

§USA, Japan, Australia and New Zealand.

Region (660,000), it is estimated that more than 40,000 deaths still occur annually in the industrialized nations.

Characteristics of Patients

There is a striking difference in 'who suffers from tuberculosis' between developing and industrialized countries due to the differences in the pathogenesis of the disease in these countries. In the industrialized countries, tuberculosis is mainly seen in the elderly and is usually the result of endogenous reactivation of infection contracted in the past. Only a small percentage of all cases are the result of recent infection and these occur mainly in ethnic minorities and migrants. In developing countries the risk of infection remains high and tuberculosis afflicts nearly all age groups. While 1.3 million cases in 450,000 deaths from tuberculosis in developing countries occur in children under the age of 15 years [3], the greatest incidence and mortality is concentrated in the economically most productive age group of the population (15–59 years). More than 80% of the tuberculosis toll in the developing world falls in this age group. Furthermore, it is estimated that tuberculosis accounts for 26% of avoidable deaths.

Table 2 The Epidemiological Pattern of Tuberculosis

Countries or areas	Annual risk of infection		Health resource availability
	Current level (%)	Annual decline trend (%)	
I Industrialized	0.1–0.01	>10	Excellent
II Middle-income in Latin America, West Asia, and North Africa	0.5–1.5	5–10	Good
III Middle-income in East and South-East Asia	1.0–2.5	<5	Good
IV Sub-Saharan Africa and Indian subcontinent	1.0–2.5	0–3	Poor

Current Levels and Past Trends of Infection

Countries can be divided into four groups in terms of the current level and past trends of the annual risk of infection and health resource availability [4] as shown in Table 2. In industrialized countries (group I), tuberculosis has been declining very rapidly as transmission, measured as the annual risk of infection, has diminished. Nevertheless, tuberculosis remains one of the most common notifiable infectious diseases. Furthermore, in many industrialized countries, the declining trend has slowed down and, in some countries (USA and Japan), it has reversed. In some middle-income developing countries (group II), tuberculosis has declined relatively rapidly and has begun to lose its status as a major public health problem. In other middle-income developing countries (group III), the decline is slow and tuberculosis remains a major public health problem. In these countries there is a higher frequency of patients with drug-resistant disease than in other countries, due to a combination of quality of treatment and the national tuberculosis control programmes in the past and uncontrolled use of anti-tuberculosis drugs in the private sector. In the majority of low-income developing countries (group IV), there has been almost no observable decline and the absolute number of cases is probably increasing due to population growth.

Current Status of Control Activities

In order to assess the current status of tuberculosis control activities in developing countries, WHO undertook another special study in 1985 [5]. The results of the study can be summarized as follows:

Monitoring

The majority of countries do not have a build-in mechanism to monitor the outcome of treatment. The WHO investigation has so far identified less than 15 countries with such a build-in monitoring system to produce, on a regular basis, crucial information on the percentage of patients who were cured or who died or absconded. Many countries, however, have partial information on the outcome of treatment based on *ad hoc* surveys in a limited number of treatment centres.

Cure Rates

In many developing countries less than half of the tuberculosis patients who started treatment were cured or completed their course of chemotherapy. However, four countries (Malawi, Mozambique, Nicaragua and Tanzania), which have built-in systems to monitor treatment outcomes, achieved cure rates of over 80%. These excellent results were obtained with technical and financial assistance of the International Union Against Tuberculosis and Lung Disease (IUATLD).

Coverage of Tuberculosis Services

It is roughly estimated that less than half of the existing tuberculosis patients in developing countries, excluding China, are covered by the treatment services. This proportion varies considerably among the different WHO regions (Table 3). There has been no significant change in the coverage rate of services in any region over the past 15 years.

Table 3 Estimate of Tuberculosis Service Coverage in Developing Countries: 1988–89

Region	Service coverage (%)
Africa	24
Americas*	42
Eastern Mediterranean	70
South-East Asia	44
Western Pacifict	88
Total	46

*Excluding USA and Canada.

† Excluding China, Australia, Japan and New Zealand.

The Impact of HIV Infection

It is estimated that more than 3 million people are duly infected with the tubercle bacillus and HIV in the world, 2.4 million in Sub-Saharan Africa alone. HIV infection is the highest risk factor so far identified which increases the chance of latent infection with tubercle bacilli progressing to active tuberculosis by reducing the protection provided by cell-mediated immunity [6]. Presently, less than 5% of cases of tuberculosis throughout the world are associated with HIV infection but the majority of these cases are concentrated in only 10 Sub-Saharan African countries. In these countries, the AIDS epidemic is having a devastating effect on tuberculosis control programmes, with up to 100% increases in reported tuberculosis cases in the last 4–5 years [7]. There are more demands for diagnostic services, anti-tuberculosis drugs, hospital beds and other supplies and services in areas where they are already in short supply. HIV infected persons have a higher frequency of extrapulmonary tuberculosis, which is more difficult to diagnose than pulmonary tuberculosis. Also, as HIV infected persons have, in certain instances, had adverse reactions to drugs, particularly to thiacetazone, patient management is becoming increasingly difficult. As the association between tuberculosis and HIV infection becomes more widely known, the diagnosis of tuberculosis will begin to carry an additional social stigma. It also creates fear among health workers who become reluctant to work in the programme. A higher mortality rate among HIV-related tuberculosis patients, together with the difficulties described above, may frustrate the workers and decreased the credibility of the programme.

Objectives and Policy at the WHO Tuberculosis Programme

The objectives of the programme are to reduce:

- i) tuberculosis mortality;
- ii) the prevalence of the disease is currently estimated at more than 20 million world-wide; and
- iii) the incidence of tuberculosis.

The basis of WHO's control policy (case-finding and treatment with priority being given to sputum smear-positive infectious cases, and BCG vaccination at birth) was formulated more than a quarter of a century ago, with the aim of achieving the above three objects. It was based on a relatively comprehensive understanding of the natural history and epidemiology of the disease, and on the availability of relatively effective and simple intervention techniques. Since then, no major policy changes have occurred, except it was realised that the epidemiological impact of mass BCG vaccination had been grossly overestimated [9]. Although BCG prevents childhood tuberculosis, particularly the most severe forms (more than 50,000 deaths in children aged 0–4 years can be prevented by increasing BCG coverage from the current 81–90%), its preventative effect on the infectious types of adult tuberculosis is limited. BCG vaccination does not therefore contribute significantly to the reduction of the transmission of infection. Otherwise, from a scientific perspective, this policy is basically sound for achieving the programme objective in countries where the risk of infection remains substantial.

This control policy was, in fact implemented in the industrialized countries and in some middle-income developing countries, leading to a rapid decrease in the incidence of tuberculosis. For example, after the implementation of modern tuberculosis control, the annual decline rate in Western European countries reached 10–15%, compared with 4–5% as a result of the general improvement in socio-economic conditions (housing, nutrition etc.) and the isolation of tuberculosis patients in sanatoria in the pre-control era [10]. While the incidence in the industrialized countries has reached a very low level, its decline rate has recently slowed down since the majority of cases now originate from the still large pool of persons infected in the past. Thus, it should be realized that these countries have reached a stage in which the once very effective tuberculosis control strategies no longer have the same impact. A new strategy is therefore needed in order to achieve the elimination of tuberculosis in the future. (The working definition of elimination of tuberculosis is the achievement of an incidence that less than one case per million of the population [13]).

On the other hand, the implementation of this policy in the majority of developing nations has not been successful. The main problem in the majority of developing nations is that not 'enough' tuberculosis patients are cured to achieve the objectives of the programme. This is probably due to a combination of the following factors:

1. Technical policies are largely concentrated on 'what should and could be done' in relatively well-developed health services systems or under special research settings, and often lack the component of 'how to do it' under different settings.

2. Some of the intervention technologies, which are effective, simple and affordable in well-developed health service systems, are not necessarily effective, simple and affordable in poorly developed health service systems.

3. Some of the technical policies appear to have been taken as dogma (e.g. tuberculosis patients should not be hospitalized) so that there

has been a tendency to discourage result-orientated [*sic*] and local innovative approaches.

Outline of the New WHO Tuberculosis Control Strategy

Given the current tuberculosis situation in the world, there is an urgent need to develop control and elimination strategies which include *specific target settings* and the identification of *key activities* and *monitoring indicators* for the following groups of countries:

i) low-income developing countries in which health infrastructures are still poorly developed;

ii) middle-income countries with relatively well-developed health infrastructures;

iii) industrialized countries with a low incidence of tuberculosis and

iv) countries with an AIDS epidemic.

Some important components of the new WHO tuberculosis control strategy, the development of which was based on a series of workshops, case studies etc. over the last 2 years, are as follows:

Improvement of the Cure Rate

The prime objective of the control programme is to improve the cure rate of tuberculosis patients under treatment, particularly sputum smear-positive patients. The proposed target rate is 85% in developing countries and 95% in industrialized countries. Experience of tuberculosis control programmes in more than a dozen countries has clearly demonstrated that both the introduction of short-course chemotherapy in place of 'standard' chemotherapy and improved systems for the management of treatment are necessary for the achievement of this 85% cure rate in developing countries which lack exceptionally well-developed or manpower-intensive health services [13]. In addition, operations research has shown that short-course chemotherapy, which at present costs US $30–40 per patient, is more cost-effective than 'standard' chemotherapy, which costs US $15. This is mainly because short-course therapy makes it much easier to achieve a high cure rate by securing patient compliance, reducing the number of patients under treatment at a given time and preventing the emergence of drug-resistant bacilli, especially when combined tablets (isoniazid/rifampicin) are used [14].

However, as experienced on many occasions, the introduction of short-course therapy does not automatically lead to an 85% cure rate without simultaneous improvement in the management of the treatment system.

Key factors for an improved management system include a regular supply of anti-tuberculosis drugs and a rigorous cohort analysis of the outcome of treatment of all sputum smear-positive patients at all treatment centres. The latter will show the health workers how well or badly they are implementing the treatment activities.

Expansion of Tuberculosis Services

The second objective, which should not be actively pursued until the first objective has been achieved, is to expand the tuberculosis services by fully utilizing the available health services network, at least down to district hospitals, in order to detect more cases, particularly sputum smear-positive cases. It should be realized that the establishment of a microscopy service below district hospital level is not necessarily effective. This is mainly because the prevalence of tuberculosis is usually much lower than that of common infectious diseases, such as diarrhoea and pneumonia, so that less than five smear-positive cases can be expected in a year at a typical health centre in a developing country covering 10,000 inhabitants. In this situation, it is not easy to maintain a high-quality examination by microscopy.

The most effective factor that increases the services coverage rate is a high cure rate of diagnosed cases, which can attract tuberculosis patients from even very remote areas. By achieving a high cure rate at all district hospitals, where tuberculosis is diagnosed by direct microscopical examination, often with the use of chest x-ray for screening, the 65% case-finding coverage rate has been achieved in Tanzania. It would be quite possible to achieve much higher services coverage rates in countries with more developed health service infrastructures. Tentatively proposed target tuberculosis services coverage rates are 60–65% in low income countries with poorly developed transport and communication systems, and 85% in middle-income countries with relatively well developed infrastructures.

The Proposed Global Target

The proposed global target of WHO's new tuberculosis control strategy is to achieve, by the year 2000, an 85% cure rate of all sputum-positive patients under treatment and 70% case detection. Different targets are set according to the health-related resource availability of the various countries. The expected impact of the control strategies is shown in Table 4. Achievement of these targets will have three significant effects. First, it is expected that the annual tuberculosis death rate will be reduced by 40%, from the present level of 2.9 million to 1.7 million. Secondly, the world-wide prevalence of tuberculosis will be reduced by 50% from the current level of more than 20 million by curing vast numbers of chronic/retreatment

Table 4 New Tuberculosis Control Strategy Targets and Expected Impact

Countries	Target cure rates (%)	Case-finding coverage rates (%)	Expected duration to achieve 50% reduction of tuberculosis incidence	Expected number of annual tuberculosis deaths prevented world-wide
Low-income developing countries with poorly developed health services	85	60–65	10–12 years	
Middle-income developing countries with relatively well-developed health service systems	85	85	8 years	1,200,000
Industrialized countries in low tuberculosis incidence countries	95	NA	Not known	

NA: Due to the lack of a method to estimate the incidence of tuberculosis when the annual rate of infection becomes low, it is impossible to monitor the case-finding coverage rate.

cases by short-course chemotherapy. The majority of this reduction will occur in countries belonging to WHO's Western Pacific and South-East Asian Regions. In some countries in these regions the prevalence of tuberculosis is 3–5 times higher than the incidence. Thirdly, in high and middle incidence countries, the incidence of tuberculosis is expected to be halved in 12 years with an 85% cure rate in the 60–65% case-finding coverage rate, and in 8 years with an 85% cure rate and an 85% case-finding coverage rate.

SOURCE

Kochi A. 1991. The global tuberculosis situation and the new control strategy of the World Health Organization. *Tubercle* 72:1–6. Copyright 1991 *Tubercle*. Reprinted with permission of Elsevier.

CHAPTER 9

HIV/AIDS

HIV does not make people dangerous to know, so you can shake their hands and give them a hug. Heaven knows they need it.
—Princess Diana of Wales (1961–1997)

Don't die of ignorance.
—AIDS publicity campaign, 1987

GAËTAN DUGAS, THE FRENCH-CANADIAN FLIGHT ATTENDANT identified as "Patient Zero" in the Acquired Immunodeficiency Syndrome (AIDS) epidemic, suffered the same infamy as did Mary Mallon ("Typhoid Mary"). As an inapparent carrier of the human immunodeficiency virus (HIV), Dugas passed on the infectious agent to others without knowing that he was infected. Such is the tragedy of infectious diseases with long latency periods. Their spread is silent but deadly.

Finding Patient Zero was important for defining the new disease entity as being sexually transmitted. At the same time it set in motion partisan politics in the United States—politics that were ugly, mean, and blind to blatant discriminatory practices. AIDS was marginalized by the political right as a "gay disease," and President Ronald Reagan and his administration found it expedient to ignore AIDS, pandering to their political base. Indeed, the founder of the Moral Majority, Jerry Falwell, called AIDS ". . . the wrath of God upon homosexuals." With each passing month the number of AIDS cases grew, yet the president was silent. As intravenous drug users and Haitians were also identified as "at risk" for AIDS, the administration found no reason to change its policy of ignoring the disease. At the beginning of 1984, the United States reported more than 4,000 cases of AIDS; by year's end there were more than 11,000. The CDC estimated that perhaps 500,000 people were infected without knowing it. This astonishing figure brought out more than 100,000 people to march at the Democratic National Convention in San Francisco in an effort to bring attention to the growing epidemic. Still, the Reagan administration did not respond.

The world was shocked when Rock Hudson, a prominent American actor, announced in July 1985 that he was a practicing homosexual and that he had AIDS. Hudson's appearance, an emaciated shadow of his former self, put a public face on the AIDS epidemic that could be recognized by all. Hudson was beloved as a leading man in many Hollywood films, and his death three months later created new AIDS activism on the part of well-known personalities such as Elizabeth Taylor. A slow change in the public's attitude toward AIDS victims began to emerge. Despite this palpable shift in attitude on the street and the specter that the epidemic was spreading rapidly into other segments of the population, Reagan still refused to speak to the issue. Whether this was homophobic on his part or purely politics, there is no doubt that the epidemic spread like wildfire because the leadership of the United States government chose not to act.

Outbreak and Chaos

The early stages of the AIDS epidemic were fraught with controversy, ranging from competing hypotheses about the cause of the disease to some groups heaping scorn upon the victims and generating public fear. The first cases of Kaposi's sarcoma (KS), a rare form of slow-growing cancer usually seen in the elderly, began appearing in young gay men in New York City in 1981. About the same time, a cluster of *Pneumocystis carinii* pneumonia (PCP) appeared in Los Angeles and New York, again among gay men. What linked these two outbreaks was that they were opportunistic diseases, striking those with compromised immune function and striking a segment of society not exactly considered mainstream: gay men. Contact tracing of cases of PCP in Southern California and New York suggested that the underlying cause of the disease might be a sexually transmitted infectious agent not yet identified.

Reports in the medical literature expanded the groups at risk beyond gay men to include injection drug users, Haitians, and hemophiliacs. When the first case of AIDS appeared in the United Kingdom, concerns grew that there might be a smoldering pandemic afoot. Yet the disease still did not have a name. The CDC referred to the outbreaks in Los Angeles and New York as "Kaposi's sarcoma and opportunistic infections" (KSOI). *The Lancet* called the new disease "gay compromise syndrome." Other groups, depending on their political agendas, called it "gay cancer," "gay-related immune deficiency" (GRID), "community-acquired immune dysfunction," or "acquired immunodeficiency disease" (AID). The term "Acquired Immune Deficiency Syndrome" (AIDS) was finally defined by the CDC on September 24, 1982. The equivalent acronym in both French and Spanish was SIDA.

Naming the new disease neither identified its causative agent nor translated to the public what the known risks were. Due to a frenzy of inaccurate information, patients with AIDS were stigmatized, often losing their jobs, health insurance, housing, and family and friends. Public health authorities in San Francisco closed bathhouses and sex clubs, and they put out the message to cease body fluid sharing, to limit the number of sex partners, and to always use a condom. The public was offended by the frank talk about sex, and rumors abounded about transmission via toilet seats and mosquitoes. In response to the lack of governmental response, AIDS activists charged the CDC and the Reagan administration with racism and homophobia. By the beginning of 1986, almost 30,000 cases of AIDS were reported in the United States. Although there were fewer than 400 cases among children under the age of 13, these were enough to cause many parents to demand that their local school boards refuse to let children with AIDS attend public school. Police departments were issued masks and gloves to deal with people who might have AIDS. School nurses were issued the same equipment to deal with the bodily fluids of children who might have the disease. In some instances, physicians and dentists refused to treat patients, until their professional societies reminded them of their oaths. Surgeons began to "double glove" (wearing two sets of surgical gloves to prevent them from being exposed to bodily fluids of patients who might have AIDS) and the concept of "universal precautions" (treating all body fluids from any patient as if they were infectious) was widely instituted.

By the end of 1986, the U.S. surgeon general felt compelled to respond—to clarify the situation for the American public. C. Everett Koop released *The Surgeon General's Report on Acquired Immune Deficiency Syndrome* in October 1986. In it, Koop described the symptoms of the disease and its modes of transmission (sexual intercourse, sharing of contaminated needles, from mother to child during pregnancy or birth, and through contaminated blood or blood product transfusions). He clearly explained that AIDS could not be spread through casual contact and reassured parents that children infected with AIDS posed no problem to other children in a school environment. In a somewhat bold political move that contrasted with the Reagan administration's policies, Koop outlined what he believed to be a realistic approach to AIDS prevention: early sex education in schools, increased use of condoms, and voluntary testing. He argued that mandatory testing would drive those who feared they might be infected underground and that this would be contrary to protecting the public's health. Conservatives were outraged and charged that Koop's plan would encourage promiscuity. They continued to push for mandatory testing. At the other end of the spectrum, AIDS activists hailed the surgeon general's report as "frank" and hoped it would open discussion of U.S. AIDS policy. Although the policy debate continued to rage with little compromise, Koop was successful in explaining to the American public that AIDS was a preventable disease and that it did not require the physical and social isolation of its victims.

THE SEARCH FOR CAUSE

The story of the discovery of HIV as the cause of AIDS is true high drama, with an overlay of international intrigue. It begins with Robert C. Gallo and his scientific team at the NIH who were investigating a link between viruses and leukemia. The group developed new methods for isolating human retroviruses throughout the 1970s. Success came when they finally isolated human T-cell lymphotropic virus type I (HTLV-I) in 1980 and linked it to adult T-cell leukemia in 1981. In 1982, Gallo's group also isolated HTLV-II, though they could not link it specifically to a malignancy.

At the Institute Pasteur, Françoise Barré-Sinoussi and colleagues reported in 1983 that they had isolated a new human retrovirus, lymphadenopathy virus (LAV), from a patient with persistent swelling of the lymph nodes, a condition present in the early stages of AIDS. The protocol used for isolating and identifying LAV was the same as that described by Gallo's team two years earlier. Some in the scientific community questioned whether LAV was the same virus as either HTLV-I or HTLV-II. Speaking for the French team in April 1984, Luc Montagnier contended that LAV was morphologically distinct from HTLV-I and II, and that it could be one, if not the only, etiological agent for AIDS.

At virtually the same time, in May 1984, Gallo's group reported isolating HTLV-III. The new retrovirus was harvested from pre-AIDS cases with a clinical presentation of lymphadenopathy, from both children and adults with AIDS, and from a homosexual blood donor who later developed AIDS. The turning point came when Gallo's group could determine the presence of HTLV-III through a screening test, the enzyme-linked immunosorbent assay (ELISA), and a confirmatory test, the Western electrophoretic blotting technique (Western blot). This meant that the blood supply could now be screened for the presence of a potential etiologic agent for AIDS for the first time. NIH promptly filed for a patent on the testing process, and it was approved quickly.

The Institute Pasteur also filed for a patent for the test, but it was delayed, setting off a patent feud between the United States and France. The feud seemed to end amicably in March 1987 when French Prime Minister Jacques Chirac arrived at the White House and signed an agreement with President Ronald Reagan to share the AIDS test patent. Their agreement, however, did not end the controversy. Only a few days later, genetic testing by a laboratory in Los Alamos showed that the viruses from both the NIH and the Pasteur laboratories were identical; thus, they had to have come from the same patient. There were outcries of fraud and scientific misconduct, setting off more than five years of investigations by multiple institutions, public and private, on both sides of the

Atlantic. Eventually, most investigators were satisfied that there was no malevolent wrongdoing. Although the NIH received samples of LAV from the Pasteur Institute in both 1983 and 1984, the samples were not the same. Montagnier agreed that the possibility existed that the 1984 sample had been contaminated. Gallo agreed that by using pooled samples, they might have inadvertently contaminated their samples with LAV. Despite the controversy, what is clear is that the isolation of human retroviruses was a hop, the connection of the retroviruses to AIDS was a skip, and the creation of a screening test was a jump in our ability to understand the HIV epidemic.

EPIDEMIOLOGIC SPREAD

Multiple research laboratories worldwide are now investigating the spread of the HIV epidemic using genetic sequencing. In general, their results show that the epidemic most likely began as a zoonosis, with perhaps two different simian viruses jumping the species barrier to infect humans in Africa, perhaps as early as the 1930s. The genome of the virus shows it has two types: HIV-1 and HIV-2. These types can be divided into groups, and many of the groups can be further divided into subgroups. Following the genetic footprint backward in time, HIV-1 seems to have moved from Africa, either through immigration or tourism, into North America (perhaps through Haiti), then into Europe, Australia, and Asia. The HIV-1 subtype found primarily among homosexuals differs from that found primarily among injection drug users (IDUs), and the footprint of the virus found among heterosexuals is similar to that found in IDUs. In other words, HIV is not a single epidemic but a least two separate ones, and maybe more.

Because there were at least two epidemics arising at about the same time among different risk groups, confusion about HIV/AIDS led to inaction, as did flat out denial of risk. In many African nations, the ABCs were implemented: 1) abstinence, 2) being loyal to your partner, and 3) condoms. Under the George W. Bush administration, this was reduced to abstinence only, which may have contributed to the further spread of the disease. Response to HIV was varied among African nations. The relative success of Uganda in stemming the epidemic due to an aggressive comprehensive campaign beginning in the early 1990s contrasts with the flat-out failure to acknowledge the disease in places such as post-apartheid South Africa. At the beginning of the twenty-first century, the prevalence of HIV in Uganda was about 6 percent of the adult population. In contrast, the prevalence in South Africa was about 20 percent, with neighboring Botswana, Lesotho, and Swaziland facing at least one-quarter of their populations infected with HIV.

TREATMENT

As soon as HIV was confirmed as the cause of AIDS, scientists at Burroughs-Wellcome Company began looking into whether azidothymidine (AZT), a drug that had previously been shown to be effective against a mouse retrovirus, could be used to treat HIV infection in humans. The company filed for a patent on AZT in 1985 after a collaborative phase I trial with the NCI showed that the drug increased CD4 cell counts in patients with AIDS. AZT was approved as a treatment (later as a preventive) for HIV by the FDA in 1987 after a placebo-controlled, randomized clinical trial showed that AZT could prolong the life of patients with AIDS. The trial required that high doses of the drug be administered every four hours around the clock. The cost of treatment was expensive, and patients endured significant toxic side effects. AIDS activists complained that the trial was unethical, that the drug company was price gouging, and that the government was complicit with big pharma in promoting an expensive, toxic, and mediocre treatment.

Over time, research showed that treatment with protease inhibitors interrupted the replication of HIV, and this, in turn, allowed CD4 cell counts to rise. This information meant that physicians could now monitor viral loads and adjust the amount of drug needed to suppress HIV so that it was less toxic for the patient. Highly active antiretroviral therapy (HAART), or triple-drug therapy, evolved in the 1990s and changed the face of the epidemic. A drug cocktail containing a protease inhibitor, a nucleoside analogue reverse-transcriptase inhibitor, and a non-nucleoside reverse-transcriptase inhibitor effectively kept those infected with HIV from progressing to AIDS and thus turned the disease into a chronic illness rather than an acute, deadly one.

The rising global epidemic of HIV/AIDS brought calls for more action, especially in sub-Saharan Africa. HAART was not the answer because it is an expensive treatment rather than a preventive measure. In the United States, a drug regimen using AZT was shown to be effective in preventing the perinatal transmission of HIV by 50 percent, but it was expensive. Finding a vaccine or a less expensive drug regimen that would prevent the transmission of HIV from mother to infant became an intense focus of research. Clinical trials were launched in developing nations around the world by both the NIH and the UN AIDS Program. There was rapid outcry about these studies being unethical, and many were shut down. The source of the problem was that in the United States all subjects in the prevention trials had access to antiretroviral treatments whereas those participating in similar trials in developing nations did not. Bioethicists charged exploitation of subjects in the developing world and called for ethical standards that could not be waived. As of this writing, such international standards have yet to be promulgated. Time and improved laboratory technology now give us a perspective on the HIV/AIDS pandemic that did not exist when the disease first burst upon the stage in the United States in the early 1980s. Genetic analysis of the virus now offers us explanations of where this emerging infectious disease came from and how it spread. We have a better understanding of how to prevent the disease and how to treat those who become infected. But these changes were a long time coming—about a quarter of a century—and have yet to extend to all countries involved in this global pandemic. Not all nations have the political will to address the problem. Sub-Saharan African nations, in particular, faces enormous challenges in providing health care and social support to large proportions of the population dealing with HIV. Millions of deaths, especially in the early phases of the epidemic, left enormous numbers of orphans and challenge the very future of some nations. World efforts to bring the disease under control are not yet secure.

SELECTED READINGS

The first reading for this chapter is a short report by M.S. Gottlieb and colleagues that appeared in the *MMWR* in 1981 about a cluster of five cases of *Pneumocystis carinii* pneumonia among young homosexual men living in California. These sentinel cases warned the world of an emerging new disease. Of particular interest is the recommendation in the editorial note that physicians should consider a new differential diagnosis, that of *Pneumocystis* pneumonia, among previously healthy homosexual men who present with difficulty breathing and pneumonia.

David M. Auerbach and others completed an epidemiologic investigation of the 19 known AIDS cases in Southern California as of 1982. Their methods of sexual contact tracing and their results appear in this second reading, except for one figure that was too large for reproduction here. Despite the fact that the etiologic agent of AIDS was still unknown at the time of their investigation, the research confirmed that the disease was infectious in origin, that it was linked to specific sexual practices, and that the mean latency period could be determined. Efforts such as these are key to the investigation of any new disease entity, and the fact that the agent is not known does not preclude developing important new information about transmission and possible etiology.

The final reading for this chapter is by Kent A. Sepkowitz. This retrospective on the first 20 years of the epidemic provides a timeline of important dates as well as a description of the politics and activism surrounding the epidemic. The work is complete except for Figure 1, which is adequately described in the text.

The piece shows that although some progress had been made in stemming the epidemic, at least in the developed world, it is far from conquered.

BIBLIOGRAPHY

Angell M. 1997. The ethics of clinical research in the third world. *N Engl J Med* 337 (12): 847–49.

Auerbach DM, Darrow WW, Jaffe HW, and Curran JW. 1984. Cluster of cases of the acquired immune deficiency syndrome: Patients linked by sexual contact. *Am J Med* 76:487–92.

Beck EJ, Mays N, Whiteside AW, and Zuniga JM. 2006. *The HIV Pandemic: Local and Global Implications.* Oxford: Oxford University Press.

Beral V, Peterman TA, Berkelman RL, and Jaffe HW. 1990. Kaposi's sarcoma among persons with AIDS: A sexually transmitted infection? *Lancet* 335:123–28.

Buchanan D, Sifunda S, Naidoo N, James S, and Reddy P. 2008. Assuring adequate protections international health research: A principled justification and practical recommendations for the role of community oversight. *Public Health Ethics* 1 (3): 146–57.

Connor EM, Sperling RS, Gelber R, Kiselev P, Scott G, O'Sullivan MJ, VanDyke R, Bey M, Shearer W, Jacobson RL, Jimenez E, O'Neill E, Bazin B, Delfraissy J-F, Culnane M, Coombs R, Elkins M, Moye J, Stratton P, and Balsley J, for The Pediatric AIDS Clinical Trials Group Protocol 076 Study Group. 1994. Reduction of maternal-infant transmission of human immunodeficiency virus type I with zidovudine treatment. *N Engl J Med* 331 (18): 1173–80.

Culliton BJ. 1990. Inside the Gallo probe (in Research News; News Report). *Science,* New Series 248 (4962): 1494–98.

Fischl MA, Richman DD, Grieco MH, Gottlieb MS, Volberding PA, Laskin OL, Leedom JM, Groopman JE, Mildvan D, Schooley RT, et al. 1987. The efficacy of azidothymidine (AZT) in the treatment of patients with AIDS and AIDS-related complex: A double-blind placebo-controlled trial. *N Engl J Med* 317:185–91.

Gilbert MTP, Rambaut A, Wlasiuk G, Spira TJ, Pitchenik AE, and Worobey M. 2007. The emergence of HIV/AIDS in the Americas and beyond. *PNAS* 104 (47): 18566–70.

Gottlieb MS, Schroff R, Schanker HM, Weisman JD, Fan PT, Wolf RA, and Saxon A. 1981. *Pneumocystis carinii* pneumonia and mucosal candidiasis in previously healthy homosexual men: Evidence of a new acquired cellular immunodeficiency. *New Engl J Med* 305:1425–31.

Herrell RK. 1991. HIV/AIDS Research and the Social Sciences (in Reports). *Current Anthropology* 32 (2): 199–203.

Jaffe HW. 2008. Universal access to HIV/AIDS treatment: Promise and problems. *JAMA* 300 (5): 573–75.

Jaffe HW. 2008. The early days of the HIV-AIDS epidemic in the USA. *Nat Immunol* 9 (11): 1201–3.

Kuiken C, Thakallapalli R, Eskild A, and de Ronde A. 2000. Genetic analysis reveals epidemiologic patterns in the spread of human immunodeficiency virus. *Am J Epidemiol* 152 (9): 814–22.

Lurie P and Wolfe SM. 1997. Unethical trials of interventions to reduce perinatal transmission of the human immunodeficiency virus in developing countries. *N Engl J Med* 337 (12): 853–56.

MacLure M. 1998. Inventing the AIDS virus hypothesis: An illustration of scientific vs. unscientific induction (in Epidemiology and Society). *Epidemiology* 9 (4): 467–73.

Merson MH. 2006. The HIV-AIDS epidemic at 25—the global response. *N Engl J Med* 354 (23): 2414–17.

Parker R. 2002. The global HIV/AIDS pandemic, structural inequalities, and the politics of international health. *Am J Public Health* 92 (3): 343–46.

Peterson L, Taylor D, Roddy R, Belai G, Phillips P, Nanda K, Grant R, Clarke EEK, Jaffe HS, and Cates W. 2007. Tonofovir disoproxil fumarate for prevention of HIV infection in women: A phase 2, double-blind, randomized, placebo-controlled trial. *PLoS Clin Trials* 2 (5): e27. doi:10. 1371/journal.pctr.0020027.

Rawling A. 1994. The AIDS virus dispute: Awarding priority for the discovery of the human immunodeficiency virus (HIV). *Science, Technology, & Human Values* 19 (3): 342–60.

Shilts, R. 1987. *And the Band Played On: People, Politics and the AIDS Epidemic*. New York: St. Martin's Press.

Simon V, Ho DD, and Abdool Karim Q. 2006. HIV/AIDS epidemiology, pathogenesis, prevention, and treatment. *Lancet* 368:489–504.

Stall R and Mills TC. 2006. A quarter century of AIDS. *Am J Public Health* 98 (6): 959–61.

U.S. Government Accountability Office (GAO). 2006. Global Health: Spending Requirement Presents Challenges for Allocating Prevention Funding Under the President's Emergency Plan for AIDS Relief. Testimony Before the Subcommittee on National Security, Emerging Threats, and International Relations, Committee on Government Reform, House of Representatives (GAO-06-1089T). Washington, DC: GPO. http://www.gao.gov/new.items/d06395.pdf (accessed June 10, 2007).

Vahlne A. 2009. A historical reflection on the discovery of human retroviruses. *Retrovirology* 6:40. doi:10.1186/1742-4690-6-40.

Vlahov D, Des Jarlais DC, Goosby E, Hollinger PC, Lurie PG, Shriver MD, and Strathdee SA. 2001. Needle exchange programs for the prevention of human immunodeficiency virus infection: epidemiology and policy. *Am J Epidemiol* 154 (Suppl. 12): S70–77.

Pneumocystis *Pneumonia—Los Angeles*
(1981)

In the period October 1980–May 1981, 5 young men, all active homosexuals, were treated for biopsy-confirmed *Pneumocystis carinii* pneumonia at 3 different hospitals in Los Angeles, California. Two of the patients died. All 5 patients had laboratory-confirmed previous or current cytomegalovirus (CMV) infection and candidal mucosal infection. Case reports of these patients to follow.

PATIENT 1: A previously healthy 33-year-old man developed *P. carinii* pneumonia and oral mucosal candidiasis in March 1981 after a 2-month history of fever associated with elevated liver enzymes, leukopenia, and CMV viruria. The serum complement-fixation CMV titer in October 1980 was 256; in May 1981 it was 32.* The patient's condition deteriorated despite courses of treatment with trimethoprim-sulfamethoxazole (TMP/ SMX), pentamidine, and acyclovir. He died May 3, and postmortem examination showed residual *P. carinii* and CMV pneumonia, but no evidence of neoplasia.

PATIENT 2: A previously healthy 30-year-old man developed *P. carinii* pneumonia in April 1981 after a 5-month history of fever each day and elevated liver-function tests, CMV viruria, and documented seroconversion to CMV, i.e., an acute-phase titer of 16 and a convalescent-phase titer of 28* in anticomplement immunofluorescence tests. Other features of his illness included leukopenia and mucosal candidiasis. His pneumonia responded to a course of intravenous TMP/SMX, but, as of the latest reports, he continues to have a fever each day.

PATIENT 3: A 30-year-old man was well until January 1981 when he developed esophageal and oral candidiasis that responded to Amphotericin B treatment. He was hospitalized in February 1981 for *P. carinii* pneumonia that responded to oral TMP/SMX. His esophageal candidiasis recurred after the pneumonia was diagnosed, and he was again given Amphotericin B. The CMV complement-fixation titer in March 1981 was 8. Material from an esophageal biopsy was positive for CMV.

PATIENT 4: A 29-year-old man developed *P. carinii* pneumonia in February 1981. He had had Hodgkins disease 3 years earlier, but had been successfully treated with radiation therapy alone. He did not improve after being given intravenous TMP/SMX and corticosteroids and died in March.

---

*Paired specimens not run in parallel.

Postmortem examination showed no evidence of Hodgkins disease, but *P. carinii* and CMV were found in lung tissue.

PATIENT 5: A previously healthy 36-year-old man with a clinically diagnosed CMV infection in September 1980 was seen in April 1981 because of a 4-month history of fever, dyspnea, and cough. On admission he was found to have *P. carinii* pneumonia, oral candidiasis, and CMV retinitis. A complement-fixation CMV titer in April 1981 was 128. The patient has been treated with 2 short courses of TMP/SMX that have been limited because of a sulfa-induced neutropenia. He is being treated for candidiasis with topical nystatin.

The diagnosis of *Pneumocystis* pneumonia was confirmed for all 5 patients ante-mortem by closed or open lung biopsy. The patients did not know each other and had no known common contacts or knowledge of sexual partners who had had similar illnesses. The 5 did not have comparable histories of sexually transmitted disease. Four had serologic evidence of past hepatitis B infection but had no evidence of current hepatitis B surface antigen. Two of the 5 reported having frequent homosexual contacts with various partners. All 5 reported using inhalant drugs, and 1 reported parenteral drug abuse. Three patients had profoundly depressed numbers of thymus-dependent lymphocyte cells and profoundly depressed *in vitro* proliferative responses to mitogens and antigens. Lymphocyte studies were not performed on the other 2 patients.

Reported by MS Gottlieb, MD, HM Schanker, MD, PT Fan, MD, A Saxon, MD, JD Weisman, DO, Div of Clinical Immunology-Allergy, Dept of Medicine, UCLA School of Medicine; I Pozalski, MD, Cedars-Mt. Sinai Hospital, Los Angeles; Field Services Div, Epidemiology Program Office, CDC.

EDITORIAL NOTE: *Pneumocystis* pneumonia in the United States is almost exclusively limited to severely immunosuppressed patients (1). The occurrence of pneumocystosis in these 5 previously healthy individuals without a clinically apparent underlying immunodeficiency is unusual. The fact that these patients were all homosexuals suggests an association between some aspect of a homosexual lifestyle or disease acquired through sexual contact and *Pneumocystis* pneumonia in this population. All 5 patients described in this report have laboratory-confirmed CMV disease or virus shedding within 5 months of the diagnosis of *Pneumocystis* pneumonia. CMV infection has been shown to induce transient abnormalities of *in vitro* cellular-immune function in otherwise healthy human hosts (2,3). Although all 3 patients tested had abnormal cellular-immune function, no definitive conclusion regarding the role of CMV infection in these 5 cases can be reached because of the lack of published data on cellular-immune function in healthy homosexual males with and without CMV antibody. In 1 report, 7 (3.6%) of 194 patients with pneumocystosis also had CMV infection; 40 (21%) of the same group had at least 1 other major concurrent infection (1). A high prevalence of CMV infections among homosexual males was recently reported: 179 (94%) of 190 males reported to be exclusively homosexual had serum antibody to CMV, and 14 (7.4%) had CMV viruria; rates for 101 controls of similar age who were reported to be exclusively heterosexual were 54% for seropositivity and zero for viruria (4). In another study of 64 males, 4 (6.3%) had positive tests are CMV in semen, but none had CMV recovered from urine. Two of the 4 reported recent homosexual contacts. These findings suggest not only that virus shedding may be more readily detected in seminal fluid than in urine, but also that seminal fluid may be an important vehicle of CMV transmission (5).

All the above observations suggest the possibility of a cellular-immune dysfunction related to a common exposure that predisposes individuals to opportunistic infections such as pneumocystosis and candidiasis. Although the role of CMV infection in the pathogenesis of pneumocystosis remains unknown, the possibility of *P. carinii* infection must be carefully considered in a differential diagnosis for previously healthy homosexual males with dyspnea and pneumonia.

SOURCE

Gottlieb MS, Schanker HM, Fan PT, Saxon A, Weisman JD, and Pozalski I. 1981. *Pneumocystis* Pneumonia—Los Angeles. *MMWR* 30 (21): 250–52.

Cluster of Cases of the Acquired Immune Deficiency Syndrome: Patients Linked by Sexual Contact
(1984, Abridged)

David M. Auerbach, M.D., William W. Darrow, Ph.D.,
Harold W. Jaffe, M.D., James W. Curran, M.D., M.P.H.

From the Field Services Division, Epidemiology Program Office, and the AIDS Activity, Center for Infectious Diseases, Centers for Disease Control, Atlanta, Georgia. This work was presented in part at the symposium "Controversies in the Management of Infectious Complications of Neoplastic Disease," Memorial Sloan-Kettering Cancer Center, New York, New York, March 17 and 18, 1983.

The possibility that homosexual men with the Acquired Immune Deficiency Syndrome (AIDS) had been sexual partners of each other was studied. Of the first 19 homosexual male AIDS patients reported from southern California, names of sexual partners were obtained for 13. Nine of the 13 patients had sexual contact with one or more AIDS patients within five years of the onset of symptoms. Four of the patients from southern California had contact with a non-California AIDS patient, who was also the sexual partner of four AIDS patients from New York City. Ultimately, 40 patients in 10 cities were linked by sexual contact. On the basis of six pairs of patients, a mean latency period of 10.5 months (range seven to 14 months) is estimated between sexual contact and symptom onset. The finding of a cluster of AIDS patients linked by sexual contact is consistent with the hypothesis that AIDS is caused by an infectious agent.

Acquired Immune Deficiency Syndrome (AIDS) was first suggested in June 1981 by a report from Los Angeles of *Pneumocystis carinii* pneumonia in five previously healthy homosexual men [1]. Subsequently, Kaposi's sarcoma [2] and a variety of opportunistic infections other than *P. carinii* pneumonia, such as chronic, progressive herpes simplex virus infection, central nervous system toxoplasmosis, cryptococcal meningitis, and disseminated cytomegalovirus infection [3–5], were also found to be manifestations of AIDS. The abnormality in cellular immune function has been indicated by cutaneous anergy, lymphopenia, and T cell deficiency [3].

AIDS appeared suddenly and almost simultaneously in several metropolitan areas of the United States. Homosexual men living in New York City, San Francisco, and Los Angeles accounted for the greatest number of reported cases [6]. A case-controlled study conducted by the Centers for Disease Control in October and November 1981 concluded that a large number of sexual partners was the most important risk factor among these homosexual men [7]. AIDS has also been found in intravenous drug users [8], Haitians living in the United States [9], and patients with hemophilia [10]. Recently, AIDS or illnesses suggestive of AIDS have been reported in a recipient of a platelet transfusion from an AIDS patient [11], in children born to mothers who are Haitian [12] or have used drugs intravenously [13], and in women who had sexual relations with men belonging to AIDS risk groups [14]. Epidemiologic information suggests that an infectious agent may cause AIDS.

If AIDS is caused by an infectious agent, evidence of person-to-person spread might be expected. None of the five homosexual men first reported from Los Angeles with *P. carinii* pneumonia gave histories of sexual contact with other patients [1]. In a subsequent series of 41 cases of Kaposi's sarcoma reported from New York City, four homosexually active men were reported to have had "transient, intimate sexual contact with other men in this Kaposi's sarcoma group" [15]. In March 1982, several persons in southern California informally reported to public health officials that some men in whom AIDS was later diagnosed had attended the same social gatherings and may have had sexual contacts with one another. Consequently, an investigation was initiated to assess the social and sexual relationships among homosexual men in whom AIDS had been diagnosed.

Patients and Methods

All 19 cases of biopsy-confirmed Kaposi's sarcoma or *P. carinii* pneumonia in previously healthy homosexual men residing in Los Angeles or contiguous Orange County and reported to the Centers for Disease Control as of April 12, 1982, were included in the initial investigation. Patients with AIDS from outside southern California were included in this study only if previously obtained information suggested their associations with another AIDS patient.

Written, informed consent was obtained from each patient or his sexual contact before interviews were conducted. Patients were interviewed in person by one or more of us and asked to name their sexual partners during the five-year period before they became ill. For those who had died, we interviewed their close companions and asked them to name the sexual partners of the deceased patient. Patients who had been interviewed during earlier studies conducted by the Centers for Disease Control were not re-interviewed for information obtained previously, but were asked to name their sexual partners.

Homosexual men with AIDS who could be linked by sexual contact were considered to belong to a cluster of AIDS patients if the sexual exposure occurred within five years of the onset of illness. Sexual contact reported by one patient (or his surviving companion) had to be confirmed (or not denied) by the other patient (or his companion).

Patients included in the cluster ("linked" patients) were compared with homosexual male AIDS patients not known to be sexual partners of other AIDS patients ("nonlinked" patients). Among the linked and nonlinked patients were groups of patients who had been interviewed in depth regarding their behavioral patterns. Two sources of data were analyzed: surveillance information on all cases reported to the Centers for Disease Control as of April 12, 1982, and interview records of all patients interviewed by Centers for Disease Control representatives as of October 12, 1982.

Tests of significance (chi-square with 1 degree of freedom) and estimates of relative risk (odd ratios for 2 X 2) derived by the method of Mantel and Haenszel [16] and by Mantel's extension [17] were used to assess differences between the linked and nonlinked patients. Ninety-five percent confidence intervals were calculated with estimates of relative risk and levels of statistical significance.

Results

Of the 19 patients with Kaposi's sarcoma or *P. carinii* pneumonia reported from southern California, eight were alive and 11 had died at the time the investigation was initiated. Interviews were conducted with the eight living patients and with the close companions of seven of the dead patients. Names of sexual contacts were obtained during 13 of the interviews. Nine of the 13 patients were found to have had sexual exposure with other AIDS patients within five years of the onset of symptoms. Four of these nine had had sexual exposures with more than one other patient. The observation that nine of 15 patients who were interviewed named at least one other reported patient as his sexual partner was not expected and seemed highly unusual (see Appendix).

AIDS developed in four men in southern California after they had sexual contact with a non-Californian, Patient 0 (Figure 1). [Figure not included to save space, Ed.] In Patient 0, lymphadenopathy developed in December 1979, and Kaposi's sarcoma was diagnosed in May 1980. He estimated that he had had approximately 250 different male sexual partners each year from 1979 through 1981 and was able to name 72 of his 750 partners for this three-year period. Eight of the 72 named partners were AIDS patients: four from southern California and four from New York City.

Because Patient 0 appeared to link AIDS patients from southern California and New York City, we extended our investigation beyond the Los Angeles-Orange County metropolitan area. Ultimately, we were able to link 40 AIDS patients by sexual contact to at least one other reported pa-

Table I Comparison of Demographic and Clinical Features for Homosexual Men with AIDS Linked and Nonlinked by Sexual Contact

Patient characteristic	Percent of patients		Odds ratio	Confidence limits	p value
	Linked (n = 40)	Nonlinked (n = 208)			
Kaposi's sarcoma only	57.5	33.7	2.7	1.4–5.2	0.004
White	87.5	72.6	2.6	1.0–6.9	0.047
Intravenous drug use	3.6	12.9	4.0	0.6–27.0	0.154
Exclusively homosexual	95.0	89.4	2.2	0.5–9.6	0.275
Resident of Manhattan	52.5	48.6	1.2	0.6–2.3	0.648
Deceased when reported	35.0	34.6	1.0	0.5–2.1	0.963
Age 35 years or older	60.0	60.1	1.0	0.5–2.0	0.991

tient. Of the 40 linked patients, 22 resided in New York City, nine resided in Los Angeles or contiguous Orange County, and another nine were living in eight other cities in North America when their illnesses were diagnosed. Twenty-four of these men had Kaposi's sarcoma, six had *P. carinii* pneumonia, eight had both Kaposi's sarcoma and *P. carinii* pneumonia, one had disseminated cytomegalovirus infection, and one had central nervous system toxoplasmosis. Thirty-six of these men were white (not Hispanic), three were Hispanic (two originally from Puerto Rico and one originally from Mexico), and one was black. Their median age was 36 years.

These 40 patients were compared with the 208 other homosexual male patients with AIDS who were reported to the Centers for Disease Control as of April 12, 1982, but not named as sexual partners of patients included in the cluster (Table I). The 40 linked patients (16.1 percent of the total reported) were significantly more likely to be white and to have only Kaposi's sarcoma than the 208 other patients. However, the two groups were not significantly different with respect to all other variables available from surveillance reports.

The 29 patients who were linked and interviewed (72.5 percent of 40 patients) and the 49 nonlinked patients who were interviewed (23.6 percent of 208 patients) were compared with respect to selected behavioral

Table II Selected Interview Variables for Homosexual Men with AIDS Linked and Nonlinked by Sexual Contact

Interview variable	Percent of patients		Odds ratio	Confidence limits	p value
	Linked (n = 29)	Nonlinked (n = 49)			
Met a sexual contact in bathhouse in year before onset	96.6	73.5	10.1	1.7–59.8	0.010
Used nitrite inhalants more than 1,000 times in lifetime	86.2	53.1	5.5	1.8–17.2	0.003
Inserted hand or fist into partner's rectum during year before onset	82.8	44.9	5.9	2.0–17.1	0.001
Received partner's hand or fist into rectum during year before onset	51.7	18.4	4.8	1.8–12 .9	0.002
Had 50 or more male sexual partners in year before onset	75.9	57.1	2.4	0.9–6.5	0.096
Had 1,000 or more sexual partners during lifetime	65.5	44.9	2.3	0.9–6.0	0.078
White	89.7	75.5	2.8	0.7–10.6	0.126
Kaposi's sarcoma only	82.8	69.4	2.1	0.7–6.6	0.191

characteristics (Table II). The 29 linked patients were significantly more likely than the 49 nonlinked patients to have met sexual partners in bathhouses, have been frequent users of inhaled amyl or butyl nitrite, and have participated in the sexual practice of "fisting" (manual-rectal intercourse). Patients in both groups tended to have large numbers of sexual partners. Use of recreational drugs other than nitrate inhalants and participation in sexual activities other than "fisting" were not significantly different for the two groups.

To estimate a possible latency period for AIDS among members of the cluster, we looked at the 20 patients who apparently had had sexual exposures with only one other reported patient. Nine of these 20 reported

Table III Possible Latency Periods for Homosexual Men with AIDS

Possible source patient	Linked patient	Date of exposure	Symptom onset	Latency (months)
LA 4	LA 5	12/80	7/81	7
FL 1	GA 2	10/80	6/81	8
Patient 0	LA 9	11/80	8/81	9
NY 18	NY 20	7/80	7/81	12
Patient 0	LA 8	2/80	3/81	13
Patient 0	NY 15	4/80	6/81	14
				$\bar{X} = 10.5$

having had sexual relations with their partners for a period lasting no longer than 30 days. Of the nine, three showed symptoms before or at about the same time as their partners, and six noted symptoms after their partners became ill (Table III). In these six patients, symptoms were first noticed a mean of 10.5 months (range of seven to 14) after having had sexual contact with one of four partners who also was a reported patient.

The four partners may have been sources of AIDS. Three of the possible sources of AIDS were asymptomatic at the time of sexual exposure. The fourth possible source was Patient 0. Lymphadenopathy had already developed in Patient 0 when he had sexual contact with two men in whom AIDS subsequently developed, and he had skin lesions of Kaposi's sarcoma at the time of sexual contact with a third.

Comments

Although the cause of AIDS is unknown, it may be caused by an infectious agent that is transmissible from person to person in a manner analogous to hepatitis B virus infection: through sexual contact; through parenteral exposure by intravenous drug abusers who share needles; through blood products, particularly in patients with hemophilia who received clotting factor concentrates; and, perhaps, through mothers who are Haitian or intravenous drug users to their infants. The existence of the cluster of AIDS cases linked by homosexual contact is consistent with an infectious-agent hypothesis.

The cluster may represent a group of homosexual men who were brought together by a common interest in sexual relations with many different partners or in specific sexual practices, such as manual-rectal intercourse. Frequent social contacts among some patients enabled them to identify other patients by name. Although these men were sexual partners of each other, nonsexual activities, such as drug use, may have contributed to the development of AIDS.

If the infectious-agent hypothesis is true, Patient 0 may be an example of a "carrier" of such an agent. He had had sexual contact with eight other AIDS patients and was the possible source of AIDS for at least three of them. Two of these three men had been his partners before he had overt signs of Kaposi's sarcoma. The existence of an asymptomatic carrier state of AIDS has been suggested by a report of AIDS-like illness in an infant who had received a platelet transfusion from a man who had no symptoms when he donated blood, but had AIDS eight months later [11]. Furthermore, abnormalities in T lymphocytes have been described among asymptomatic homosexual men in New York City [18] and among persons with hemophilia [19, 20]. Whether these immune abnormalities are a reflection of "asymptomatic AIDS" or are unrelated to AIDS is not yet known.

The estimated mean latency period of 10 to 11 months for the six AIDS patients described in this study is similar to the estimated mean latency period for the development of Kaposi's sarcoma among renal transplant recipients. Kaposi's sarcoma developed in 15 renal allograft transplant recipients an average of 15 months following renal transplantation (range three to 46 months) in one study [21], and 20 Kaposi's sarcoma patients showed signs of Kaposi's sarcoma an average of 16 months after transplantation (range four to 53 months) in another [22].

The observation of the cluster formed on the basis of reported sexual exposures reinforces case-control study findings [7] regarding the importance of sexual activities in the development of AIDS among homosexual men. Sexual partners of AIDS patients appear to be at increased risk for AIDS. This conclusion is reflected in the interim Public Health Service recommendations for the prevention of AIDS: "Sexual contact should be avoided with persons known or suspected to have AIDS. Members of high-risk groups should be aware that multiple sex partners increase the probability of developing AIDS" [23].

[Acknowledgments deleted to save space, Ed.]

Appendix

The problem is determining the likelihood that nine of 15 homosexual men with AIDS would name at least one other homosexual man with AIDS as his sexual partner can be approached in a variety of ways. A simple approach is presented here. Start with any sexual partner of any one of the patients interviewed in southern California. Observe each partner to determine if he has been reported as a patient or not. Count the number of patients who were interviewed and the number who named at least one other patient as his sexual partner. Nine of 15 patients said that they had had sexual contact with at least one other patient. For this observation to be insignificant at the 95 percent level of confidence, we note that, following the formula for binomial expansion,

$$\sum_{x=9}^{15} (x^{15}) p^x (1 - p)^{15-x} > 0.05.$$

The iteratively estimated value of p is 0.3597. A greater value of p would make the observation in southern California less significant. Since p is approximately equal to 0.3597, then it follows that the probability of no contact $(1 - p)$ would be 0.6403. Since we were concerned with the large number of sexual partners of patients, the probability of no contact can be evaluated with the Poisson distribution. In the Poisson distribution, the probability of no contact is evaluated by $e^{-\theta n} = 0.6403$, which implies that $\theta = \log e(0.6403)/n$. Among the 15 patients interviewed, we find that the average number of sexual partners over a period of five years is 610. Now, when n is equal to 610, the contact parameter, θ, is equal to 0.000731. If there are exactly 19 patients with AIDS in southern California, in the homosexual population in southern California, estimated by $19/\theta$, would be approximately 26,000. On the other hand, if we estimate the homosexual male population in southern California to be at least 250,000, then we would expect to find the number of AIDS cases in southern California, estimated at 250,000 (θ), to be 183. Finally, if there are only 19 patients had at least 250,000 homosexual men, then the average number of sexual partners for a five-year period would have to be about 6,000, almost 10 times as many as the average reported by the 15 patients who were interviewed. From this exercise, we conclude that the observation of nine of 15 patients in southern California naming at least one other patient as a sexual partner would be highly unusual.

—Dennis J. Bregman and Kung–Jong Lui

SOURCE

Auerbach DM, Darrow WW, Jaffe HW, and Curran JW. 1984. Cluster of cases of the Acquired Immune Deficiency Syndrome: Patients linked by sexual contact. *Am J Med* 76:487–491. Copyright 1984 *The American Journal of Medicine*. Reprinted with permission of Elsevier.

AIDS—The First 20 Years
(2001, Abridged)

Kent A. Sepkowitz, M.D.

The disease now known as the acquired immunodeficiency syndrome, or AIDS, was first reported 20 years ago this week in the *Morbidity and Mortality Weekly Report* under the quiet title *"Pneumocystis* pneumonia—Los Angeles."[1] The description was not the lead article; that distinction went to a report of dengue infections in vacationers returning to the United States from the Caribbean.

Not even the most pessimistic reader could have anticipated the scope and scale the epidemic would assume two decades later. By December 2000, 21.8 million people worldwide have died of the disease, including more Americans (438,795), than died in World War I and World War II combined.[2] This article reviews the many important developments in the first 20 years of AIDS.

[References from here on are not chronologic, but reflect the original Ed.]

Early Years: Free Fall

The initial report describes five young homosexual men in whom a rare disease, *Pneumocystis carinii* pneumonia, and other unusual infections have developed. Each had abnormal ratios of lymphocyte subgroups and was actively shedding cytomegalovirus. This report was followed quickly by more series, and within a few months, the basic outline of the epidemic was established (Table 1). Although the disease was first encountered in homosexual men and injection-drug users, the risk groups soon included Haitians,[5] transfusion recipients, including those with hemophilia,[6,10] infants,[11] female sexual contacts of infected men,[8,12] prisoners,[13] and Africans.[15]

Additional opportunistic complications were soon described, including mycobacterial infections, toxoplasmosis, invasive fungal infections, Kaposi's sarcoma, and non-Hodgkin's lymphoma. A working definition for AIDS, developed by the Centers for Disease Control,[21] has required just a single revision in the past decade.[22]

Causation

In the early years, there were numerous theories regarding the cause of AIDS, many of which now seem eccentric. The evidence that the disease was caused by cytomegalovirus, as posited in the early reports,[1,23] was straightforward: groups with the new immunodeficiency had extremely high rates of infection with cytomegalovirus, a potentially immunosuppressive virus. Some hypothesized that the virus had inexplicably become more virulent. Yet this theory failed to account for all cases, and attention turned elsewhere.

A case was made for attributing causality to amyl nitrite, a prescription drug, and to isobutyl nitrite, a closely related chemical marketed as a room deodorizer.[24] Both were used as sexual stimulants but were also known immunosuppressive agents. This theory had scientific plausibility and suggested a simple solution. But soon cases were reported among nonusers.

A sophisticated theory developed around the notion that repeated exposure to another's sperm could trigger an immune response, resulting in a condition resembling chronic graft-versus-host disease and, ultimately, opportunistic infections.[25] Another hypothesis invoked the general overloading of the immune system—a sort of physiological battle fatigue in which the immune system simply wore out.[26,27] Outside the scientific community, there were suggestions that the disease was a punishment for homosexual men and injection-drug users.[28]

A novel viral cause of the disease was only one of many plausible theories in the early years. It was favored by those familiar with the epidemiology of hepatitis B infection,[8,29,30] which affected the same groups, and by those who worked with animal retroviruses. Feline leukemia virus had been described in the 1970s as a cause of general immunodeficiency (the "fading-kitten syndrome") and was associated with lymphoma and leukemia as well.[31,32] For the researchers in this field, the notion that human retroviruses may cause a similar syndrome was a simple intellectual leap.

Nonetheless, doubt about a viral cause persisted until the actual virus was detected,[16] confirmatory studies were performed,[18] and the reports of transmission through blood and blood products became too numerous to ignore.[6,9] The complicated and rivalrous story that culminated in the isolation of the virus has been well described. High-stakes scientific inquiry has seldom been placed in a less attractive light.

The delay on the part of some in accepting a novel viral cause may appear puzzling now, but investigators may have been intimidated by the enormous implications that a new virus would carry for blood banking, the safety of health workers, and the overall public health. There was also a hesitancy, particularly among those outside the medical community, to acknowledge that the infection could be spread through heterosexual contact. Indeed, many preferred to invoke any but the obvious cause. The spread of the disease in Haiti, for example, was postulated to be the result of voodoo practices rather than heterosexual sex.[33] Today, most human

Table 1 Important Dates in the First Decade of the AIDS Epidemic*

Date	Reported event	Comment†
June 5, 1981	5 Cases of *Pneumocystis carinii* pneumonia in homosexual men[1]	Initial report
July 3, 1981	26 Additional cases of new immunodeficiency syndrome[3]	Cases in New York and California
June 18, 1982	Cluster in southern California[4]	First report that "infectious agents [may be] sexually transmitted"
July 9, 1982	Initial cases in 34 Haitians[5]	Mode of transmission of unclear
July 16, 1982	Initial cases in 3 persons with hemophilia[6]	Possibility of tainted blood supply
September 24, 1982	Term "acquired immune deficiency syndrome" (AIDS) used for first time[7]	Term coined at July 1982 meeting, replacing "gay-related immune deficiency" (GRID)
October 1982	5 Cases in women reported, including 1 with only heterosexual exposure[8]	First possibly heterosexually transmitted case
November 5, 1982	Precautions published for clinical and laboratory staff[9]	"Patterns resembled the distribution and modes of spread of hepatitis B"
December 10, 1982	Initial transfusion-related case, in an infant[10]	Further evidence of tainted blood supply
December 17, 1982	Initial vertically transmitted cases reported in 4 infants[11]	Reported as "Possible that these infants had AIDS"
January 7, 1983	Report of heterosexual transmission to 2 female partners of injection-drug users[12]	"Supports infectious agent hypothesis"
January 7, 1983	Initial cases in 16 prisoners[13]	Given known risk groups, occurrence in prisoners "might have been anticipated"

Date	Reported Event	Comment
March 4, 1983	CDC releases prevention recommendations[14]	Groups at risk advised not to donate blood
March 19, 1983	Initial cases and 5 persons from Central Africa[15]	"Black Africans may be another group predisposed to AIDS"
May 20, 1983	Isolation of the virus from a patient with AIDS[16]	Retrovirus belongs to HTLV group, but is "clearly distinct from each previous isolate"
July 15, 1983	Report of 4 possibly occupational cases among health care workers[17]	Occupational transmission suspected but not proven
September 22, 1983	Infection-control guidelines published for care of patients with AIDS[18]	"Measures consistent with those suggested for prevention of hepatitis B should be followed"
January 13, 1994	AIDS tabulated as "notifiable disease" for first time[19]	25 Cases reported in first week
May 4, 1984	Frequent detection of HTLV-III in patients at risk[20]	"HTLV-III may be the primary cause of AIDS"
March 1985	FDA approves commercial test to detect HIV	Tremendous impact on patients at risk and blood supply
1986	CDC provides working definition of AIDS[21]	Updated in 1993[22]
1986	AIDS Clinical Trials Group established by NIH	Now largest clinical trials group in the United States
March 1987	FDA approved AZT (zidovudine)	First drug active against HIV

*CDC denotes Centers for Disease Control, FDA Food and Drug Administration, HIV human immunodeficiency virus, HTLV human T-cell lymphotropic virus, and NIH National Institutes of Health.

† Each quoted statement is from the reference cited under the corresponding Reported Event.

immunodeficiency virus (HIV) infections in the world derive from heterosexual transmission—a fact that is still overlooked by many.

In some quarters, doubt persists that HIV causes AIDS. One prominent dissident has theorized that the disease occurs because of long-term use of recreational drugs and is exacerbated by nucleoside analogues given as treatment.[34] The improvements that have been made in antiviral therapies for HIV disease have, paradoxically, only intensified the debate.[35,36]

Treatment

Recent advances in therapy have obscured the difficult and often demoralizing character of the early years of therapies for HIV. As the 1980s wore on, a hard-boiled fatalism settled in. Although patients and physicians did their best, they were all just playing out the same grim script.

Many of the agents that were studied in the first years of the epidemic are shown in Table 2. The list is incomplete; dozens and possibly hundreds of other concoctions were tried. The story for most was remarkably similar: a few patients in San Francisco, Los Angeles, or New York took a certain medication; some felt better; a few had improvements in CD4 cell counts. With the first whisper of encouragement, others joined in, a clinical trial was organized, and another great hope was born.

After the intense excitement came tempered optimism, then fading expectations, and finally an unsentimental assignment of the treatment to the scrap heap. Two agents, compound Q (Chinese cucumber plant root)[37] and peptide T,[38] are particularly representative. Each was briefly the darling of the emerging community of patients and activists seeking an effective therapy, but each moved slowly into formal clinical trials, prompting patients to criticize the medical–industrial complex as uncaring and uncooperative.[46] When studied, neither drug proved to be effective.

The growing sense of despair and frustration opened the door for charlatans. A typical fraudulent therapy was MM-1, promoted by an Egyptian rectal surgeon with "unbelievable claims of cure," but support for the claims was never presented.[47] The cost of the therapy, however, was presented: $75,000, including the trip to Zaire, where the treatment was administered.

The Late 1980s: Slow Progress

Once a retrovirus had been identified, the search began for agents that might act on reverse transcriptase, the enzyme necessary for transcribing HIV RNA to DNA. To study potential therapies, the National Institute of Health (NIH) organized the AIDS Clinical Trials Group (ACTG) in 1986.

Table 2 Early Therapies for the Management of HIV Infection

Drug	Source	Possible mechanism	Findings	Comment
Putative antiviral drugs				
Compound Q	Chinese cucumber root	Enters macrophage to eradicate virus	Ineffective[37]	Increase of 1 CD4 cell per cubic millimeter per month
Peptide T	Synthetic	Competitive receptor blockade[38]	Never published	Trials continue for HIV-related cognitive impairment
AL 721 (active lipids at 7-2-1 ratio)	Hen's-egg yolks	Destabilizes cell membrane	Ineffective[39]	Transient weight gain
Soluble CD4	Synthetic	Competitive receptor blockade	Ineffective[40]	No oral form
Dextran sulfate	Synthetic	Anticoagulant, blocks attachment	Ineffective[41]	Not absorbed orally
Putative immune modulators				
Isoprinosine	Synthetic	Immune stimulation, possible antiviral activity	Minimally effective[42]	Prolonged controversy regarding efficacy
Imuthiol	Metal chelator similar to disulfiram	Modulates T-cell differentiation	Ineffective[43]	Investigators reported, "Use of [drug] should be discontinued"
Ampligen	Antisense RNA	Enhancement of killer cells	Ineffective[44]	Prolonged controversy regarding efficacy
Imreg-1	Synthetic	Enhanced production of interferon, interleukin-2	Minimally effective[45]	Prolonged controversy regarding efficacy; slower CD4 cell decrease with drug

Since its inception, the ACTG has systematically studied dozens of candidate therapies in adults and children. This research, along with trials sponsored by pharmaceutical companies, has led to the current guidelines that advocate triple-drug therapy.[48]

Zidovudine (earlier known as azidothymidine, or AZT) was among the earliest compounds tested[49] and, in 1987, became the first drug approved for the treatment of AIDS. After initial exuberance, many in the community of AIDS patients turned against the drug.[46] They came to see its promotion as an almost hostile act on the part of the NIH, Burroughs Wellcome, and treating physicians. Accusations abounded that cheap and simple treatments had been overlooked in favor of a mediocre, costly, and toxic agent. Patients soon claimed that everyone they knew who took zidovudine was dead—still a familiar lament.

This was the time of greatest tension between the community of patients and the medical establishment.[50] There was discord about access to study drugs, protocol selection, design, and interpretation, and perhaps most of all, the overall pace and sincerity of scientific investigation. Even the bedrock concepts of the placebo-controlled trial became a point of contention, because it struck many as unethical.

Progress was very slow in the years after the approval of zidovudine, further fraying the relationship between physicians and the community. Additional nucleosides were identified and compared in numerous trials, and incremental differences were noted. Real advances were made in the area of prophylaxis against opportunistic infections, especially *P. carinii* pneumonia and *Mycobacterium avium* complex infection.[51,52]

The Mid-1990s: High Hopes

In the 1990s, highly active antiretroviral therapy (HAART) first became available, and it fundamentally altered the epidemic in the United States (Fig. 1) [Not shown, Ed.]. By this time, the community of patients and the medical community had begun a productive collaboration that remains the hallmark of AIDS care today.

The potential effectiveness of the new drugs was evident long before the confirmatory clinical trials had been performed (Table 3). First came a new understanding of the dynamics and pathophysiology of HIV infection.[54] Patients with chronic infection who were treated with the protease inhibitor ritonavir had a precipitous drop in HIV RNA level, reflecting an abrupt interruption of high-grade replication of HIV (billions of copies daily). They also had an increase in the CD4 cell count, which revealed the regenerative capacity of the CD4 cell population. The establishment of these two principles profoundly influenced clinicians' subsequent approach to antiviral therapy.[54]

Table 3 Important Dates in the Second Decade of the AIDS Epidemic*

Date	Reported event	Comment[†]
1991	Approval of didanosine and zalcitabine	Second and third approved drugs; combination therapy used increasingly
1993	AIDS becomes leading cause of death of Americans 25–44 years old[53]	AIDS surpasses unintentional injuries as cause of death in this group
January 12, 1995	Dynamics of HIV replication redefined[54]	"Primary [therapeutic] strategy ought be to target virally mediated destruction"
May 4, 1995	Identification of viral cause of Kaposi's sarcoma[55]	Human herpesvirus 8 isolated
July 15, 1995	First Public Service guidelines to prevent opportunistic infections[51]	Two subsequent revisions
August 1995	First protease inhibitor, saquinavir, approved[56]	Within 18 months, 3 additional protease inhibitors approved
1996	U.S. AIDS death rate decreases[57]	"For the first time, deaths among persons with AIDS have decreased substantially"
May 24, 1996	Prognostic power of viral-load determination established[58]	Important laboratory determination for routine management
1997	President Bill Clinton seeks AIDS vaccine in 10 years	HIV Vaccine Trials Network established
May 7, 1998	First public report of lipodystrophy syndrome[59]	Lipodystrophy, hyperlipidemia, diabetes, and other metabolic abnormalities described with increasing frequency in patients with AIDS
June 1998	Efavirenz approved[60]	"Protease-sparing" regimens introduced
January 10, 2000	UN Security Council discusses AIDS[61]	"AIDS threatens our security"
December 2000	WHO estimates 36.1 million had HIV–AIDS, with an additional 21.8 million already dead[2]	5.3 million new infections in 2000; 14,500 new infections per day
March 2001	U.S. pharmaceutical companies substantially reduce prices and may allow generic drugs for Africa[62,63]	Cost will be 1–10% of U.S. price

*UN denotes United Nations, and WHO World Health Organization.

[†] Each quoted statement is from the reference cited under the corresponding Reported Event.

A crucial study examined the fate of 180 homosexual men from whom serial plasma specimens had been collected for more than 10 years.[54] In this group, the viral load proved to be a significantly more powerful predictor of long-term survival than the CD4 cell count, which had been used since the start of the epidemic. Thus, the viral load became a central new piece of information for decisions about beginning and modifying treatments.

Armed with these new insights, investigators confidently initiated a series of landmark clinical trials.[56,60] Most studies have shown dramatic and durable responses for at least two thirds of patients with minimal previous antiviral exposure who adhere to a regimen of triple-drug therapy. In the United States, 15 agents have been approved in three classes of drugs: nucleoside analogue reverse-transcriptase inhibitors, nonnucleoside reverse-transcriptase inhibitors, and protease inhibitors. With the use of these potent medications, there have been sharp and sustained declines in the incidence of AIDS and in AIDS-related mortality (Fig. 1).[64] Although this type of treatment is expensive, the cost is offset by savings in other areas, particularly hospital and home care charges.[65]

Current efforts focus on simplifying the drug regimens to improve adherence, developing alternatives for those in whom the current medications have failed, and managing a wide range of side effects, particularly the metabolic disorders, including lipodystrophy.[59] The optimal time in which to initiate therapy remains controversial, as it has been throughout the epidemic. But recently, experts have suggested that the risk of long-term side effects from the current regimens argues against routine early therapy, in contrast to the "hit early, hit hard" strategy that had been favored since the introduction of the protease inhibitors.[48] The complete eradication of infection, particularly latent virus, remains the focus of intense investigation.[66]

The Late 1990s: Global Crisis

Despite these advances, there is a gathering sense of doom in the face of the scale of the global epidemic. The numbers are familiar but bear repeating: 36.1 million persons worldwide are infected with HIV; an additional 21.8 million have died; and 13.2 million children have become "AIDS orphans," having lost their mother or both parents to the disease.[2] More than 14,000 new infections occur daily—5.3 million in 2000 alone, including 600,000 in children younger than 15 years old. Approximately 70 percent of cases occur in sub-Saharan Africa, where, in some regions, the seroprevalence of HIV among adults exceeds 25 percent.[2] The Caribbean, Southeast Asia, and eastern Europe are also struggling with substantial rates of new infection.

In these areas, AIDS has evolved into two distinct epidemics: a horizontal epidemic in adults, spread by sexual contact or shared needles, and a vertical epidemic in which infected mothers give birth to infected children. Each requires a different approach to control and management, and each raises different sets of complex issues. For example, women are advised to abstain from breast-feeding to prevent transmission through breast milk, but a mother who does not breast-feed is immediately assumed to be HIV-infected and may be shunned by neighbors.

The high seroprevalence of HIV in some countries has raised concern that AIDS may represent a threat to the political stability of entire nations.[61] In 2000, the Security Council of the United Nations began to address the possibility that, by devastating a country's entire population of young adults, AIDS now threatens the world's security. This marked the first time that a medical illness had received the attention of this important deliberative body.

Recent events in Africa appeared to herald a profound change in the way antiretroviral drugs are distributed in the developing world. In response to local and international pressure, some pharmaceutical companies will offer expensive agents to African patients at a fraction of their cost in the United States.[62] In addition, there are efforts to allow generic-medication companies to produce antiretroviral agents for local sale,[63] as is done in Brazil.[67] The sharply reduced price will still be too high for most infected persons.

Despite recent developments, control of AIDS still awaits a vaccine. In 1997, President Bill Clinton challenged scientists to provide an effective vaccine within 10 years. Toward this end, a national HIV Vaccine Trials Network has been established to develop and test possible compounds. Among the difficulties confronting researchers are viral heterogeneity, uncertainty about how to achieve optimal immunogenicity, the lack of a practical animal model, and the ethical dilemmas involved in conducting primary prevention trials in the United States and abroad.

The Blood Supply and AIDS Activism

AIDS has had lasting effects on several areas separate from HIV-infected patients and those who care for them. These include the challenges the epidemic has brought to blood banking and activism by patients.

Blood Banking

The first alarm about the safety of the blood supply was sounded in July 1982, when the newly described immunodeficiency syndrome developed in three persons with hemophilia.[6] Those with hemophilia are at particular risk for transfusion-related infections, since a single dose of cryoprecipitate contains products from between 1,000 and 20,000 donors.

Disagreement arose because of the competing priorities of the professional groups that were involved. On the basis of the three reported cases of the disease, the public health community sensed an impending disaster. Hemophilia specialists, on the other hand, had witnessed the enormous benefit cryoprecipitate had provided their patients and thought that this gain dwarfed the theoretical concern that the blood supply might contain a possible transmissible virus that would take years to cause disease. And the blood-banking community, wrestling then as now with a barely adequate blood supply, was concerned about scaring off donors.

The debate intensified, and various solutions were rejected is either too costly (testing for surrogate markers) or too stigmatizing (the exclusion of members of various risk groups from donation). Finally, the virus was isolated, and in March 1985, a screening test became available. By then, HIV had been transmitted to at least 50 percent of the 16,000 persons with hemophilia in the United States and to an additional 12,000 recipients of blood transfusions.[68]

In its investigation, the Institute of Medicine criticized the blood-banking community.[68] It found that the safety measures that had been adopted were "limited in scope" and that opportunities for more effective interventions had been lost. Screening to rule out the presence of infectious agents that would require rejection of blood products now requires 10 tests on each donated unit of blood, as compared with the 2 (for syphilis and hepatitis B surface antigen) that were required in 1981.

The lessons from the AIDS epidemic influence decisions regarding blood-banking procedures today. A recent example is the scramble to develop guidelines to prevent the possible introduction into the blood supply of the agent of bovine spongiform encephalopathy, a prion disease that has not yet been demonstrated to be transmissible through blood.[69]

New Drugs and Disease-Related Activism

AIDS has radically altered the development of drugs. Before the AIDS epidemic, the Food and Drug Administration (FDA) was often viewed as a remote bureaucracy. With the advent of AIDS and the community that formed around it, numerous innovative approaches were developed to expedite the development of new drugs and patients' access to investigational drugs.[46] The FDA became substantially more efficient: in 1986, the average interval between a drug application and the granting of FDA approval was 34.1 months; by 1999, it had decreased to 12.6 months.[70]

Activism related to diseases has also evolved remarkably.[46] In the 1970s, Washington-based, organized advocacy groups that focused on particular diseases were few; now, at least 150 such organizations exist (Trull FL, National Association for Biomedical Research: personal communication). Activism by patients with AIDS has influenced advocates for patients with other diseases, including breast cancer, Parkinson's disease, Alzheimer's disease, and juvenile diabetes.[46] Using creative approaches rather than following the established rules of lobbying, AIDS activists created a new model. New techniques ranged from drug buyers' clubs and red ribbons pinned to the lapel to aggressive civil disobedience and telephone "zaps," wherein the telephone switchboard of a specific company was jammed by a coordinated barrage of incoming calls. Today, patients are routinely consulted regarding the design of studies, and community-based research is conducted across the country.

The success of AIDS activists led to criticism by the public and Congress alike that federal dollars were not being apportioned according to the burden of disease, but according to a more political set of criteria. The Institute of Medicine has recommended broader public input into decisions about the allotment of funds.[71]

Conclusions

In 20 years, the AIDS epidemic has grown from a series of small outbreaks in several risk groups scattered throughout the United States and western Europe into a global public health calamity. Tremendous strides have been made in understanding the disease, from the molecular level to the broadest perspective of public health. In addition, important advances in antiretroviral therapy and blood-supply safety have been achieved. During the 1990s, the disease was transformed for many patients in industrialized nations from a predictably fatal infection to a chronic condition requiring daily medication and occasional visits to the doctor's office.

Despite these gains, however, the epidemic threatens to spin completely out of control in many of the world's poorest nations. Until a vaccine is available, two humble but effective interventions have been shown to limit the horizontal spread of HIV: sex education and the use of condoms that results from it,[72,73] and drug-abuse treatment, including the provision of clean needles.[74] Widespread implementation of these interventions, however, continues to be hampered by personal, social, and political barriers in almost all countries and governments.[75] To some extent, the disease has continued to spread horizontally because of an unwillingness to use effective control measures, rather than because of the lack of a vaccine or other remedy.

Given these difficulties, improved control of HIV infection in the next decade looms as a daunting task. An effective vaccine is not imminent, and most governments are unlikely to initiate frank public discussions about sexual intercourse and injection-drug use, despite the glaring need. Nonetheless, patients and health care workers alike should find solace and inspiration in the remarkable achievements of the past 20 years. Not so long ago, the hope that a cause of AIDS would be found and that effective therapies for the disease would be developed seemed as unlikely as global control of the disease seems today.

SOURCE

Sepkowitz KA. 2001. AIDS—The first 20 years. *N Engl J Med* 344 (23): 1764–72. Copyright 2001 *New England Journal of Medicine*. Reprinted with permission of Massachusetts Medical Society.

CHAPTER 10

VACCINE-PREVENTABLE DISEASES

... Declares solemnly that the world and its peoples have won freedom from smallpox, which was a most devastating disease sweeping in epidemic form through many countries since earliest time, leaving death, blindness and disfigurement in its wake and which only a decade ago was rampant in Africa, Asia and South America.
     —Resolution of the 33rd World Health Assembly (WHA 33.3)
     Geneva, Switzerland, May 8, 1980

WHEN THE WORLD HEALTH ASSEMBLY MADE ITS HISTORIC 1980 declaration that the world was free of smallpox, the vast majority of physicians in the developed world had never seen a case of the disease. The announcement came at a time when there was a general belief that many of the vaccine-preventable diseases would soon be eradicated. Indeed, American families had lined up their children to be "Polio Pioneers" in the 1950s, convinced that protection from the scourge was finally at hand. Believing their actions to be patriotic, they had their children vaccinated against multiple diseases for school and summer camp attendance. Given the enormous efforts for vaccine research and development put forth by mid century, as well as mass immunization campaigns, why have we not eliminated more of these persistent infectious afflictions?

The story of vaccines and their antecedents began centuries ago. Most Western public health texts begin with the story of Edward Jenner's 1796 trial of cowpox as a preventive for smallpox (see Volume I, Chapter 6). Although Jenner was not the first to try this technique, his experiments were successful and fully documented. Despite his success, it took more than 50 years for Jenner's technique of vaccination to be widely adopted. In 1839, a smallpox epidemic raced through England and killed more than 22,000 people. At the time, Parliament condemned the use of the inoculation with live smallpox particles (known as variolation), a Turkish technique designed to give a controlled and hopefully mild case of the disease. More cases, reasoned Parliament, could break into yet another epidemic. In 1853, however, Parliament took action against smallpox, this time mandating that all English citizens be vaccinated with Jenner's cowpox vaccine to prevent future epidemics. Anyone refusing to be vaccinated was

Table 1 Vaccines, by Year of Development, First Successful Use in Humans, or Licensure

Disease	Year	Comment
Smallpox	1100	Variolation—China
	1600	Variolation—Turkey
	1706	Variolation—Boston
	1721	Variolation—Britain
	1798	Vaccination—Britain
Rabies	1885	
Plague	1897	
Cholera	1917	
Typhoid	1917	Parenteral
	1990	Oral
Diphtheria	1923	
Pertussis	1926	
Tuberculosis (BCG)	1927	
Yellow Fever (17D)	1935	
Tetanus toxoid	1937	
Typhus	1938	
Influenza A/B	1945	Parenteral
	2003	Nasal mist
Diphtheria, Pertussis, and Tetanus (DPT)	1949	
Tetanus and Diphtheria (Td)	1953	
Poliomyelitis	1955	Inactivated
	1961	Monovalent oral
	1963	Trivalent oral
Measles	1963	
Mumps	1967	
Rubella	1969	
Anthrax	1970	
Measles, Mumps, and Rubella (MMR)	1971	
Meningitis	1975	

Table 1 *(continued)*

Disease	Year	Comment
Pneumonia	1977	
Adenovirus	1980	
Hepatitis B	1981	
Haemophilus influenzae type b	1985	
Japanese encephalitis	1992	
Hepatitis A	1995	
Varicella	1995	
Lyme disease	1998	
Rotavirus	1998	Withdrawn 1999
	2006	Oral
Human papilloma virus	2006	
Herpes zoster	2006	
Avian influenza (H5N1)	2007	
Swine influenza (H1N1)	2009	

Sources:
Centers for Disease Control. 1999. Achievements in public health, 1900–1999: Impact of vaccines universally recommended for children—United States, 1990–1998. *MMWR* 48 (12): 243–8.

Red Book® Online. http://aapredbook.aappublications. org/news/vaccstatus.shtml (accessed May 15, 2008 and September 28, 2009).

punishable by a fine. Although 98 percent of the English population was vaccinated against smallpox by the beginning of the twentieth century, the effort was not without its critics. In response, a "conscience clause" was added to the mandatory vaccination legislation to deal with these vocal opponents. Public adversity toward mandatory vaccination programs has never disappeared. Voluntary vaccination against diseases, however, is widely accepted, especially in times of outbreaks.

In the 1880s, Louis Pasteur's laboratory in Paris developed a live rabies vaccine by taking spinal cord tissue from rabid animals and drying it. The drying process did not kill the virus but attenuated it. Healthy animals were then injected with the weakened virus and, amazingly, did not die. When the same animals were later given injections of virulent rabies virus, they still did not die, thus proving that an attenuated vaccine could protect against a more virulent form of disease.

In 1885, Joseph Meister, a nine-year-old boy from Alsace, was bitten by a rabid dog. It took Joseph's mother two days to get him to Paris whereupon she pleaded with Louis Pasteur for the new vaccine. Pasteur originally declined but yielded to the argument that without the vaccine Joseph would surely die. Treatment consisted of 13 daily injections of attenuated vaccine made from rabid rabbit neurologic tissue. Joseph survived, becoming the first known survivor of a rabid animal bite. Three months later, Pasteur treated Jean-Baptiste Jupille, a 14-year-old shepherd boy who had fought off a rabid dog attack six days before. Again, the patient survived. In October 1885, Pasteur announced his treatment of rabid animal bites to the French Academy of Sciences. His fame spread rapidly, and patients began flocking to his laboratory for treatment. By the end of 1886, Pasteur reported his results of treating 726 subjects exposed to rabies, only one of whom died because the treatment had been started too late after the bite had taken place (11 days). Today, deaths from rabies are rare, with newer vaccines and protocols that require only three-to-five intramuscular injections.

The bacteriologic revolution that occurred at the end of the nineteenth century (see Volume I, Chapter 17 on Robert Koch) thrust the development of vaccines into high gear. Table 1 shows the development of vaccines during the course of the twentieth century. Some brought with them significant challenges and controversy.

Polio

At the beginning of the twentieth century, poor sanitation and ingestion of contaminated food and water were widespread in the Western world. These resulted in most individuals contracting multiple *Enterovirus* infections, including polio, before their first birthdays. At the time, physicians considered polio a disease of infancy, because those who recovered developed immunity. Water treatment, refrigeration, and legislation ensuring food safety changed that epidemiologic pattern. As the age of exposure and development of immunity to polio shifted upward, so did the ages of polio victims.

In 1921, Franklin Roosevelt was 39 years old and vacationing at Campobello Island in Canada when he contracted a paralytic disease that multiple physicians diagnosed as polio. His condition was somewhat surprising given his advanced age. The future president of the United States refused to believe there was no cure for his condition and became convinced that hydrotherapy would restore his health. After hearing about the therapeutic mineral baths in Warm Springs, Georgia, Roosevelt began vacationing there regularly in 1924. Two years later, he bought the facility and enlisted his friend and law partner, Basil

O'Connor, to run it. Together they established the Georgia Warm Springs Foundation, a nonprofit entity. Although he remained paralyzed below the waist for the remainder of his life, Roosevelt never lost faith that there a cure for polio would be found.

As a fundraising mechanism for the Warm Springs facility, O'Connor organized Birthday Balls across the United States on January 30, Roosevelt's birthday. These became so successful after Roosevelt became president that they were merged into a national organization, the National Foundation for Infantile Paralysis (NFIP). Shortly afterward, comedian Eddie Cantor suggested that the name of the fundraising effort be changed to "The March of Dimes." Cantor made his first fundraising radio announcement for the March of Dimes in early January 1938. In it he requested that Americans send dimes directly to the White House to support the effort against polio. By the target date of January 30, the White House received a flood of mail with $268,000 in dimes. This successful fundraising campaign set in motion the more than $25 million raised by the foundation for grants to develop the first polio vaccine. To honor the leading role he took in defeating polio, the U.S. Congress voted to place Franklin Roosevelt's face on the dime beginning January 30, 1946.

It took almost half a century for scientists to understand that polio was transmitted by one of three different viruses: poliovirus type 1 (PV1), type 2 (PV2), or type 3 (PV3). Until this information was established in the late 1940s, creating an efficacious vaccine against the disease was impossible. Physician and virologist Jonas Salk first developed a means of growing poliovirus in a culture medium composed of monkey kidney cells. He then combined the three types of poliovirus grown in various cell cultures and chemically inactivated the mixture using formalin.

To test the new vaccine in the field, Salk engaged the services of his former mentor, Thomas Francis, Jr. of the School of Public Health at the University of Michigan. In 1953, Francis designed two studies. The first design called for the vaccination of second-graders at selected schools whose parents agreed to let their children participate (the treatment group). Their rate of polio was compared to that of first- and third-graders at the same schools who did not receive the vaccination (the control group). This design was called the observed control experiment, and it was roundly challenged by statisticians as suffering from selection and diagnostic bias. The second design was that of a randomized controlled trial. In it, all children whose parents agreed that they could participate were enrolled in the trial. They were then randomly divided into two groups. One group was given the polio vaccination, and the other was given a placebo. The study was double-blind in that neither the child nor the person administering the injection knew whether the inoculation was the vaccine or a placebo. To

Francis's credit, he insisted that all children be monitored in the same way regardless of which group they were in and that there be no interference from the foundation funding the effort.

The polio field trials, the largest in history, included more than 20,000 physicians and public health officers, 64,000 school personnel, and 220,000 volunteers to inoculate and monitor more than 1.8 million children from 217 communities in the United States, Canada, and Finland. In total, 444,000 children received the vaccine, 210,000 received a placebo, and 1.2 million more served as noninoculated controls. The results were published as The Francis Report in 1955 and documented that the vaccine was 60 to 70 percent effective against PV1 and more than 90 percent effective against PV2 and PV3. Although there were some breakthrough cases of the disease, the Salk vaccine was quickly licensed in 1955, and a plan for a massive immunization campaign developed. To provide sufficient vaccine for the campaign, multiple laboratories applied for licenses to produce it. One of these, Cutter Laboratories in Berkeley, California, mistakenly produced a batch of 120,000 doses containing particles of live poliovirus. Of the children who received a dose of the Cutter vaccine, about 40,000 developed nonparalytic poliomyelitis and 56 developed paralytic poliomyelitis, 5 of whom died of the infection. The Cutter incident brought widespread attention to the need for quality control in vaccine production and spurred an effort to find a safer alternative to the "killed" Salk vaccine, which required multiple injections and booster shots every five years.

Physician and immunologist Albert Bruce Sabin at the University of Cincinnati began his quest to find a live virus vaccine for polio about the same time as Salk. He figured that a live vaccine would confer lifelong immunity to the disease. Sabin determined that polio was transmitted through the gut, not the respiratory tract as had previously been assumed, and an oral preparation of the virus might be able to confer lifelong immunity. Although it took some time to obtain weak live virus of all three types and to prepare dilutions that could still stimulate antibody production in chimpanzees, Sabin was ready to test his "attenuated" live oral vaccine in the field in 1958 and 1959. Unable to muster funding in the United States because of the availability of the Salk vaccine, Sabin went to the WHO for political approval and to the Health Ministry of the Soviet Union for vaccine testing in a massive field trial. After vaccination of more than two million people during the course of two years, the Sabin vaccine was demonstrated to be safe and as easy to administer as a drop on a lump of sugar. The United States granted approval for manufacture of the Sabin vaccine in 1960.

The battle between the killed Salk and the live attenuated Sabin polio vaccines persisted throughout the 1970s. Eventually the WHO became convinced that the Sabin vaccine, which conferred lifelong immunity, would be the tool that could eradicate the disease. Because polio is similar to smallpox in that it has no animal or environmental reservoirs, once immunity was achieved, polio would be eradicated. Indeed, the WHO declared that wild polio was eradicated in the Americas in 1994 and from the Western Pacific region in 2000. Globally, less than 3,000 cases of wild polio were reported in 2000, down 99 percent from just a decade before. Rotary International and the Bill and Melinda Gates Foundation sponsored a fundraising campaign to help finish the job as early as possible. Unfortunately, a major disadvantage of the Sabin vaccine is that it cannot be given to immunocompromised individuals, and many areas where polio remains endemic have large numbers of people with HIV/AIDS. This means the oral Sabin vaccine, the one most easy to use in the field, cannot be targeted toward those populations, and in these cases, the Salk vaccine is the treatment of choice.

Influenza

The 1917–1918 influenza pandemic (known as Spanish flu) left humanity in shock after it infected one-third of the world's population and killed between 50 and 100 million individuals. As a matter of national security, the United States created the Commission on Influenza of the U.S. Armed Forces Epidemiological Board and supported multiple efforts to create a vaccine. The commission sponsored a number of vaccine trials in closed communities, such as in children's institutions, army and navy units, and medical schools. Different preparations of vaccine against influenza A, the most dangerous type of the virus for humans, were tested, including some with adjuvants for improving the vaccine response. By 1943, trials of army units in colleges across the United States showed that the risk of epidemics of influenza A could be reduced due to the presence of vaccinated individuals; today this is what we call herd immunity. By 1945, all U.S. Army personnel were vaccinated, and efforts began to find a vaccine for influenza B, a common but less virulent form of the disease.

In 1951, the MRC followed suit to find a vaccine against influenza A in Great Britain, creating the Council on Clinical Trials of Influenza Vaccine. Four variants of influenza A vaccine were created, and a field trial of the best vaccine option was carried out in the winter of 1951–1952. Despite that year being a low-incidence flu season, the trial did establish that the vaccine was able to confer significant protection from the disease.

Influenza virus is notorious for mutating, or undergoing an "antigenic shift". This is precisely what happened in 1968 when it became clear that an outbreak of influenza A in Hong Kong would likely strike the United States, perhaps in epidemic proportions. Although a vaccine was available, the supply was limited.

Therefore, it was decided to try a technique that had been suggested in 1920 by epidemiologist Wade Hampton Frost but never tested in the field. All school-children in Tecumseh, Michigan, were vaccinated, and the flu rate in that com-munity was compared to that of a neighboring community where the school-children remained unvaccinated. Flu-related illness in the vaccinated community was only one-third that of the unvaccinated community, which showed that mass immunization of schoolchildren is not only a feasible strategy for reduc-ing illness among schoolchildren, but also a way to reduce the impact of a com-municable disease on an entire community.

There are three types of influenza viruses (A, B, and C), which can be classified by their protein composition: H (hemagglutinin) and N (neuraminidase). Influ-enza type A is the most pathogenic to humans; it caused the major epidemics of the twentieth century (1918, 1957, and 1968). Influenza A, which infects ducks, chickens, pigs, and whales, as well as humans, has 16 H subtypes and 9 N sub-types. In contrast, type B and C influenza viruses have no subtypes. Influenza A also mutates easily, which makes the next potential influenza A epidemic difficult to predict and a reliable vaccine to fight it difficult to produce in a timely manner. For example, the 2009 appearance of H1N1 created a flurry of activity to produce enough vaccine to protect the public from another 1917–1918 pandemic.

RUBELLA

A U.K. physician, George Maton, first reported in 1814 that a mild childhood ill-ness with a three-day rash and little or no fever was a disease separate from measles (rubeola) and scarlet fever (caused by Group A β-hemolytic *Streptococ-cus*). Most physicians considered rubella a routine childhood infection until 1941, when Australian ophthalmologist Norman Gregg noticed that women who were exposed to rubella in the first trimester of pregnancy often had infants born with cataracts (see Chapter 7). Gregg's observations, however, were not verified until an epidemic is Sweden in 1951 reported not only cataracts, but also deaf-ness, congenital heart disease, and other birth anomalies in infants with mater-nal rubella exposure. Rubella epidemics swept Europe and the United States from 1963 to 1965, and epidemiologic studies estimated that congenital rubella syndrome affected about 1 percent of all pregnancies in some regions. The rush was then on to isolate the virus and create an effective vaccine.

In the late 1960s, two types of attenuated rubella vaccine were developed and licensed in United States and the United Kingdom, respectively. Not only the types of vaccine but also the strategies for using them were different. The United States focused on vaccinating all infants, and the United Kingdom tar-geted all adolescent girls, the upcoming cohort it was important to protect during pregnancy. Both strategies left currently pregnant women in nonvaccinated populations potentially exposed to cases of rubella. Eventually, the U.K. vaccine was adopted as preferable, and both countries determined the best strategy for vaccination was universal immunization of infants, as well as immunization of adolescent girls and women, military recruits, and health care workers. Later, rubella vaccine was combined with measles and mumps vaccines in the MMR immunization. The effort for global measles eradication has aided somewhat in the reduction of cases of rubella. At the twentieth century's end, cyclic rubella epidemics continued to occur every four to seven years, primarily among children ages two to eight years in developing countries, similar to those that occurred in the prevaccine era.

Vaccine Controversies

Since the beginning of vaccines, there has been controversy. This is easy to understand as the concept of purposefully infecting oneself or one's children to the agent of disease, killed or otherwise, may be terrifying. Additionally, when a vaccine is mandated for a population rather than voluntary for each individual, there tends to be resistance to complying without complaint. Critics of vaccines often argue that they simply do not work, that they are dangerous or contain dangerous contaminants, that their use is against religious doctrine, that the rate of disease is so low the vaccine is no longer needed, or that other preventive measures such as alternative medicines are just as effective for preventing disease. In the twentieth century, several major antivaccine efforts took root, such as in the 1970s when reactions attributed to pertussis (whooping cough) vaccine caused sufficient fear in the populations of the United Kingdom and Sweden that immunization rates fell and epidemics quickly followed. Outbreaks of disease, especially measles, occurred during that time among unvaccinated religious groups, even where herd immunity of the general population was reached, as in the United States, Ireland, and The Netherlands.

A second controversy erupted over hepatitis B vaccine in the 1980s. Hepatitis B is a virus that causes 80 percent of all liver cancers worldwide. It follows that a vaccine that protects against hepatitis B infection also protects those who get it from developing liver cancer. The virus was discovered serendipitously by physician and medical anthropologist Baruch Blumberg in his quest to find differences in inherited susceptibility to diseases in indigenous populations around the world. Blumberg found an unknown antibody reaction to an antigen found in a blood sample from an Australian Aborigine. This antigen was eventually determined to be the cause of "serum hepatitis," and its etiology was hepatitis B. In 1969, Blumberg teamed with microbiologist Irving Millman to develop a vaccine against hepatitis B virus. By 1979, three placebo-controlled, random-ized, double-blind clinical trials were proposed to assess the efficacy of an in-activated hepatitis B vaccine in high risk groups—dialysis patients, dialysis clinic staff, and male homosexuals. The trials all indicated that the vaccine was close to 100 percent effective for those who received all three doses. Significant con-troversy erupted over the use of the third group because male homosexuals were at risk for both hepatitis B and HIV exposure through the same modes of transmission. Among the homosexual study subjects, those without HIV infec-tion had a seroconversion rate (i.e., they developed immunity) of about 90 percent. Those with HIV infection, however, had a seroconversion rate of less than 50 percent, and many became chronic carriers of hepatitis B. Thus, vacci-nation for hepatitis B was indicated only for individuals without HIV infection to provide long-term protection against hepatitis B and liver cancer. Because the vaccine was not covered by insurance, many homosexual men did not get vaccinated, and there was a rumor in the gay community that the vaccine was part of a conspiracy to pass the infection rather than prevent it.

The most high-profile controversy regarding vaccines is arguably that sur-rounding the use of an organomercury compound, thimerosal (or thiomersal), as a preservative beginning in the 1930s. In 1997, the FDA Modernization Act required that all mercury-containing food and drugs be reviewed and the risk of mercury exposure assessed. As a result, the CDC and the American Academy of Pediatrics determined that the vaccination schedule for the first six months of life might cause mercury exposure to exceed that which would be considered safe for infants. The agencies strongly suggested that thimerosal be removed from vaccines as quickly as possible as a precaution.

Many parents of children with autism, a disease under scrutiny for its increas-ing prevalence, held that thimerosal was to blame. Thousands of lawsuits were filed for alleged toxicity from vaccines containing thimerosal. Congressional hear-ings were held on the matter, and the CDC empanelled a scientific review by the IOM to consider the evidence that thimerosal might be a causative agent for autism. Although the hearings on Capitol Hill concluded that there was cause for alarm, the scientific community rejected a causal relationship between thimerosal-containing vaccines and autism. Three large observational studies, one in Den-mark, one in the United Kingdom, and one in the United States, followed and found no connection between autism and thimerosal-containing vaccines. De-spite the findings of these studies, some parents of children with autism remain convinced that thimerosal vaccines were indeed responsible for their plight, with more than 5,000 seeking vaccine compensation from the courts.

Vaccines have been spectacularly successful in reducing epidemics from some communicable diseases. Smallpox has been eradicated globally, and polio is no longer found in the Western hemisphere, Europe, the Indo-West Pacific, and the Western Pacific, including China. Eradicating measles may be the next success, with the disease now eliminated from the Western hemisphere, Europe, and the Western Pacific. Despite these successes, challenges remain. For example, we are just beginning to understand how best to use vaccines to protect against some cancers, such as hepatitis B vaccine to protect against liver cancer and human papilloma virus (HPV) vaccine to protect against cervical cancer. Other vaccines currently in development target cancers of the skin, lung, and prostate.

A major challenge for global public health is creating adequate and effective vaccine stocks against seasonal influenza viruses. The WHO estimates that in nonpandemic years there are about one billion cases of seasonal influenza, leading to 300,000 to 500,000 deaths worldwide. The WHO Global Influenza Surveillance Network selects three influenza virus strains—the ones thought most likely to cause significant human suffering in the coming season—for seasonal flu vaccine each year. Once the decision is made, vaccine manufacturers struggle to produce adequate vaccine stocks. Should a novel influenza virus arise, it is hoped that seasonal influenza vaccines will offer some protection against severe disease and moderate the impact of a global epidemic.

SELECTED READINGS

Although Gregg reported the first cases of congenital cataracts among the offspring of Australian women exposed to rubella in the first trimester of pregnancy, it took some time for his findings to be validated. A few studies followed, but none was as comprehensive to date as that reported by Rolf Lundström on the rubella epidemic in Sweden in 1950. In this reading, Lundström describes an almost complete case series of congenital rubella syndrome from population-based reporting (95 percent of maternity hospitals). His report gave urgency to the importance of finding the virus and creating a vaccine to protect infants from congenital rubella syndrome. Unfortunately, the virus was not identified until 1962, and a vaccine did not become available until 1969. During that period, a rubella pandemic began in Europe and spread to the United States between 1963 and 1965, leaving a trail of damaged infants in its wake. In one year in the United States alone, there were 12.5 million cases of rubella reported with more than 20,000 affected infants. Of these infants born with congenital rubella syndrome, 2,100 died, 12,000 were deaf, 3,580 were blind, and 1,800 were mentally retarded. Some cities, such as New York, had 1 percent of all births affected. Today, the developed world is largely protected from congenital rubella syndrome by the use of the rubella vaccine. In the developing world, however, the WHO estimates that about 100,000 infants are born with congenital rubella syndrome each year.

Our second reading, by K. Ehresman and colleagues, addresses a serious adverse event, intussusception associated with the introduction of a vaccine against rotavirus. Rotavirus is a major cause of diarrhea and gastroenteritis among children. Although the rotavirus vaccine may not have had the potential for dramatically reducing hepatocellular carcinoma as did the hepatitis B vaccine, it would greatly reduce a major cause of morbidity among the young. Thus, the vaccine was initially hailed as a major public health advance in the United States. There were 15 reports of intussusception during the vaccine's first nine months of availability, which raised concerns regarding the vaccine's safety. Further investigation disclosed a strong association between receipt of the vaccine and subsequent intussusception. In some cases, the intussusception required surgical intervention. In response to these findings, the vaccine was subsequently removed from the market, and reports of intussusception among the young returned to baseline (i.e., before introduction of the vaccine) levels. It is clear that although vaccines have great potential for preventing infectious diseases, they (like all medicines) also have the unintended potential of doing harm. Thus, the need for careful testing before a vaccine comes to market, along with instituting a broad-based adverse events reporting program, is clearly demonstrated.

The third paper, by John P. Fox and colleagues, lays out an important public health concept: herd immunity. Herd immunity is defined as the threshold proportion of people in a population that are not susceptible to a disease and thus can stop an outbreak from becoming an epidemic. Each disease has a different threshold for herd immunity, depending on the virulence of the disease agent, the efficacy of the vaccine, and the social network of contacts in the population. Thus, it is herd immunity that allows public health officials to plan and implement immunization campaigns. The reading clearly shows the importance of identifying the group with the most social contacts to immunize in order to maximize a vaccine program. It is presented here in an abridged form, with the statistical appendices removed to save space.

BIBLIOGRAPHY

Allen A. 2007. *Vaccine: The Controversial Story of Medicine's Greatest Lifesaver.* New York: W.W. Norton & Co.

Baer, GM, ed. 1991. *The Natural History of Rabies,* 2nd ed. Boca Raton, FL: CRC Press.

Bodian D. 1976. Poliomyelitis and the sources of useful knowledge. *Johns Hopkins Medical Journal* 138:130–36.

Burke DS. 2004. Lessons learned from the 1954 field trial of poliomyelitis vaccine. *Clin Trials* 1 (1): 3–5.

Centers for Disease Control. 1994. Certification of poliomyelitis eradication—the Americas, 1994. *MMWR* 43:720–22.

Centers for Disease Control. 1997. Paralytic poliomyelitis—United States, 1980–1994. *MMWR* 46:79–83.

Centers for Disease Control. 1999. Achievements in Public Health, 1900–1999: Impact of vaccines universally recommended for children—United States, 1990–1998. *MMWR* 48 (12): 243–48.

Committee on Clinical Trials of Influenza Vaccine. 1953. Clinical trials of influenza vaccine: A progress report to the Medical Research Council by its Committee on Clinical Trials of Influenza Vaccine. *Br Med J* 2 (4847): 1173–77.

Dawson L. 2004. The Salk polio vaccine trial of 1954: Risks, randomization and public involvement in research. *Clin Trials* 1 (1): 122–30.

Fenner F, Henderson DA, Arita I, Jezek Z, and Ladnyi ID. 1988. *Smallpox and Its Eradication.* Geneva: WHO.

Francis T Jr. 1953. Vaccination against influenza. *Bull World Health Org* 8:725–41.

Francis T Jr., Korns RF, Voight RB, Boisen M, Hemphill FM, Napier JA, and Tolchinsky E. 1955. *An Evaluation of the 1954 Poliomyelitis Vaccine Trials.* Ann Arbor, MI.: The Poliomyelitis Vaccine Evaluation Center, University of Michigan. Reprinted 1955 in *Am J Public Health* 45 (5, Part 2): 1–63.

Francis T Jr., Napier JA, Voight RB, Hemphill FM, Wenner HA, Korns RF, Boisen M, Tolchinsky E, and Diamond EL. 1957. *Evaluation of the 1954 Field Trial of Poliomyelitis Vaccine: Final Report.* Ann Arbor, MI: Poliomyelitis Vaccine Evaluation Center, University of Michigan.

Gangarosa EJ, Glazka AM, Woldfe CR, Phillips LM, Gangarosa RE, Miller E, and Chen RT. 1998. Impact of anti-vaccine movements on pertussis control: The untold story. *Lancet* 351:356–61.

Gregg, NM. 1941. Congenital cataract following German measles in the mother. *Trans Opthal Soc Aust* 3:35–46.

Hurwitz ES, Schonberger LB, Nelson DB, and Holman RC. 1981. Guillain-Barré syndrome and the 1978–1979 influenza vaccine. *N Engl J Medicine* 304 (26): 1557–61.

Knox EG. 1980. Strategy for rubella vaccination. *Int J Epidemiol* 9 (1): 13–23.

Lambert SM and Markel H. 2000. Making history: Thomas Francis, Jr., MD, and the 1954 Salk Poliomyelitis Vaccine Field Trial. *Arch Pediatr Adolesc* 154 (5): 512–17.

Lustbder ED, London WT, and Blumberg BS. 1976. Study design for a hepatitis B vaccine trial. *P Natl Acad Sci USA* 73 (3): 955–59.

Monto AS, Davenport FM, Mapier JA, and Francis Jr. T. 1969. Effect of vaccination of a school-age population upon the course of an A2/Hong Kong influenza epidemic. *Bull World Health Org* 41:537–42.

Mullaney L. Considerations for implementing a new combination vaccine into managed care. 2002. *Am J Manag C* 9:S23-S29.

Nathanson N. 2005. David Bodian's contribution to the development of poliovirus vaccine. *Am J Epidemiol* 161 (3): 207–12.

Nathanson N and Langmuir AD. 1963. The Cutter incident: Poliomyelitis following formaldehyde-inactivated poliovirus vaccination in the United States during the spring of 1955. II. Relationship of poliomyelitis to Cutter vaccine. *Am J Hyg* 78:29–60. Reprinted in 1995 *Am J Epidemiol* 142 (2): 109–40; discussion 107–8.

Offit PA. 2005. The Cutter incident, 50 years later. *N Engl J Med* 352 (14): 1411–12.

Offit PA, Quarles J, Gerber MA, Hackett CJ, Marcuse EK, Kollman TR, Gellin BG, and Landry S. 2001. Addressing parents' concerns: Do multiple vaccines overwhelm or weaken the infant's immune system? *Pediatrics* 209:124–29.

Plotkin SA and Orenstein WA. 1999. *Vaccines*, 3rd ed. Philadelphia: WB Saunders.

Reingold A, Cutts F, Kamau T, Levine O, O'Brien K, Ignacio Santos Preciado J, and Schrag S. 2006. Detailed Review Paper on Pneumococcal Conjugate Vaccine. Presented to the WHO Strategic Advisory Group of Experts (SAGE) on Immunization, November 2006, p. 69. http://www.who.int/immunization/SAGE_wg_detailedreview_pneumoVaccine. pdf (accessed August 30, 2009).

Robbins FC. 1993. Eradication of polio in the Americas. *JAMA* 270 (15): 1857–59.

Sabin AB. 1950. Antipoliomyelitic substance in milk of human beings and certain cows. *Am J Dis Child* 80 (5): 866–67.

Sabin AB. 1951. Paralytic consequences of poliomyelitis infection in different parts of the world and in different population groups. *Am J Public Health* 41 (10): 1215–30.

Salk JE. 1955. Vaccination against paralytic poliomyelitis performance and prospects. *Am J Public Health* 45:575–96.

Sporton RK and Francis S-A. 2001. Choosing not to immunize: Are parents making informed decisions? *Family Practice* 19 (2): 181–88.

Zhou F, Santoli J, Messonnier ML, Yusuf HR, Shefer A, Chu SY, Rodenwald L, and Harpaz R. 2005. Economic evaluation of the 7-Vaccine routine childhood immunization schedule in the United States, 2001. *Arch Pediatr Adolesc Med* 159:1136–44.

FROM THE STATE BACTERIOLOGICAL LABORATORY
(HEAD: PROF. G. OLIN) STOCKHOLM

Rubella during Pregnancy

(1952)

Its Effects upon Perinatal Mortality, the Incidence of Congenital Abnormalities and Immaturity.
A Preliminary Report

by Rolf Lundström

In order to estimate the risk of injury to the child from rubella during pregnancy, it is necessary to study as large a number as possible of cases of rubella during pregnancy, with regard to the condition of the child at birth and subsequent development. The occasion is only provided by large epidemics and involves certain difficulties. In the majority of countries, only a small proportion of cases are notified: the disease is mild and does not, as a rule, necessitate a visit to a physician for diagnosis. No large investigation of the above mentioned kind has hitherto been made.

In the spring of 1951, a widespread epidemic of rubella broke out in Sweden. Its extent was confirmed by reports from the majority of the military units and by the large number of cases reported by the schools (see Table 1).

Inquiries addressed to the maternity welfare centres throughout the country disclosed that a not inconsiderable number of pregnant women had contracted rubella during their current pregnancy. The Royal Medical Board therefore instructed all the maternity hospitals in Sweden to question all the women who were delivered there, or who aborted spontaneously, on the following points: 1. Whether they had been in contact with any person suffering from rubella.—2. Whether they had contracted rubella during their current pregnancy.

Those who replied in the affirmative to either of these questions were also requested to state whether they had previously suffered from the disease. A questionnaire containing the following points was drawn up: name, date and place of birth, diagnosis of parturition and disease, date of last menstrual period, date of exposure to rubella and, when applicable, date of onset, date of earlier attack of rubella, whether rubella had been diagnosed by a physician on either occasion, date of parturition, data regarding earlier childbirth and/or abortions. The following data were requested with regard to

Table 1   Number of Cases of Rubella in Swedish Schools Reported to the Board of Education in January—June 1951

	No. of pupils	No. of cases of rubella	Percentage
Stockholm	61,228	5,560	9.1
Remainder of Sweden	97,593	13,729	14.1
Total	158,821	19,289	12.1

the child: sex, birth weight and length, condition at birth, with detailed information regarding possible developmental defects and, when applicable, the cause of death.

A similar questionnaire was addressed to each of the parturient women with the case-note number immediately before each of the aforementioned women; they comprised the control series.

These data were assembled quarterly between July 1, 1951 and June 20, 1952.

It may be mentioned that the majority of pregnant women in Sweden, i.e., 94.1 per cent in 1950, were delivered at the maternity hospitals in question.

Table 2 shows the distribution of the material assembled in this way. Seven pregnant women given convalescent serum when the illness was detected were not included in the series. This also applies to about 100 women who were given such serum prophylactically after contact with cases of rubella. In connexion with the epidemic, 275 women underwent legal abortion after rubella during the first four months of pregnancy (in 3 cases during the fifth to sixth month). A number of these foetuses were preserved for a future investigation. The total number of legal abortions in Sweden in 1951 amounted to 6,328.

The series assembled was classified into the following groups:

1. Cases of rubella during the 1st up to and including the 4th month of pregnancy, counted from the first day of the last menstrual period.

2. Cases of rubella from the beginning of the 5th month of pregnancy until its termination (delivery).

3. Cases of contact with rubella during the 1st up to and including the 4th month of pregnancy but without contracting the disease, although there was no knowledge of a previous attack of rubella. The

majority of these women may be assumed, with some degree of probability, not to be immune to the disease.

4. As in group 3, but contact with rubella during the 5th or subsequent months of pregnancy.

5. Cases of contact with rubella during the 1st up to and including the 4th month of pregnancy without contracting the disease, and with knowledge of a previous attack of rubella. These women may be regarded as probably immune to the disease.

6. As in group 5, but contact with rubella during the 5th or subsequent months of pregnancy.

7. Parturient women, selected at random, who had not contracted rubella during pregnancy and who had not, to their knowledge, been in contact with cases of rubella during this time.

If rubella had a pathogenic effect on the foetuses during the 1951 epidemic in Sweden, the following conditions could be anticipated. There would be a higher incidence of abnormal results of pregnancy in group 1 (rubella during the first 4 months of pregnancy) than in the control group. Those in group 3 (non-immune women exposed to rubella during the same period) may—since they did not contract the disease—be assumed to have escaped infection. This group may, however, contain women who contracted rubella in an inapparent form. In this case, a higher incidence of abnormal results of pregnancy could be expected in this group as well. Group 5 (women exposed to infection during the same period) may contain cases that should rightly be referred to group 3 on the grounds of an earlier erroneous diagnosis of rubella. Others may have escaped contact with the virus altogether. Presumably, however, a number of the women were actually infected, and if—as Béla Schick assumed (1949)—the virus can pass through the immune mother and have a pathogenic effect on the foetus, a higher incidence of abnormal results of pregnancy would be found in this group as well. Rubella, or contact with it, after the 5th month of pregnancy (groups 2, 4 and 6) should result in incidence figures in agreement with those in the control group.

The object of the present investigation was twofold: firstly, to estimate the incidence of abnormal results of pregnancy in the groups enumerated and, secondly, to analyze the differences between these incidence figures.

Any of the following conditions of the infant[1] were counted as an abnormal result of pregnancy:

---

[1] In accordance with the official Swedish statistics, an infant denotes a liveborn child or a stillborn infant at least 35 cm long. A liveborn infant is one that has breathed.

A. Stillbirth or neonatal death.

B. Congenital abnormalities discernible at birth, *i.e.*, all the pathological conditions recorded in the living infants. They consisted of anatomical malformations, blood diseases, birth injuries and other pathological conditions of unknown origin. Thus, in addition to severe malformations—such as encephalocele, myelomeningocele, deformities of the extremities of various kinds, heart disease and cataract—hypospadias, hydrocele testis and naevus were included. Such conditions as melaena, anaemia gravis, cerebral haemorrhage and asphyxia neonatorum were also referred to this category, whereas cephalohaematoma and pemphigus neonatorum were not included, as they were unimportant in the present connexion.

C. Immaturity, *i.e.*, birth weight of 2,500 grams or below.

Among those women who contracted rubella during pregnancy, the incidence of foetal defects was found to be highest when this occurred in the 2nd month and to decrease successively until the 7th month. The group with rubella during the 1st to 5th month of pregnancy exhibited a higher incidence of foetal abnormalities than the control group. On the other hand, the incidence was higher in the control group than those who contracted rubella during the 7th month of pregnancy or later.

Table 2 shows the number of women with 0, 1, 2 or several earlier childbirths, respectively.

The table discloses fairly appreciable differences. For example, primiparae predominated in the group of those who contracted rubella; this is particularly apparent in the first four months of pregnancy, whereas this tendency was not so marked in the control group. The opposite applied to those who did not contract the disease after exposure to infection. It was also found (the figures are not given here) that there was a marked tendency to a higher incidence of immatures among the primiparae. This is a strong indication for taking into consideration the selection with respect to the incidence of immaturity associated with the parity number.

The duration of pregnancy may also have a similar selective effect. An analysis (not recorded here) showed that the duration of pregnancy was practically the same in those who contracted rubella and in the controls.

Certain diseases in the mother (for example, diabetes or thyrotoxicosis) or complications during childbirth have no relationship to rubella. For this reason, and in order to illustrate the effect of rubella more clearly, they were not recorded in Table 3.

The weighted means for the relative incidence of foetal abnormalities are shown in the lower part of Table 3. The weighting was performed as

Table 2 Distribution of the Material According to the Number of Childbirths Preceding the Current Pregnancy. The Figures Denote the Number of Children in Each Group

| No. of earlier childbirths | Contracted rubella | | Contact but no attack of rubella | | | | Controls |
| | 1st–4th months of pregnancy | Subsequent months of pregnancy | No earlier attack | | Earlier attack | | |
			Contact 1st–4th mths. of pregnancy	Contact subseq. mths. of pregnancy	Contact 1st–4th mths. of pregnancy	Contact subseq. mths. of pregnancy	
0	295	184	106	146	52	70	1,035
1	131	102	105	154	44	80	746
≧2	183	172	163	228	58	97	671
Total	609	458	374	528	154	247	2,452

Table 3 Distribution of the Material According to the Number of Childbirths Preceding the Current Pregnancy. Cases of certain diseases other than rubella in the mother and complications during childbirth, respectively, are excluded. The weighted means were obtained from the arithmetical means formed by the percentage figures for the three groups 0, 1 and 2 or more childbirths, respectively. For definitions of groups D, D+M and D+M+I, see text to Fig. 1.

| Group | Contracted rubella | | Contact but no attack of rubella | | | | Controls |
| | 1st–4th months of pregnancy | Subsequent months of pregnancy | No earlier attack | | Earlier attack | | |
			Contact 1st–4th mths. of pregnancy	Contact subseq. mths. of pregnancy	Contact 1st–4th mths. of pregnancy	Contact subseq. mths. of pregnancy	
D	5.9 %	2.1 %	3.5 %	3.1 %	4.4 %	1.6 %	1.8 %
D+M	10.4 %	5.5 %	5.3 %	4.4 %	9.8 %	2.3 %	3.2 %
D+M+I	16.6 %	7.2 %	7.3 %	7.7 %	11.0 %	4.6 %	5.8 %
Total	579	450	344	508	153	240	2,226

follows. The material was grouped according to the number of previous childbirths (0, 1 and 2 or more); the relative incidence for each of these three groups was then calculated. The figures recorded in the table are the arithmetical means for the respective incidences.

Results

The investigation showed that rubella during the earlier part of pregnancy was associated with an increased incidence of stillbirths, neonatal mortality, congenital abnormalities and immaturity. This did not apply when the disease was contracted during the later months of pregnancy.

Contact with cases of rubella also increased the incidence of abnormal results of pregnancy. This increase was slight and not statistically significant for the children of non-immune mothers, whereas it was more marked—and significant—in those who might be considered as immune when they were exposed to infection, on the grounds of an earlier attack of rubella.

Discussion

The results of this investigation—made in connexion with an epidemic in Sweden in 1951—confirm the observation that rubella contracted during the early part of pregnancy has a pathogenic effect on the foetus.

A slight increase in the incidence of abnormal results of pregnancy was noted in the group of women who were presumably not immune and who were exposed to infection during the first four months of pregnancy, but did not have rubella. A possible explanation is that some of them contracted the infection but failed to recognize it as rubella. The increase is not significant; there is therefore a reason to presume that the majority of these women escaped infection on the grounds of insufficient exposure to the virus.

The rise in the aforementioned incidence was more marked in the group of immune women exposed to rubella during the 1st to 4th months of pregnancy. This indicates that the observation mentioned by Béla Schick was not necessarily an isolated phenomenon and that the prophylactic use of serum should be extended to all women exposed to rubella during early pregnancy.

Spontaneous abortions were not taken into account, since they were not recorded systematically. Those defects in the children that were not observed at birth were not recorded. A number of cases of cataract, cardiac defects and deaf-mutism may be mentioned. The results will be completed by a later follow-up examination.

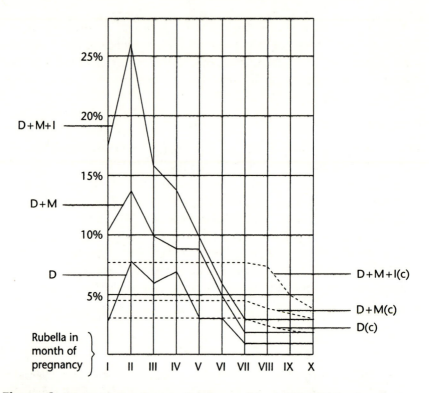

Figure 1 The incidence of congenital abnormalities: 1,067 children of mothers having had rubella during pregnancy compared to 2,452 control children.

Rubella during pregnancy (solid lines)
Curve D: Stillbirths and neonatal deaths including those of the immature infants and those with congenital abnormalities.

Curve D+M: Incidence of deaths according to the aforegoing, and of living malformed infants (including malformed immatures).

Curve D+M+I: Total incidence of dead, malformed and immature infants.
The cases of rubella in the 7th–10th months of pregnancy have been combined and the smoothed curve gives the mean incidence for these cases.

Controls (broken lines)
Curves D(c), D+M(c) and D+M+I(c): Corresponding relative incidence curves for pregnancies of the duration given on the abscissa. Because the incidence of immaturity in particular decreases for pregnancies that have lasted for 8 months and longer, the curve falls after the 8th month.

Month of pregnancy I denotes the first 30 days after the beginning of the last menstrual period; *II* denotes 31–60 days after the beginning of the last menstrual period, etc.

The diagnosis of rubella might have been incorrect. It was obtained in somewhat more than 80 per cent of the cases from the case-histories and was verified in the remainder by a medical certificate. The cases diagnosed by a physician showed no increased incidence of the foetal abnormalities in question. This fact strengthens the reliability of the diagnosis.

The time of onset might have been recalled incorrectly and referred to the wrong month of pregnancy. Thus, rubella actually occurring during the 5th month could have been referred to the 4th month and *vice versa*. This would have resulted in too low an incidence of abnormal results of pregnancy in the women who contracted rubella. With regard to the 1st month, it should be borne in mind that a number of women might have contracted the infection before conception, which may be calculated to take place—on the average—15 days after the beginning of the last menstrual period. This would explain the fact that the incidence of abnormal results of pregnancy was lower in the group of women who contracted rubella during the 1st month of pregnancy than in the corresponding group with the onset in the 2nd month (Fig. 1).

In every instance, any effect of the aforementioned sources of error would have been that the recorded figures for the incidence and foetal abnormalities would have been lower than in actual fact.

Summary

1. An investigation has been started to ascertain the pathogenic effects on the foetus of rubella in the mother during pregnancy. A preliminary report is given of these effects, as assessed at birth and shortly afterwards, in a series of 1,067 cases of rubella during pregnancy.

2. Rubella during the first 4 months of pregnancy is found to have a demonstrable effect in the form of stillbirth, neonatal death, anatomically demonstrable abnormalities and immaturity. The total incidence is approximately 17 per cent as compared to approximately 6 per cent in a concurrent control series.

3. A higher incidence (11 per cent) of abnormal foetuses than in the controls is also recorded in the following group: women who had earlier suffered from rubella, had been exposed to infection by the virus during the first 4 months of pregnancy, and had not contracted rubella on this occasion.

4. Women who had not had rubella earlier and who were known to have been in contact with rubella during their pregnancy but did not contract the disease show a slightly higher incidence (approximately 7 per cent) of abnormal foetuses than the control series. This difference is not significant.

5. After the 5th month of pregnancy, neither an attack of rubella nor exposure to the infection without contracting it is found to result in any significant difference as compared to the control series.

6. The investigation is being continued, both with regard to the further development of the children and to the results of the administration of convalescent serum.

Acknowledgements

The investigation was aided by a grant from the Swedish Medical Research Council. The statistical analyses were performed with the assistance of G. Eklund and A. Raud, of the Institute of the Statistics of the University of Uppsala. I wish to express my sincere thanks to the doctors at the maternity hospitals for their help in assembling the material.

[French, German, and Spanish translations follow but are not included here to save space, Ed.]

SOURCE

Lundström R. 1952. Rubella during pregnancy: Its effects upon perinatal mortality, the incidence of congenital abnormalities and immaturity. A preliminary report. *Acta Paediatrica* 41:583–94. Copyright 1952 *Acta Paediatrica*. Reprinted with permission of John Wiley & Sons, Ltd.

Intussusception among Recipients of Rotavirus Vaccine—United States, 1998–1999
(1999)

On August 31, 1998, a tetravalent rhesus-based rotavirus vaccine (RotaShield®*, Wyeth Laboratories, Inc., Marietta, Pennsylvania) (RRV-TV) was licensed in the United States for vaccination of infants. The Advisory Committee on Immunization Practices (ACIP), the American Academy of Pediatrics, and the American Academy of Family Physicians have recommended routine use of RRV-TV for vaccination of healthy infants (1,2). During September 1, 1998–July 7, 1999, 15 cases of intussusception (a bowel obstruction in which one segment of bowel becomes enfolded within another segment) among infants who had received RRV-TV were reported to the Vaccine Adverse Event Reporting System (VAERS). This report summarizes the clinical and epidemiologic features of these cases and preliminary data from ongoing studies of intussusception and rotavirus vaccine.

VAERS

VAERS is a passive surveillance system operated by the Food and Drug Administration (FDA) and CDC (3,4). Vaccine manufacturers are required to report to VAERS any adverse event reported to them, and health-care providers are encouraged to report any adverse event possibly attributable to vaccine. Vaccine recipients and their families also can report adverse events to VAERS. For this report, VAERS case reports of intussusception following rotavirus vaccination were reviewed, and health-care providers, parents, or guardians of patients were contacted by telephone for additional clinical and demographic information. Data on RRV-TV distribution were obtained from the manufacturer. To estimate the expected rate of intussusception among infants aged <12 months, hospital discharge data from New York for 1991–1997 were reviewed.

Of the 15 infants with intussusception reported to VAERS, 13 (87%) developed intussusception following the first dose of the three-dose RRV-TV series, and 12 (80%) of 15 developed symptoms within 1 week of receiving any dose of RRV-TV (Table 1). Thirteen of the 15 patients received concurrently other vaccines with RRV-TV. Intussusception was confirmed radiographically in all 15 patients. Eight infants required surgical reduction, and one required resection of 7 inches (18 cm) of distal ileum and proximal colon. Histopathologic examination of the distal ileum indicated

---

* Use of trade names and commercial sources is for identification purposes only and does not imply endorsement by CDC or the U.S. Department of Health and Human Services.

Table 1   Reported Cases of Intussusception among Recipients of Tetravalent Rhesus-based Rotavirus Vaccine (RRV-TV) (RotaShield®*), by State—United States, 1998–99

State	Age (mos)	Sex	No. doses received of RRV-TV	No. days from dose to symptom onset
California	7	M	2	4
California	4	F	2	14
California	3	M	1	3
California	5	M	1	59
Colorado	4	F	1	4
Colorado	3	M	1	5
Kansas	2	F	1	5
Missouri	11	M	1	5
New York	3	F	1	5
New York	2	M	1	3
North Carolina	4	F	1	5
Pennsylvania	6	M	1	3
Pennsylvania	2	M	1	4
Pennsylvania	2	M	1	29
Pennsylvania	3	M	1	7

* Use of trade names and commercial sources is for identification only and does not imply endorsement by CDC or the U.S. Department of Health and Human Services.

lymphoid hyperplasia and ischemic necrosis. All infants recovered. Onset dates of reported illness occurred from November 21, 1998, to June 24, 1999 (Figure 1). The median age of patients was 3 months (range: 2–11 months). Ten were boys. Intussusception among RRV-TV recipients was reported from seven states (Table 1). Of the 15 cases reported to VAERS, 14 were spontaneous reports and one was identified through active postlicensure surveillance.

The rate of hospitalization for intussusception among infants aged <12 months during 1991–1997 (before RRV-TV licensure) was 51 per 100,000 infant-years[†] in New York (95% confidence interval [CI]=48–54 per 100,000). The manufacturer had distributed approximately 1.8 million doses of RRV-TV as of June 1, 1999, and estimated that 1.5 million doses (83%) had been administered. Given this information, 14–16 intussus-

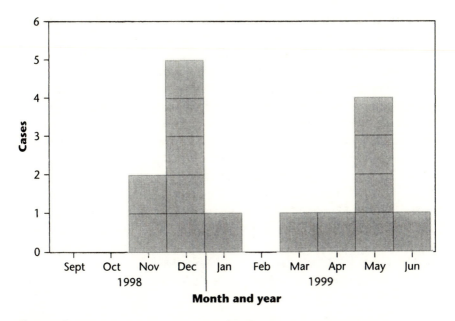

Figure 1 Number of confirmed intussusception cases among recipients of tetravalent rhesus-based rotavirus vaccine (RotaShield®*) reported to the Vaccine Adverse Event Reporting System, by month of onset—United States, September 1988–June 1999.

* Use of trade names and commercial sources is for identification only and does not imply endorsement by CDC or the U.S. Department of Health and Human Services.

ception cases among infants would be expected by chance alone during the week following receipt of any dose of RRV-TV. Fourteen of the 15 case-patients were vaccinated before June 1, 1999, and of those, 11 developed intussusception within 1 week of receiving RRV-TV.

Postlicensure Studies of Adverse Events Following RRV-TV

As part of a preliminary analysis of ongoing postlicensure surveillance of adverse events following vaccination with RRV-TV, cases of intussusception during December 1, 1998–June 10, 1999, were identified among infants aged 2–11 months at Northern California Kaiser Permanente (NCKP) by review of hospital discharge diagnoses, admitting diagnoses for the records for which discharge summaries were not yet complete, and computerized records of all barium enemas performed on children

---

† An infant-year is a unit of measurement combining infants and time used as a denominator in calculating incidence. In this report, it is the sum of the individual units of time (days, weeks, or months) converted to years that the infants in the study population have been followed.

aged <1 year. Relative risks were age-adjusted because of differences in the ages of vaccinated and unvaccinated infants, and p values were calculated by Poisson regression.

At NCKP, 16,627 doses of RRV-TV were administered to 9,802 infants during December 1, 1998–June 10, 1999. Nine cases of intussusception among infants were identified with onset during that same period, all of which were radiographically or surgically confirmed. Three were among vaccinated children, with intervals of 3, 15, and 58 days following vaccination. The rate of intussusception among never-vaccinated children was 45 per 100,000 infant-years, and among children who had received RRV-TV was 125 per 100,000 infant-years (age-adjusted relative risk [RR] = 1.9, 95% CI = 0.5–7.7, p = 0.39). The rate among children who had received RRV-TV during the preceding 3 weeks was 219 per 100,000 infant-years (age-adjusted RR = 3.7, 95% CI = 0.7–19, p = 0.12). Among children who had received RRV-TV during the previous week, the rate was 314 per 100,000 infant-years (age-adjusted RR = 5.7, 95% CI = 0.7–50, p = 0.11).

Minnesota

In Minnesota, intussusception cases were identified among infants aged 30 days–11 months who were born after April 1, 1998, and were hospitalized with radiographically or surgically confirmed intussusception with onset during November 1, 1998–June 30, 1999. During October 1, 1998–June 1, 1999, 62,916 doses of vaccine were distributed. Eighteen cases of intussusception were identified, five of which were among infants who had received RRV-TV. Vaccinated children had a median age of 4 months (range: 3–5 months), and unvaccinated children had a median age of 7 months (range: 5–9 months). Four of the five RRV-TV recipients with intussusception required surgical reduction, and five of 13 unvaccinated children required surgical reduction. Intussusception occurred after receipt of dose one (two children), dose two (two children), and dose three (one child). The five RRV-TV recipients developed intussusception within 2 weeks of receipt of vaccine; intervals were 6 days (two children), 7 days, 10 days, and 14 days after receipt of vaccine. Assuming 85% of RRV-TV doses distributed in Minnesota were administered, the observed rate of intussusception within 1 week of receipt of RRV-TV was 292 per 100,000 infant-years.

Reported by: K Ehresman, MPH, R Lynfield, MD, R Danila, PhD, Acting State Epidemiologist, Minnesota Dept of Health. S Black, MD, H Shinefield, MD, B Fireman, MS, S Cordova, MS, Kaiser Permanente Vaccine Study Center, Oakland, California. Div of Biostatistics and Epidemiology, Food and Drug Administration. Viral Gastroenteritis Section, Respiratory and Enteric Viruses Br, and Office of the

Director, Div of Viral and Rickettsial Diseases, National Center for Infectious Diseases; Vaccine Safety Datalink Team; Statistical Analysis Br, Data Management Div; Vaccine Safety and Development Activity; Child Vaccine Preventable Diseases Br, Epidemiology and Surveillance Div, National Immunization Program; and EIS officers, CDC.

Editorial Note

Rotavirus is the most common cause of severe gastroenteritis in infants and young children aged <5 years in the United States, resulting in approximately 500,000 physician visits, 50,000 hospitalizations, and 20 deaths each year. Worldwide, rotavirus is a major cause of childhood death, accounting for an estimated 600,000 deaths annually among children aged <5 years. Rotavirus vaccines offer the opportunity to reduce substantially the occurrence of this disease (1).

In prelicensure studies, five cases of intussusception occurred among 10,054 vaccine recipients and one of 4,633 controls, a difference that was not statistically significant (5). Three of the five cases among vaccinated children occurred within 6–7 days of receiving rotavirus vaccine. On the basis of these data, intussusception was included as a potential adverse reaction on the package insert, and the ACIP recommended postlicensure surveillance for this adverse event following vaccination (1).

Because of concerns about intussusception identified in prelicensure trials, VAERS data were analyzed early in the postlicensure period. The number of reported intussusception case-patients with illness onset within 1 week of receiving any dose of vaccine is in the expected range; however, because reporting to VAERS of adverse events following vaccination is incomplete (6), the actual number of intussusception cases among RRV-TV recipients may be substantially greater than that reported.

In response to the VAERS reports, a preliminary analysis of data from an ongoing postlicensure study at NCKP was performed, and a multistate investigation was initiated to determine whether an association exists between administration of RRV-TV and intussusception in infants. Preliminary data from Minnesota and from NCKP also suggest an increased risk for intussusception following receipt of RRV-TV. Observed rates of intussusception among recently vaccinated children were similar in both studies. However, the number of cases of intussusception among vaccinated children is small at both NCKP and in Minnesota, and neither study has adequate power to establish a statistically significant difference in incidence of intussusception among vaccinated and unvaccinated children. Available data suggest but do not establish a causal association between receipt of rotavirus vaccine and intussusception, and additional studies are ongoing.

Although neither these studies nor the VAERS reports is conclusive, the consistency of findings from these three data sources raises strong concerns. Because more data are anticipated within several months and rotavirus season is still 4–6 months away in most areas of the United States, CDC recommends postponing administration of RRV-TV to children scheduled to receive the vaccine before November 1999, including those who already have begun the RRV-TV series. Parents or caregivers of children who have recently received rotavirus vaccine should promptly contact their health-care provider if the infant develops symptoms consistent with intussusception (e.g., persistent vomiting, bloody stools, black stools, abdominal distention, and/or severe colic pain). Health-care providers should consider intussusception in infants who have recently received RRV-TV and present with a consistent clinical syndrome; early diagnosis may increase the probability that the intussusception can be treated successfully without surgery. Vaccine providers, parents, and caregivers should report to VAERS intussusception and other adverse events following vaccination.

Information on reporting to VAERS and case report forms can be requested 24 hours a day by telephone, (800) 822–7967, or the World-Wide Web, http://www.nip.gov/nip/vaers.htm.

Source

Ehresman K, Lynfield R, Danila R, Black S, Shinefield H, Fireman B, and Cordova S. 1999. Intussusception among recipients of rotavirus vaccine—United States, 1998–1999. *MMWR* 48:577–81.

Herd Immunity: Basic Concept and Relevance to Public Health Immunization Practices
(1971, Abridged)

John P. Fox, Lila Elveback, William Scott, Lael Gatewood, and Eugene Ackerman

Specific immunization has long been a basic tool in medical practice and in local, state, national and international public health. However, the protection afforded by such immunization has been largely limited to persons immunized because: 1) the usual sources of infection are extra-human (tetanus, yellow fever); 2) spread is primarily by indirect means (typhoid); or 3) those immunized may remain at least partially susceptible to infection and, hence, continue as potential links in the future spread of agents transmitted by contact (diphtheria, pertussis, Salk-type inactivated polio vaccine). An important exception has been vaccination against smallpox which does induce solid though temporary resistance to infection. Presumably as the result of systematic vaccination, endemic smallpox has disappeared from large areas including the United States and major efforts are now in progress to eliminate the disease in developing countries as in West Africa (1).

The advent of live virus vaccines against poliomyelitis, measles and, most recently, rubella, has raised realistic hopes that, as with smallpox, these diseases also can be made to disappear from large populations by means of large-scale immunization programs. Whether in developing or developed countries, the planning of such programs, if they are to be of maximum effectiveness, requires full understanding of the principle of herd immunity and of all the factors which influence its operation.

That the factors influencing the operation of herd immunity are not fully understood by many people was well illustrated during the 1969 meetings of the American Public Health Association. A report on measles epidemics in West Africa (2), where over 90 per cent of the population is immune, including virtually all those over two years of age, was followed by a number of questions from the floor concerning the fact that epidemics continue to occur despite the large proportion of immunes. These questions stemmed from the currently prevailing concept that, as defined in a medical dictionary (3), herd immunity is "the resistance of the group to attack by a disease to which a large proportion of the numbers are immune, thus lessening the likelihood of a patient with a disease coming into contact with the susceptible individual."

This concept is directly applicable only to randomly mixing populations. However, truly random mixing can be assumed only for certain small closed populations and never occurs in open populations. In his treatise on the mathematical theory of epidemics, Bailey (4) states: "it is well known that epidemics in a large population can often be broken down into smaller epidemics occurring in separate regional subdivisions. These smaller epidemics are in general not in phase but interact with each other to some extent. We could hardly assume even a small town to be a single homogeneously mixing unit. Each individual is normally in close contact with only a small number of individuals, perhaps of the order of 10–15. The observed figures are therefore pooled data for several epidemics occurring simultaneously in small groups of associates. In reality such groups overlap and interact."

In his review article on epidemic theory (5), Serfling notes that as early as 1906 it was recognized that "the progress of an epidemic is regulated by the number of susceptibles and the rate of contact between infectious cases and susceptibles." While the literature on epidemic theory since 1906 contains excellent expositions of the concept of herd immunity, these are usually embedded in rather mathematical discussions of the validity of various epidemic models. Hence, it seems appropriate to offer a simple and minimally mathematical presentation which explicitly identifies and illustrates the factors which favor the spread of infection in populations containing many immunes and those which restrict such spread.

Crucial to our presentation is the recognition that open populations are made up of innumerable definable but often interlocking subgroups which differ in respect to proportions of immunes and intimacy of contact. In particular, we will try to show how variations of these population characteristics may affect "the rate of contact between infectious cases and susceptibles" and, hence, determine whether epidemic spread will occur.

Some Basic Assumptions

For the sake of simplicity, we will confine our discussion and illustrations to agents restricted to man and spread only by person-to-person contact. Also, we assume that the following postulates are generally applicable.

1. Individuals are either susceptible or fully immune, and immunity is durable.

2. The period of infectiousness is short, and is of approximately the same length for all who become infected.

3. There is no need to allow for "removals," that is for the withdrawal from circulation of infectives who become ill. (This may be because

many infections are silent and those illnesses which do occur are mild, or because the period of greatest infectivity precedes the onset of illness as in measles.)

Since the purpose of an immunization program is to halt the spread of the agent, and our purpose here is to study herd immunity, we will confine ourselves entirely to infection and will not consider illness. The word "case" throughout will refer to a person who is infectious to others, or more simply, to an infective.

First we will consider the importance, or lack of importance, of the proportion immune in a randomly mixing population. We will, by considering the simplest of models, develop the tools which will enable us to tackle the more complex problems of the multiple and overlapping mixing groups which exist in all societies.

Randomly Mixing Populations—The Reed-Frost Model

A randomly mixing population is one in which the probability of contact within any time interval is the same for every choice of two individuals in the population. Epidemic models based on random mixing have been used in connection with small closed populations such as those of orphanages, boarding schools or companies of military recruits (5–7).

One of the simplest models, and one with which most persons in public health work are acquainted, is that which Reed and Frost taught for many years at Johns Hopkins. For demonstration, they used a mechanical model in which random mixing was illustrated by stirring up a collection of colored balls. The Reed-Frost model involves consideration of discrete equal intervals of time (such as days or weeks) which, in our illustrations, we will take as equal to the length of the period of infectivity. Then, if a person becomes infected during the interval from t to $t + 1$ (the first week) he becomes infectious to others at $t + 1$ (the beginning of the second week), ceases to be infective and becomes permanently immune at $t + 2$ (the beginning of the third week).

The Reed-Frost model and its application in one extended example are described in some detail in the Appendix. Two definitions are particularly important to understanding this model: 1) *adequate contact* between two individuals is that sufficient to allow transmission of the infecting agent from an infectious person to a susceptible; and 2) the *contact rate, p,* is the probability that *any* two persons in the population will make adequate contact during any interval. This contact rate thus summarizes both the infectivity of the agent and the social habits of the population. It also is important to understand that the *expected number of contacts during any interval* for any member of the population is the product of the contact rate, p, and a number of potential contacts (the total population or N minus one) and that these contacts will be distributed between susceptibles, immunes and infective cases in the proportions in which each are present in the population during the specified time interval.

A simple, first example begins with the play group of 11 children of whom 10 are susceptibles and one is an infective and examines the consequences of increasing the size of the play group by adding five immunes. These are summarized in the following tabulation. [see table on next page, Ed.]

It can be seen that, if the contact rate (p) is unchanged, addition of the immunes does not alter the probability of no spread. Although the expected total number of contacts by case (m) is increased, the additional contacts are wasted on immunes. However, if m is held constant at 2 when the immunes are added, the contact rate decreases as does the expected number of contacts with susceptibles (m') and the probability of no spread increases.

A second example extends the Reed-Frost model to the introduction of a single infected case into larger populations ranging in size from 400 to 10,000 while one of the six pairs of specified characteristics are held constant and others are allowed to change. In practice the average number of contacts per person per interval (m) will be relatively constant as the total population size (N) increases. However, examples in which p is constant and m or $p(N-1)$ increases with N are included in example 2 for the sake of completeness and to stress the underlying principles. The results expected in each of these situations are shown in some detail and table 2 (Appendix) but our interest centers in the columns indicating number of susceptibles, average number of contacts with susceptibles, probability of no spread and epidemic size. The important relations shown can be summarized as follows:

1. The expected number of contacts by the case with susceptibles during the first interval, pS_0 completely determines the probability of no spread, $P(A)$;
   a. if pS_0 is constant, so is $P(A)$ (sets 1 and 2),
   b. if pS_0 is increases, $P(A)$ declines (sets 3 and 4),
   c. if pS_0 falls, $P(A)$ rises (sets 5 and 6).

2. Given constant pS_0 and $P(A)$, the median epidemic size increases with the number of susceptibles (set 2).

3. Population size, proportion immune and contact rate influence the probability of spread and median epidemic size *only* when, under the conditions postulated, their change necessarily causes changes in number of susceptibles (sets 2, 3 and 6) or in average number of contacts with susceptibles (sets 3, 4, 5 and 6).

Play group composition at beginning of the first interval				Contact rate	Expected number of contacts by case in first interval			Probability of no spread
Size	Cases	Susceptibles	Immunes		with susceptibles	with immunes	Total	
N	C	S	I	p	$m'=pS$	$w=pI$	$m=p(N-1)$	$(1-p)^S$
11	1	10	0	0.2	2	0	2	.107
16	1	10	5	0.2	2	1	3	.107
16	1	10	5	1.33	1.33	0.67	2	.239

In brief summary, the application of the Reed-Frost model in the fore-going examples demonstrates that, over a wide range of variations, the number of susceptibles and the rate of contact between them determine epidemic potentials in randomly mixing populations. If these are held constant, changes in population size and, therefore, in the proportion immune do not influence the probability of spread.

Populations with Complex Mixing Structure

As noted already, random mixing serves as an adequate approximation of contacts between individuals only in certain small closed populations. In this section we will consider the more complex mixing structures of real-life, free-living populations as typified by a large city. In a typical city in the United States there may be a densely populated central area surrounded by various residential neighborhoods of differing population density and also differing in respect to economic, occupational and educational characteristics. Superimposed are school districts, the pediatrician's office, health department clinics, shopping areas, entertainment or recreational centers, transportation systems and occupational or business groups. Some of these may be heterogeneous with respect to cultural and socioeconomic factors and all may play a role in creating paths along which infection may spread from one otherwise isolated subgroup to another.

Important Mixing Groups

The *basic unit*, social and epidemiologic, is the *family or household*, within which the contact rate between members is high, whether they be of the same or quite different age groups. In some countries or cultures the effective household may be quite large, consisting of several related families living in one compound.

In general, the between-family contacts will be higher for neighborhoods in the same *geographic neighborhood*. The role of neighborhoods in the spread of infection may be quite variable from one society to another. The habit common to American children of running in and out of neighboring houses, having lunch or "sleeping over" with Johnny is obviously of real importance as a type of population mixing, as are the "coffee klatch" and neighborhood events such as picnics and Christmas parties. Also, common recreational interests, membership in the same religious group or social club and similarity in ages of children will result in the definition of *clusters of families* between which contact will be more intimate than that with other families in the same neighborhood.

The *schools* serve to bring together subgroups of the population defined by age, by broad area of residence and, in many cases, by socioeconomic status. They bring together children from different families and different immediate neighborhoods. Further, in rural and suburban areas, the school bus service is a particularly effective exposure chamber for respiratory agent spread. Since schoolchildren are characterized by high susceptibility rates for many infectious diseases, the schools provide potentially important paths of spread from one part of the population to another. Hence, whether or not the school is open may be of major importance as in the occurrence of an epidemic (as in influenza).

The largest proportion of susceptibles is usually found among *preschool children*. The preschool child, according to the social habits of his society, will be exposed to the other members of his family, school age sibs and parents, and to the preschool children in other families through the naturally occurring neighborhood play groups. In addition, preschool children from birth on are apt to accompany their mothers to the market place (as in West Africa where the mothers carry their small children on their backs) and on other errands. In such societies, as is evident from the epidemic occurrence of measles in West Africa despite the high proportion of immunes, this practice alone may create high contact rates among large groups of susceptible infants and preschool children. In other societies the nursery school (or day care center), church school, or community playgrounds may serve this purpose.

The Distribution of Immunes

In general, the most important stratification of the community by immune status is that by age. The proportion immune increases with age and, for highly infectious agents, will approach unity at some point in life. In developed countries this may be in early adulthood, e.g. measles in the USA, while in developing countries this may be very early in childhood, e.g. measles in West Africa. However, within the population of a community, there may be pockets of susceptibles, either because prior epidemics have failed to spread into the group or because they have not accepted immunization. Current important examples in the USA relate to measles and poliomyelitis, both of which continue to occur in small outbreaks among unvaccinated groups characterized by low economic and educational status.

A Community Mixing Model

In this example we will consider 100 susceptible children and one infected child whose opportunities for contact with each other depend on various types of social mixing groups. These may be considered as part of a much larger community of families. Although it is not necessary to specify the total community size or the proportion immune, important

Table 1 Distribution by Size of Epidemics among 100 Susceptible Children in a Community of Families, Play Groups, and a Nursery School*

Mixing groups	Within group contact rate	No. of epidemics with indicated nos. of cases										Medium epidemic size	Mean no. of cases	Maximum no. of cases
		1	2	3	4	5-9	10-19	20-29	30-39	40-59	60-79			
Total community	.002	82	15	2	1							1	1.2	4
Total community	.002	22	18	34	8	17	1					3	3.3	16
Families	.500													
Total community	.002													
Families	.500	11	6	26	23	23	9	1	1			4	5.6	33
Play groups	.100													
Total community	.002													
Families	.500	23	4							28	45	58	45	73
Play groups	.100													
Nursery school	.100													

*Observed distributions of epidemics size from computer simulations of an extension of the Reed-Frost model to allow for multiple mixing groups, based on 100 simulated epidemics per situation. The 100 susceptible children and the case were in 62 families containing 1 to 3 children (average 1.6) and in 24 play groups containing up to 10 children (average 4.2). The case was in a 3-child family and a 5-child play group. Although the case did not attend nursery school, his two younger siblings did.

aspects of the distribution of these children are noted in the footnote to table 1.

The Reed-Frost model will apply here only as it pertains to within subgroup mixing, that is to a single family, a single nursery school, or a small neighborhood preschool play group. It will, however, provide a useful framework of terms and definitions.

Four situations will be considered. In the first there is no contact beyond the total community mixing at a very low level (a random mixing case); in the second we allow also for high contact rates within the family or household; in the third we add small play groups in which children of neighboring families come in contact; and in the fourth we add a nursery school which is attended by 40 of the 100 susceptible children. The purpose is to show that, with a fixed number of susceptibles, as we allow more and more opportunity for contacts between susceptibles, the epidemic potential increases *whether or not* the proportion immune remains constant.

Table 1 presents the results in terms of the distribution by size of 100 computer-simulated epidemics per situation using a model (8) in which each separate group (family, play group, nursery school, total community) is randomly mixing but with differing contact rates prevailing in each. With contact depending entirely on total community mixing, 82 per cent of the trials resulted in no spread and the maximum epidemic size was four cases. When contacts within families were taken into account, only 22 per cent of the trials resulted in no spread but 74 per cent had three or fewer cases. With play group mixing added, 34 per cent of the epidemic trials resulted in more than five cases and in only 11 did spread fail to occur. Finally, when the nursery school of 40 children was opened, 73 per cent of the epidemics spread through more than one half of the susceptibles, the median epidemic size was 58, and the largest epidemic reached 73 of the 100 susceptibles. It also is of interest that the distribution of epidemic size has assumed the bimodality typical of contact rates high enough to permit large epidemics but not high enough to insure them. Here the introduction of a single case resulted in virtually no spread in 27 per cent of the trials, in large epidemics in the remaining 73 per cent and in no outbreaks of moderate size. The effective contact rate was high enough that, in every case in which three or more persons were infected, the epidemic caught fire and continued to more than 40 cases.

Discussion

The foregoing examples should have made it clear that for a given infectious agent, epidemic potential is determined by the number of susceptibles and the nature and frequency of their contacts with each other. If these characteristics of the population are held constant, other characteristics such as the size of the total population and the proportion immune have no influence on the epidemic potential. In this light, the question "what proportion of the population should be immunized to prevent an epidemic?", is not answerable in absolute terms. First, the question must be restated to allow for the element of chance, e.g. "What proportion of the population must be immunized to lower the probability of an epidemic of more than 10 cases below 5 per cent?" To reach even an approximate answer we must consider:

1. The infectivity, method of spread and viability of the infectious agent.

2. The season, and what effect this has on population mixing (school open or closed) and the viability of the agent.

3. The number of susceptibles and their distribution by age, geographic area, economic status, etc.

4. The social habits of the society with respect to mixing groups which provide the type of contacts involved in the transfer of infection.

5. Some estimates of the subgroup contact rates among susceptibles.

Considerable information concerning items 1 and 2 ordinarily will exist and information concerning item 3 usually can be developed. Items 4 and 5 pose real difficulties. We can differentiate broadly between West Africa and the United States in terms of social habits, we can recognize important differences between urban and rural areas, and we can define populations linked by specific schools. Unfortunately, precise definition of the multitude of interlocking mixing groups in large populations and estimation of their respective contact rates are not possible to achieve. Nonetheless, recognition of the dominant influence of these factors on agent spread can help assure that an immunization program will be maximally effective. It is not enough to know how non-immunes are distributed in the total population by age alone. We also should know how they are distributed in population subgroups defined by such other attributes as place of residence, economic status, ethnic origin, and religious affiliation.

This concept is hardly novel in that recurrent, usually small, outbreaks of such generally well-controlled diseases as diphtheria, measles and poliomyelitis continue to occur in population subgroups characterized by their reluctance to accept immunization and which, typically, also can be defined in terms of race, though educational and economic level and even, as described in the following, religious preference. This latter is dramatically illustrated by a small outbreak of smallpox which lingered on for several months in the unusually well immunized community of Abakalike in Eastern Nigeria (9). Investigation revealed that it was confined entirely to members of a small religious sect who refused vaccination and who, despite dispersal throughout the community, maintained both close social ties within the group and relative segregation from the rest of the population. This experience, together with the theoretical considerations herein presented, suggest that, to reduce the probability of epidemic spread to the minimum, an immunization program should be preceded whenever possible by surveys to identify particularly susceptible population subgroups and be characterized by special efforts to reach groups so identified. In effect, this is a strategy to increase to the maximum the number of susceptibles immunized which, in view of the inescapable but important uncertainties described, must be the goal of every immunization program.

The foregoing considerations are most relevant to programs and systematic immunization such as those directed against polio, measles and, more recently, rubella in the United States which have as their ultimate goal elimination of the causative agent from the country. A different strategy uses probability of exposure rather than susceptibility to guide administration of vaccine. Thus, in countries previously freed of smallpox, reintroduction is followed by strenuous efforts to contain the disease, including intensive vaccination to build a wall of immunes about the newly recognized focus. This strategy also has been employed in West Africa since 1968 to supplement the program of general mass immunization now underway. Dubbed "eradication escalation," this new effort represents "a specific attack on transmission of smallpox when the disease is at its seasonal low ebb." As an intensive nationwide search leads to the recognition of new cases and epidemiologic investigations reveal their sources and contacts, intensive vaccination is employed to contain the focus. This strategy is believed to have greatly accelerated the very dramatic progress made in eradicating smallpox from this region (1).

Summary

Examples demonstrate that the potential for contact spread of an agent depends entirely on the number of susceptibles and their opportunities for contact with each other. The purpose of an immunization program is to reduce the supply of susceptibles to such an extent that the probability of spread is very small.

Free living populations of communities are made up of multiple and interlocking mixing groups, defined in such terms as families, family clusters, neighborhoods, playgroups, schools, places of work, ethnic and socioeconomic subgroups. These mixing groups are characterized by differing contact rates and by differing numbers of susceptibles. The optimum

immunization program is one which will reduce the supply of susceptibles in all subgroups. No matter how large the proportion of immunes in
the total population, if some pockets of the community, such as low economic neighborhoods, contain a large number of susceptibles among
whom contacts are frequent, the epidemic potential in the neighborhoods
will remain high.

Success of a systematic immunization program requires knowledge
of the age and subgroup distribution of the susceptibles and maximum
effort to reduce their concentration throughout the community, rather
than aiming to reach any specified overall proportion of the population.

Addendum

Since this paper was submitted, a particularly appropriate illustration of
the thesis presented has come to attention. Scott (10) has described epidemic measles in Rhode Island in 1968 which was virtually confined to
an "ethnic Island" (Portuguese, chiefly recent immigrants) in a highly vaccinated general population. In this episode, the agent was introduced from
Portugal via a three-year-old child who was developing disease as he
arrived.

Appendix

The Reed-Frost Model

A full discussion of this model is given elsewhere (6, 7). [The remainder
of the appendix is statistical and not included here, Ed.]

SOURCE

Fox JP, Elveback L, Scott W, Gatewood L, and Ackerman E. 1971. Herd immu-
nity: Basic concept and relevance to public health immunization practices.
Am J Epidemiol 94:179–89. Copyright 1971 *American Journal of Epidemiology*.
Reprinted with permission of Oxford University Press.

CHAPTER 11

CANCER

We are here today for the purpose of signing the Cancer Act of 1971. I hope that in the years ahead that we may look back on this day and this action as being the most significant action taken during this administration. It could be, because when we consider what cancer does each year in the United States, we find that more people each year die of cancer in the United States than all the Americans who lost their lives in World War II.

—Richard M. Nixon (1913–1994), president of the United States
Remarks upon signing the National Cancer Act, 1971

On March 21, 1973, John Dean, White House Counsel, informed President Richard M. Nixon, "There's a cancer growing on the presidency." The use of cancer as an analogy was apt, as two years before, the Nixon administration had declared a "war on cancer." Nixon sought to make "conquest of cancer a national crusade." Indeed, for the final three decades of the twentieth century, cancer held primacy in terms of both public attention and U.S. dollars for health research.

The high fatality rate of the disease, the seeming randomness in its occurrence, and the prevalence of malignancies in the developed world resulted in unusually strong public support for cancer research. Yet the biological complexities of cancer have confounded intense efforts to discern how and why cancerous cells develop. Considerable advances in our understanding of occupational, environmental, and other causes of cancer have not translated to improved treatment strategies. They have, however, led to the development of stricter exposure limits for workers handling carcinogenic materials. Also, decline in the prevalence of cigarette smoking in many countries in the developed world has been matched by a fall in cancer incidence, particularly lung cancer incidence. The cancer story in the twentieth century began with three simultaneous efforts: to define what is meant by the term "cancer," to create an organizational infrastructure to facilitate cancer research, and to establish whether cancer incidence was increasing.

What Does "Cancer" Mean?

The effort to define what was meant by the term "cancer" began with the work of James Ewing, one of the first academic pathologists in the United States and founder of the Memorial Sloan-Kettering Cancer Center in New York City. Although his work touched on every major area of pathology, Ewing is best known for his work in cancer. He identified a particular malignancy of the bone that has come to be known as Ewing's sarcoma, he advocated early for the use of radium to treat cancer, and he postulated the role of trauma in the etiology of cancer. This last contribution influenced thinking about the origin of cancer for almost four decades. Although many organic carcinogens were identified in the 1920s and 1930s, Ewing's seminal observation that trauma led to the development of all cancers meant that any etiologic factor for cancer had to be explained in terms of injury. It was not until the 1940s that carcinogenic mechanisms not involving injury began to appear in the medical literature.

Ewing was not the only advocate for radiation therapy for cancer. Francis Carter Wood, a leading physician at St. Luke's Hospital in New York City, also campaigned for the use of radiation in the treatment of cancer. Wood also recognized the need for accurate data on cancer incidence and campaigned for active surveillance of cancer in the population. He thought that through such data, cancer control efforts, such as screening for breast cancer, might be better focused. Wood also understood the role of professional societies in the development of a field such as cancer medicine; he was not only a member of the American Association for Cancer Research but also its president twice and the editor of its journal for a decade.

The creation of an organizational infrastructure to facilitate cancer research was also a key development in the first part of the twentieth century. In the United States, the American Association for Cancer Research was formed in 1907, and the American Society for Cancer Control (which became the American Cancer Society) was formed in 1913. The Imperial Cancer Research Fund was founded in 1902 as the Cancer Research Fund, changing to its current name in 1904. Other organizations developed globally in the first quarter of the twentieth century, all with a focus on cancer research. Through the meetings of such societies, considerable information was exchanged by scientists and clinicians.

A key focus of early cancer research challenged whether the incidence of cancer was increasing. Many cancer researchers held that it was, but other members of the community suggested the incidence was constant and the perceived increase reflected better detection. The arguments raged on both sides from 1910 through about 1930, and much effort was expended to assess whether better diagnosis alone could explain the newly collected data suggesting increased occurrence of the disease. In 1925, for instance, the American Public Health Association (APHA) investigated the feasibility of population-based cancer registries; APHA was unable to recommend such surveillance after considering the costs involved and the low likelihood of sufficient funding to support those efforts. Such registries were initiated in the 1930s and early 1940s in the United States and elsewhere, but it would not be until the 1960s and 1970s that cancer registries became one of the cornerstones of cancer control and prevention programs.

One of the key developments during the early part of the twentieth century was the acceptance that cancer was not one disease but rather a collection of diseases with similar underlying pathophysiological processes. Cancer cells displayed uncontrolled growth; they invaded adjacent tissue; and they sometimes spread to other parts of the body via lymph or blood. With this change in thinking, it was no longer a question of whether cancer in general was increasing; the issue was whether cancer for a given organ was increasing. Moreover, the question of how much cancer there was challenged policymakers. One of the first activities of the NCI (founded in 1937 with Francis Carter Wood on its National Cancer Advisory Board) was the First National Cancer Survey. The survey established the extent to which cancer was a burden on the U.S. population, and it suggested where prevention efforts could best be focused.

Lung Cancer

By the late 1930s, increasing lung cancer mortality in the United States and Britain caught the attention of public health officials. A number of hypotheses were advanced as possible explanations for these increases, including tobacco use, air pollution, industrial pollutants, and tuberculosis. Some preliminary investigations into air pollution generally and industrial pollutants in particular suggested that these were not the agents for the increase in lung cancer. Because tobacco smoking was seen as one variant of air pollution, it, too, was excluded as a source of the increase, though such exclusion was controversial (see Chapter 2). Tuberculosis was seen as a potential explanation by some researchers, but the evidence was neither consistent nor compelling. By World War II, tuberculosis had effectively been eliminated as a source of the increase in lung cancer.

In Nazi Germany during the 1930s, a strong national effort against cancer resulted in the identification of several potent carcinogens, including asbestos and tobacco smoke. Lung cancer was a targeted disease, and controls were sought that would minimize exposures to identified lung carcinogens. The German government implemented a strong antismoking campaign that lasted until the end of World War II. Although the effort did not completely escape notice by the medical community outside of Germany, it also did not influence health policy in either the United States or Britain.

With the onset of World War II, researchers' endeavors focused on the immediate task of supporting military activities, and cancer research efforts declined. Although some seminal research continued, such as that on the relationship between asbestos and lung cancer (see Chapter 5), further investigations would await the end of hostilities. In the United States in 1947, the Second National Cancer Survey disclosed that cancer in general was not increasing markedly in the population but the incidence of lung cancer had increased. That same year in Britain, concern with the rising lung cancer death rate led the MRC to sponsor a variety of investigations, including one into the potential for air pollution as a cause of the increase, and another that was a case-control study of lung cancer and tobacco smoking. The results from the latter showed a strong relationship between smoking and lung cancer (Doll and Hill, 1950), one of the three major publications that defined the tobacco–lung cancer association (see Chapter 2).

THE ENVIRONMENT

The publication of the case-control results from a variety of researchers, all associating lung cancer with cigarette smoking, set the stage for three cohort studies: the British Doctors Study, the U.S. VA Life Insurance Study, and the American Cancer Society Study. Although these studies were important for the evolving understanding of the role of smoking in the development of lung cancer, they also showed that smoking might be associated with the development of cancer at sites other than the lungs. However, they also demonstrated that other factors in the general environment and in personal habits might be causal for cancer. For example, Ernst Wynder, in the wake of his 1950 paper with Evarts Graham, undertook a series of case-control studies into cancers of every organ. Although he determined that many cancer sites were associated with smoking, he also identified factors in the general environment and among personal habits as being associated with specific cancers. At the same time, the relationship between occupational exposure and various cancers began to emerge. The notion of cancer as a genetically mediated disease began to give way to one in which factors in the general environment, including personal habits, were seen as causal for these diseases.

A second offshoot of the 1950 publication of the results of the case-control studies on lung cancer and smoking was the realization of the global need for cancer incidence data. Although there were independent national and local efforts to establish population-based cancer registries, by the 1970s the WHO came to view such activities as part of its global cancer-control program. Comparison of cancer incidence data among the various registries yielded many testable etiological hypotheses, many of which were the focus of research efforts during the last two decades of the twentieth century. These data also provided a strong base for the activities of the International Agency for Research on Cancer (IARC), founded in 1965 as an extension of the WHO. By the end of the century, the global geographical extent of cancer could be assessed for each of the various sites at which it develops.

One successful strategy that emerged during the middle part of the twentieth century to better understand the etiology of cancer was investigating groups with particularly intense exposures to potential carcinogens. For example, asbestos workers were studied to determine which organ systems might be most vulnerable to the carcinogenic properties of asbestos. Similarly, other occupational groups were examined, some more successfully than others. For instance, studies of rubber workers established the carcinogenic potential associated with exposure to benzene. This model of special exposures was exploited to great success among the survivors of the atomic bombings of Hiroshima and Nagasaki. Shortly after the bombings, the United States and Japan organized the Atomic Bomb Casualty Commission to study the long-term effects of radiation exposure among the survivors. Now known as the Radiation Effects Research Foundation, this effort provided much of the information used for constructing exposure thresholds for ionizing radiation (such as might be encountered during an x-ray).

Exposure to environmental radiation emerged as a focal point of popular concerns during the latter portion of the twentieth century. Residents near the Sellafield nuclear facility in England grew anxious about the effects of the plant's radiation on their health. Several studies suggested that the effects were minimal, but the public was not assuaged. In the United States, similar concerns—occupational and environmental—arose for the Hanford, Washington, nuclear facility. Although the U.S. government reported many studies suggesting there was no danger, nongovernmental scientists such as British physician and radiation expert Alice Stewart argued otherwise. The degree to which an elevated risk exists is still a point of contention within the public health community.

A prominent component of the investigations into the environment as a source of cancer appeared in the late 1970s with the development of geographical mapping programs. One result was the county-level mapping of mortality for selected cancer sites in the United States over a 20-year period. This led some areas to be labeled as dangerous; for example, the media dubbed New Jersey "Cancer Alley." The scale of the data was problematic, and it became clear that potential sources of carcinogens had been overlooked, such as shipyards in which asbestos had been used during World War II activity. This approach of identifying populations at risk for specific cancers has since been widely adopted, including by many of the cancer registries, to develop hypotheses about the origins of human cancers. Many observational studies have been undertaken in recent decades to test these hypotheses.

A major component of our environment is sunshine. Its effects on cancer have been examined in terms of the direct development of cancer cells (particularly for malignant melanoma and also for basal cell and squamous cell cancers of the skin) as well as its role as an indirect influence (through vitamin D, though the data supporting such a relationship are preliminary). With the identification of sun exposure as a causal agent of cancer have come recommendations on exposure reduction through sunscreens and protective clothing. However, the impact of such knowledge has yet to be discerned in cancer incidence data.

Screening

The promise of screening as a means to reduce the toll of cancer on the health of the population dates back to the early part of the twentieth century when it was difficult to diagnose the disease prior to metastases becoming apparent. Screening, it was thought, might catch the disease in an early stage of development, when excision of the tumor would be curative. Several screening tests were created and introduced into practice during the latter half of the twentieth century. The first successful cancer screening approach was the Pap smear, developed in the 1940s by George Papanicolaou to detect cancer cells in vaginal and cervical smears (see Chapter 6). Indeed, in some countries where Pap screening has been implemented, cervical cancer deaths have declined by 99 percent. Further progress against cervical cancer was made in the 1980s with the discovery of the role of the human papilloma virus as an etiologic factor for cervical cancer. This discovery carried with it the potential for a new vaccine against the virus.

Advances in cancer screening during the twentieth century significantly affected cancers other than that of the cervix. The emergence of mammography after World War II carried with it the potential for the early detection of breast cancer. However, it also carried the potential for causing breast cancer as a result of radiation exposure. The Health Insurance Plan of New York (HIP) decided to conduct a randomized trial to determine if mammography resulted in a net reduction in breast cancer mortality. The study found that for woman in their 50s, the procedure did reduce mortality, but for those in their 40s, the effect was not as clear. As a result, women began getting mammograms in their 50s. However, controversy persists about the practice, particularly for women in their 40s. Further research will hopefully provide sufficient data to resolve these issues.

DIET

The role of diet in the development of cancer and the potential for cancer prevention and control by dietary means have been matters of debate for much of the second half of the twentieth century. Although efforts aimed at determining the dietary origins of gastric and colon cancer produced useful findings during the 1960s and 1970s, it was not until Richard Doll and Richard Peto examined the broad range of cancer incidence in the United States that estimates of the extent to which cancer might be avoided was first placed before the scientific community. A major conclusion from the Doll and Peto study was that dietary habits provided an opportunity to reduce cancer incidence, an area which had not been well explored. To evaluate the role of diet, an instrument was needed that could systematically collect dietary intake information. The response from the nutritional public health community was the food frequency questionnaire (FFQ). Different versions of FFQs have been developed, but all seek to convert the consumption of various foodstuffs into nutrients, the effects of which can then be analyzed.

Although the Doll and Peto publication was generally well received, some researchers raised questions regarding the rigor of its analyses and the soundness of its conclusions. In particular, the extent to which environmental sources, as opposed to dietary ones, contribute to cancer incidence has remained a bone of contention. The NIH, however, used the opportunity of the Doll and Peto work to investigate diet as a means of preventing cancer occurrence. Several large trials were initiated into dietary modifications and how these might affect diverse cancer sites, but none was able to unequivocally establish a reduction in cancer risk. Indeed, the noted health journalist Gary Taubes reported the lack of effect observed in these dietary studies. Taubes has suggested that future prevention efforts should focus on factors other than diet.

VIRUSES

The potential role of viruses as among the etiological factors for the development of cancer has tempted scientists for a good portion of the twentieth century. In the 1960s, the Epstein-Barr virus was associated not only with infectious mononucleosis but also with Burkitt's lymphoma. However, this was the extent of demonstrating a direct connection. Much of the 1970s intramural research program at the NCI focused on viruses as a major cause of cancer. Although the knowledge gained proved useful with the appearance of AIDS in the early 1980s, it did little to improve our understanding of the development of cancer. AIDS demonstrated that cancers might be associated with a dysfunctional immune system, but it was unlikely that the disease was associated with only one virus. For example, a herpes virus, HSV-8, is now considered causal for Kaposi's sarcoma. Further searching for causal viruses continues, but these efforts have not produced additional knowledge to date.

UNDERSTANDING AND PREVENTING CANCER

During the course of the twentieth century, the developed nations underwent a demographic transition—a shift in death rates from primarily infectious causes to death rates from primarily chronic ones. Cancer mortality paralleled this phenomenon for two reasons, the first of which can be described as competing mortality. As individuals age, they are more likely to have mutations during routine cell division, some of which may result in cancers. Thus, as entire populations age, as they did in the developed world during the twentieth century, cancer mortality increases, replacing competing causes of death.

A second reason cancer mortality paralleled the demographic transition is that manufactured cigarettes replaced pipe and cigar tobacco (see Chapter 2) at the same time that population structures in the developed world shifted. Cigarettes were affordable, accessible, and addictive. As cigarette smoking increased, lung cancer followed suit 20 to 30 years later. By mid century, lung cancer became the most commonly diagnosed of all cancers.

Radiation was confirmed as an etiologic factor for cancer during the twentieth century. Environmental exposures and diet were both identified and challenged as etiologic factors. The knowledge base about cancers grew and continues to expand, but information about prevention remains limited. Beyond minimizing exposures to ionizing radiation and tobacco and developing and implementing anticancer vaccine programs, we still have much to learn.

SELECTED READINGS

The first reading, by Jarrett H. Folley and colleagues, reports on the incidence of leukemia among survivors of the atomic bombs dropped on Hiroshima and Nagasaki, Japan, in 1945. The immediate results from the bomb blast were devastatingly apparent, but questions remained about the residual effects on the survivors. President Harry S Truman requested that the National Academy of Sciences examine the health of the survivors and determine whether there were genetic effects on their children born after the blast. The survivors represented all ages, both genders, and varied levels of exposure. The risk of leukemia appeared within five years in a clear dose-response relationship, and these results paved the way for understanding the long-term effects of ionizing radiation on humans. The piece is abridged in that one table of primary data has been removed to save space, but we do not believe it detracts from the text.

The second selected reading, by R. Palmer Beasley et al., describes the results of a prospective study of Taiwanese men and their likelihood of developing hepatocellular carcinoma if infected with hepatitis B virus. This study is the first to conclude that a chronic viral infection could be causal for cancer, thus spurring the search for the first anticancer vaccine. Today, we know that hepatitis B virus has seven subtypes that infect more than 350 million people worldwide. What we still need to learn is how the subtypes and their viral loads affect the development of liver cancers.

Our third reading, by B. K. Armstrong and C. D. J. Holman, summarizes results from global epidemiologic studies on malignant melanoma and sunlight, with results from Australia in particular. Armstrong and Holman's conclusions that fair-skinned individuals are at risk for melanoma, that intermittent recreational exposure increases risk, and that screening and behavioral change are needed were widely heeded. In Australia, melanoma was identified as epidemic during the 1970s. In 1981, the government began the "Slip, Slop, Slap" national health education campaign (slip on a shirt, slop on sunscreen, and slap on a hat) to try to change behaviors and reduce sun exposure. The campaign later made its way to New Zealand and Canada and became second nature to those populations. Dermatologists in the United States and Europe warned against too much sun exposure and recommended that sunscreen be applied every time an individual went outdoors. "Skin checks" became part of routine preventive care. Cosmetic companies began including sunscreen in their formulations.

Behavioral change did occur, and individuals began reducing their and their children's sun exposure and using ever-increasing amounts and strengths of sunscreens. This led some researchers to hypothesize that the excessive use of sunscreen could actually increase cancer risk. Several large studies have yielded conflicting results on this issue. Additionally, pediatricians have begun counseling parents that their children should have a few minutes of sun exposure per day before being covered in sunscreen. If not, they should provide their children with vitamin D supplementation.

BIBLIOGRAPHY

Adami H-O, Balker B, Rutqvist L-E, Persson I, and Ries L. 1986. Temporal trends in breast cancer survival in Sweden: Significant improvement in 20 years. *JNCI* 76 (4): 653–59.

Ames BN. 1983. Dietary carcinogens and anticarcinogens. *Science* 221:1256–64.

Armitage P and Doll R. 1954. The age distribution of cancer and a multi-stage theory of carcinogenesis. *Br J Cancer* 8 (1): 1–12. Reprinted in 2004 *Int J Epidemiol* 33 (6): 1174–79.

Bud RF. 1978. Strategy in American cancer research after World War II: A case study. *Social Studies of Science* 8 (4): 425–59.

Burkitt DP. 1971. Epidemiology of cancer of the colon and rectum. *Cancer* 28 (1): 3–13. Reprinted in 1987 *Nutr Rev* 45 (7): 212–14.

Doll R and Peto R. 1981. *The Causes of Cancer.* New York: Oxford University Press.

English DR, Armstrong BK, Kricker A, and Fleming C. 1997. Sunlight and cancer. *Cancer Causes Control* 8:271–83.

Faguet GB. 2005. *The War on Cancer: An Anatomy of Failure, A Blueprint for the Future.* Dordrecht, The Netherlands: Springer.

Graham GG, Armstrong BK, Curton RC, Staples MP, and Thursfield VJ. 1996. Has mortality from melanoma stopped rising in Australia? Analysis of trends between 1931 and 1994. *BMJ* 312:1121–25.

Greenwald P. 1984. Epidemiology: A step forward in the scientific approach to preventing cancer through chemoprevention. *Public Health Rep* 99 (3): 259–64.

Haenszel W. 1961. Cancer mortality among the foreign-born in the United States. *J Natl Cancer Inst* 26:37–132.

Haenszel W and Correa P. 1971. Cancer of the colon and rectum andenomatous polyps: A review of epidemiologic findings. *Cancer* 28 (1): 14–24.

Hueper WC and Conway WD. 1964. *Chemical Carcinogenesis and Cancers.* Springfield: Charles C. Thomas.

Lerner BH. 2001. *The Breast Cancer Wars: Hope, Fear, and the Pursuit of a Cure in Twentieth-Century America.* New York: Oxford University Press.

Luinsky W and Zeiger E.1983. Carcinogenic risk (letter). *Science,* New Series 221 (4613): 810.

Marx J. 1993. New colon cancer gene discovered (in Research News). *Science,* New Series 260 (5109): 751–52.

Mills CA and Porter MM. 1957. Tobacco smoking, motor exhaust fumes and general air pollution in relation to lung cancer incidence. *Cancer Res* 17 (10): 981–90.

Proctor RN. 1999. *The Nazi War on Cancer.* Princeton, NJ: Princeton University Press.

Richards E. 1988. The politics of therapeutic evaluation: The vitamin C and cancer controversy. *Social Studies of Science* 18 (4): 653–701.

Shapiro S. 1977. Evidence on screening for breast cancer from a randomized trial. *Cancer* 39 (6): 2772–82.

Smith T. 1979. The Queensland Melanoma Project—An exercise in health education. *Brit Med J* 1:253–54.

Taubes G. 2007. *Good Calories, Bad Calories: Fats, Carbs, and the Controversial Science of Diet and Health.* New York: Alfred A. Knopf.

Vessey, MP and Gray, M. 1985. *Cancer Risks and Prevention.* New York: Oxford University Press.

Ward HW. 1973. Anti-oestrogen therapy for breast cancer: A trial of tamoxifen at two dose levels. *Brit Med J* 1 (5844): 13–14.

Wingo PA, Ries LA, Giovino GA, Miller DS, Rosenberg HM, Shopland DR, Thun MJ, and Edwards BK. 1999. Annual report to the nation on the status of cancer, 1973–1996, with a special section on lung cancer and tobacco smoking. *J Natl Cancer Inst* 91:675–90.

Woolf SH. 1995. Screening for prostate cancer with prostate-specific antigen: An examination of the evidence. *N Engl J Med* 333 (21): 1401–5.

Incidence of Leukemia in Survivors of the Atomic Bomb in Hiroshima and Nagasaki, Japan*
(1952, Abridged)

Jarrett H. Folley, M.D.,[†] Wayne Borges, M.D.[‡] *and*
Takuso Yamawaki, M.D.[§] *Hiroshima, Japan*

The concept of irradiation as a leukemogenic agent is not a new one. A considerable amount of experimental work in animals has been done concerning the effects of irradiation and its possible relationship to the development of leukemia. There is general acceptance of the experimental evidence that leukemia may be produced in susceptible species of animals by exposure to roentgen irradiation.[1] Reports suggesting that man may be similarly affected have appeared since 1911 but the evidence has been less convincing.[2] Martland in 1931 reported agreement among authorities that contact with radioactive substances and x-rays produces alterations of which the principal objective symptoms are leukopenia, more rarely a leukemia, and an anemia of the aplastic type.[3] Recently, March has reported that leukemia has occurred as a cause of death more than nine times as frequently in radiologists as in non-radiologic physicians in the United States.[1]

In 1948 the Atomic Bomb Casualty Commission initiated the first survey of the incidence of leukemia in whole human populations exposed to high energy radiation by the explosion of an atomic bomb. The aim of the investigation has been to obtain information concerning all individuals in Hiroshima and Nagasaki having onset of symptoms of leukemia or dying of the disease since the atomic explosion in 1945. It was found that data previous to late 1947 were unreliable and insufficient due to the destruction of records and the general medical conditions prevailing.

*Sponsored by the Atomic Bomb Casualty Commission, National Research Council, with funds supplied by the United States Atomic Energy Commission. The Atomic Bomb Casualty Commission was authorized by directive of the President of the United States in 1946. It was established in the same year under the auspices of the National Research Council, with the support of the Atomic Energy Commission for the purpose of studying long-term medical effects of the atomic bombs exploded in Japan.

†Medical Director, Atomic Bomb Casualty Commission. On leave of absence from the Hitchcock Clinic, Hanover. New Hampshire.

‡Atomic Bomb Casualty Commission, 1949–1950. The Children's Center, Boston, Massachusetts.

§Department of Pediatrics, Hiroshima Red Cross Hospital, Hiroshima, Japan.

The purpose of this report is to present data on the incidence of leukemia and deaths from leukemia in the survivors of the bombing in Hiroshima and Nagasaki during the years 1948, 1949 and 1950 and to compare the incidence and death rate from leukemia in individuals exposed to radiation at various distances from the hypocenter.

Case Material

In all cases of leukemia from all sources an attempt has been made to establish the location of the individual at the time of the explosion of the atomic bomb, to determine the presence or absence of symptoms of radiation injury and to confirm the diagnosis of leukemia by objective criteria. The sources of material in Hiroshima were (1) patients referred by physicians to the Commission with the diagnosis of leukemia or suspected leukemia; (2) patients admitted to hospitals of the city with the diagnosis of leukemia or suspected leukemia; and (3) cases discovered by a review of the death certificates on file with the Health Center of the city in which leukemia was listed as a cause of death.

The patients seen at the Commission's laboratory were given complete medical histories, including a history concerning symptoms of radiation injury, complete physical examinations, peripheral blood studies and, in many cases, bone marrow aspirations or biopsies.

Patients in outside institutions were examined by the commission's personnel whenever possible. In all cases the hospital records of this group were received and blood smears and bone marrow preparations, when available, were examined.

Cases which were discovered by death certificate were investigated by means of contact with immediate family, the physician of the deceased and, in patients who had been hospitalized, the review of hospital records, laboratory data and autopsy material. Information obtained from death certificates was personally checked by the Commission.

Data on the cases of leukemia in Nagasaki were largely obtained from investigation of individuals dying from the disease since January, 1948. The initial source of material was death certificates on file in the Nagasaki Health Center. The same procedure of investigation was followed as in Hiroshima.

The Commission investigated a total of ninety cases of leukemia. Insufficient information concerning possible exposure to the atomic bomb, residence in another city and onset of symptoms of leukemia previous to August, 1945, eliminated six of this total number. Table I shows the distribution of these eighty-four cases and the deaths from leukemia in each group.

Table I Accepted Cases of Leukemia Investigated by the Commission in the Exposed and Non-Exposed Population and the Number of Deaths in These Groups

	Exposed		Non-Exposed	
	Cases of leukemia	Deaths from leukemia	Cases of leukemia	Deaths from leukemia
Hiroshima	31	22	23	19
Nagasaki	16	15	14	14
Total	47	37	37	33

Table II [Not shown, Ed.] lists the forty-seven exposed cases of leukemia with the method of diagnostic confirmation available. In only four cases located by means of a death certificate could no objective confirmation be made. The entire series of cases is available for analysis by age and sex distribution and the type of leukemia. However, only those patients having onset of symptoms or dying of the disease during the years 1948, 1949 and 1950 in the cities of Hiroshima and Nagasaki have been used in the analysis of the incidence of the total numbers of that population. The figures for the exposed population presently residing in the cities of Hiroshima and Nagasaki used in the incidence calculations of this report were obtained from the Commission's survivor questionnaire circulated with the Japanese National Census of October 1, 1950. The accuracy, within 10 per cent, of the figures from this source has been confirmed by population estimates obtained from the Public Health and Welfare Section of SCAP, a sample census by the Commission in 1950 and the Commission census file.

Distribution of the exposed population of the two cities by distance from the hypocenter was established by a radiation census in which the location of the individual at the time of the bombing was determined by trained interviewers.

Comparative Incidence

Table III shows the incidence of leukemia in all of Japan and the Untied States for 1940. Data for Japan are not available for the war years and the immediate postwar years of 1941 through 1947. No data for the cities of Hiroshima and Nagasaki are available as the records were destroyed in 1945.

It becomes apparent from a comparison of the available statistics in Japan with those of the United States that the reported incidence of

Table III Official Figures on the Incidence of Leukemia in All Japan
Including Okinawa for the Years 1935–1940, 1948, 1949* and the
Incidence in the United States for the Year 1940**

Year	Population	Total deaths	Leukemic deaths	Leukemic deaths per 10^6 living	Leukemic deaths per 10^4 total deaths
1935	69,254,148	1,161,936	969	14.0	8.3
1936	70,258,200	1,230,278	991	14.1	8.1
1937	71,252,800	1,207,899	930	13.1	7.7
1938	72,222,700	1,259,805	911	12.6	7.2
1939	72,875,800	1,268,760	930	12.8	7.3
1940	73,114,308	1,186,595	939	12.8	7.9
1948	80,200,000	950,610	956	11.9	10.1
1949	82,200,000	945,444	1,120	13.6	11.8
UNITED STATES					
1940	131,669,000	1,417,285	5,135	39	36.2

*The Division of Health and Welfare Statistics, Welfare Minister's Secretariat, Tokyo.

**Based on a publication of the United States Department of Commerce—Vital Statistics Rates in the United States 1900–1940, by Linder, F.E. and Grove, R.D.

leukemia in Japan averages only one-third of that in the United States in terms of per million living population and about one-fourth in terms of per 10,000 total deaths. Sacks and Seeman reported that the death rate from leukemia in the United States has risen continuously since 1900, with an accelerated rate of increase since 1920. They pointed out that the increase is not due to changes in the age distribution of the population and that improved diagnostic techniques and greater use of medical facilities must be considered in determining the cause for the rising death rate.[4] The lower incidence of leukemia, as reported in Japan, may be due to a relative lack of medical facilities available and the ratio of physicians to a large rural population. The available figures suggest that the incidence in Japan may actually be lower than in the United States.

In the absence of a satisfactory basis for predicting an expected incidence and death ratio it has been considered desirable to compare the incidence and death rate from leukemia in the exposed and non-exposed populations of the cities of Hiroshima and Nagasaki. Further, a comparison of the incidence and death rate from leukemia is made between the population exposed under 2,000 meters and 2,000 meters and over.

Principal Findings and Their Interpretation

INCIDENCE OF LEUKEMIA. Table IV lists the cases with onset of leukemia and deaths from leukemia during the years 1948, 1949 and 1950 in the cities of Hiroshima and Nagasaki.

A total of thirty cases and twenty-four deaths were recorded in Hiroshima as compared with nineteen cases and nineteen deaths in Nagasaki. An analysis by the Chi square and interaction method shows no significant difference between the two cities.

In the total exposed population of the two cities twenty-nine cases and twenty deaths are recorded as compared with twenty cases and twenty deaths in the non-exposed population. This is a highly significant increase in the incidence from leukemia in the exposed population as shown by the Chi square analysis.

In Table V the cases of leukemia and deaths from leukemia for 1948, 1949 and 1950 in the exposed population are presented according to distance from hypocenter of the atomic explosion. A total of twenty-two cases and eighteen deaths from leukemia were recorded in the population exposed under 2,000 meters as compared with seven cases and five deaths in the population exposed at 2,000 meters or over. A comparison of these data by the Chi square test reveals a highly significant increase in both the incidence and deaths from leukemia in the group exposed at a distance of less than 2,000 meters from hypocenter.

The data for deaths from leukemia in Table V are graphically represented by Figure 1 in which the per cent of total deaths, occurring in the combined cities, contributed by the various segments of the exposed population is compared to per percent of the total exposed population comprised by each segment. The population exposed at distances up to 1,999 meters contributed 78 per cent of all deaths from leukemia although it comprises only 20 per cent of the total exposed population. The population at 2,000 meters or over contributed only 22 per cent of the leukemic deaths although it comprises 80 per cent of the total exposed population.

Figure 2 represents the number of deaths from leukemia in the subjects at various distances from the hypocenter expressed as deaths per 10^6 living persons in each group. Table VI presents a calculated death rate from leukemia in the exposed populations of the two cities by distance from the hypocenter. The death rate per 10^6 living persons in the population exposed at distances less than 2,000 meters is high as compared with the death rate in the population exposed at 2,000 meters or over.

Table IV Cases with Onset of Symptoms or Death from Leukemia during 1948–1950 Inclusive in the Population of the Cities of Hiroshima and Nagasaki

	Exposed			Non-Exposed			Total		
	Population	Cases 1948–1950	Deaths 1948–1950	Population	Cases 1948–1950	Deaths 1948–1950	Population	Cases 1948–1950	Deaths 1948–1950
Hiroshima	98,265	19	13	187,447	11	11	285,712	30	24
Nagasaki	96,962	10	10	144,843	9	9	241,805	19	19
Total	195,227	29	23	332,290	20	20	527,517	49	43

Summary of Comparison

Comparison	D/F	Number of cases of leukemia		Deaths from leukemia	
		X^2	P	X^2	P
Hiroshima vs Nagasaki	1	0.99		0.05	
Expose vs unexposed	1	10.34	0.002	5.01	0.03
Interaction	1	3.30		0.47	

Table V Case of Leukemia with Onset of Symptoms or Death from Leukemia during 1948–1950 Inclusive in the Cities of Hiroshima and Nagasaki According to Distance from Hypocenter

Distance from hypocenter (meters)	Hiroshima city			Nagasaki city			Totals (combined areas)		
	Exposed population	Cases of leukemia	Deaths from leukemia	Exposed population	Cases of leukemia	Deaths from leukemia	Exposed population	Cases of leukemia	Deaths from leukemia
0–999	1,400	3	1	671	1	2	2,071	4	3
1,000–1,499	10,596	8	5	3,227	4	4	13,823	12	9
1,500–1,999	19,002	4	3	4,361	2	3	23,363	6	6
Under 2,000	30,998	15	9	8,259	7	9	39,257	22	18
2,000–over	67,267	4	4	88,703	3	1	155,970	7	5
Totals	98,265	19	13	96,962	10	10	195,227	29	23

Comparison of Incidence in Combined Cities of Cases and Deaths from Leukemia Exposed under 2,000 Meters vs 2,000 Meters or Over

	Cases of leukemia	Deaths from leukemia
X^2	56.12	48.42
D/F	1	1
P	<.001	<.001

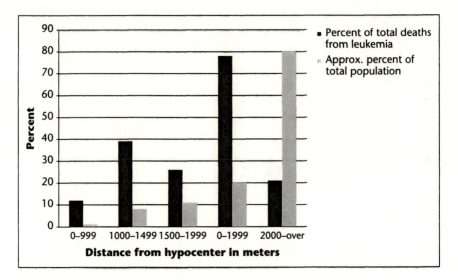

Figure 1 Comparison of per cent of total deaths from leukemia in the cities of Hiroshima and Nagasaki during 1948, 1949 and 1950 contributed by various segments of the exposed population compared with the per cent of total exposed population comprised by each segment.

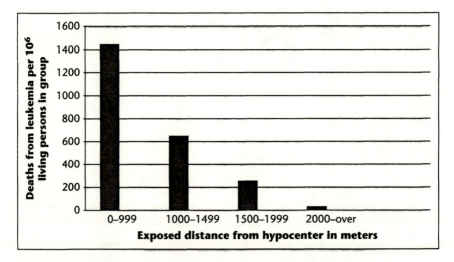

Figure 2 Number of deaths from leukemia in Hiroshima and Nagasaki cities 1948–1950 occurring in the exposed groups expressed as deaths per 10^6 living persons in that group.

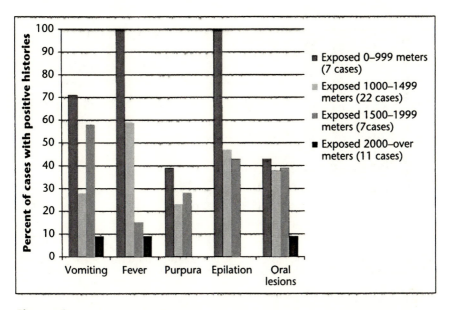

Figure 3 Incidence of symptoms and signs of radiation injury at time of atomic bomb in forty-seven subjects exposed in Hiroshima and Nagasaki in whom leukemia subsequently developed.

ACUTE RADIATION SYMPTOMS. It should be recognized that due to shielding, and perhaps other factors such as individual resistance, a significant percentage of the survivors exposed to radiation at distances less than 2,000 meters gives no history of acute radiation illness following the exposure.* A positive radiation history in the population exposed beyond 2,000 meters is unusual. It becomes significant in comparing the incidence of leukemia in the exposed populations according to distance from the hypocenter to document actual exposure to radiation injury.

Data are available on forty-seven exposed patients who developed leukemia with reference to symptoms of radiation injury following the bombing. (Fig. 3.) Epilation, purpura and oropharyngeal lesions are reliable signs of acute radiation effect. It has been recognized that fever and vomiting may be non-specific symptoms unrelated to radiation. However, all radiation histories were taken by physicians and the symptoms and signs were evaluated as to the time of appearance, relationship to other portions of the medical history and the accuracy and intelligence of the informant before being recorded. The radiation histories represent signs and symptoms based on the etiologic factor of radiation as well as can be determined.

---

*Atomic Bomb Casualty Commission unpublished data

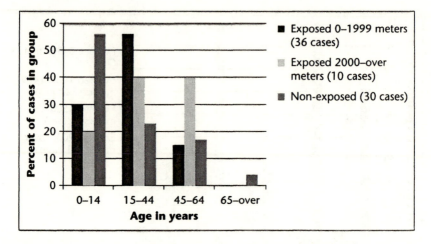

Figure 4 Age distribution based on age at onset of symptoms in seventy-six cases of leukemia developing in Nagasaki and Hiroshima areas since the atomic bomb.

While the case numbers are small and the incidence of the symptoms varies somewhat from group to group, fever and epilation show a striking progressive diminution of occurrence as distance from the hypocenter increases. Epilation, which occurred in all of the patients with leukemia exposed at distances less than 1,000 meters, was also more severe in this group, being complete in 75 per cent of the cases. The symptoms and signs of radiation injury appeared to diminish in the patients exposed beyond 2,000 meters. Whereas epilation of some degree occurred in 70 per cent of the patients exposed under 2,000 meters it was not observed in the eleven patients exposed beyond this point. Purpura also was not found in the latter group, and a positive history of the other symptoms listed was found only in a single case.

The presented data in the cases of leukemia exposed at distances less than 2,000 meters documents the actual exposure to radiation injury by a high incidence of symptoms and signs indicative of a severe radiation insult. This is again evidence supporting the concept of radiation exposure as a leukemogenic agent in man.

AGE DISTRIBUTION. In the United States leukemia affects persons in the older age groups, fifty-five years and older, with the greatest frequency and the death rate from leukemia is lowest in the intermediate ages.[4] Forty-six cases of leukemia, developing since 1945, in the exposed population and thirty cases in the non-exposed population of Hiroshima and Nagasaki in whom the age at onset of symptoms could be determined are presented in Figure 4.

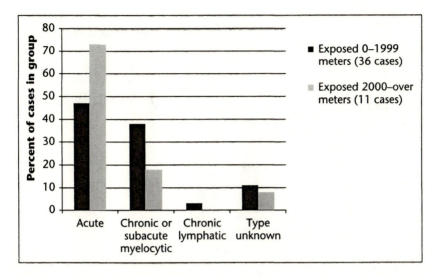

Figure 5 Distribution by type of leukemia of the forty-seven exposed patients with leukemia in Hiroshima and Nagasaki areas since the atomic bomb.

In the thirty-six patients exposed at distances less than 2,000 meters approximately 86 per cent (thirty-one patients) had onset of symptoms before the age of forty-five years and in no patients has leukemia been observed to develop after the age of sixty-five. In ten patients exposed beyond 2,000 meters 60 per cent (6 cases) occurred before the age of forty-five, 40 per cent (4 cases) between ages forty-five and sixty-four and none after the age of sixty-five years. The cases found in the non-exposed population show a roughly comparable distribution, 80 per cent (24 cases) being observed in the 0 to 44 age group and only 3.3 per cent (one case) after the age of sixty-five years. In the non-exposed populations of Hiroshima and Nagasaki a higher incidence is noted in the 0 to 14 age group than in the exposed population. It should be recognized that in the exposed population there was, for example in 1950, no individual under the age of five years. Since the incidence of leukemia is relatively high in the first two years of life, the advancing years have removed a segment of the 0 to 14 age group in exposed subjects which in a normal population would be expected to contribute some cases of leukemia.

It is tempting to read into these figures a possible shift in the age of onset of leukemia to a younger than average group and to speculate as to the possible role of radiation as a causative agent. However, it appears that a similar incidence of leukemia in younger age groups is present in the non-exposed group and the cases exposed beyond 2,000 meters as well. Since this latter group showed no increase in the incidence of leukemia,

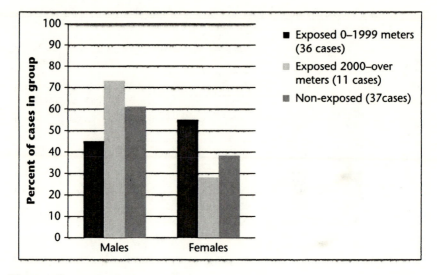

Figure 6 Distribution by sex of the cases of leukemia occurring in Hiroshima and Nagasaki areas since the atomic bomb.

there is no support in the present data for speculation concerning the acceleration of the appearance of leukemia by exposure to radiation.

TYPE OF LEUKEMIA. The distribution by type of leukemia in forty-seven cases in the combined populations of Hiroshima and Nagasaki is illustrated in Figure 5. A high proportion of acute leukemia is found in both the group under 2,000 meters, presumably most heavily exposed to radiation, and the group exposed at distances greater than 2,000 meters in which no increase in the incidence of leukemia is found. It has already been pointed out that the age of onset of leukemia in these cases is early and acute leukemia and myelocytic leukemia are more common in the younger age groups. No statement concerning the role of radiation in the determination of the type of leukemia which develops is warranted on the basis of the present data.

SEX DISTRIBUTION. Figure 6 indicates the distribution by sex of all known cases of leukemia in both the exposed and non-exposed populations of Hiroshima and Nagasaki. The cases involved here are obviously too few from which to draw conclusions and are presented only as a matter of record.

Summary

Data have been presented concerning the incidence and death rate from leukemia for the years 1948, 1949 in 1950 in the populations of Hiroshima and Nagasaki, Japan, which were exposed to radiation effects of the atomic bombs exploded in 1945.

The incidence and death rate from leukemia has been compared in the exposed and non-exposed populations of Hiroshima and Nagasaki and also within the exposed population by distance from the hypocenter.

The daily show an increase in the incidence of leukemia in the total exposed populations compared with the total non-exposed populations of the two cities. A highly significant increased incidence of leukemia is found in the subjects exposed to radiation at distances of less than 2,000 meters as compared with those exposed beyond 2,000 meters.

Analysis of medical radiation histories in exposed subjects with leukemia presents evidence of severe radiation injury in a high proportion of the cases exposed under 2,000 meters. There is little evidence, by this same analysis, of severe radiation injury occurring beyond 2,000 meters.

The same pattern of findings of the collective analysis is present in the data obtained separately in Hiroshima and Nagasaki.

Leukemia in the cases exposed both under 2,000 meters and over 2,000 meters occurs most frequently in the early and intermediate age groups.

Acute leukemia and myelocytic leukemia have dominated in all cases irrespective of the individual's distance from hypocenter at the time of the bomb explosion. Chronic lymphatic leukemia was observed in only a single case. The number of cases is small and the types of leukemia observed are not inconsistent with the age distribution in which they occurred.

Comparative differences in the sex distribution in the cases of leukemia are slight and the total numbers too small to warrant any conclusions.

Conclusions

1. There is a significant increase in the incidence of leukemia in the exposed populations of Hiroshima and Nagasaki as compared with the non-exposed populations of the two cities.

2. There is a significant increase in the incidence of leukemia within the exposed population of Hiroshima and Nagasaki in subjects exposed at distances less than 2,000 meters from the hypocenter.

3. The concept that radiation from the atomic bomb explosions in Hiroshima and Nagasaki is a leukemogenic agent in man is supported.

4. No conclusions can be drawn concerning the relationship of radiation to the possible acceleration of the appearance of leukemia or the type of leukemia which may develop in the exposed subjects.

5. The present study should continue and emphasis should be placed on the position of these data relative to a curve of increased incidence of leukemia in the exposed population under 2,000 meters, and the

presence or absence of an increased incidence of leukemia occurring at a later date in the populations exposed to radiation beyond 2,000 meters.

ACKNOWLEDGMENT: The material presented in this report is from a survey by the Atomic Bomb Casualty Commission with the cooperation of the Japanese physicians, medical institutions and municipal health agencies. Dr. Yoshimichi Yamasowa was responsible for some of the early aspects of the survey. The medical department of the Commission in Hiroshima under the direction of Dr. Paul G. Fillmore and in Nagasaki under Dr. James N. Yamazaki have contributed greatly. The advice of Dr. John S. Lawrence and Dr. William N. Valentine, consultants in medicine to the Atomic Bomb Casualty Commission, was most helpful. Dr. Valentine's assistance in the final collection and analysis of the material was invaluable. Finally, this report could not have been written without the generous cooperation and assistance of all departments of the Atomic Bomb Casualty Commission.

SOURCE

Folley JH, Borges W, and Yamawaki T. 1952. Incidence of leukemia in survivors of the atomic bomb in Hiroshima and Nagasaki, Japan. *Am J Med* 13 (3): 311–21. Copyright 1952 *The American Journal of Medicine.* Reprinted with permission of Elsevier.

Hepatocellular Carcinoma and Hepatatis B Virus
(1981)
A Prospective Study of 22,707 Men in Taiwan

R. Palmer Beasley, Chia-Chin Lin,
Lu-Yu Hwang, and Chia-Siang Chien

University of Washington Medical Research Unit, Taipei;
Institute of Public Health, College of Medicine,
National Taiwan University; and Government Employees'
Clinic Centre, Taipei, Taiwan

SUMMARY A prospective general population study of 22,707 Chinese men in Taiwan has shown that the incidence of primary hepatocellular carcinoma (PHC) among carriers of hepatitis B surface antigen (HBsAg) is much higher than among non-carriers (1,158/100,000 *vs* 5/100,000 during 75,000 man-years of follow-up). The relative risk is 223. PHC and cirrhosis accounted for 54.3% of the 105 deaths among HBsAg carriers but accounted for only 1.5% of the 202 deaths among non-carriers. These findings support the hypothesis that hepatitis B virus has a primary role in the aetiology of PHC.

Introduction

Primary hepatocellular carcinoma (PHC) is the most common malignant neoplasm in China, in much of Asia, and in Africa,[1-5] but it is uncommon in the U.S.A. and Europe. It ranks 22nd among malignancies in White men in the U.S.A., accounting for less than 1% of all malignancies.[3] Many possible aetiological factors have been implicated, but most of these (for instance, androgenic steroids or hepatic parasites) do not occur widely enough or do not show the same geographical distribution as PHC and can explain only a small proportion of cases. Two implicated factors, aflatoxins and hepatitis B virus (HBV), occur widely; it is possible that they may have major aetiological roles in PHC and macronodular cirrhosis, in which PHC arises.[1,6,7]

Early case-control studies showed poor correlation between PHC and HBV. [8,9] Later, more sensitive techniques for the detection of hepatitis B surface antigen (HBsAg) showed that HBsAg appeared in the serum of patients with PHC substantially more frequently than in serum from controls.[10-12] Epidemiological studies have revealed a very strong correlation between the geographical frequency of the HBsAg-carrier state and prevalence of PHC.[1] Several other observations have strengthened the association between PHC and the chronic HBsAg-carrier state, and there is widespread awareness that HBV may have a major role in the aetiology of PHC. [13,14] Our large-scale cohort study started in 1974 when there was little awareness or acceptance of the possible association between HBV and PHC, in order to establish prospectively the incidence and the relative risk of PHC among HBsAg carriers and to determine whether the HBsAg-carrier state is antecedent to the development of PHC. This report is the first on this prospective general population study of 22,707 Chinese men, 15.2% of whom are HBsAg carriers.

Subjects and Methods

Study Population and Recruitment

The study is being conducted among male Chinese government employees (civil-servants) in Taiwan because their life and health insurance system provides almost total ascertainment of the fact of death with excellent determination of cause of death. The study was restricted to men for the following reasons: prevalence of PHC is three to four times higher in men than women; there are more male government employees; their average age is higher; and they stay in government service longer. Initially, enrolment was restricted to men aged 40 to 59 years; later, because of general popularity of the project, men of all ages were recruited. Study participants were recruited through two sources:

1. Government Employees' Clinic Centre (GECC) men were enrolled during routine free physical examinations or selected other clinics (e.g., dental, ear, nose, and throat, and ophthalmology) where it was considered likely that a sample unbiased for liver disease could be obtained.

2. Cardiovascular Disease Study (CVDS) men had been recruited from the GECC ten years earlier, when they were 40–59 years old, for a prospective study of cardiovascular disease risk factors; they had been kept under active surveillance since then.

Potential participants from the GECC group were given a written description of the study while they were waiting for their clinic appointment. Those willing to participate (99.99%) signed a consent form and completed a brief health questionnaire. A portion of serum from the sample taken as part of the subject's routine examination was procured for our study. We wrote to participants from the CVDS group, explaining the study and inviting those interested (89.6%) to come to our clinic, where a blood sample was obtained and a similar health questionnaire was completed. There were 1,480 men in the CVDS group and 21,227 men in the GECC group. The CVDS and GECC groups are almost identical in most respects but the CVDS group is older. We believe the study participants are representative of male government employees in Taiwan as regards health but, compared with the general population, government employees have higher educational backgrounds and better health care, and enjoy better living conditions and health. The frequencies of HBV infections, cirrhosis, and PHC are similar in government employees to those in the general population. The HBsAg carrier rate is the same as that in other groups of men of the same age, and the mortality rate from PHC and cirrhosis is approximately the same as that in the general population.

Detection of PHC

PHC is detected through the health and life insurance which is mandatory for all government employees and is provided by a single large government bureau operating exclusively for this purpose. Insurance is usually retained after retirement and can be cancelled only at the request of the retired person. Substantial financial benefits are paid by the insurance system irrespective of cause of death and there are few, if any, deaths for which no claim is filed. Thus, all deaths of active government employees and deaths of most retired government employees are known to the insurance bureau: we receive from the bureau monthly lists of recent deaths and newly retiring employees who have cancelled their insurance. Each government employee has a unique number which is retained even after retirement and is never duplicated. Death and retirement lists are compared by computer with the study population and verified.

We contacted by letter or telephone newly retired men who cancelled their insurance, to find out about their state of health. To date only 643 men have cancelled their insurance (2.8% of study subjects). To verify the completeness of the insurance system for the ascertainment of deaths, we actively followed all HBsAg-positive men and controls matched for age and province of origin with each HBsAg-positive man. Province of origin represents the historical origin of the man's family in China and in all but a few men corresponds to place of birth. This active surveillance involved annual completion of a health questionnaire and retesting for HBV markers. Adherence to follow-up has averaged 95% annually. The state of health of those who failed to return for follow-up was determined by telephone or home visit. We lost contact with only 74 men and could not verify that they were still alive. From this active surveillance we were able to verify that among men retaining their insurance all deaths are known to us.

We contacted 569 of the 643 men who cancelled their insurance (88.5%) leaving only 0.3% of the original recruits whose possible deaths would not be known to us.

Diagnosis of Cause of Death

The causes of death of all study subjects are investigated through the records of preceding periods in hospital. Most deaths, other than sudden deaths, among government employees occur in hospital or very soon after discharge and most patients have been admitted to large well-equipped and well-staffed hospitals so that clinical parameters relating to cause of death are usually well established; necropsies, however, are not common. Among the 41 deaths due to PHC that we report, 19 (46.3%) were confirmed histologically. 19 of the remaining patients had had raised serum alpha fetoprotein (AFP) levels and changes on a liver scan, or angiography, or both, interpreted as PHC; 1 more patient had had scans interpreted as PHC but AFP was not measured, and the remaining 2 patients had had raised AFP levels and their clinical picture was interpreted as PHC. The clinical picture, liver scan, and angiographic patterns did not differ between histologically confirmed and unconfirmed cases. In fact, for the patients we report as having PHC the diagnoses were clear and there appeared no likely alternatives. Deaths attributed to cirrhosis all showed unequivocal clinical evidence of chronic hepatic failure in the presence of portal hypertension and other classical evidence of cirrhosis.

Laboratory Tests

All recruitment and follow-up specimens are tested for HBsAg, alanine aminotransferase, and AFP. Anti-HBs and anti-HBc (hepatitis B core antigen) testing were too expensive to undertake on all 19,253 HBsAg-negative subjects. All 1,020 HBsAg-negative men from the CVDS group and controls matched for age and province of origin with each HBsAg-positive subject in the GECC group were selected from among the HBsAg-negative subjects for anti-HBs testing. 3,661 men were tested for anti-HBs. From these, all the 615 who were anti-HBs-negative were tested for anti-HBc. The anti-HBs and anti-HBc rates derived from the above sample were then used to project the frequency of these markers for the entire study population. HBV markers are tested by radioimmunoassay (RIA) with standardised commercial kits ('AUSRIA', 'AUSAB, and 'CORAB', Abbott Diagnostics, North Chicago). AFP levels are also measured by RIA with a commercial kit, ('AFP-PEG', Dianabot, Tokyo).

Results

Between Nov. 3, 1975, and June 30, 1978, 22,707 men were enrolled in the study; 81.6% were aged between 40 and 59 years. Within this age range our sample constitutes 12.8% of male government employees and 1.4% of all males in Taiwan. Among the 22,707 men, 3,454 were HBsAg-positive (15.2%), and 19,253 were HBsAg-negative (84.8%). From sample testing we estimate that 15,570 (68.6%) would be anti-HBs positive, 2,248 (9.9%) would be anti-HBc positive only, 1,272 (5.6%) would be negative for all three HBV markers, and in 163 (0.7%) the anti-HBc results would be borderline. By Dec. 31, 1980, 307 study subjects had died, and 74 had retired and cancelled their insurance and could not be traced (0.3%). We had carried out approximately 75,000 man years of follow-up, an average of 3.3 years per man.

Of the 307 deaths, 41 were due to PHC and 19 to cirrhosis. Thus, PHC and cirrhosis together accounted for 19.5% of all deaths. The next most common causes of death were accidents (11.4%), ischaemic heart disease (10.7%), and lung cancer (9.1%).

There was a very pronounced excess of deaths from PHC and cirrhosis in those who were HBsAg-positive on recruitment (table I). Of the 41 men who died of PHC, 40 were in the group of 3,454 men who were HBsAg-positive and only 1 was in the group of 19,253 HBsAg-negative subjects, a relative risk of 223.

There was also a large excess mortality from cirrhosis among HBsAg-positive men. 17 of 19 men who died from cirrhosis were HBsAg-positive. PHC and cirrhosis together accounted for 57 of 105 deaths among the HBsAg-positive subjects (54.3%) compared with 3 of 202 deaths among the HBsAg-negative subjects (1.5%). There was a slight excess of mortality from other causes among the HBsAg-positive men, but the difference was not significant. Together PHC and cirrhosis accounted for 19.5% of all deaths in the total study population.

Table I Deaths by Cause and HBsAg Status on Recruitment

HBsAg status on recruitment	Cause of death			Population at risk	PHC incidence*
	PHC	Cirrhosis	Other		
HBsAg-positive	40	17	48	3,454	1,158
HBsAg-negative	1	2	199	19,253	5
Total	41	19	247	22,707	181

*Incidence of death from PHC per 100,000 during the time of the study.

Table II Deaths by Cause, Previous History of Cirrhosis, and HBsAg Status

Status on recruitment	Cause of death			Population at risk	PHC incidence*
	PHC	Cirrhosis	Other		
Previous cirrhosis:					
HBsAg-positive	5	7	0	40	12,500
HBsAg-negative	0	0	0	30	0
No cirrhosis:					
HBsAg-positive	35	10	48	3,414	1,025
HBsAg-negative	1	2	199	19,223	5
Total	41	19	247	22,707	181

*Incidence of death from PHC per 100,000 during the time of the study.

Of the 3 HBsAg-negative men who died of PHC (1) and cirrhosis (2), 1 of the cirrhosis patients was anti-HBs-positive and the others were positive for anti-HBc only. Thus, the risk of dying from PHC or cirrhosis was much lower in HBsAg-negative men even if they were positive for other HBV markers. If anti-HBc-positive men had the same risk of PHC as those who were HBsAg-positive, approximately 26 anti-HBc-positive men would have died instead of only 1 ($p < 0.00001$).

PHC frequently coexists with cirrhosis, and patients with cirrhosis are at increased risk of PHC. The frequency of underlying cirrhosis in this study population is of course unknown. All 22,707 men were asked on recruitment if they had ever had liver disease and to give details of such disease. 70 reported they had previously been told they had cirrhosis; we were able to confirm this by examining their medical records. Of the 40 HBsAg-positive men with a history of cirrhosis on recruitment, 12 have died (table II), 5 from PHC and 7 from cirrhosis (30% combined). None of the 30 HBsAg-negative men with a history of cirrhosis on recruitment have died (table II).

1,257 men gave a history of having had "hepatitis" on recruitment. 390 were HBsAg-positive (31%); 8 of the 390 men have subsequently died of PHC (2.1%), whereas there were no PHC deaths among 867 HBsAg-negative men with a history of "hepatitis" on recruitment.

The incidence of death from PHC during the study period was 181/100,000 for the entire group and for HBsAg-positive men only it was 1,158/100,000. These figures convert to annual incidence figures of 55/100,000 and 351/100,000, respectively. Whether calculated for the whole group or for HBsAg-positive subjects only, the incidence of PHC deaths rose as a direct function of age (table III).

Table III PHC Incidence by Age at Recruitment

| Age* | Subjects | | | PHC incidence per 100,000[†] | |
	Total	HBsAg-positive no. (%)	PHC deaths	Total	HBsAg-positive
20–29	647	130 (21.1)	0	0	0
30–39	1,814	398 (21.9)	1	55	251
40–49	8,338	1,415 (17.0)	4+1 [††]	60	283
50–59	9,949	1,303 (13.1)	28	281	2,149
60–69	1,920	206 (10.7)	7	364	3,398
≥ 70	39	2 (5.1)	0	0	0
Total	22,707	3,454 (15.2)	40 + 1[††]	181	1,158

* Age when HBsAg status first determined.

[†] Incidence from PHC per 100,000 during the time of the study.

[††] HBsAg-negative.

To verify that this prospective study is measuring the continuing incidence of new liver carcinomas (not subclinical tumours present at the time of enrolment) we analysed the PHC deaths according to time since recruitment. As expected, the incidence was almost constant over time (table IV).

There were subjects in the study who come from most of China's 35 provinces. The 16 most populated provinces were each represented by 100 or more subjects who made up 93% of the study participants. The prevalence of HBsAg varied from 4.7% to 20.1% in the subjects from these 16 provinces. There were cases of PHC among participants from 13 of the 16 provinces. There were no significant differences in the incidence of deaths from PHC among HBsAg carriers by province.

Discussion

This study shows that the risk of PHC is much higher in HBsAg carriers than in non-carriers. The results support the hypothesis that HBV has a

Table IV PHC Incidence and Length of Follow-up

| Year of follow-up | HBsAg-positive | | PHC incidence* |
	Men in follow-up	PHC deaths	
1	3,454	15	434
2	3,426	11	321
3	3,397	7	206
4	2,275	6	264
5	309	1	324

*Incidence of death from PHC per 100,000 at the time of the study.

role in the aetiology of PHC. In this large prospective study, the present relative risk estimate of PHC is 223 for HBsAg carriers compared with non-carriers. However, since all but 1 of the subjects who died from PHC were HBsAg-positive, the 95% confidence interval for the relative risk is quite wide (28 to 1,479). Irrespective of the eventual value for the relative risk, it is clear that it is very high. This study establishes beyond any doubt that the HBsAg carrier state commonly precedes PHC in Chinese men. The primary contributions of a prospective study are to establish the prior occurrence of a factor or agent in relation to the disorder in question, to verify increased relative risk estimates made from case-control studies, and to establish or verify the incidence of the disease. Our study strongly supports the hypothesis that HBV has a role in the aetiology of PHC because it establishes a very much increased risk of PHC among persons who were HBsAg carriers before they developed PHC.

Although this study strengthens the argument that HBV may be a cause of PHC, it does not prove it. Alternative explanations of the very high relative risk among HBsAg carriers are that HBV is a cofactor with another aetiological agent or is simply a risk factor. The very high relative risk found in this study and many case-control studies in various parts of the world, however, suggests that HBV is closely associated with the process leading to PHC and is not simply a risk factor. This association is in fact the strongest ever established between a virus and a human neoplasm.

Case-control studies have repeatedly shown that PHC does occur in HBsAg-negative subjects. This finding can be taken to mean either that HBV is not sufficient to cause PHC or that there are several independent causes. The fact that some cases of PHC are not associated with HBV is a weak argument against its aetiological role, for many diseases have multiple independent aetiologies.

Before the strong association between HBV and PHC was established, aflatoxins in foodstuffs were thought to be the most probable cause of PHC. Aflatoxins are established hepatic carcinogens in many animal species,[6,15] and many studies have shown that aflatoxins are frequently present in human foods in areas of the world with high incidences of PHC. [16-19] A study in Africa showed a geographical correlation between the amount of aflatoxin in food and the incidence of PHC.[20] Aflatoxin-feeding experiments in monkeys, however, suggest that primates are much less sensitive to the carcinogenic effects than many other species.[21] Aflatoxins have been demonstrated in foodstuffs in Taiwan but there are insufficient data regarding distribution, frequency, or concenrration.[22] No effort in this study was made to study aflatoxins mainly because there is no way to measure previous aflatoxin exposure; and because the Chinese diet is so complex, food sampling for aflatoxins is a formidable task. All we can say is that the currently available data are consistent with HBV having a role as an independent aetiological agent for PHC or as a cofactor with aflatoxin. The very high relative risk among HBsAg-positive men in this study, however, suggests that HBV is an almost essential factor, whereas the aflatoxin in the food in Taiwan is not likely to be an independent inducer of PHC among Chinese men.

PHC usually occurs in cirrhotic livers.[23,24] Prospective studies of patients with clinical cirrhosis have shown a considerably higher risk of PHC among HBsAg-positive than HBsAg-negative cirrhosis patients.[14] The data from our study also show a close relationship between PHC and cirrhosis; 30 of the 41 (73%) men who died of PHC also had cirrhosis. Since necropsies were not done, this figure might be considered an underestimate of cirrhosis in PHC; however, cirrhosis was found in a similar proportion (14 of 19; 74%) of histologically confirmed PHC cases. Thus, our study suggests that HBsAg carriers are at increased risk of PHC even if they do not have underlying cirrhosis. It is not possible to find out whether the risk of PHC is greater in HBsAg carriers with cirrhosis since most subclinical cirrhosis cannot be diagnosed in a population study. The data from this study, however, show that an HBsAg carrier with clinical cirrhosis is at considerably greater risk of dying from PHC than a carrier with no suspicion of liver disease. PHC did not develop in any of 30 HBsAg-negative men who were known to have cirrhosis when they joined the study but did develop in 5 of 40 HBsAg-positive men with clinical cirrhosis when they were recruited. This finding indicates that HBV rather than cirrhosis promotes PHC, as suggested by the prospective study by Klatskin[25] of subjects with chronic active hepatitis in the U.S.A.; among the 24 HBsAg-positive patients PHC developed in 3, whereas none of the 67 HBsAg-negative patients developed PHC.

Death-certificate data from Taiwan show that PHC is the most common malignant neoplasm, accounting for 20% of all malignancies for both sexes combined and for 25.4% of malignancies among men only. Our study, in which cause of death is generally well established and which is more reliable than figures derived from death certificates, suggests that the death-certificate data have underestimated the frequency of PHC in Taiwan. Together PHC and cirrhosis in this study accounted for 20% of all deaths and 54% of all deaths among HBsAg-positive male carriers. PHC accounted for 37% of malignancies in our study compared with 25.4% of malignancies in men from death-certificate data. The death certificate data give the ratio of PHC deaths to cirrhosis deaths as 0.78%, whereas in our study the ratio is 2·6. This pronounced difference suggests that many deaths due to PHC are attributed to cirrhosis on death certificates.

Although this study contributes substantially to the understanding of the relation between HBV and PHC, it leaves many unsolved questions: what is the role of cirrhosis in the aetiology and pathogenesis of PHC; do HBV carriers of other races and in other places have the same risk of PHC as Chinese men in Taiwan; and what factors determine which HBV-infected persons will develop PHC? Where feasible, prospective studies should be carried out in other populations.

We thank all the UWMRU staff, in particular nurses Maggie Huang and Marie Ao, who conducted the recruiting and follow-up for the GECC and CVDS groups respectively, all the nurses and nurses' assistants, and the teams of technicians headed by T.Y. Lin. We also thank the many GECC employees who helped in recruiting, follow-up, and record searches. The study was supported by the National Cancer Institute of the U.S. National Institutes of Health (contract No. YO1 CP 60502 and grant No. CA 25327-03), and by the China Foundation and National Science Council of Taiwan (award NSC- 69B-0412-02[17].

SOURCE

Beasley RP, Lin C-C, Hwang L-Y, and Chien C-S. 1981. Hepatocellular carcinoma and hepatitis B virus: A prospective study of 22,707 men in Taiwan. *Lancet* 1981 (Nov 21): 1129–33. Copyright 1981 *The Lancet*. Reprinted with permission of Elsevier.

Malignant Melanoma of the Skin
(1987)

B. K. Armstrong & C. D. J. Holman

Ultra-violet radiation (UVR) in sunlight is thought to be the main cause of malignant melanoma in lightly-pigmented populations. Individuals with fair skin, fair hair, blue eyes and/or a tendency to burn rather than tan when exposed to the sun are at particularly high risk of melanoma and should be given special attention in primary prevention programmes. Intermittent exposure to the sun, as in recreational exposure, may be a more potent cause of melanoma than more continuous exposure. Primary prevention offers the best prospects for a substantial reduction in mortality from malignant melanoma. However, there is little evidence available to judge the effectiveness of primary prevention of melanoma through reduction of exposure to the sun. Education for reducing exposure to the sun is common in high-risk populations but has never been evaluated adequately. Mortality from melanoma could also possibly be reduced by earlier diagnosis through education or screening of high-risk groups. Regular screening of patients with the familial dysplastic naevus syndrome should reduce their mortality from melanoma.

Etiology

Constitutional Factors

RACE. Racial differences in skin pigmentation and the skin's response to sunlight are known to be the predominant factor affecting the incidence rate of melanoma. On average, melanoma is some 3–4 times more common in lightly-pigmented than heavily- pigmented races (1). These differences in pigmentation are due to variation in melanogenesis and the skin content of melanin, and not to the density of melanocytes (2). Melanin exerts a photoprotective effect in skin by acting as a neutral density filter, attenuating radiation by scattering, and absorbing the ultraviolet radiation (UVR) energy. In addition, it can undergo immediate oxidation and, as a stable free radical, can act as a biological exchange polymer (3). These latter effects, while not influencing UVR penetration into the skin, may block chemical reactions leading to carcinogenesis.

Among heavily-pigmented races there is appreciable variation in the incidence of melanoma. Thus, for example, the rates are twice as high in black Africans as in U.S. Blacks; the latter, in turn, have rates three times higher than those in most Asian populations (1). Since Asians are less heavily pigmented than black Africans, factors other than skin pigmentation, which are correlated with race, must influence the risk at this lower end of the incidence distribution. It may be relevant to note that melanoma of the foot (mainly sole) comprises about 30% of all melanomas in the Japanese, but 40–75% of melanomas in U.S. Blacks or black Africans (4).

INDIVIDUAL PIGMENTARY CHARACTERISTICS. Within predominantly lightly-pigmented populations, the incidence of melanoma is influenced by individual pigmentary characteristics. Several studies have shown that incidence is least in those with black hair, olive or dark skin and brown eyes, and highest in those with red hair, fair or light skin and blue eyes (4). In addition, those who tend to burn or freckle in response to sunlight are at greater risk than those who tend to tan (5). These relationships are supported by direct measurement of the sensitivity of skin to sunlight (6).

SPECIFIC GENETIC PREDISPOSITION. Increased risk of melanoma in some families is well recognized (4). Independently of pigmentary characteristics and number of naevi, a family history of melanoma has been found to be associated with a 2.4 times increased risk of melanoma (5). The dysplastic naevus syndrome (7) is now recognized as associated with familial melanoma in a high proportion of cases. The familial dysplastic naevus syndrome may be present in from 6% to 10% of all melanoma patients (8).

The incidence of melanoma and other skin cancers is increased greatly in patients with xeroderma pigmentosum, an autosomal recessive condition characterized, in most cases, by a defect in the capacity to repair UVR-induced DNA damage (9), and in albino subjects who lack normal skin pigmentation.

BENIGN NAEVI. The number of benign melanocytic naevi that a person has on the skin is a very strong predictor of subsequent risk of melanoma (5, 10). Number of naevi is arguably a constitutional factor; whether benign naevi are predominantly genetically determined or are due to an environmental agent is uncertain.

Environmental Factors

SUNLIGHT. Short-wave UVR in sunlight is thought to be the main environmental factor responsible for melanoma and other skin cancers (4). In this context, short-wave means wavelengths of from about 290 nm (the shortest which reaches the earth's surface) to 315 or 320 nm (so called ultraviolet B radiation). The same wavelength band is mainly responsible for sunburn.

The main effects of UVR are to produce pyrimidine dimers (particularly thymine dimers), cross-linkages between DNA bases and nucleoproteins, and breakages in polynucleotide chains (11). UVR alone can induce sarcomas and squamous cell carcinomas of the skin in mice (*12*) but not melanoma. It may also promote melanoma development in strains of mice prone to spontaneous melanoma (*13*).

The associations between the incidence of melanoma and racially determined skin pigmentation, individual pigmentary characteristics, and skin reaction to sunlight in lightly-pigmented races provide strong circumstantial evidence of an etiological role of sunlight in this disease. Evidence is also provided by the increased incidence of melanoma and other skin cancers in patients with xeroderma pigmentosum (see above).

More direct evidence comes from the association between incidence of melanoma in light-skinned populations and proximity to the equator both within and among countries (*14*). There are, however, exceptions to this pattern. For example, in Australia the incidence of melanoma varies inversely with the latitude between States but within Queensland and Western Australia, both of which have a high incidence, the latitude gradient is reversed. In Europe the latitude gradient is also reversed, with high rates in Nordic countries and the lowest rates in the south. This inconsistency may be explained, at least in part, by greater degrees of constitutional skin pigmentation in southern European populations. Other inconsistencies could be due to supervening climatic factors, as latitude is not the only determinant of UVR flux. A positive association can be shown, in some situations, between melanoma incidence and the mean number of hours of sunshine daily, but this is generally weaker than the association with latitude (*15*).

The incidence of melanoma also varies with the seasons, with a summer-time peak, and between years apparently in association with sunspot activity (which may influence the atmospheric ozone content, a major absorber of short-wave UVR) (*4*) or the extent of summer sunshine (*16*). The latter effects have a lag period of 2 to 5 years, thus suggesting an action of UVR with short latency, more consistent with cancer promotion than cancer initiation.

Attention has been drawn to aspects of the epidemiology of melanoma which are inconsistent with the solar hypothesis (*17*). For example, the distribution of melanoma on the body surface favours relatively unexposed sites—the trunk is the commonest site in males and the legs in females. This distribution contrasts with the distribution of non-melanocytic skin cancers which favours the face and upper limbs (*18*). Melanoma also differs from other skin cancers, for which the evidence of a solar etiology is more clear cut (*18*), in its higher incidence in females than males and the early rise and middle-age peak in its incidence. Non-melanocytic skin cancers are substantially commoner in males (who are more likely to work outdoors) than females, and their incidence rises more or less exponentially with age (as would be expected from continuing accumulation of exposure to the sun). Also against the solar hypothesis for the etiology of melanoma is evidence that the incidence is greater in indoor than outdoor workers and, at least sometimes, in urban than rural populations (4). The opposite is true, in each case, for non-melanocytic skin cancer (18).

Several hypotheses have been advanced to explain these inconsistencies, the most recent being the intermittent exposure hypothesis (19). It suggests that the risk of non-melanocytic skin cancers and possibly also melanoma of the Hutchinson's melanotic freckle type (which appears to be epidemiologically similar to non-melanocytic skin cancers) varies with the total accumulated dose of UVR, however received, whereas other melanomas are more likely to arise if sun exposure is received in intermittent, intense bursts (as in the recreational exposure of body sites not usually exposed to the sun). If true, this theory could explain most if not all the inconsistencies referred to above.

A number of recent studies of individuals provide evidence for the effects of both cumulative and intermittent exposure to the sun on the incidence of melanoma. In a study in Western Australia, the incidence of melanoma was lower in immigrants (who generally came from areas of low sun exposure) than in native-born Australians, had a direct correlation with the annual hours of bright sunlight averaged over all places of residence in the native-born, and was positively associated with an objective measure of sun damage in the skin (20). These observations suggest that the total accumulated sun exposure has a bearing on melanoma etiology. The same study failed to find convincing effects from intermittent exposure to the sun as measured by the proportion of all outdoor exposure that was recreational (21). Incidence of melanoma, however, did increase with frequency of participation in waterside recreations, particularly boating and fishing, and melanoma of the trunk was increased substantially in incidence in women who usually wore a two-piece bathing suit at the beach in summer or bathed nude (21). In a similar study from western Canada, positive associations were observed between melanoma and the number of hours of beach activities in summer and the number of sunny vacations per decade (22).

OTHER FACTORS. A variety of other environmental factors have been suggested as increasing the risk of melanoma. They include female sex hormones (both endogenous and exogenous), diet, alcohol drinking, use of certain medications, use of hair dyes, exposure to fluorescent light, occupational exposure to petroleum products and other hydrocarbons, trauma and X-irradiation. The evidence for most of them is limited at present (4, 23). It is doubtful whether any could explain more than a small proportion of melanomas in any general population.

Therapy and Outcome

Therapy

Surgical excision of the primary lesion is the treatment of choice for all but advanced malignant melanoma. Traditionally, wide local excision of the primary lesion has been recommended but there is little evidence that *wide* excision is especially beneficial (*24*). Recent recommendations for stage I disease require an excision margin of no more than 1.5 cm for a lesion with a good prognosis and a 3.0 cm margin for all other lesions (*25*). Therapeutic block dissection of draining lymph nodes is beneficial when, on clinical evidence, the nodes are the site of metastases. Prophylactic block dissection in stage I disease probably does not confer a survival advantage (*26*).

Outcome

The prognosis of melanoma depends mainly on sex, clinical stage, and the site and thickness of the primary lesion. Females have a better prognosis than males; stage lesions (local disease only) do better than stage II (nodes involved) and stage III lesions (distant metastases); lesions of the extremities tend to have a better prognosis than lesions of the trunk; and thin lesions have a better prognosis than thick lesions (*25, 27*). Preinvasive melanomas (Clark's level I) and invasive melanomas less than 0.76 mm in thickness show 100%o disease-free survival at 5 years (*28*).

The prognosis of melanoma has improved substantially over the past 20 to 30 years. Thus, for example, in the U.S. National Cancer Institute's End Results Surveys the relative 5-year survival increased from 41% in melanomas diagnosed in 1940–49 to 67% in melanomas diagnosed in 1965–69 (*29*) and to 76% in 1973–79 in the US SEER (Staging, Epidemiology and End Results) Registries (*30*). In some populations a parallel trend towards diagnosis of less-advanced lesions has been documented. For example, in Queensland (Australia) in 1966 some 70% of melanomas were diagnosed at level III or higher, whereas in 1977 this proportion had fallen to 50% (*31*).

The improving prognosis of melanoma has paralleled increasing incidence rates (see below). To illustrate again from the experience in Queensland, the estimated crude incidence of invasive melanoma (level 2 or deeper) rose from 11.4 per 100,000 in males and 14.1 per 100,000 in females in 1963–69 to 24.9 per 100,000 in males and 25.4 per 100,000 in females in 1977 (*31,32*). The estimated crude incidence of preinvasive (level 1) melanoma rose proportionately more from 1.3 per 100,000 in males and 1.5 per 100,000 in females to 8.4 per 100,000 and 8.7 per 100,000, respectively. Over the same period mortality from melanoma in Queensland was almost constant (32), thus implying an improving prognosis.

In addition to a temporal association there is a geographical association between incidence and prognosis of melanoma (28). Australia has the highest incidence of melanoma and the best prognosis; patients with invasive melanoma diagnosed in Western Australia in 1975 and 1976 had relative 5-year survival rates of 85% in males and 89% in females. By way of comparison the 5-year survival rates from melanomas diagnosed in Iowa (USA) (which has one sixth the incidence rate of Western Australia) in 1970–74 were 58% in males and 71% in females (28). Differences in distributions of tumour thickness probably underlie this geographical variation in prognosis (33).

While behavioural factors leading to earlier diagnosis in high-incidence populations are generally thought to be responsible for these temporal and geographical associations between incidence and survival, the possibility that a high incidence of melanoma is associated with a less aggressive form of the disease cannot be excluded. Alternatively, or as well, the association of a high incidence of melanoma with increased public and professional awareness of the disease may lead to increased diagnosis of lesions which, if left, would not lead to death. It should be noted, however, that in Queensland at least, as described above, the incidence of invasive, as well as preinvasive, melanoma increased while mortality was constant.

A near 100% cure rate could be achieved for melanoma if all patients were diagnosed in the preinvasive stage, or with lesions less than 0.76 mm in thickness, and treated surgically (28). Currently some 30% of melanomas diagnosed in Western Australia are preinvasive and 4,870 of invasive melanomas are less than 0.76 mm thick. As indicated above, this comparatively favourable distribution could be due as much to the nature of the underlying disease as to awareness of the need for early diagnosis. It cannot be assumed, therefore, that similar or better distributions could be obtained elsewhere by education for early diagnosis or screening.

Size of the Worldwide Problem

Geographical Variation in Incidence

Melanoma varies some 300-fold in incidence between different populations. The highest incidence rates, 39.6 per 100,000 person-years in males and 31.3 per 100,000 person-years in females (standardized to the age distribution of the "world" population), were reported from Queensland (Australia) in 1979–80 (34). The lowest recent rates, 0.2 per 100,000 in both sexes, came from Osaka (Japan) in 1973–75 (35). In Australia the disease is essentially confined to the white population, in whom it is the fourth most common cancer in incidence (after lung, breast and colon) and the fourth most common cause of loss of life before the age of 70 years (*36*).

Between the extremes of Australia and Asia lie the populations of New Zealand, North America and Scandinavia towards the top end of the range, although with rates one half or less than those in Australia (4 to 18 per 100,000); other northern European populations (2 to 4 per 100,000); black Africans, whether resident in Africa or not (0.5 to 2 per 100,000); populations in Spain and of Mediterranean origin in South America (0.3 to 2 per 100,000); and, finally, other Asian populations (0.2 to 1 per 100,000) (*35*). This distribution, which is highly skewed to the right, is determined almost certainly by a combination of constitutional susceptibility and environmental exposure to, mainly, UVR. Differences in the availability of health services and diagnostic evaluation of preinvasive melanomas may also contribute to variation between populations in the recorded incidence rates. The median incidence of melanoma in a survey of 53 populations was 1.2 per 100,000 in males and 1.5 per 100,000 in females (*35*).

Like melanoma, non-melanocytic skin cancer varies very widely in incidence. In the same survey of 53 populations the highest incidence was in Manitoba, Canada (97 per 100,000 in males and 67 per 100,000 in females) and the lowest in Osaka, Japan (1.4 per 100,000 in males and 0.6 per 100,000 in females) (*35*). The crude incidence in the white population of Queensland, Australia has been reported at 265 per 100,000 in males and 156 per 100,000 in females (*37*). There is a rough positive correlation between the incidence of non-melanocytic skin cancer and melanoma, with the former usually substantially higher (10-fold or more in males and 5-fold or more in females) than the latter. Like melanoma also, non-melanocytic skin cancer is rare in most Asian populations for which incidence data are available (*35*), and uncommon in heavily pigmented populations in comparison with lightly pigmented populations living in the same area. In heavily-pigmented populations non-melanocytic skin cancer has a predilection for the lower limbs where it commonly occurs in burn scars or at the site of chronic infection or ulceration (*18*) [(*38*), Ed.]. In most populations mortality from melanoma is higher than that from non-melanocytic skin cancer; in a few, in which mortality from both is low, the opposite is true (*39*).

Trends in Incidence with Time

Almost all white populations have experienced an increase in incidence of melanomas, averaging from 1.5% to 20% per year (*40*), since at least 1950 (*4*). No similar increase has been seen in black populations. Where it has been studied, a birth-cohort effect has usually been evident in the increases with a peak incidence and/or mortality in those born between about 1920 and 1930 (40). This suggests that the increase will level off and then end shortly after the year 2000 in the absence of introduction of any new causal or protective agent.

Most of the increase in melanoma incidence has been on the trunk in males and legs in females. There has been little change in melanoma of the head and neck (40). The increase has been attributed to increasing recreational exposure to the sun.

Prospects for Reduction in Incidence

On present evidence it would be reasonable to suggest that the difference in melanoma incidence between the white population of Australia and the populations in their countries of origin (predominantly the United Kingdom and Ireland) is attributable largely to their difference in exposure to sunlight. The potential exists, therefore, by control of such exposure, to reduce the incidence rates in Australia from between 10 and 40 per 100,000 (depending mainly on latitude of residence) to the levels of 2 to 4 per 100,000 as in the United Kingdom, or even lower. Reduction to these levels should also be possible in other high-incidence white populations (e.g., in New Zealand, USA and Scandinavia).

A reduction in incidence does not promise the same relative reduction in mortality. Mortality from melanoma varies only 20- to 30-fold, from about 2 to 3 per 100,000 in Australia and New Zealand to 0.1 per 100,000 in Japan. Median levels of mortality in a survey of 26 populations were 0.8 per 100,000 in males and 0.9 per 100,000 in females (41). The distribution of mortality from melanoma is therefore much less skew than that of incidence, the difference probably being due to the association between incidence and survival (see above, p. 247). By use of the reasoning applied to incidence rates (see above), mortality from melanoma in Australia and New Zealand could be reduced from 2–3 to 0.7–0.8 per 100,000 by control of sun exposure.

Prevention

Primary Prevention

On present evidence, only control of exposure to sunlight warrants serious attention as a measure for the primary prevention of melanoma. Attention in controlling such exposure can be directed towards readily identifiable high-risk groups—generally lightly-pigmented populations living in areas where average UV flux is high, and specifically fair-skinned people whose predominant reaction on exposure to the sun is to burn rather than tan.

The process of prevention has so far been through education towards the following behaviour:

(i) reducing the total time spent out of doors, particularly in summer;

(ii) limiting outdoor activities, again particularly in summer, to before 10h00 and after 14h00 solar time; about 66% of UV energy from the sun in any 24-hour period is received during these four hours (42);

(iii) wearing a wide-brimmed hat whenever in the sun;

(iv) covering the skin as much as possible in the sun; different clothing materials may allow passage of as little as none to as much as 50% of the UVR that would otherwise reach unclothed skin (42);

(v) making maximum use of available shade out of doors; in seeking shade, consideration must be given to skylight, light scattered from clouds, dust and moisture, and reflected light as well as direct sunlight; as much as 50% of UVR may be received as skylight and appreciable amounts of UVR are reflected from fresh snow and, to a lesser extent, dry, white sand (42);

(vi) using highly protective sunscreen lotions or creams correctly on all skin not protected in any of the above ways.

Educational programmes based on the above principles are conducted regularly in Australia (43) and have been implemented elsewhere. There has been little research into their likely effects (knowledge, attitudes, acceptability, etc.) and no evaluation of their ultimate effectiveness has been reported. There are limited indications that such programmes might work. Experimentally, paraaminobenzoic acid (an effective sunscreen) applied topically one hour before exposure to UVR can block the production of squamous cell carcinoma of the skin in hairless mice first given dimethylbenzanthracene (44). In patients with xeroderma pigmentosum, a programme of protection against UVR, similar to that described above, has slowed or halted the development of solar keratoses and other skin cancers, including melanoma (45).

Secondary Prevention

Theoretically early detection, as well as incidence reduction, has the potential to reduce mortality from malignant melanoma although, as stated above (see above), there is no certainty that recent improvements in prognosis of melanoma have been due to earlier recognition of suspicious lesions. Efforts at early detection have been based on education of the public and the medical profession regarding features of a pigmented lesion that should excite suspicion (46).

The effectiveness of education for early diagnosis has not been evaluated. In Queensland, however, following the Queensland Melanoma Project, which was accompanied by a substantial amount of public education (43), mortality from melanoma has remained comparatively steady although the incidence has risen, while mortality has continued to rise in the other States of Australia (32). This is suggestive of an effect of early diagnosis on incidence and mortality.

Specific screening of skin for suspicious lesions by a trained observer has been advocated and practiced in a desultory fashion but never evaluated as to effectiveness or cost. It is most likely to be justified in patients with the dysplastic naevus syndrome (see above, page 245), whether familial or sporadic, and might be considered in subjects with large numbers of naevi even if none appears to be dysplastic. It has been recommended that patients with the dysplastic naevus syndrome be subject to regular photographic surveillance for change in the appearance of their pigmented naevi (7). Change suggestive of progression to melanoma would be followed by excision of the lesion. This approach has been successful in reducing the average thickness of melanomas diagnosed in individuals with the familial dysplastic naevus syndrome (47).

Conclusions

Ultraviolet radiation (UVR) in sunlight is thought to be the main cause of malignant melanoma in lightly-pigmented populations. Individuals with fair skin, fair hair, blue eyes and/or a tendency to burn rather than tan when exposed to the sun are at particularly high risk of melanoma and should be given special attention in primary prevention programmes. Intermittent exposure to the sun, as in recreational exposure, may be a more potent cause of melanoma than long continued exposure. There is little evidence available to judge the effectiveness of primary prevention of melanoma through reduction of exposure to the sun. Education for reduction in sun exposure is common in high-risk populations but has never been evaluated adequately.

Mortality from melanoma could possibly be reduced by earlier diagnosis through education or screening of high-risk groups. Regular screening of patients with the familial dysplastic naevus syndrome should reduce their mortality from melanoma.

No research aimed directly at evaluating the effectiveness of primary or secondary prevention of melanoma in known to be in progress. However, primary prevention offers the best prospects for a substantial reduction in mortality from malignant melanoma. There is a need for evaluation of the effectiveness of the measures detailed above in reducing the incidence of and mortality from melanoma. This could be done best by a multi-centre, collaborative controlled trial of these or related measures. Effectiveness would be assessed, in the short term, as behaviour change and, in the long term, as change in the incidence rate of melanoma.

SOURCE

Armstrong BK and Holman CDJ. 1987. Malignant melanoma of the skin. *Bull World Health Organ* 65 (2): 245–252. Reprinted with permission of WHO Press.

CHAPTER 12

HEART DISEASE AND STROKE

Disease and ill health are caused largely by damage at the molecular and cellular level, yet today's surgical tools are too large to deal with that kind of problem.
　　—Ralph C. Merkle (b. 1952), American inventor (nanotechnology)

Medical science has proven time and again that when the resources are provided, great progress in the treatment, cure, and prevention of disease can occur.
　　—Michael J. Fox (b. 1961), Canadian actor

On Monday, September 26, 1955, the Dow Jones Industrial Average plunged 32 points (from 487), a one-day decline of 6.5 percent. The cause of this drop, which destroyed $14 billion (the largest single day financial market loss up to then), was the hospitalization of President Dwight David Eisenhower with a myocardial infarction (heart attack) two days prior. At the time, coronary heart disease mortality in the United States and in other Western countries was in ascendancy. Spurred by the epidemic of cigarette smoking (see Chapter 2) and dietary factors, coronary heart disease became the No. 1 killer in the United States during the first two-thirds of the twentieth century. In its wake, epidemiologic innovations such as the Framingham, Seven Countries, Whitehall, and American Cancer Society Million Person Studies (among others) took place, and clinical interventions including antihypertensives, statins, coronary artery bypass graft surgery (CABG), and stents were developed and entered into the popular lexicon.

CARDIOVASCULAR DISEASE

Cardiovascular disease (CVD) encompasses many conditions, including coronary heart disease, hypertension (high blood pressure), peripheral artery or vascular disease (PAD, PVD), cerebrovascular disease (stroke), hypertensive kidney disease, congestive heart disease, and valvular heart disease (including rheumatic heart disease). Concurrent with the rise in coronary heart disease mortality were increases in stroke mortality and in the prevalence of hypertension, as well as declines in rheumatic heart disease. To some degree, the observed increases reflected improved disease ascertainment; not until the mid twentieth century was increasing blood pressure during the lifespan understood as a cardiovascular condition requiring treatment. However, there were also increases in the incidence and prevalence of these diseases, likely reflective of increased exposure to risk factors (e.g., cigarette smoking) and, in the latter third of the twentieth century, improvements in medical care leading to enhanced survivorship.

The medical and public health communities responded to the increase in cardiovascular disease mortality with the establishment of cohort studies to determine which risk factors were associated with specific diseases. They created specialized research networks to better define the clinical and biochemical characteristics of cardiovascular diseases and instituted international collaborations to standardize both clinical and epidemiologic methods for studying these now epidemic chronic disease entities. The Framingham Heart Study is perhaps the best known of these investigations, and it continues six decades later with ongoing studies of second-generation offspring of the members of the original cohort. Although the study is limited in diversity, it has the strength of examining narrowed variables in a large population to give clear information about risk.

Framingham is not the only continuing cohort study, however, and the many rich data sets collected in the course of these investigations continue to be mined for new insights into the occurrence and prevention of cardiovascular disease. For example, studies into the role of sex hormones, particularly oral contraceptives, ensued, and cardiovascular risks associated with their use were defined. In addition, post-menopausal estrogen use was investigated from the perspective of providing protection against cardiovascular disease. Standardized methods were also developed from these research efforts—from how to read electrocardiograms (EKGs) to how to conduct population surveys. As information burgeoned about how cardiovascular disease develops, several interventions to reduce exposure to risk factors emerged; improved therapeutic modalities to treat those persons demonstrating clinical manifestations of the disease emerged as well.

INTERVENTIONS

Cardiovascular disease mortality peaked in the United States in 1968; stroke mortality peaked about a decade before. However, it was in the cerebrovascular arena, with the Veterans Administration Acute Stroke Study (VASt), that intervention showed its first promise. This early randomized clinical trial demonstrated the efficacy of antihypertensive therapy in the prevention of strokes.

The study was significant in establishing the concept of secondary prevention in the cardiovascular field, and it provided a template for investigators seeking to undertake similar efforts. For instance, in the early 1970s, the National Heart, Lung, and Blood Institute of the NIH initiated the Multiple Risk Factor Intervention Trial (MRFIT), which sought to reduce exposure to smoking, high blood pressure, and high serum cholesterol through behavioral modifications recommended by physicians in their usual course of patient care. In the early 1980s, the MRFIT Study Group reported no statistically significant effect of the interventions on cardiovascular mortality.

Concurrent with efforts focused on cardiovascular risk reduction in individual patients, a pioneering community-based intervention effort was launched by John W. Farquhar and colleagues at Stanford University in California. Between 1972 and 1976, the Stanford Three-Community Study found that community-based interventions (advertising and other mass media messages implemented in towns of about 20,000 people) could successfully reduce cardiovascular risk factor exposures and the toll of disease from these conditions. Subsequent efforts with the Stanford Five Cities Study, the Pawtucket (Rhode Island) Heart-Health Program, the Minnesota Heart-Health Program, and similar efforts in North Karelia, Finland, sought to validate these results; they were not successful.

During the latter third of the twentieth century, as cardiovascular disease mortality continued to fall in the United States, efforts to explain the decline repeatedly demonstrated the considerable impact of medical interventions, such as CABG, transcutaneous angioplasty, implantation of stents, and similar invasive procedures. Not all interventions were efficacious. For example, the Extracranial-Intracranial Bypass Study found that the popular surgery did not reduce stroke risk, contrary to the contentions of its advocates. Identifying effects of the interventions was challenging, and direct efficacy could not be established. However, the need for risk-factor reduction was understood to be essential in order to attain further progress in cardiovascular disease prevention.

New classes of antihypertensive drugs were developed and opened the possibility that mortality could be reduced not only from coronary heart disease but also from the associated conditions of chronic kidney disease and congestive heart failure. In the last two decades of the twentieth century, statins became available and promised to reduce the effect of hyperlipidemias, as well as that of cardiovascular inflammation, a newly defined risk factor. International cardiovascular disease prevention efforts did not begin with the appearance of pharmacological interventions, however. They began in the middle of the twentieth century, in the wake of World War II and the founding of the WHO.

INTERNATIONAL EFFORTS

During the 1950s, the rising tide of coronary heart disease morbidity and mortality caught the attention of the WHO, which sponsored by creating a standard ascertainment tool called the Rose Questionnaire (RQ). The RQ facilitated the identification of people at risk for cardiovascular diseases for whom intervention efforts might have greater impact than if applied to the population as a whole. It also facilitated estimation of the degree to which cardiovascular disease was present in a community, assisting health policy makers in the allocation of resources. As cardiovascular epidemiology studies in the United States and England (particularly the Whitehall Study) proceeded, they enumerated new risk factors, including dimensions such as socioeconomic status. The Seven Countries Study identified a reduced risk of coronary heart disease associated with the "Mediterranean diet," which was low in animal fats and high in mono- and polyunsaturated fats.

The North Karelia Project in Finland took place at the same time as U.S. intervention efforts to reduce cardiovascular disease risk. The province of North Karelia had been observed to have a notably high mortality rate from cardiovascular diseases. Further investigation disclosed that the North Karelia population had high rates of cigarette smoking, hypercholesterolemia, and hypertension. An interventional program was developed to address the prevalence of these risk factors. As part of the assessment of the effectiveness of the interventional effort, changes in risk factor prevalence and cardiovascular disease mortality were compared in a province with a population similar to North Karelia's. Subsequent analyses demonstrated the benefit of the project's interventions, and the Finnish government quickly moved to expand the project to the entirety of Finland.

At the same time, the WHO developed a global cardiovascular surveillance network: the multination monitoring of trends and determinants in cardiovascular disease (MONICA) Project. The 26-country monitoring effort evolved into interventional initiatives to reduce exposure to cardiovascular disease risk factors and to monitor the occurrence of cardiovascular disease at 39 collaborative centers. The WHO's sponsorship of the MONICA Project continues into the twenty-first century as a coordinated global effort to combat cardiovascular disease mortality.

Although cardiovascular disease no longer captivates Western populations as it did five decades ago, it remains a prominent cause of morbidity and mortality. And with the development of a global economy, it seems likely this health problem will be exported to the developing world along with jobs and affluent lifestyles.

PEDIATRIC ATHEROSCLEROSIS

During the Korean War, pathologists examining the bodies of soldiers returned for burial noted that the bodies of what should have been healthy young men exhibited an increased incidence of coronary atherosclerosis. At the time, the focus of research efforts was on adults, as they were the ones experiencing the clinical effects of cardiovascular disease such as angina pectoris, myocardial infarction, strokes, and so on. More than a decade later, a similar observation by pathologists examining the bodies of soldiers killed in the Vietnam War was made, raising the possibility that cardiovascular disease begins in childhood. If this possibility were to be validated in epidemiologic studies, cardiovascular prevention efforts would need to begin earlier in life, that is, during or prior to adolescence.

The Bogalusa Heart Study was mounted in an effort to discern if and how cardiovascular disease developed in children. It established several cohorts of children in Bogalusa, Louisiana, who were followed to track the behavior of cardiovascular risk factors during childhood. In so doing, the study established that children with the greatest exposure to high serum cholesterol and high blood pressure maintained those elevated cardiovascular risk profiles into adulthood. It then extended its analyses to include obesity and suggested that obese children with these risk profiles grew into the obese adults constituting the initial wave of the developing epidemic of diabetes mellitus. Anatomic changes indicative of atherosclerosis were documented in the Bogalusa cohorts as early as five to eight years of age. Data from the Bogalusa Heart Study stimulated efforts to intervene during childhood to reduce risk factor exposure, including changes in diet, prevalence of cigarette smoking, and exercise.

Although the Bogalusa Heart Study continued to follow subjects into the twenty-first century, by the early 1980s, it was clear that cardiovascular disease did not begin in adulthood and that our understanding of the pathophysiologic process leading to it was at best incomplete. As a bridge between the accruing data in children from Bogalusa and the established understanding of overt disease in adults, the Coronary Artery Risk Development in Young Adults (CARDIA) study began in 1986 with four cohorts of young adults (ages 18 to 30) followed for the development of subclinical atherosclerosis. With Bogalusa and CARDIA, the importance of beginning cardiovascular risk factor intervention in childhood has become clear, as the children with the greatest risk become the adults who subsequently manifest both subclinical and overt cardiovascular disease.

Primary, Secondary, and Tertiary Prevention

In the mid 1940s, Ancel Keys from the University of Minnesota described the Mediterranean diet in Salerno, Italy (low consumption of meat and meat products; moderate consumption of dairy products, fish, and wine; and high consumption of olive oil, fruits, vegetables, and unrefined cereals) and linked it to normal body weight and longevity. Unfortunately, the Mediterranean diet was not common among Westernized populations, and obesity increased. With obesity came elevated serum triglycerides and insulin resistance. By the early 1990s, the occurrence of insulin resistance, obesity, hypertension, and elevated serum cholesterol in the same individual, termed "Metabolic Syndrome," was associated with markedly elevated risk of cardiovascular disease. At the close of the twentieth century, insulin resistance alone, and as part of Metabolic Syndrome, loomed as a public health threat in Westernized populations and was spreading worldwide.

It took the media to make dietary intervention for heart disease fashionable, despite the fact that several large cardiovascular clinical trials showed that changing diet, increasing exercise, and taking certain types of drugs could all reduce morbidity and mortality from cardiovascular disease. Specifically, MRFIT showed that lipid profiles predict the development of cardiovascular disease, hypertension is related to stroke, and amputations are influenced by arterial calcification and duration of diabetes. The Nurse's Health Study showed that cardiovascular mortality rates among women who smoked were higher than among those who did not smoke. The Physician's Health Study showed that taking aspirin for the primary prevention of cardiovascular disease reduced the risk of myocardial infarction. The Scandinavian Simvastatin Survival Study (4S) showed that statins reduced mortality in cardiovascular disease patients by 30 percent, though they were not effective for primary prevention. Despite these findings, we have far to go in the prevention and treatment of cardiovascular disease.

Selected Readings

The first reading, by Thomas R. Dawber, Gilcin F. Meadors, and Felix E. Moore, Jr., describes the 1951 design of the Framingham Study. The authors explain the logic behind the selection of the community, the way in which subject recruitment was done, the variables collected for analysis, and the types of questions that were expected to be addressed from this massive endeavor after five years or more of data accumulation. In 1980, Dawber outlined the following research hypotheses based on the Framingham data: 1) CVD increases with age and occurs earlier and more frequently in males; 2) Persons with hypertension develop

CVD at a greater rate than those who are not hypertensive; 3) Elevated blood cholesterol level is associated with an increased risk of CVD; 4) Tobacco smoking is associated with an increased occurrence of CVD; 5) Habitual use of alcohol is associated with increased incidence of CVD; 6) Increased physical activity is associated with a decrease in the development of CVD; 7) An increase in thyroid function is associated with a decrease in the development of CVD; 8) A high blood hemoglobin or hematocrit level is associated with an increased rate of the development of CVD; 9) An increase in body weight predisposes to CVD; 10) There is an increased rate of the development of CVD in people with diabetes mellitus; and 11) There is higher incidence of CVD in people with gout.

Our second reading, by Geoffrey Rose, is based on his Adolf Streicher memorial lecture given at the North Staffordshire Medical Institute in 1980. In it, Rose argues that there is a "regrettable separation" between the therapeutic and preventive roles played by physicians and that most doctors only tend to those in their care after they are already sick. Prevention, he argues, is the key to reducing the adverse outcomes associated with CVD. Rose argues for a "mass strategy" rather than simply targeting high-risk individuals, an approach he considers far more effective, safe, and acceptable. The work appears here without several graphs that we have determined as unnecessary for the overall readability of the text.

Finally, the paper by Alfred McAlister and colleagues describes the North Karelia Project, a community health intervention to reduce high rates of cardiovascular disease in Finland. The authors describe the program objectives and how health promotion programs were shown to be effective at the time of the five-year evaluation. Of particular interest is the estimate that Finland had already saved $4 million in disability payments, compared to the less than $1 million expended on the North Karelia Project itself. The reader will find the discussion of the limitations of the project clear and should note that the authors admit the project might not be easily replicated in the United States or other countries where the health care system is not easily shifted toward prevention.

BIBLIOGRAPHY

Anderson GF and Chu E. 2007. Expanding priorities—confronting chronic disease in countries with low income. *N Engl J Med* 356 (3): 209–11.

Barritt DW and Jordon SC. 1960. Anticoagulant drugs in the treatment of pulmonary embolism: A controlled trial. *Lancet* 275 (7138): 1309–12.

Belanger CF, Hennekens CH, Rosner B, and Speizer FE. 1978. The Nurses' Health Study. *Am J Nurs* 78:1039–40.

Belanger C, Speizer FE, Hennekens CH, Rosner B, Willett W, and Bain C. 1980. The Nurses' Health Study: Current findings. *Am J Nurs* 80:1333.

Blackburn H. 1983. Research and demonstration projects in community cardiovascular disease prevention. *J Public Health Policy* 4 (4): 398–421.

Centers for Disease Control. Achievements in Public Health, 1900–1999: Decline in deaths from heart disease and stroke—United States, 1900–1999. *MMWR* 48 (30): 649–56.

Chen H-J and Pan W-H. 2007. Probable blind spot in the International Diabetes Federation definition of metabolic syndrome. *Obesity* 15:1096–1100.

Data Monitoring Board of the Physicians' Health Study (Cairns J, Cohen L, Colton T, DeMets DL, Deykin D, Friedman L, Greenwald P, Hutchinson GB and Rosner B). 1991. Issues in the early termination of the aspirin component of the Physicians' Health Study. *Ann Epidemiol* 1:395–405.

Dawber TR. 1980. *The Framingham Study: The Epidemiology of Atherosclerotic Disease.* Cambridge, MA: Harvard University Press.

Dawber TR and Kannel WB. 1958. An epidemiologic study of heart disease: the Framingham study. *Nutr Rev* 16 (1): 1–4.

Dawber TR, Moore FE, and Mann GV. 1957. Coronary heart disease in the Framingham study. *Am J Public Health* 47 (4 Part 2): 4–24.

Dawber TR and Stokes JI. 1956. Rheumatic heart disease in the Framingham Study. *N Engl J Med* 255 (26): 1228–33.

De Lorgeil M, Salen P, Paillard F, Laporte F, Boucher F, and de Leiris J. 2002. Mediterranean diet and the French paradox: Two distinct biogeographic concepts for one consolidated scientific theory on the role of nutrition in coronary heart disease. *Cardiovasc Res* 54:503–15.

Diet and all-causes death rate in the Seven Countries Study. *Lancet* 1981 (July 11); 2 (8237): 58–61.

Enos WF, Holmes RH, Beyer J, and the U.S. Army. 1953. Coronary disease among United Sates soldiers killed in action in Korea: preliminary report. *JAMA* 152:1090–93. Reprinted in 1986. *JAMA* 256 (20): 2859–62.

Epstein FH. 1992. Contribution of epidemiology to understanding coronary heart disease. In: Marmot M and Elliott P, eds. *Coronary Heart Disease Epidemiology: From Aetiology to Public Health.* New York: Oxford University Press.

Ernst ND, Sempos ST, Briefel RR, and Clark MB. 1997. Consistency between U.S. dietary fat intake and serum total cholesterol concentrations: The National Health and Nutrition Examination surveys. *Am J Clin Nutr* 66: 965S–72S.

Fogel RW. 2004. Changes in the process of aging during the twentieth century: Findings and procedures of the early indicators project (in History, Biology, and Disease). *Population and Development Review* 30 (Suppl: Aging, Health, and Public Policy): 19–47.

Fries JF. 1980. Aging, natural death, and the compression of morbidity. *N Engl J Med* 303 (3): 130–35. Reprinted in 2002 *Bull World Health Organ* 80 (3): 245–50.

Fries JF. 2005. The compression of morbidity. *Milbank Q* 83 (4): 801–23.

Fries JF. 2005. Frailty, heart disease, and stroke: The Compression of Morbidity paradigm. *Am J Prev Med* 29 (5 Suppl 1): 164–68.

Gordon T. 1957. Mortality experience among the Japanese in the United States, Hawaii, and Japan. *Public Health Rep* 72:543–53.

Kempler P. 2005. Learning from large cardiovascular clinical trials: Classical cardiovascular risk factors. *Diabetes Res Clin Pract* 68 (Suppl. 1): S43–47.

Keys A. 1951. The cholesterol problem. *Voeding* 13:539–55.

Keys A, ed. 1970. Coronary heart disease in seven countries. *Circulation* 41 and 42 (Suppl. I): 1–211.

Keys A and Aravanis C. 1980. *Seven Countries: A Multivariate Analysis of Death and Coronary Heart Disease.* Cambridge, MA: Harvard University Press.

Keys A, Karvonen MJ, and Fidanza F. 1958. Serum-cholesterol studies in Finland. *Lancet* 2:175–78.

McCully KS. 1998. Homocysteine, folate, vitamin B6, and cardiovascular disease. *JAMA* 279 (5): 392–93. Comment in 1998 *JAMA* 280 (5): 417; author reply 418–19.

McNamara JJ, Molot MA, Stremple JF, and Cutting RT. 1971. Coronary artery disease in combat casualties in Vietnam. *JAMA* 216 (7): 1185–87.

Medical Research Council Working Party. 1988. Stroke and coronary heart disease in mild hypertension: Risk factors and the value of treatment. *Brit Med J* 296:1565–70.

Multiple risk factor intervention trial (MRFIT). 1976. A national study of primary prevention of coronary heart disease. *JAMA* 235 (8): 825–27.

National Institutes of Health. 1997. *The Sixth Report of the Joint National Committee on Prevention, Detection, Evaluation, and Treatment of High Blood Pressure* (NIH 98-4080). Rockville, MD: U.S. Department of Health and Human Services, NIH, and the National Heart, Lung, and Blood Institute.

Olshansky SJ and Ault AB. 1986. The fourth stage of the epidemiologic transition: The age of delayed degenerative diseases. *Milbank Q* 64 (3): 355–91.

Phillips KA, Shlipak MG, Coxson P, Heidenreich PA, Hunink MG, Goldman PA, Williams LW, Weinstein MC, and Goldman L. 2000. Health and economic benefits of increased beta-blocker use following myocardial infarction. *JAMA* 284 (21): 2748–54. Comment in 2001 *JAMA* 285 (8): 1013.

Puska P, Vartiainen E, Laatikainen T, Jousilahti P, and Paavola M, eds. 2009. *North Karelia Project: From North Karelia to National Action.* Helsinki: Terveyden ja hyvinvoinnin laitos. http://www.thl.fi/thl-client/pdfs/731beafd-b544-42b2-b853-baa87db6a046 (accessed November 10, 2007).

Rimm EB, Willett WC, Hu FB, Sampson L, Colditz GA, Manson JE, Hennekens C, and Stampfer MJ. 1998. Folate and vitamin B6 from diet and supplements in relation to risk of coronary heart disease among women. *JAMA* 279 (5): 359–64.

Rodríguez T, Malvezzi M, Chatenoud L, Bosetti C, Levi F, Negri E, and La Vecchia C. 2006. Trends in mortality from coronary heart and cerebrovascular diseases in the Americas: 1970–2000. *Heart* 92:453–60.

Rose G. 1982. Incubation period of coronary heart disease. *Brit Med J* 284:1600–1601.

Rose GA and Blackburn H. 1969. Cardiovascular survey methods. *East African Medical Journal* 46 (5): 220–26.

Rose G, Hamilton PJS, Keen H, Reid DD, McCartney P, and Jarrett RJ. 1977. Myocardial ischemia, risk factors and death from coronary heart-disease. *Lancet* 1 (8003): 105–9.

Rose G and Shipley M. 1990. Effects of coronary risk reduction on the pattern of mortality (Review). *Lancet* 335 (8684): 275–77.

Rothstein WG. 2003. *Public Health and the Risk Factor: A History of an Uneven Medical Revolution.* Rochester, NY: University of Rochester Press.

Schroeder HA. 1960. Relation between mortality from cardiovascular disease and treated water supplies. *J Am Med Assoc* 192:1902–8. Reprinted in 1984 *Nutr Rev* 42 (6): 226–29.

Stallones RA. 1980. The rise and fall of ischemic heart disease. *Scientific American*, November, 53–59.

Stamler J. 1992. Established major coronary risk factors. In: Marmot M and Elliott P, eds. *Coronary Heart Disease Epidemiology: From Aetiology to Public Health.* New York: Oxford University Press.

Steering Committee of the Physicians' Health Study Research Group. 1989. Final report on the aspirin component of the ongoing Physicians' Health Study. N Engl J Med 321 (3): 129–35.

Trichopoulou A and Lagiou P. 1997. Worldwide patterns of dietary lipids intake and health implications. *Am J Clin Nutr* 66 (Suppl.): 961S–64S.

Tunstall-Pedoe H. 1985. Monitoring trends in cardiovascular disease and risk factors: The WHO "Monica" project. *WHO Chronicle* 39 (2): 3–5.

Veterans Administration Cooperative Study Group on Antihypertensive Agents. 1970. Effects of treatment on morbidity in hypertension II: Results in patients with diastolic blood pressure averaging 90 through 114 mm Hg. *JAMA* 213 (7): 1143–52.

Epidemiological Approaches to Heart Disease: The Framingham Study
(1951)

Thomas R. Dawber, M.D., Gilcin F. Meadors, M.D., M.P.H., and Felix E. Moore, Jr.

National Heart Institute, National Institutes of Health, Public Health Service, Federal Security Agency, Washington, D.C.

The use of the word "epidemiology" and the concept of what epidemiology as a discipline may encompass has varied widely since the days of Peter Panum and John Snow. There are today many differing definitions of the word, but nearly all workers in the field will agree on one element of the definition: The word "epidemiology" by etymology refers to the study of something "which is thrust upon the people." There are still some who insist that epidemiology deals only with epidemics of infectious diseases, but current usage suggests that most workers would now agree that epidemiology deals with "the fundamental questions as to where a given disease is found, when it thrives, where and when it is not found . . . in other words it is the ecology of disease"[1] without regard to whether the disease is believed to be infectious.

Frost gave an analytical definition when he wrote that epidemiology "includes the orderly arrangement of facts into chains of inference which extends more or less beyond the bounds of direct observation."[2] His definition might be called the essence of the "epidemiological method" except for the fact that it has been used by the physician since the time of Hippocrates to arrive at his clinical diagnosis. Thus, today, the epidemiological approach is used to explore certain relationships in health and disease which, with present technological methods, cannot be observed directly. In addition to the many studies of the infectious diseases, there have been epidemiological studies in the field of nutritional imbalance, metabolic disorders, occupational hazards, accidents, cancer, and rheumatic fever—to mention only a few.

In the field of cardiovascular diseases, studies using the epidemiological method have led to findings of considerable practical importance for prevention and treatment. Mention may be made, for example, of the studies of nutritional diseases, such as beriberi, pellagra, and scurvy, and of the infectious diseases such as syphilis, hemolytic streptococcal infections, and streptococcus viridans bacteremia. Rubella and other virus diseases have been implicated as etiological factors in congenital malformations of the heart, but further epidemiological study is still required to establish these relationships beyond the possibility of reasonable doubt.[3] Even in rheumatic fever, where fundamental etiology is still obscure, epidemiological studies have helped to demonstrate the relationship of streptococcal infection to subsequent rheumatic activity, and this has led to the adoption of control measures which show great promise.[4]

It should be pointed out, however, that except for rheumatic fever, the diseases mentioned above account for only a very small proportion of morbidity or mortality from cardiovascular disease. Of the epidemiology of hypertensive or arteriosclerosis cardiovascular disease almost nothing is known, although these two account for the great bulk of deaths from cardiovascular disease. The scanty epidemiological knowledge of these diseases which does exist is based either on a study of mortality statistics, which in the investigation of long-term diseases are often not very revealing, or on clinical studies, which have the disadvantage from the epidemiologist's point of view of being based on the study of those who already have the disease. Clearly, what is required is the epidemiological study of these diseases based on populations of normal composition, including both the sick and the well as they are found in the community.

These facts have long been recognized. Sir James Mackenzie, one of the great pioneers in cardiology, over 30 years ago began what was intended to be a long-term study of disease in the entire population of the town of St. Andrews, Scotland.[5] Because of Mackenzie's retirement a few years after the start of the study, it was never completed, however, and since that time there have been no other attempts to study heart disease in a large population of normal composition over any long period of time. The expense of such a study and the necessity of guaranteeing its operation for a span of many years puts it beyond the capabilities of the individual investigator. If such a study is to be done, it is clear that it must be carried out by the community health agencies. In the light of the situation, and with the growing interest in chronic diseases, the U.S. Public Health Service began in 1947 to lay plans for setting up an epidemiological study of the cardiovascular diseases in coöperation [*sic*] with state and local health agencies.

At this point it is well to present in outline the principal considerations which guided the development of the study, and led ultimately to its location in Framingham, Mass.

The study is focused on arteriosclerotic and hypertensive cardiovascular disease, because these are the most important of the cardiovascular diseases and the least is known about their epidemiology. As a working hypothesis it is assumed that these diseases do not each have a single cause (as is the case in most infectious diseases), but that they are the result of multiple causes which work slowly within the individual. It is recognized that, for the most part, specific and unambiguous tests for precise diagnosis of the early stages of these diseases are lacking.

Based on these general considerations the following research plan was developed. A group of randomly selected persons in the ages where arteriosclerotic and hypertensive cardiovascular disease are known to develop is selected for study. Based on as complete a clinical examination as feasible, there are selected out of this initial group those persons who are free of definite signs of these diseases. These persons will be termed the normals, and they will be observed over a period of years until a sizable number are found to have acquired the diseases. At that time a search is made for the factors which influenced the development of disease in the one group and not in the other.

As one by-product of this investigation it will also be possible to study the efficiency of various diagnostic procedures in fighting heart disease or as indicators of the subsequent development of heart disease. (These findings, of course, have important bearing on the question of including tests for heart disease in mass screening programs.) A second by-product will be data on prevalence and incidence of cardiovascular diseases.

With these aims set up, it was then necessary to define the population on which this study would be carried out. Ideally, perhaps, epidemiological investigations of cardiovascular disease should be set up in a number of widely separated areas simultaneously, so that various racial and ethnic groups will be represented, and a variety of geographic, socio-economic, and other environmental factors can be considered. The results of the study of a single area will have generality only in so far as the population of the area is representative of some larger population. Many thousands of persons should be included to allow for numerous axes of analysis, and it would be profitable to follow a cohort of individuals from birth to death. Because of the expense of examination and follow-up, however, it is not practicable to carry on studies simultaneously in several areas, nor to observe more than a few thousand persons for a limited number of years. It was concluded, therefore, that the study should be set up in a single area, and that coverage would have to be limited to approximately 6,000 persons in a limited age range, who would be observed for a period up to 20 years. A town of 25,000 to 50,000 population will supply this number of adults, and it was felt that a town this size would be more desirable than a larger city for the type of community approach required to secure full coöperation and coverage. This limitation in geographic coverage clearly limits the generality of conclusions which can be reached. There is, however, reasonable basis for the belief that the distribution of arteriosclerosis and hypertension in the white race in the United States is such that within-community variance is very much greater than between-community variance, and a wide range of type-situations influencing development of these diseases may be found in any community. This hypothesis can only be tested, of course, by similar studies in other communities.

In mid-1947, Dr. Vlado A. Getting, State Commissioner for Massachusetts, offered to coöperate with the U.S. Public Health Service in setting up the study in that state, and after consideration of a number of possible areas the Town of Framingham was selected. Framingham, lying 21 miles west of Boston, is an industrial and trading center of 28,000 population, and is almost independent of Boston from the standpoint of providing suburban residence for the city. As is true of New England towns, it includes not only the built-up business and residential areas but also the outlying rural area within the town limits. Other points of interest are that Framingham has the town-meeting form of government and the people are accustomed to and well-versed in the group approach to their problems. It was in Framingham that the first community study of tuberculosis was undertaken—a program sponsored by the National Tuberculosis Association and the Metropolitan Life Insurance Company, which began in 1917 and continued successfully for six years.[6] This latter fact, together with an indication of interest in response to the initial approach influenced to some extent the selection of the town.

The problems involved in setting up the study fell into four categories: professional, administrative, organizational, and technical, and all will be discussed in some detail. A program which involves medical examination of large numbers of people requires the respect, endorsement, and support of the medical profession. The plans of the project were given the endorsement of the Massachusetts Medical Society.[7] In Framingham the medical groups which center around the two local hospitals offered their active support to the program as proposed.

From an administrative standpoint it was necessary to secure clinic facilities and recruit a professional and technical staff. A centrally located residential building was remodeled for clinic and laboratory space, and diagnostic equipment installed. A staff was organized, including the examining physicians; a clinic nurse; x-ray, electrocardiography and laboratory technicians; statisticians; interviewing and administrative clerks; a health educator; and visiting consultants in the fields of cardiology, electrocardiography, roentgenology, pathology, and biochemistry.

The organizational problems are those involved in bringing into the study the cross-section of the population which it is desired to study. The mechanics of selecting the cross-section are described in a later section; at this point the focus of interest is the method of bringing about community participation. The work of building a community organization began months before the start of clinic operation.

At the start, a health educator was placed in the Health Department with the assignment of studying the community. This meant not only learning about the history, resources, and government of the town but, more important, getting to know the people—their national origins, economic conditions, and lines of social stratification; their religious, fraternal, and civic organizations; and their recognized and potential leaders. From this study grew plans for the appointment, by the Town Health Officer, of the Executive Committee of 15 persons for the study—a committee which was broadly representative of the various groups in the community. Parallel to, and integrated with, the lay Executive Committee, there was organized a Professional Committee of physicians and dentists under the chairmanship of a cardiologist. Together, the Executive Committee and the Professional Committee accepted the following responsibilities:

1. To assist in planning a program which would be acceptable to the community as a whole.

2. To interpret the aims and objectives of the study in a way which would be understandable to all elements of the community.

3. To bring recognized and potential leaders of the community into active participation in the organizational aspects of the study.

After analysis of the community organization requirements of this study by the Executive Committee, six subcommittees were set up: Arrangements, Publicity, Industry, Business, Civic Organizations, and Neighborhood Organization. The Arrangements Committee has assisted in the operation of the study by providing clerical assistance and transportation. The Publicity Committee, composed of residents who are specialists in areas of press, radio, advertising, and associated fields developed a plan for publicity media to be used in placing the program before the community. The Industry, Business, and Civic Organizations Committees brought the study to the attention of their special publics.

Perhaps the most important of the committees, however, is the Neighborhood Organization Committee. It has been the aim that every participant in the study should come into it on the basis of an invitation from someone he knows, and in whom he has confidence, and further that the invitation should come from a person who has been through the clinic. At the start, therefore, examinations in the clinic were offered to all members of the committees and these, in turn, passed word of the study on to other members of the community who were encouraged to volunteer for examination. From these volunteers a set of neighborhood committees has been selected. To those committees falls the all-important job of inviting the initial participation of the selected individuals and later stimulating coöperation in return for follow-up observation.

Up to the present time, use has been made of standard publicity channels to inform the people about the program. However, as we discovered from sampling of opinion of persons volunteering for the study, the most valuable public information has come through word-of-mouth. The community has accepted the program as its responsibility, and recognizes that when people participate they make a real contribution to medical research. It should be added that the nature of the examinations provides a service to the selected individuals, and this has undoubtedly motivated many in the community to participate. It should be noted parenthetically at this point, however, that the service aspects of the study are limited to diagnostic information which is furnished only to the personal physician of the person examined. Where there are abnormal findings, the individual is referred to his own physician for interpretation of the findings and treatment if necessary. The clinic staff does not provide treatment, nor offer advice on treatment.

The technical problems of this study may be considered under two headings: medical and statistical. The medical problems involve selection of diagnostic procedures and methods of measuring the various characteristics of the people, and the establishment of criteria for interpretation of these tests. Statistical problems include the development of a method for sampling the population, and of methods for recording and analyzing the data obtained.

To determine the presence or absence of cardiovascular diseases and to record those items in the patient's past history that may have a bearing on the development of disease requires a rather extensive study of each selected individual. Within the framework of this type of study, it is also necessary that the examination be organized in such a way that the whole procedure can be done in a reasonable length of time and without discomfort or risk for the person being examined.

All medical planning for this study was done in consultation with a Technical Advisory Committee appointed by the State Health Commissioner and made up of eleven physicians from the Boston area expert in the fields of cardiology and public health. This committee aided in setting up the broad outlines of the study by proposing hypotheses as to suspected etiological factors for testing. The committee assisted also in suggesting specific items for examination and laboratory study, and in advising on criteria for evaluating these criteria. The procedures which are carried out on each person admitted to the study may be summarized briefly as follows:

1. An extensive medical history including:
    a. Family history of cardiovascular disease in mother and father, siblings, and children.

b. A detailed past medical history of diphtheria, scarlet fever, sore throat, rheumatic fever, various chronic diseases, operations, thyroid diseases, presence of transient or permanent hypertension, heart murmurs, and "heart attacks"; previous diagnoses of angina pectoris, limitation of activity due to heart disease, congenital heart disease, heart failure, vascular disease of any kind, enlarged heart, "nervous heart," pericarditis; and the history of any previous kidney disease, renal or hypertensive complications of pregnancy, or of any menopausal symptoms.

c. Careful questioning for any current symptoms of heart or pulmonary diseases including cough, dyspnea, hemoptysis, smothering sensation, palpitation, chest pain and discomfort, edema, and phlebitis, etc.

d. Personal habits of the individual, including number of hours of sleep, amount of tobacco and alcohol consumed.

e. Average weight at five year intervals, beginning at age 25.

f. History of peptic ulcer, chronic colitis, nervousness, headache, and other symptoms suggestive of emotional upset.

g. Use of drugs or medicines.

2. A careful, detailed physical examination performed independently by at least two physicians, aimed at detecting cardiovascular abnormalities or diseases related to the cardiovascular system, and measurement of characteristics which may be related to such disease including:

a. Height, sitting and standing, weight, and anterio-posterior diameter of chest, chest circumference, waist circumference, vital capacity, estimate of body build, color of eyes and hair, and distribution of hair and degree of baldness.

b. Skin color and degree of freckly, the presence or absence of sweating, clubbing of fingers and toes, cyanosis, exopthalmos, arcus senilia, xanthelasma, thyroid enlargement or tumors, chest deformity, and evidence of pulmonary disease.

c. Examination of the heart itself, including description of heart sounds, murmurs, abnormal rhythm, blood pressure determinations on admission and at time of discharge, and at intervals during the examination by each of the examining physicians.

d. Examination of abdomen for tumors, liver enlargement, or palpable spleen.

e. Examination of the extremities for presence or absence of femoral pulse, dorsalis pedis and posterior tibial pulsations, ankle edema, varicose veins, and phlebitis.

3. X-ray examinations, teleoroentgenogram on 14" x 17" film and on 70 mm. film with two meter target distance.

4. Electrocardiogram using twelve leads.

5. Electrokymographic tracing at 12 points on the cardiac silhouette.

6. Examination of blood sample for:
    a. Hemoglobin
    b. Serum cholesterol
    c. Serum phospholipid
    d. S_f 10–20 fraction (of Gofman)
    e. Uric acid
    f. Glucose level
    g. Serologic test for syphilis

7. A routine urinalysis.

The aim of securing information on all of these items of history, physical examination or laboratory test is twofold. First, it is desired to record, in as full detail as possible, the characteristics of each individual which are considered relevant to the presence or absence, or the potential development of cardiovascular disease. Second, it is desired on the basis of this examination as a whole to classify the populations studied into two groups: (1) those with definite signs of arteriosclerotic or hypertensive cardiovascular disease, and (2) those apparently free of these diseases (who may be termed "normal" for the purpose of this discussion).

It is the "normals" who are the principal focus of interest of the study. They will be brought back for reëxamination [sic] biennially for a period which it is hoped to extend for as long as 20 years. If they move from Framingham, an attempt will be made to bring them under a comparable examination elsewhere. If they die, an attempt will be made to secure autopsy data, and, at the very least, complete description of cause of death, and data as to the existence of cardiovascular diseases at time of death.

The choice of the sampling plan for this study was dictated by a number of considerations, some of which have already been suggested. The number of cases which could feasibly be studied—6,000—was much smaller than the adult population. Therefore, some method had to be introduced to select persons and avoid the unknown biases of self-selection. The total sample had to be allocated in such a way as to yield the maximum information over the period that the study was to be carried out. And the plan had to be such that it would be acceptable to the community, and could be carried out through the community organization.

One important decision which had to be reached concerned the age range of the study population. Clearly, if only a very young group was studied, only a very small number would develop arteriosclerotic or hypertensive cardiovascular disease even in 10 to 20 years' time. On the other hand, in a very old group there would be too large a proportion with preëxisting [*sic*] cardiovascular disease. To balance these two effects, the age group 30 through 59 was selected for study. The population in this age range was approximately 10,000. If 6,000 of this group were taken into the study, with the age-sex distribution existing in the town, it could be predicted (on the basis of the criteria of this study and tentative data available from a small volunteer group) that roughly 5,000 would be free of cardiovascular disease at the time of initial examination. Of these 5,000 it was estimated that approximately 400 would be found to have cardiovascular disease at the end of the 5th year, and 2,150 at the end of the 20th year. (These numbers include, of course, persons who would be dead of the disease at the end of the specified period.) These numbers appear to be large enough to ensure statistically reliable findings, though it is recognized that even this number of cases will not be sufficient to carry out all of the detailed analyses which will suggest themselves in the course of the study.

There remained the problem of securing an actual listing of persons who would form the sample. Under ordinary circumstances, it would probably have been desirable to use some form of area sampling. The Town of Framingham, however, publishes annually a listing of all residents 20 years of age and over, based on a local census, and it has been possible to use this list as a basis for sampling. (An independent check of the completeness of the listing is being made by the Bureau of the Census.)

The Executive Committee advised that it would be desirable not to break up families—that is, if one member of the family was to be brought into the sample, all other family members resident in the same household should also be brought in, provided they were within the eligible age limits. This has been arranged, and the sample has been drawn in systematic fashion from a list which is first stratified by family size and by precinct of residence, and then arranged in serial order by address.

The sampling ratio is two-thirds, which will yield approximately 6,600 names. This is 10 per cent over the number required for this study in order to provide for losses through refusal or by moving out of town before examination.

As the description of the examination suggests, a formidable mass of data will be available when the initial examinations have been completed early in 1952, and this will increase as follow-up examinations are carried out through the years on the normal group. Analysis of the data will proceed at each stage of data collection. When initial examinations have been completed, it will be possible to extract prevalence data of considerable interest. It will also be possible to proceed with a study of the contribution which various elements of the total examination make in the determination of the final diagnostic impression. Analysis of this type will, for example, give a basis for determining the relative efficiency of the miniature chest x-ray, or of certain electrocardiographic leads, as diagnostic tools as compared with the total examination. In this area, some tentative data based on the group of volunteers already examined will shortly become available. Another important type of information will be data on the range of values of various diagnostic tests for "normal" populations, which have not hitherto been available in medical literature.

The more truly epidemiological parts of the analysis are essentially retrospective and must wait the passage of time. At the end of 5 years a portion of the base population, which was normal at the time of initial examination with respect to the diseases studied, will have passed the borderline into definite abnormality, and a few will have died. At that point it will be possible to study the differences, as of the time of the initial examination, between those who remained essentially normal, and those who subsequently became abnormal (or diseased). From this study it should be possible to test a number of hypotheses with respect to factors associated with the development of arteriosclerotic or hypertensive cardiovascular disease. As the abnormal group increases in size with the passage of time, such differences as are found to exist can be determined with increasing statistical reliability. For the group which becomes abnormal, the rate of progression of disease can be measured, and from the entire group there will be data which will yield estimates of incidence of arteriosclerotic and hypertensive cardiovascular disease for a more representative population group than has hitherto been studied.

SOURCE

Dawber TR, Meadors GF, and Moore FE Jr. 1951. Epidemiological approaches to heart disease: The Framingham Study. *Am J Public Health* 41 (3): 279–86. Copyright 1951 *American Journal of Public Health*. Reprinted with permission of American Public Health Association.

Strategy of Prevention: Lessons from Cardiovascular Disease
(1981, Abridged)

Geoffrey Rose

If an obstetrician had a case of eclampsia he would ask, "What went wrong?" The occurrence of a preventable disaster is a threat to his professional reputation, for an obstetrician accepts prevention as an integral part of his normal professional responsibilities. Antenatal care is in fact largely preventive, and the integration of prevention with treatment has led to an excellent fall in maternal and perinatal mortality rates. In paediatrics too there are no demarcation disputes between prevention and treatment; and a similar trend is now also appearing in general practice. If the stroke occurs in an untreated or badly treated hypertensive patient, a good general practitioner asks, "What went wrong?" For, in middle age at least, strokes are largely preventable. When one occurs it suggests a possible failure of practice organisation.

Clinician and Prevention

Unfortunately, in other branches of medicine there is a continuing and regrettable separation of the therapeutic and preventive roles, and doctors generally continue to see the care of the sick as their whole responsibility.

Coronary Heart Disease Is Preventable

Figure 1 shows the recent trends in mortality from coronary heart disease in various countries of the world [Not shown, Ed.]. In Japan the rates have throughout this period been extremely low. In Australia and the United States at the start of the period they were high, but they have fallen by some 25%. In England and Wales they started a little short of the American and Australian rates and have shown little change. The Japanese owe their low rates not to their genes but to their way of life: when they move to America they rather quickly acquire American rates. The large recent declines in Australia and the United States must surely be due to a declining incidence of disease, since only a limited part of that large decline can be attributed to therapeutic advances. These patterns show that coronary heart disease is largely preventable.

In Britain, then, we are failing to prevent a preventable disease. If we had shared in the Australian and American decline each year in England and Wales there would be upwards of 25,000 fewer coronary deaths. One can imagine the outcry if some shortcoming in therapeutic services were to cause even a tiny fraction of this number of unnecessary deaths. Why then, one may ask, do we not as a profession evince a corresponding alarm at the failure of prevention? Why do we not feel that it is our fault? Why is so large a part of our research devoted to the "mechanics of dying," and so little to the scientific, social, and economic basis of prevention?

The answers to these questions are satisfactorily complex. We do not know why the Australians and the Americans have done well in their control of coronary heart disease, or whether (if we did know) we could have shared their good fortune. Yet surely, as a profession, we should at least feel deeply disturbed by the problem and involved in it. We have a professional responsibility for prevention, both in research and in medical practice. When ordinary doctors do not accept that responsibility then prevention is taken over (if at all) by uncritical propagandists, by cranks, and by battling commercial interests.

"High-risk" Strategy

As doctors we are trained to feel responsible for patients—that is, to care for the sick; and from that position accepting responsibility for those with major risk factors is not too difficult a transition. They are almost patients. A general practitioner, say, makes a routine measurement of a man's blood pressure and finds it raised. Thereafter both the man and the doctor will say that he "suffers" from high blood pressure. He walked in a healthy man but he walks out a patient, and his new-found status is confirmed by the giving and receiving of tablets. And inappropriate label has been accepted because both public and profession feel that if the man were not a patient the doctor would have no business treating him. In reality the care of the symptomless hypertensive person is preventive medicine, not therapeutics.

Absolute and Relative Risk

Life insurance experts concerned with charging the right premiums taught us that "high risk" meant "high relative risk," and in this until recently they have been abetted by the epidemiologists. Figure 2(a) [Not shown, Ed.], taken from life insurance data,[1] shows for each of four age groups the relation of blood pressure to the relative risk of death, taking the risk for the whole in each age group as 100. The relative risk is seen to

Table I Cardiovascular Risk in Users of Oral
Contraceptive[2]

	Age (yr)	
	30–9	40–9
Relative risk	2.8	2.8
Attributable risk (per 100,000 a year)	3.5	20.0

increase with increasing pressure, but the gradient gets a little steep as age advances. That is perhaps not surprising, because a systolic pressure of 160 mm Hg is common in older men, and we would not expect it to be so unpleasant as at younger ages, when it is rare.

In figure 2(b) [Not shown, Ed.] the same data are shown but with a scale of absolute instead of relative risk. The pattern now appears quite different. In particular, the absolute excess risk associated with raised pressure is far greater in older men. A systolic pressure of 160 mm Hg may be common to these ages, but common does not mean good. To identify risk and relative units rather than absolute units may be misleading.

To take another example, at any given age a woman taking oral contraceptives has the risk of cardiovascular death about 2.8 times that of her contemporary who is not taking the pill. This relative risk is more or less independent of age, and it is the same in smokers and non-smokers.[2] But although relative risk does not change, the absolute excess or *attributable risk* is profoundly different (table I). We are nowadays discouraging the use of oral contraceptives in older women, especially those with any coronary risk factor, because we recognize that advice must relate to absolute not relative risk.

Absolute and Relative Benefit

The same argument applies in assessing the benefits of preventive action. In the Veterans Administration trial of antihypertensive treatment[3] the effectiveness of treatment expressed in relative terms was around 50–60% regardless of age or the presence of cardiovascular-renal abnormality (table II). The final column of the table, however, expresses treatment effectiveness in absolute units; and again we now see a quite different pattern. The absolute benefit received from this form of preventive action is nearly five times greater in the older age group with risk factors than in the younger age group without risk factors. To express the results of trials only in terms of percentage effectiveness is to conceal what the user really needs to know.

Table II   Relative and Absolute Benefits from the Treatment of Hypertension, According to Age and the Presence of Cardiovascular-Renal Abnormality[3]

Age (yr)	Cardiovascular renal abnormality	Treatment effectiveness (%)	Lives saved per 100 treated
50	–	59	6
	+	62	14
50	–	50	15
	+	60	29

Population Risk

If we are to take decisions, then, we need to measure risks and benefits in absolute rather than relative terms. Nevertheless, although such measures will describe the situation for individuals they tell us next to nothing about the effects on the whole community of the strategy based on identifying and caring for high-risk individuals. Unfortunately the effects of a "high-risk strategy" may be more limited than we imagine, for the community benefit depends not only on the benefit that each individual receives but also on the prevalence of the risk factor. If a large benefit is conferred on only a few people then the community as a whole is not much better off. In familial hypercholesterolaemia affected men have a risk of premature coronary death of more than 50%; but fortunately it is rare. Consequently, serious though the disease is for affected individuals, the deaths resulting from it make up less than 1% of all coronary death. What we may call *population attributable risk*—the excess risk associated with a factor in the population as a whole—depends on the product of the individual attributable risk (the excess risk in individuals with that factor) and the prevalence of the factor in the population.

Figure 3 [Not shown, Ed.] illustrates the relation in the Framingham Study[4] between coronary mortality and the concentration of serum cholesterol when men entered the study. The risk rises fairly steeply with increasing cholesterol concentration; but out on the right, where the risk to affected individuals is high, the prevalence is fortunately low. If we want to ask, "How many excess coronary deaths is the cholesterol-related risk responsible for in this population?," we simply multiply the excess risk at each concentration by the number of people with that concentration who are exposed to that risk. In fig 3 these attributable deaths are shown as the numbers on top of the bars. They add up to 34 extra deaths

Table III Population Attributable Mortality from Coronary Heart Disease and Stroke Arising at Different Levels of Blood Pressure[5]

Diastolic BP (mm Hg)	Cumulative % of excess deaths attributable to hypertension	
	Coronary heart disease	Stroke
<80	(0)	(0)
<90	21	14
<100	47	25
<110	67	73
≥ 110	100	100

per 1,000 of this population over a 10-year period, of which only three arise at concentrations at or above 310 mg/100 ml (8 mmol/1)—which would be called high ("outside the normal range") by conventional clinical standards. The rest (90%) arise from the many people in the middle part of the distribution who are exposed to a small risk.

This illustrates a fundamental principle in the strategy of prevention. A large number of people exposed to a low risk is likely to produce more cases than a small number of people exposed to a high risk. In business the same principle underlies the mass market: profits are larger when small amounts are taken from the masses than when large amounts are taken from the few rich people; and this principle of the mass market applies to many community health hazards.

In our Whitehall Study[5] we examined some 20,000 middle-aged male civil servants in London, noting among other things their blood pressures. Follow-up shows that mortality rises rather steeply with increasing pressure. One may calculate (just as with the Framingham cholesterol data) the numbers of deaths attributable to the different levels of raised blood pressure (table III). Two-thirds of the attributable coronary deaths and three-quarters of the attributable deaths from stroke occur in men with diastolic pressure is below 110 mm Hg, and about half the attributable coronary deaths and a quarter of the attributable deaths from stroke occur below 100 mm Hg.

In the "high-risk" preventive strategy we go out and identify those at the top end of the distribution and give them some preventive care—for example, control of hypertension or hyperlipidaemia. But this "high-risk" strategy, however successful it may be for individuals, cannot influence that large proportion of deaths occurring among the many people with slightly raised blood pressure and a small risk. Hypertension clinics, lipid clinics, diabetic clinics—excellent though they may be for the individuals who receive their benefits—offer only a limited answer to the community problem of heart disease.

Mass Strategy

We are therefore driven to consider mass approaches, of which the simplest is the endeavour to lower the whole distribution of the risk variable by some measure in which all participate. Supposing that some dietary measure, such as moderation of salt intake, were able to lower the whole blood pressure distribution, we may estimate how the potential benefits might compare with what is currently achieved by the "high-risk" strategy of detecting and treating hypertension. From the Whitehall study data one can consider two strategies whose effects might be expected to be equivalent. The first predicates a 100%-effective treatment for high blood pressure given to and accepted by everyone with a diastolic (phase 4) pressure of 105 mm Hg or more. We can estimate how many lives that would save, assuming a commensurate fall in risk. On the same assumption, a similar benefit might follow a mass lowering of the whole blood pressure distribution of the population by 7–8 mm Hg. In practice, however, treatment is not completely effective, all cases are not detected, and the people who are detected will often not take our treatment. Making allowance for the shortcomings, we may estimate that all the life-saving benefits achieved by current antihypertensive treatment might be equaled by a downward shift of the whole blood pressure distribution and the population by a mere 2–3 mm Hg. The benefits from a mass approach in which everybody receives a small benefit may be unexpectedly large.

The Individual Gains Little

The mass approach is inherently the only ultimate answer to the problem of a mass disease. But, however much it may offer to the community as a whole, it offers little to each participating individual. When mass diphtheria immunisation was introduced in Britain 40 years ago, even then roughly 600 children had to be immunised in order that one life would be saved—599 "wasted" immunisations for the one that was effective. If all male British doctors wore their car seatbelts on every journey throughout their working lives, then for one life thereby saved there would be about 400 who always take that preventive precaution: 399 would have worn a seatbelt every day for 40 years without benefit to their survival. This is the kind of ratio that one has to accept in mass preventive medicine. A measure applied to many will actually benefit few.

Table IV Estimated Proportion of Men and Women Who Might Avoid Clinical Coronary Heart Disease before Age 55 If They Had Reduced Their Serum Cholesterol Concentration by 0.65 mmol/l (25 mg/100 ml) throughout Adult Life, Based on Framingham Estimates of Risk[4]

	Men	Women
Average risk*	1 in 50	1 in 400
High risk†	1 in 25	1 in 150

*Serum cholesterol 6.1 mmol/l (235 mg/100 ml), systolic BP 120 mm Hg, non-smoker.

†Serum cholesterol 6.7 mmol/l (260 mg/100 ml), systolic BP 150 mm Hg, smoker.

Table IV presents some estimates made from the Framingham data.[3] If we supposed that throughout their adult life, up to the age of 55, Framingham men were to modify their diet in such a way as to reduce their cholesterol levels by 10%, then among men of average coronary risk about one in 50 could expect that through this preventive precaution he would avoid a heart attack (if change in a risk factors leads to commensurate reduction in risk): 49 out of 50 would eat differently every day for 40 years and perhaps get nothing from it. For the same preventive measure in a higher-risk group (those with a little hypertension and a slightly raised cholesterol concentration and smoking cigarettes), the ratio rises to one in 25. For women the prospects for individual benefit from this preventive measure are much smaller.

The "Prevention Paradox"

We arrive at what we might call the prevention paradox—"*a measure that brings large benefits to the community offers little to each participating individual.*" It implies that we should not expect too much from individual health education. People will not be motivated to any great extent to take our advice, because there is little in it for each of them, particularly in the short and medium term. Change in behaviour has to be for some the larger and more immediate reward.

Social Motivation

There has been a gratifying decline in smoking by male doctors in Britain in the past 20 years. In most cases the motivation has probably not been the intellectual argument that in the end some will obtain health benefits; it has been social pressure. Being a smoking doctor is uncomfortable these days for your colleagues either pity you or despise you. Not smoking may be easier. Social pressure brings immediate rewards for those who conform.

Few doctors are optimistic about their ability to achieve weight reduction in obese patients and to maintain it. But many young women make strenuous, sustained, and successful efforts to control their weight, not for medical reasons but because thinness is socially acceptable and obesity is not. So in health education our aim should perhaps be to create more social pressure that makes "healthy behaviour" easier and more acceptable, thereby earning immediate social rewards for those who conform.

Another major determinant of behaviour is the force of economics and convenience. In the United States and Australia, and more latterly in Britain, there has been a large market shift away from butter towards soft margarine. Though the medical argument has helped, the main reason has probably been the price, and the fact that butter when kept in the refrigerator goes hard and soft margarine does not. Thus the friends of butter, quite apart from the bad scientific basis for their case, have little chance of making much headway. To influence mass behaviour we must look to its mass determinants, which are largely economic and social.

Safety Is Paramount

The recent World Health Organisation controlled trial of clofibrate produced disturbing results.[6] In the treated group non-fatal myocardial infarction was reduced by 26% (about the effect predicted from the fallen cholesterol concentrations). Mortality from non-cardiac causes, however, increased by one-third, an effect rather unlikely to be due to chance. This finding is important to the strategy of prevention. Clofibrate has been in use for many years and has been given to enormous numbers of patients. Until the results of this trial appeared there was no suspicion that it might kill. Indeed, by clinical standards it can still be called a relatively safe drug, since the estimate of excess mortality works out at only about one death per 1,000 patient-years. In patients with severe hyperlipoproteinaemia we would be prepared to take such a risk if it was thought that the drug might reduce their very high death rate.

Intervention for prevention where the risk is low is totally different. I suggested earlier that a large number of people exposed to a small risk might yield more cases in the community than a small number exposed to a big risk. There is a counterpart to that in regard to intervention. As a preventive measure exposes many people to a small risk, then the harm it does may readily—as in the case of clofibrate—outweigh the benefits, since these are received by relatively few. Unfortunately we cannot have many trials as large as the clofibrate study, nor are we able to keep such trials going for longer than a few years, usually five at the most. We may thus be unable to identify that small level of harm to individuals from long-term intervention that would be sufficient to make that line of prevention unprofitable or even harmful. Consequently we cannot accept long-term mass preventive medication.

Conclusions

In chronic diseases the clinician's first contact with the patient comes late in the natural history of the disease, usually after a catastrophe or major complication and when there is already much irreversible pathological change. Indeed, in some 20% of cases of coronary heart disease there is no contact with physicians at all, the first recognised occurrence being sudden death. It follows inexorably that prevention is essential. With coronary heart disease, the recent experience of Australia and the United States shows also that prevention is possible, at least in part.

The preventive strategy that concentrates on high-risk individuals may be appropriate for those individuals, as well as being a wise and efficient use of limited medical resources; but its ability to reduce the burden of disease in the whole community tends to be disappointingly small. Potentially far more effective, and ultimately the only acceptable answer, is the mass strategy, whose aim is to shift the whole population's distribution of the risk variable. Here, however, our first concern must be that such mass advice is safe.

Addition and Removal

We may usefully distinguish two types of preventive measure. The first consists of the removal of an unnatural factor in the restoration of "biological normality"—that is, of the conditions to which presumably we are genetically adapted. For coronary heart disease such measures would include a substantial reduction in our intake of saturated fat, giving up cigarettes, avoiding severe obesity and the state of permanent physical inactivity, maybe *some* increase in the intake of polyunsaturated fat, and maybe avoidance of those occupational and social conditions that are conducive to so-called "type A" behaviour. Such normalising measures may be presumed to be safe, and therefore we should be prepared to advocate them on the basis of a reasonable presumption of benefit.

The second type of mass preventive measure is quite different. It consists not in removing a supposed cause of disease but in adding some other unnatural factor, in the hope of conferring protection. The end result is increased biological abnormality by an even further removal from those conditions to which we are genetically adapted. For coronary heart disease such measures include a *high* intake of polyunsaturates and all forms of long-term medication. Long-term safety cannot be assured, and quite possibly harm may outweigh benefit. For such measures as these the required level of evidence, both of benefit and (particularly) of safety, must be far more stringent.

SOURCE

Rose G. 1981. Strategy of prevention: Lessons from cardiovascular disease. *Brit Med J* 282:1847–51. Copyright 1981 *by British Medical Journal*. Reprinted with permission of BMJ Publishing Group Ltd.

Theory and Action for Health Promotion: Illustrations from the North Karelia Project
(1982)

Alfred McAlister, PhD, Pekka Puska, MD, PhD,
Jukka T. Salonen, MD, PhD, Jackko Tuomilehto, MD, PhD,
and Kaj Koskela, MD, MPolSc

ABSTRACT: The North Karelia Project in Finland illustrates the fundamental goals of health promotion. Specific activities of the project serve as examples of how concepts from the social and behavioral sciences can be applied to achieve estimated reductions in predicted risk of disease. The results in North Karelia are not conclusive, but they are encouraging, and the investigation conducted there is an essential reference for future research in health promotion and disease prevention.

Introduction

The prevention of chronic diseases has emerged as a major focus of modern public health.[1,2] Present knowledge indicates that adoption of healthy life-styles and environments are key elements of such preventive action. "Health promotion" is the effort designed to reduce unhealthy behaviors, improve preventive services, and create a better social and physical environment.[3,4] The obvious potential for prevention of several major chronic diseases has led to many campaigns and actions. Disappointment with the frequently marginal or unsatisfactory results has increased demand for a sounder theoretical basis for these health promotion activities. There is also a need for more communication between those involved with action and experts in the behavioral sciences. We believe that "nothing is as practical as a good theory,"[5] and that a comprehensive framework of theorization is urgently needed to guide research and development activities in this important field.

The North Karelia Project[6] is a comprehensive community program for health promotion in North Karelia, a rural county with 180,000 inhabitants in Eastern Finland. Most of the inhabitants of the region reside in very small villages. The largest population center, Joensuu, is a small town. Chief occupations in North Karelia are farming and forestry. The Project was started in 1972 after a petition by the local population requesting the government to do something to reduce high cardiovascular disease (CVD) rates in the area.[7] The aims of the program have been to improve detection and control of hypertension, to reduce smoking, and to promote diets lower in saturated fat and higher in vegetables and low-fat products. The following sections provide conceptual and theoretical analyses of these goals with reference to activities of the North Karelia Project.

Activities of the Project were based on practical ideas of how to improve services and change behaviors and environments. However, most of the sub-programs that were conducted demonstrate the fundamental goals of health promotion in the straight theoretical principles in action. This paper is not intended as a description of the North Karelia Project and its results; a comprehensive report has been published by the World Health Organization.[7] The aim here is to present a framework of general goals and theoretical principles for health promotion, and to illustrate their application with examples from the North Karelia Project. A chronological listing of selected publications in English is included as an Appendix to this report. [Not included, Ed.]

Program Objectives

There are several general models that may be applied to the design of health promotion programs.[8-11] The general framework presented here is comparable with these models, but our schemata emphasizes planning and analysis based on the classification of objectives:

- *Improved preventive services* to identify persons at abnormal risk of disease and provide appropriate medical attention;
- *Information* to educate people about their health and how it can be maintained;
- *Persuasion* to motivate people to take healthy action;
- *Training* to increase skills of self-control, environmental management, and social action;
- *Community organization* to create social support and power for social action;
- *Environmental change* to create opportunity for healthy actions and improve various unfavorable conditions.

The following sections provide conceptual and theoretical analyses of these goals with reference to activities of the North Karelia Project.

Improved Preventive Services

Provision of preventive services is a key function of any health care system. Detection and treatment of hypertension as a means of preventing cardiovascular disease is one of the best examples of this kind of activity.[12] Large-scale detection and control of hypertension has proven to be difficult. The greatest problems are accomplishing widespread blood pressure screening and inducing adequate adherence to indicated treatment and follow-up.[13, 14]

The North Karelia Project approached these problems with the notion that it would be more feasible to reorganize preventive services than to induce the population to use existing services more effectively. The Finnish health care system provides primary health care through community health centers serving and largely governed by local populations. Only a small minority receive routine care from private physicians. Sponsored by the National Board of Health, the North Karelia Project worked together with the County Health Administration and local municipal authorities to change the way in which hypertension was detected and treated.[15]

The central features of this reorganization were a sharp increase in the responsibility assigned to the local public health nurse and the establishment of new offices at each of the 12 community health centers in North Karelia. To provide the data base for the new activities a county-wide hypertension register was established. Screening for hypertension was integrated into routine contacts with the health center and also provided through mass screening programs at county fairs and village centers. Public health nurses were trained to refer those with elevated blood pressure to a physician for definite diagnosis and possible initiation of appropriate pharmacological regimens. Then the public health nurse was given responsibility for long-term surveillance of those patients' blood pressure through regular follow-up, including personal instructions on adherence to the treatment and on necessary modification of dietary and other habits. The public health nurse paid special attention to the individuals who seemed to experience difficulty in bringing their blood pressure under control. Meanwhile, media and community organizations were spreading the message that control of hypertension is an important goal and that individuals should cooperate with the new activities of the public health nurses. Regular mailings of highly salient reminders of follow-up visits were sent to all the persons recorded in the hypertension register maintained by the public health nurse.

At the baseline survey in 1992, the proportion of male hypertensives (systolic > 175 mm Hg or diastolic > 100 mm Hg) receiving anti-hypertensive drug treatment was about 13 per cent in both Karelia and a neighboring province which was used as a reference for comparison. In the 1977 survey conducted after five years of reorganized preventive health services in North Karelia, the proportion of male hypertensives under appropriate drug treatment had increased to 45 per cent.[16] In the neighboring province, where services for hypertension detection and treatment were beginning to be modeled after the new procedures in North Karelia, the corresponding change was from 14 per cent to 33 per cent. The proportion of hypertensives dropped sharply among North Karelian middle-aged man (30–64 years) while it increased slightly in the reference area. These findings are more completely described elsewhere.[7]

Information

Cooperation with any program or service designed to prevent disease depends on the extent to which the community is informed about the purposes and importance of the program. Thus a major objective of health promotion is to educate people about their health and how it can be maintained. Examples of this kind of activity are informing the public that cardiovascular disease may be prevented through appropriate measures and explaining the purpose and nature of these measures. However it is not always easy to adequately communicate new and somewhat complex ideas in a large population which is subject to information, sometimes conflicting, from many sources.

The design of effective information campaigns can be facilitated by the application of practical principles derived from communication research and theory. For example, research shows that mass media, especially news, powerfully influence what people talk and think about and how they judge the importance of various social problems or issues.[17] Theory suggests that new ideas must often travel through several steps of interpersonal communication to reach the general population.[18] The messages must be simple and frequently repeated if they are to be comprehended and retained.[19]

The North Karelia Project offers several illustrations of the implementation of these principles. Project staff were able to attract intense and frequent attention from the news media in the region, especially from newspapers and radio. Between 1972 and 1977, a total of 1,509 articles related to cardiovascular risk factors, their management, and the program activities were printed in the local newspapers. This was three times as many articles as appeared in the reference area papers. During that same period, over one-half-million bulletins, leaflets, posters, signs, stickers and other educational materials were distributed. To stimulate further interpersonal communication, many different groups and organizations were contacted and asked to distribute materials in their everyday work or to cooperate in organizing health education meetings. A total of 251 general meetings, reaching over 20,000 community members, were held. The community groups and organizations that were involved in these activities included worksites, schools, shops and places of commerce, clubs, and voluntary organizations.

Information about the program and its aims was disseminated rapidly.[7] According to population surveys, over a five-year period understanding of the risk factors for cardiovascular disease increased in both North Karelia and a reference area, but somewhat more in North Karelia. There were sharp baseline differences in knowledge between different educational and occupational groups, but members of all the different groups in North Karelia showed 10 to 15 per cent increases in the proportion of correct responses to survey questions designed to measure knowledge, awareness, and understanding of cardiovascular disease risk factors. However, there were no significant differences between such changes in North Karelia and in the reference area, probably because of increasing attention from the national media serving both countries.

Persuasion

It is well known that behavior cannot always be changed simply by providing information.[20] People need to be persuaded to act on the information that they have been given, to be convinced that new ideas are socially acceptable, that new foods are tasty, and that new life-styles are enjoyable.[22] Thus, in order to promote health effectively, we must accept responsibility for shaping attitudes and behavior in what we believe to be the proper direction. Much has been written concerning the ethical issues that arise in persuasive health promotion.[21,22] Debate has been centered on the right of public health activists to interfere with existing processes and on the question of whether individuals or groups should be held responsible for their own health.[23] The promotion of change in lifestyle or environment is a natural outgrowth of an improved understanding of the epidemiology of disease and injury. Given the many forces which already exert persuasive influences on individuals in our society, those concerned with public health should not shirk the duty of prudent advocacy. To do otherwise is to leave attitudes and behaviors to be shaped by the short-term contingencies of our market economy.

We are products of our environment, but we can change our environment through concerted action. Thus, we may be held collectively responsible for public health, and we must learn to use our political system more effectively to create a favorable environment for all segments of society if we hope to limit the current burden of disease. Efforts to persuade those whose options are limited and whose values are distorted by economic and social problems to accept responsibility for their own health may be futile. Yet many public health activists seeking basic social or economic change are acutely aware of the difficulty of winning popular support for their views and recommendations.

There is a broad accumulation of research and theory concerning the social psychology of persuasion.[24] Three general approaches can be described:

- The "communication" approach focuses on basic parameters of communication; it emphasizes the credibility of the source of the persuasive message and how the message form or content influences cognitive processes in a human receiver.

- The "affective" approach to persuasion concentrates on creating emotional associations.

- The "behavioral" approach centers on achieving a minor behavioral commitment with the expectation that attitudes and beliefs will follow.[25] Although attitude change was not a stated objective of the program in North Karelia, several basic principles were taken into account when different activities were conducted.

In communicating new ideas, Project staff arranged for their messages to be disseminated from many different sources—deliberately seeking a mix which would maximize perceived credibility. Explicit endorsements were obtained from prestigious organizations such as the World Health Organization. In addition, opinion leaders from both formal and informal groups were involved.[26] These individuals were targets of especially intense persuasive communication from respected medical and other experts and were then encouraged to spread and support the new ideas in the community. The physicians and public health nurses were an important part of the communication system. The surveys showed that during a five-year period both of these professional groups distributed more information and were much more involved in active contacts with decision-makers in various community organizations in North Karelia than in the reference area: eight per cent of the decision-makers in the reference area and over 20 per cent in North Karelia had been explicitly advised by a public health nurse to change dietary habits.[7]

The content of the messages was carefully constructed to anticipate and suppress counter-arguments. Since many local people, engaged in active occupations, strongly believed that a diet high in meat fat was necessary for hard-working individuals, messages aimed at decreasing fat intake often pointed out that there were hard-working vegetarian lumberjacks and that one of the most famous distance runners from Finland, H. Kolemainen, was a vegetarian. Reference was also repeatedly made to the fact that the recommended low-fat diet was more "traditional" for North Karelia than the present high-fat diet. Comparisons of changes in dietary habits in North Karelia and the reference area revealed that sizable and significantly greater reductions were observed in reported intake of fat in North Karelia than in the reference area.[7]

Realizing that any fear-provoking messages must be accompanied by clear and attainable recommendations for reducing that fear, the Project was careful with the "high-risk" concept. People with elevated blood pressure or serum cholesterol were told that their condition was potentially serious, but that simple steps could be taken to alleviate the problem. Practical dietary advice was given, and the high-risk individuals were systematically reassured at the follow-up. No distinction was made between "pathological" and "safe" levels of risk, and public health nurses and educators repeatedly pointed out that the general risk in the population was high—that everyone had reason to change. The surveys showed that the behavior changes were similar among population groups with varied initial risk levels, and that there was no tendency toward increased anxiety or psychosomatic complaints as a result of the efforts to identify and influence those with exceptionally elevated risk factors.[27]

The "emotional" approach to persuasion relies upon emotional association rather than argument. There was conscious effort by the Project to associate the goals of the project with the pride and provincial identity of the population. People were urged to participate and to make changes not only for themselves, but for "North Karelia." For instance, signs reading "Do not smoke here—we are in the North Karelia Project" were everywhere and fostered a kind of local patriotism.

The "behavioral" approach to persuasion also does not rely on rational argument. The Project staff became acquainted with hundreds of local influential people with whom problems of varying nature were discussed. Almost everyone directly contacted was asked to make at least some minor behavioral commitment in favor of the Project. Thousands of citizens cooperated with small actions such as the display of stickers and posters. Such actions undoubtedly influenced the involved individuals to take a more favorable view of the Project and its recommendations.

Training

Information and persuasion are often sufficient to permit simple behavioral change such as choices among similar, equally accessible consumer products like butter and margarine. But when complex change in habit or life-style is recommended, it is not always easy to translate intention into action. For example, adding of more vegetables to the family diet may require the homemaker to change long-standing patterns of shopping and preparation. Even when the family is persuaded that such changes should be made, they may find the transition difficult. The cessation of cigarette smoking provides another example of the difficulty of some actions.[28]

There is a fairly well-articulated body of research and theorization that can guide the creation of training programs to facilitate the learning of new habits and skills.[20] Four basic steps appear necessary for optimal training: 1) modeling or demonstration of new responses and action patterns; 2) guided and increasingly independent practice in those thoughts and behaviors; 3) feedback concerning the appropriateness or accuracy of responses; 4) reinforcement in the form of support and encouragement that can be gradually withdrawn if the new habit or skill leads to naturally reinforcing consequences. Illustrations of these steps can be drawn from the training course in dietary change that was conducted in the North Karelia Project.

Especially in rural Finland, most women occupy the traditional role of homemaker and in Eastern Finland many women belong to a local housewives' association known as the "Martha" Organization. In order to teach new cooking and food preparation skills and thus to change family diet, the North Karelia Project worked in cooperation with Martha leaders. A major practical activity here was the introduction of "Parties for a Long Life." Housewives of the village gathered in the afternoon to learn how to cook a healthier type of meal with actual demonstration and participation. For example, women were shown how potatoes and other roots can replace meat fat in soups, while still producing acceptable appearance and consistency. Guidance and feedback was presented by the course leaders as the new skills were practiced. The rest of the families were invited in the evening to enjoy the meal with them, creating good opportunities for natural reinforcement. A pleasant social program was then organized in conjunction with the meal. To increase the perception of natural incentives, participants were shown that the cost of the meal was less than that of their traditional way of preparing those dishes.

Three hundred forty-four of these sessions were held with approximately 15,000 participants. At the 1976 follow-up survey, 9 per cent of the men and 18 per cent of the women in North Karelia had been involved at least once. Since then, the "Party for a Long Life" has become part of the activities of the Martha Association on a national basis. A variety of other forms of training were conducted, including smoking cessation classes and special coronary rehabilitation groups. These are more completely described elsewhere.[7]

Community Organization

No matter how effectively a person has been educated, persuaded, and trained to make healthy changes in behavior, it is unlikely that the change will be maintained unless it is reinforced in the social environment. One of the central ideas, and probably the most important concept, of the Project in North Karelia was to involve the whole community in a broad effort to prevent cardiovascular disease. A variety of supportive activities were organized. They provide examples of how members of the community can be trained and organized to reinforce the changes that were being recommended.

Support within the family was created by involving the complete family unit whenever possible, e.g., inviting husbands and children to share the results of cooking class, or enlisting the support of wives in their husbands' adherence to smoking cessation courses, anti-hypertensive regimens, or coronary rehabilitation courses. Wives of smokers were informed about how to deal with nervousness on the part of a recent ex-smoker and how to be patient and reinforcing as their husband learned to live without cigarettes.

Special efforts were made to create general support within the community, based upon the well known sociological phenomenon of natural leadership in social networks of the community.[29] The Project staff, jointly with the Heart Association, identified local leaders by informally interviewing shopkeepers and other knowledgeable persons. They inquired about individuals who regularly have influential contacts with the large number of practical activities. Those who agreed to participate in the "lay leaders" program were invited to a weekend of training which included basic information about risk factors for cardiovascular disease and suggestions on how to encourage positive changes in day-to-day contacts with people. Participants in these brief courses were also educated about the new activities that were being conducted by the health centers and given advice on how to encourage cooperation among their families, friends, and acquaintances. Finally, these natural leaders were told that they were models for the rest of the community and urged to be positive examples by following the various recommendations themselves. This activity was started toward the end of the five-year period and was continued after that. Over a four-year period more than 1,000 of the most influential members of the local communities in North Karelia were involved in this local organizational work.

Environmental Change

The environment is often a determining influence on behavior and may be a direct influence on health. Thus a very important goal of health promotion is the achievement of appropriate environmental changes. Community organization is an important element of such change. Both governmental and economic organizations tend to be most responsive to organized, collective actions.[30,31] Various concepts and theories of social influence and change suggest both direct influence and advocacy among decision-makers[32] and indirect influence through the organization of "grass-roots" support and action.[33]

The major environmental goals of the North Karelia Project were to increase the availability of low-fat foodstuffs and to introduce restrictions on smoking in many indoor spaces such as restaurants. Direct advocacy of those goals was accomplished through individual meetings with crucial individuals. For example, shop proprietors were individually asked to display signs which prohibited smoking in their shops. Management of a local sausage factory was particularly interested in cardiovascular disease prevention after two managers suffered heart attacks. The Project staff took advantage of their offer of cooperation by helping to create a new sausage product which replaced some meat and fat with mushrooms. Especially important was the assistance of the main county dairy in promoting the consumption of low-fat dairy products. Through this cooperation some entirely new products were created.

Indirect influence was organized out of the many contacts between North Karelia Project staff and influential members of the community. The weekend courses for natural community leaders involved discussions of how useful environmental changes could be accomplished, and participants in these meetings were asked to accomplish specific objectives. For example, local restaurants and shops were visited by local leaders, who asked the proprietors to offer additions to the food products on sale, to prohibit or restrict smoking, and to remove tobacco advertisements.

A particularly powerful form of indirect influence on environmental change is the creation of consumer demand for new products or services. The educational and persuasive activities of the North Karelia Project stimulated increased demand for low-fat food products. When a survey showed that more than half of the population of North Karelia would buy low-fat milk if it were available, that fact was persuasively communicated to those responsible for the production and distribution of dairy products. In response, the dairy agreed to produce nonfat milk and other new products and joined with the Project in promoting those new products. Dairy sales were sustained without increasing costs.

The proportion of people in North Karelia who regularly drink high-fat milk dropped almost 40 per cent. However, this development took place in the whole country, so that in the reference area similar but smaller shifts away from high-fat milk consumption were observed. Other internal changes that were stimulated by the North Karelia Project also spread throughout Finland. A special soft butter (mixed butter and vegetable oil), introduced by the Project in connection with the "Parties for Long Life," was made available to all Finns as a result of legislative actions in 1978. The voluntary restraint on tobacco promotion that was evoked in North Karelia became a national law in 1977 with the passage of national legislation prohibiting the promotion of tobacco products.

Summary of Five-Year Results

Selected examples of the results achieved in North Karelia have been mentioned throughout this paper and full report of intermediate and primary outcomes are available elsewhere.[7] Only a brief summary of the risk factor changes that were observed will be presented here. Because of the tendency for longitudinal study of cohorts to exaggerate estimates for change in the whole community,[34] the project evaluation relied upon independent surveys of population samples drawn from the national population register. In 1972, a baseline survey was conducted in which a total of 5,115 men and women between the ages of 25 and 59 were sampled in North Karelia and 7,348 were sampled in the reference area (neighboring county). Excluding those who had died or migrated out of the area, well over 90 per cent of those asked to respond were studied. In 1977, a five-year follow-up survey was made in which 4,728 new persons were sampled from North Karelia and 6,776 were sampled in the reference area. Response rates were again around 90 per cent. Both of these surveys included similarly structured questionnaires and direct risk factor measurement using standardized techniques. Smoking was measured by a set of questions; the reported answers were validated at the terminal survey by analyzing the serum thiocyanate levels of a random half of subjects. Casual blood pressure was measured in sitting position using standardized techniques; the fifth phase was used as diastolic blood pressure. Serum cholesterol assessments were made in one central laboratory standardized against the WHO reference laboratory in Atlanta. An overall risk score was computed for each subject using a multiple logistic function based on their smoking, serum cholesterol and systolic blood pressure values.[7]

Changes in risk estimates for smoking, serum cholesterol, blood pressure, and total risk are presented in Table 1, showing significant reductions in North Karelia when compared to the reference area. A more detailed discussion of the evaluation efforts of the project can be found in the WHO report.[7]

Five years is obviously not a long enough period of time to reduce cardiovascular morbidity and mortality, but some changes have been observed.[35] There are good data from national records of pension disability payment and a clear relative reduction in cardiovascular disease pension was observed in North Karelia as compared to the reference area.[7] Estimates from pension disability data already suggest that payment of over $4 million (US) dollars in disability payments may have been avoided by the less than $1 million expended on the Project's intervention activities.

We realize that the observation of only two statistical units (counties) and the absence of random assignment of the intervention limit the certainty of inferences that may be drawn from this study. Given the origin

Table 1 Mean Risk Factor Levels for Men and Women in North Karelia and Reference Area in 1972 and 1977

Assessment areas	Men	1972	1977	Change
Cholesterol	North Karelia	269.3	259.0	−10.3*
	Reference	260.4	261.2	+0.8
Cigarettes/day (total sample)	North Karelia	9.9	8.1	−1.8*
	Reference	8.9	8.1	−0.8
Systolic BP	North Karelia	147.3	143.9	−3.4*
	Reference	145.0	146.8	+1.8
Diastolic BP	North Karelia	90.8	88.6	−2.2*
	Reference	92.4	92.8	+0.4
Risk Score	North Korea	4.1	3.4	−0.7*
	Reference	3.7	3.7	0.0
	Women	**1972**	**1977**	
Cholesterol	North Karelia	265.3	258.2	−7.1
	Reference	259.2	255.1	−4.1
Cigarettes/day (total sample)	North Karelia	1.3	1.1	−0.2
	Reference	1.4	1.3	−0.1
Systolic BP	North Karelia	149.4	143.5	−5.9*
	Reference	144.1	145.4	+1.3
Diastolic BP	North Karelia	90.7	86.8	−3.9*
	Reference	90.0	89.5	−0.5
Risk Score	North Karelia	3.3	2.9	−0.4*
	Reference	3.0	2.9	−0.1

*Significant difference (p<.01) between change in North Karelia and reference area (one-tailed t test).

of the Project, randomization was clearly out of the question. However, the reference area was chosen in a "matched" way. Because the possible impact of the Project on the reference area is not taken into account, and a new medical school was opened in the reference area in 1972, the true impact of the Project may have been greater than estimated. Socioeconomic development was equivalent in both areas. Health services increased considerably. There was negligible in or out migration among citizens above the age of 30.

Because the objective was to serve the entire province of North Karelia, different components of intervention were not differentially applied within North Karelia. Thus, we cannot state secure conclusions about the unique or relative contributions of different programs, sub-programs, or channels of action. The observed changes may have been due to any one or all of the several actions toward each specific objective. Furthermore, the changes that took place in North Karelia were at least partly the result of more general international trends toward cardiovascular risk reduction which are difficult to disentangle from the specific events of the North Karelia Project. In spite of that, a few comments about the feasibility and coverage of different activities can be made.

The new preventive services developed gradually and required a fair amount of organizational effort and training of local personnel. Trading was expensive but at times the number of participants was restricted because of conflicts with work duties or other meetings. Environmental changes were certainly affected, but their extent was limited by national legislation, other national rules, or economic realities. The extent and coverage of general anti-smoking advice certainly matched with initial expectations. Health personnel were attentive to patients' smoking, but the success of more intensive group support in smoking cessation was not great. The nutrition program resembled these experiences. General nutrition information and counseling was extensive and had wide coverage. Less developed was the system to provide intense individual nutrition counseling for the overweight or those with very high cholesterol levels. On the other hand it was felt that mass intervention to change nutrition habits was probably a better strategy in the situation where practically everybody had an elevated cholesterol level relative to world norms. The hypertension subprogram succeeded with what proved to be clear and practical programs to screen, treat, and follow the approximately 10–15 per cent of the adult population with hypertension. The reorganization of preventive services and organization of community support and action were probably the most effective aspects of the overall project.

Although the final epidemiological results concerning mortality-reducing effects of the program in North Karelia are still to be shown, the goals of health promotion were met to the satisfaction of those who initially requested the action. The general perception of "success" had led to rapid national adoption of innovations that originated in North Karelia. For example, a major smoking cessation television program was based upon the Project experiences and methods,[36] and a more comprehensive risk factor reduction program on national television has now been conducted. As mentioned previously, several of the new dairy products and health service models that were developed in North Karelia are now available throughout Finland. The North Karelia Project has become popular as a practical and positive example that health promotion and control of modern chronic disease epidemics is feasible.

North Karelia is a fairly large administrative area, and Finland is a relatively small country where public health resources are as scarce as they are elsewhere. The expenditures for an extensive investigation have been limited to a single geographic unit, with only one other unit provided as a matched reference. We feel that the North Karelia Project must be viewed as a promising case study rather than a critical test of the effects of health promotion. That test will depend upon further studies. Only by using the different resources available for intervention and measurement in different countries can enough experience be gained to draw final conclusions on the value of health promotion in modern public health work.

Implications

It is difficult to estimate the potential impact of similar activities in the United States. Stunkard and his colleagues in Pennsylvania are attempting an approximate replication of the North Karelia Project in a rural setting and several other research teams have begun parallel investigations of community health promotion for cardiovascular disease prevention.* The Stanford-Three-Community-Study[37] demonstrated significant risk reduction in a cohort study in rural California. However there are critical differences between the Finnish and North American cultures that probably make health promotion easier to implement in Finland. United States citizens do not uniformly perceive governmental agencies as credible sources of information, whereas Finns are generally more willing to accept public recommendations and to cooperate with community health workers. Thus, public health interests in Finland find it easier to regulate promotion and marketing of products such as tobacco cigarettes. The governmental regulation of medicine in Finland undoubtedly increases the extent to which preventive services can be shaped to serve the interests of

---

*Personal communication from J. Farquhan, Stanford University, A. Stunkard, University of Pennsylvania, July 1980; H. Blackburn, University of Minnesota, February 1981; and R. Carlton, Pawtucket Memorial Hospital, (Pawtucket, RI), June 1980.

public health. Cultural acceptance of the notion that health is a public responsibility in Finland facilitates perception of the wisdom of shifting investments toward the prevention of disease. Thus the North Karelia Project serves not only to demonstrate objectives of health promotion but also to illustrate the cultural setting favorable for the development of innovations in public health and preventive medicine.

[The Acknowledgments and Appendix are not included here to save space, Ed.]

SOURCE

McAlister A, Puska P, Salonen JT, Tuomilehto J, and Koskela K. 1982. Theory and action for health promotion: Illustrations from the North Karelia project. *AJPH* 72(1): 43–50. Copyright 1982 *American Journal of Public Health*. Reprinted with permission of American Public Health Association.

PART III

Improving Public Health

The twentieth century will be remembered chiefly, not as an age of political conflicts and technical inventions, but as an age in which human society dared to think of the health of the whole human race as a practical objective.

—Arnold Toynbee, English historian (1889–1975)

CHAPTER 13

MEDICAL AND PREVENTIVE CARE

If you live to be one hundred, you've got it made. Very few people die past
that age.
—George Burns (1896–1996), American comedian

People without insurance have a tendency to ignore symptoms until they
develop a more acute disease, then they use the emergency room and the
hospital has a non-paying customer.
—David R. Obey (b. 1938), U.S. Congressman (D–Wisconsin)

MEDICAL AND PREVENTIVE CARE UNDERWENT A REVOLUTION during the twentieth century, beginning with great emphasis on public health solutions, such as providing potable water and controlling infectious diseases, and ending with medical
attempts to stem the impact of chronic diseases. At the century's beginning,
tuberculosis, pneumonia, smallpox, and typhoid fever presented major infectious
disease challenges. Although some public health measures against these diseases
were effective, improved nutrition also facilitated improved host response to
infections. Surgical interventions were just becoming practical due to the widespread use of anesthesia and aseptic technique at the beginning of the century;
however, physicians could do little about localized infections other than incise
and drain abscesses. Major advances in medical care would have to await better
scientific understanding of how to counter pathophysiologic processes.

In the 1930s, sulfa drugs were introduced into medical practice, and with
their appearance, physicians had one means of fighting infections. In the 1940s,
in short order, the arrival of penicillin, streptomycin, and chloramphenicol her-
alded the golden age of antibiotics. However, these miracle drugs presented
problems in terms of side effects and safety issues.

Cardiovascular disease and cancer emerged as leading causes of death in the
United States and Europe by mid century, requiring new and sometimes costly
treatments. With increasing health care costs came questions about the need,
efficacy, and effectiveness of treatments. Eventually, the United Kingdom established the National Institute for Clinical Excellence (NICE) as a means of
evaluating whether its National Health Service (NHS) should cover costs for

specific treatments based on the evidence of effectiveness. Globally, the field of outcomes research epidemiology developed to provide both methods and analyses to address these issues.

Preventive care also witnessed tremendous advances during the century. Vaccines became widely disseminated, eradicating smallpox and greatly reducing other diseases, including polio, measles, mumps, pertussis, diphtheria, hepatitis B, and rubella. Tuberculosis control began with the introduction of BCG vaccination and then, after World War II, streptomycin. The successful prevention and treatment of infectious diseases brought many to believe that chronic diseases should be tackled as well. Cancer registries were established, and efforts to identify the causes of cancer, heart disease, and stroke were begun. With the development of antihypertensives, major campaigns against high blood pressure were initiated. Tobacco control, too, figured prominently in the activities of most public health agencies, particularly during the latter half of the century. By century's end, public health interventions were waning in much of the developed world, with prevention being taken on by the medical establishment, big pharma, and, in the United States, the insurance industry.

HEALTH SYSTEMS

During the twentieth century, both the place and the systems within which medical and preventive care were provided changed considerably. These changes reflected the confluence of advances in medical care as well as the creation of population social welfare systems to address a variety of social problems that developed as a consequence of industrialization, particularly in (though not limited to) Western Europe. The seeds of these changes were planted by two revolutions: the French Revolution and the Industrial Revolution. Both events made clear the impoverished nature of the laboring class in Western Europe generally and in England in particular.

Karl Marx and Frederick Engels responded to this impoverishment by offering communism (or Marxism) as the solution. They fully expected an armed insurrection by the laboring classes to lead to the creation of a communist state. However, ignoring Marx and Engels and taking their cue from the French Revolution, members of the Western European laboring and middle classes fomented their own uprisings in 1848. In their wake, Western Europe's middle class as well as social democratic-laboring class political parties emerged.

The health consequences of industrialization also required redress. Although Germany hardly exemplified a socialist state, Prussia had been active in setting some physicians fees since the early seventeenth century, and all German mine workers participated in obligatory sickness insurance as of 1854. In 1856, Krupp, the German armaments manufacturer and one of the largest employers in the country, began offering health insurance to its workers, with the company paying half the premium. Germany was not alone in establishing insurance schemes; by the early twentieth century, the English Liberal Party under Lloyd George gained a mandate to implement some form of national health insurance. Although some English unions and the medical community opposed a national health insurance plan, George was determined to create a national system. The National Insurance Act of 1911 provided, among other things, for the creation of a governmental national health insurance system for individuals (but not their dependents) employed in designated industries in England and Wales. Workers in those industries were required to pay their health insurance premiums as part of their withheld taxes. By the onset of World War I, almost 15 million civilians in the United Kingdom had their health care provided under the aegis of the 1911 legislation. France, the remaining economic power in Europe, began implementing national health insurance in 1928, with initial coverage for workers in low-wage industries. In 1945, the French government expanded coverage to include all workers in French commerce and industry. Farmers joined in 1961; professionals joined five years later. Universal health care access in France was mandated in 1974.

During World War II, as part of its quid pro quo for joining a Conservative-led national unity government, the British Labor Party exacted a commitment for implementing national health insurance for all residents of the United Kingdom. In 1946, legislation creating the NHS passed. Implementation began in 1948, and little changed for almost five decades. Then, in 1994, the British government established NICE to examine the cost-effectiveness of various therapies prior to their initial use by the NHS. If NICE deemed a modality cost-effective, the NHS would adopt it; otherwise, the NHS would not pay for it. As Britain entered the twenty-first century, the NHS remained the principal health care provider for the British public.

In the United States, the health care delivery system developed in a less centralized manner. For the first two-thirds of the twentieth century, government-paid health care was limited to the members of the military and veterans. In 1965, Medicare was implemented to pay for health care provided to those in the Social Security system, primarily to those who are retired and at least 62 years old. In theory, the system is paid for by the beneficiaries, but since its implementation, the system has run on a "pay as you go" basis. At the time of Medicare's founding, the elderly were the poorest demographic group in the United States. By the close of the century, they had become the wealthiest. At the same time, Medicare-funded health care was half of all health care provided in the United States. Medicare did not cover the costs of pharmaceuticals at the end of the twentieth century, but it began to do so in 2005.

Care of the elderly is not the only function of Medicare; in 1972, Medicare began covering the costs associated with health care provided to those in the American Social Security system who had end-stage renal disease regardless of their age. Among the covered costs are dialysis treatments. Should the individual also have private health insurance, the law provides for appropriate payments by the private health insurer. The Medicare system is administered by the Centers for Medicare and Medicaid Services (CMS) within the United States Department of Health and Human Services. The CMS also administers the Medicaid system.

Begun at the same time as Medicare, Medicaid is the system implemented in the United States to pay for the health care received by those who cannot afford such services. The system is administered by each state for its residents. Participation in the system is means tested, meaning a person must be below a given income bracket to receive benefits. In contrast to Medicare, Medicaid has always covered the costs of pharmaceuticals, subject to the restrictions of individual states. It has also always covered nursing home care, again in contrast to Medicare.

Until the mid 1990s, the U.S. health care system operated predominantly as fee-for-service, whereby patients selected their physicians and then paid for each service provided. Different mechanisms were developed to provide for the payment of those services. Employer-based health insurance plans were created; the largest of these plans, Blue Cross and Blue Shield, developed from efforts to cover the hospital costs for teachers in Dallas (Blue Cross) and similar efforts to cover the physician fees for lumberjacks in the Pacific Northwest (Blue Shield).

Employer-paid health insurance arose in the United States as a result of a wage freeze during World War II. Employers desperate for workers began offering health insurance as a benefit separate from wages and not subject to government approval. During the post-World War II economic boom, employer-paid health insurance became increasingly prevalent as employers competed for workers.

By the late 1980s, problems presented by fee-for-service health care sent health care costs soaring. Employers seeking to hold down health insurance costs sought alternative approaches, and health maintenance organizations (HMOs) and managed care organizations (MCOs) became prevalent though they were not new.

For example, the Ross-Loos Medical Group began offering prepaid care to workers in the Los Angeles Department of Water and Power early in the twentieth century. By the early 1950s, the organization covered 35,000 industrial workers, teachers, and other government employees in the Southern California area.

In an attempt to curb soaring health care costs, the U.S. government passed the 1973 HMO Act, legitimizing these entities as conduits of health care. During the early 1980s, the state of Minnesota fostered HMO development, with a record proportion of care delivered by HMOs. The largest HMO on the West Coast, Kaiser Permanente, also began spreading its influence across the nation.

The Kaiser Permanente organization began in 1933, when Kaiser created an insurance company to deal with worker's compensation claims during a construction project in the Mojave Desert. The insurance company, Industrial Indemnity, contracted with a physician fresh out of his residency training, Dr. Sidney Garfield, who would build a hospital to provide the needed care. The arrangement worked well, though Garfield and his hospital were losing money on the deal. Industrial Indemnity responded to the situation with a suggestion that workers contribute a fixed fee per month to provide for medical care not related to the job. The additional fees enabled Garfield to continue running the hospital and providing health care. In 1938, when the Grand Coulee Dam project began, Kaiser approached Garfield to reproduce in the state of Washington what he had done in California. Garfield agreed. Because the Grand Coulee workers brought their families with them, Garfield had to care for the families in addition to the workers. The result was the formation of the Kaiser Permanente system. In time, Kaiser Permanente grew to be the largest HMO in the nation, with a presence in both Northern and Southern California. With the age of managed care beginning in the 1990s, Kaiser Permanente's prosperity seemed assured.

Health Economics and the RAND Study

After World War II, health care delivery systems began to be analyzed from a variety of dimensions, one of which was health economics. That field was generally considered to have developed from a 1963 paper by future Nobel laureate Kenneth Arrow. Health economists attempted to find the optimal means of delivering health care and controlling demand. The RAND Corporation, an independent think tank, designed and conducted the Health Insurance Experiment (HIE) to assess whether free medical care leads to better health than having insurance plans that require the patient to shoulder part of the cost. Conducted from 1974 to 1982, the HIE found that co-insurance (or "cost sharing") significantly reduced utilization of health services. Among those with health insurance, the impact on health status was minimal, but among those without such insurance, essential care was missed because of the cost barrier. In the United States, the HIE results were thus integrated into almost all schemes for financing health care.

MEDICAL CARE AND TREATMENT

The twentieth century opened with the medical profession increasingly focused on the use of the hospital as a means of providing both acute and chronic care to the sick. In having the patients in one place, the combined resources of the medical community could be brought to bear on any given case. As medicine advanced, particularly in the century's latter half, the costs associated with providing inpatient care would drive restrictions on the use of hospitals. First, chronic care was moved out of hospitals, particularly for the mentally ill. With the discovery of drugs such as chlorpromazine (Thorazine) to treat schizophrenia and bipolar disorder, state mental health facilities emptied. Some continued to operate through the century's end, but they no longer had the community impact present in the early 1900s.

Until the appearance of the AIDS epidemic in the early 1980s, the trend in the United States had been to reduce inpatient stays across all conditions. Driven by the increasing costs of hospital-provided services, third-party payers steered patients to receive as much care out of hospital as possible. Procedures previously performed only on an inpatient basis, such as a mastectomy as treatment for breast cancer, were now performed on day admissions or in outpatient settings. It was during this period that the term "drive-through mastectomy" was coined to describe the phenomenon. However, the complexities presented by AIDS, particularly the multitude of acute complications from the disease, forced increased use of hospitals as places for treatment of acutely ill individuals. Only with the development of HAART did hospital utilization for AIDS patients begin to conform to the trends for patients with other conditions (see Chapter 9).

Technology and Medicines

Changes in the practice of medicine during the twentieth century reflected an epochal advance in the availability and application of technology. X-ray technology moved from flat-screen views of the body to complex imaging involving contrast media. Cross-sectional assessments became available through computerized axial tomography (CT or CAT) and nuclear magnetic resonance (NMR) scans; visualization of physiological and pathophysiological processes became available through positron emission tomography (PET) scans. For the first time, extent of disease could be visualized, and interventions could interrupt pathophysiological processes. For example, by the end of the twentieth century, the extent of coronary atherosclerosis could be assessed radiologically, and, if warranted, interventions could be undertaken, either by placement of a stent or by a CABG procedure. Indeed, advances in radiology afforded surgeons a view of disease not previously available, and innovations, such as the development of an artificial kidney, allowed surgical interventions to leap forward. Advances in the laboratory during the course of the latter part of the century provided better tests of physiological functions and allowed health care providers to better assess a patient's status, either acutely or during the progression of a chronic condition. Congenital anomalies could be diagnosed *in utero* for the first time.

Improved understanding of pathophysiological processes facilitated the development of drugs to treat various diseases. For example, insulin was identified, its components determined, and synthetic versions marketed. Infections were the early focus of the pharmaceutical industry, first with sulfa drugs and then antibiotics such as penicillin, chloramphenicol, and streptomycin. These successes would catapult the pharmaceutical industry into the forefront of scientific medicine.

The second half of the twentieth century would see a wealth of anti-inflammatory drugs enter the marketplace. Cortisone was synthesized and used in patients with Addison's disease, as well as other chronic inflammatory conditions. Chemotherapeutic agents to use against cancer were developed, and means of controlling blood pressure and other cardiovascular risk factors entered the clinic. New methods of contraception were developed. In the case of oral contraceptives, the result would be major social and economic change (see Chapter 6). For other contraceptive techniques, such as the Dalkon Shield, the result would be the creation of new areas of legal study (See Chapter 14). With all of these advances came increased costs of care, spurring health economics and outcomes research investigators to assess the perceived advantages to these new technologies from the patient's perspective.

Not surprisingly, advances in technology sporadically focused on concerns about patient safety. In 1902 for example, diphtheria antitoxin was collected from a horse with tetanus, resulting in several deaths of persons. The result was U.S. legislation creating the Biologics Control Act. The FDA was created in 1906 to focus on food safety, but it had only minimal impact on the emerging pharmaceutical industry. Until the 1930s, drug safety efforts in all countries essentially remained unchanged. Then in 1937, the use of ethylene glycol as a solvent for sulfanilamide led to an epidemic of renal failure and more than 100 deaths in the United States. The FDA ordered a product recall on the basis of false labeling, but it could not address the issue of drug safety. The 1938 Food, Drugs, and Cosmetics Act called for toxicological testing of new products before marketing, but it did not give the FDA authorization to recall drugs that were unsafe. That did not happen until after World War II, when an epidemic of aplastic anemia, a rare hematological condition, was associated with use of chloramphenicol.

During the early 1950s, the son of California surgeon Albe Watkins was treated for strep throat with one of the new antibiotics of the era, chloramphenicol. The first time young Watkins was treated, the infection cleared rapidly; the second time, he developed aplastic anemia and died. The medical community was unsure whether chloramphenicol caused aplastic anemia, but the AMA was sufficiently concerned that it planned a conference on the matter in Chicago. A couple of months before that conference, the elder Watkins packed his family into their car and set out from California for Chicago. At each city or town the family stopped in along the way, Watkins called the local physicians and asked if they had seen any cases of aplastic anemia since chloramphenicol had arrived on the market. If so, Watkins asked what drugs the patient was given. He kept a list of all such cases reported to him. Upon reaching the AMA conference in Chicago, Watkins reported his methods and results. The AMA thought Watkins' idea innovative and during the 1950s established a system for compiling similar data for all diseases and all medications used in the United States. It then provided tabulations of the data to all physicians, hospitals, and medical schools. The FDA eventually took over the AMA database, and it is this database, essentially unchanged in the more than half century from Watkins's pilot study, that today constitutes the Spontaneous Reporting System and its successors. In the United Kingdom, a different approach using a cohort of new users, the Yellow Card system, was developed as an alternative approach to assessing the safety of newly marketed products.

The thalidomide episode also significantly changed drug safety regulations in the United States and Europe. During the 1950s, thalidomide was found to be an effective tranquilizer and antiemetic drug useful for the treatment of morning sickness. At the time the drug was released, it was believed that no drug could pass from the mother across the placenta to harm the fetus. Thus, thalidomide was prescribed to thousands of pregnant women from 1957 until 1961. During that time, between 10,000 and 20,000 children were born with significant birth defects (phocomelia) before the drug was withdrawn from the market. As a result of the thalidomide tragedy, pharmaceutical companies were forced to demonstrate the safety and efficacy of a product before it could be marketed. In Europe, national drug authorities now oversee drug development activities to assure that a repeat of the thalidomide episode does not occur.

In the late 1960s, Europe was challenged by the appearance of a pulmonary hypertension epidemic traced to an appetite suppressant, or anorexigen (Aminorex). In Japan, during the same time, an outbreak of subacute myelo-opticoneuropathy (SMON) was traced to clioquinol, an antifungal, antiprotozal drug. These outbreaks, coupled with the cardiovascular effects of oral contraceptives first noted in the 1960s, helped to establish the field of pharmacoepidemiology.

The mixed blessings of pharmaceuticals became clear during the 1970s as the intergenerational effects of diethylstilbestrol (DES), a drug prescribed during pregnancy to prevent miscarriages or premature deliveries, was discovered as linked to a rare form of vaginal cancer.

The appearance of HIV in the early 1980s resulted in many complaints, particularly from HIV activists, that the FDA had become overly slow in approving new products. Some reform of the FDA approval process ensued; however, outbreaks of pulmonary hypertension and valvulopathy in the United States that appeared to be related to a combination anorexigen drug (Phen-fen) led the FDA to tighten its approval procedures further.

HEALTH INFORMATION SYSTEMS

For the better part of the twentieth century, getting health information meant contacting a physician or other health care provider with a specific question about treatment of a disease. Changes in technology during the course of the century radically changed what health information was and how it could be obtained. Much of this change happened first in the United States, perhaps because it was the sole major industrial power with an economy untouched by two world wars. Accordingly, it could more readily afford the investments in health information technology than could other industrial nations. Today, the United Nations defines a health information system as "a data system, usually computerized, that routinely collects and reports information about the delivery of services, costs, demographic and health information, and results status." Health information systems are aided by the field of health informatics, generally defined as the effort to standardize data vocabularies and platforms in order to facilitate the exchange of information for clinical, research, scheduling, and billing purposes.

In the early twentieth century, it was common practice for physicians to keep a record of all patient visits by entering them into a chronologic ledger system. Each patient would have to remember the dates they were seen in order to piece together their medical history. On July 1, 1907, at the Mayo Clinic in Rochester, Minnesota, Dr. Henry Plummer instituted the single patient system whereby each patient had a single chart that included all clinical and hospital visits, laboratory and other test results, and physician notes about the patient's condition. Plummer thus created the medical record system that is now the standard used around the world. The paper system has given way in some instances to computerized medical records, also called electronic health records (EHRs) or electronic medical records (EMRs). However, considerable legal, technological, and economic issues continue to impede the widespread use of such technologies.

In 1836, U.S. Surgeon General Joseph Lowell began ordering medical books for his office. Over time, the library expanded, setting a goal to "contain every medical book published in this country and every work relating to public health and state medicine." Under the library's director, Dr. John Shaw Billings, the library began to publish an index of its holdings in 1879— the *Index Medicus*. This resource soon became the database to which those desiring to locate a particular paper on a topic or by a specific author could turn. With the rise of computer technology in the 1960s, the *Index Medicus* was transitioned into Medline, a computer-based index maintained by the National Library of Medicine (NLM), a component of the U.S. Library of Congress (with additional oversight from the NIH).

Although Medline was extremely successful at facilitating user access to the medical literature, the Presidential Commission on Heart Disease, Cancer, and Stroke released a 1965 report calling for further investment in health information technology and the creation of a decentralized health information system. With the advent of the personal computer and the Internet, the NLM created a portal into the Medline database, PubMed. This portal is freely accessible to anyone able to gain access to the Internet. It has greatly aided the medical community's efforts to remain abreast of new developments in the medical literature and to undertake reviews of that literature. By century's end, multiple search engines (such as Pub Med, Web of Science, Scopus, and Google Scholar) allowed researchers to access thousands of journals and other medical resources, as well as to utilize searchable health-related data sets (such as vital statistics, fatal accidents, or cancer registry data). Electronic medical records, enlightened databases, and websites such as WebMD allowed consumers to take control of their health and health care.

Another benefit of the Internet age was the creation of telemedicine, in which health care providers in one location can interact with patients at another location. Although it is not difficult to imagine how such a system might be advantageous in an emergency, it has also been implemented to support more routine interactions between providers and patients. There are potential legal limitations to the growth of telemedicine, but the promise of such systems to support activities as simple as discussions with patients and as complex as direction of a robotic surgeon suggests the potential for telemedicine to greatly alter the practice of medicine as the twenty-first century advances.

Selected Readings

The first reading, by Kenneth Arrow, is considered a classic in that it directly addresses a primary concern of public health—defining the role of the market when it comes to health care. The work is included here in total except for the appendix, which consists of five pages of optimization models. Arrow cautions that rationing care, by restricting the number of incoming medical students to medical schools or trying to reduce the number of physicians by restricting licensing, will not be effective in controlling costs. Rather, it will only serve to increase the incomes of currently practicing physicians. When Arrow wrote this paper in 1963, the boom in medical technology had not yet occurred, and only a small proportion of the U.S. population was covered by medical insurance. The pressures for a public system for medical coverage for elderly (Medicare) and poor Americans (Medicaid) were only at a rudimentary stage. As this is written, tensions about the overuse of medical care and the ability of either individuals or governments to pay for it are higher than ever. Thus, Arrow's work, a foundation of health economics, remains relevant today.

John Wennberg, Director of the Center for the Evaluative Clinical Sciences at the Dartmouth Medical School, and his colleague, Dartmouth statistician Alan Gittelsohn, provide the second reading for this chapter. It appears intact except for the removal of one map of the civil divisions of Vermont, which we judged to be unnecessary for the understanding of the work. In this piece, considered a classic by *Science*, the authors document that patients with similar illnesses received different types and amounts of health care based on their geographic location in the various hospital service areas of Vermont. During the course of 30 years, Wennberg continued to show that areas spending more on health care and providing more services often demonstrated worse outcomes compared to others providing less intensive care for lower costs. His findings eventually led to the field of outcomes research, and Wennberg was selected the "Most Influential Policy Maker of the Past 25 Years" by *Health Affairs* in 1997.

The last reading, by C. J. L. Murray, discusses the concept of the disability-adjusted life year (DALY). In 1990, the WHO launched the Global Burden of Disease (GBD) study out of Harvard University, and Murray headed the effort. A new metric was developed for the study, which measured the gap between an ideal health situation, where the entire population lives to an advanced age, free of disease and disability, and current health realities. This metric was called the DALY, and it combines years of life lost due to premature mortality and years of life lost due to time lived in states of less than full health. It allows the burden of disease to be measured consistently across diseases, risk factors, and regions. Richard Feacham, chairman of the World Development Report of 1993, claims the DALY "broke new ground. . . ." Although the DALY was roundly criticized for its flaws, it has rapidly become a standard measure to compare the health of nations used especially by the WHO and the World Bank.

BIBLIOGRAPHY

Adams S. 1963. The Medlars System. *Fed Proc* 22:1018–21.

Aday LA, ed. 2005. *Reinventing Public Health: Policies and Practices for a Healthy Nation.* San Francisco: Jossey-Bass.

Armitage P. 1995. Before and After Bradford Hill: Some Trends in Medical Statistics. *Journal of the Royal Statistical Society.* Series A (Statistics in Society) 158 (1): 143–53.

Arnesen T and Kapiriri L. 2004. Can the value choices in DALYs influence global priority-setting? *Health Policy* 70:137–49.

Arrow KJ. 1963. Uncertainty and the welfare economics of medical care. *American Economic Review* 53 (5): 941–73.

Bachrach CA and Charen T. 1978. Selection of MEDLINE contents, the development of its thesaurus, and the indexing process. *Med Inform* (Lond) 3 (3): 237–54.

Baker MG and Fidler DP. 2006. Global public health surveillance under new international health regulations. *EID* 12 (7): 1058–65.

Banta D. 2003. The development of health technology assessment. *Health Policy* 63 (2): 121–32.

Blumenthal D and Glazer JP. 2007. Information technology comes to medicine. *N Engl J Med* 356 (24): 2527–34.

Breslow L. 2006. Health measurement in the third era of health. *Am J Public Health* 96 (1): 17–19.

Brook RH, Ware JE, Rogers WH, Keeler EB, Davies AR, Sherbourne CD, Goldberg GA, Lohr KN, Camp P, and Newhouse JP. 1984. *The Effect of Coinsurance on the Health of Adults Results from the RAND Health Insurance Experiment.* Santa Monica, CA: RAND Corporation, R-3055-HHS, http://www.rand.org/pubs/reports/R3055/ (accessed June 1, 2009).

Cochrane AL. 1972. *Effectiveness and Efficiency: Random Reflections on Health Services.* London: Nuffield Provincial Hospitals Trust.

Cueto M. 2004. The origins of primary health care and selective primary health care. *Am J Public Health* 94 (11): 1864–74.

Doran T, Fullwood C, Gravelle H, Reeves D, Kontopantelis E, Hiroeh U, and Roland M. 2005. Pay-for-performance programs in family practices in the United Kingdom. *N Engl J Med* 355 (4): 375–84.

Drazen JM and Kurfman GD. 2004. Public access to biomedical research (editorial). *N Engl J Med* 351 (13): 1343.

Drummond M and Sculpher M. 2005. Common methodological flaws in economic evaluations. *Med Care* 43 (7 Suppl.): 5–14.

Dublin LI. 1926. *Population Problems in the United States and Canada.* Boston: Houghton Mifflin Company.

Dublin LI. 1943. *A Family of Thirty Million: The Story of the Metropolitan Life Insurance Company.* New York: The Metropolitan Life Insurance Company.

Dublin LI. 1965. *Factbook on Man from Birth to Death,* 2nd ed. New York: Macmillan.

Dublin LI. 1966. *After Eighty Years: The Impact of Life Insurance on the Public Health.* Gainesville, FL: University of Florida Press.

Dublin LI and Lotka AJ. 1946. *The Money Value of a Man.* New York: Ronald Press Company.

Falk IS. 1934. The present and future organization of medicine. *Milbank Quarterly* 12 (2): 115–25.

Falk IS. 1936. *Security Against Sickness: A Study of Health Insurance.* Garden City, NY: Doubleday.

Falk IS, Rorem CR, and Ring MD. 1933. *The Costs of Medical Care: A Summary of Investigations on the Economic Aspects of the Prevention and Care of Illness.* Chicago: University of Chicago Press.

Fries JF. 1983. The compression of morbidity. *Milbank Quarterly* 61 (3): 397–419.

Foege W. 1994. Preventive medicine and public health. *JAMA* 271 (June): 1704–5.

Garfield E. 1964. Science Citation Index—A new dimension in indexing. *Science,* New Series 144 (3619): 649–54.

Haenszel W. 1950. A standardized rate for mortality defined in units of lost years of life. *Am J Public Health Nations Health* 40 (1): 17–26.

Harrington JA. 2007. Law, globalization and the NHS. *Capital & Class* 92:81–104.

Harris RW. 1946. *National Health Insurance in Great Britain: 1911-1946.* London: George Allen and Unwin Ltd.

Lehoux P. 2006. *The Problem of Health Technology: Policy Implications for Modern Health Care Systems.* New York: Routledge, Taylor & Francis Group.

Hung DY, Rundall TG, Tallia AF, Cohen DB, Halpin HA, and Crabtree BF. 2007. Rethinking prevention in primary care: Applying the chronic care model to address health risk behaviors. *Milbank Quarterly* 85 (1): 69–91.

Karel L, Austin CH, and Cummings MM. 1965. Computerized bibliographic services for biomedicine. *Science,* New Series 148 (367): 766–72.

Keeler EB. 1992. Effects of cost sharing on use of medical services and health. *Medical Practice Management* (Summer): 317–21 http://www.rand.org/pubs/reprints/RP1114/ (accessed June 1, 2007).

Kendall DB and Levine SR. 1998. Pursuing the promise of an information-age health care system. *Health Affairs* 1998 (Nov.-Dec.): 41–43.

Kuper H, Nicholson A, and Hemingway H. 2006. Searching for observational studies: What does citation tracking add to PubMed? A case study in depression and coronary heart disease. *BMC Medical Research Methodology* 6:4.

Langmuir AD. 1963. The surveillance of communicable diseases of national importance. *N Engl J Med* 268:182–92.

Lindberg DAB and Humphreys BL. 2005. 2015—the future of medical libraries. *N Engl J Med* 352 (11): 1067–70.

McCarn DB and Leiter J. 1973. On-Line Services in Medicine and Beyond. *Science,* New Series 181 (4097): 318–24.

Michaud CM, Murray CJL, and Bloom BR. 2001. Burden of disease—implications for future research. *JAMA* 285 (5): 335–39.

Miller W, Robinson LA, and Lawrence RS, eds. 2006. *Valuing Health for Regulatory Cost-Effectiveness Analysis.* Washington, DC: National Academies Press.

Murray C and Lopez A. 1996. *The Global Burden of Disease.* Cambridge, MA: Harvard University Press.

Murray CJL. 2007. Towards good practice for health statistics: Lessons from the Millennium Development Goal health indicators. *Lancet* 369:862–73.

Newhouse JP and the Insurance Experiment Group. 1993. *Free for All? Lessons from the RAND Health Experiment.* Cambridge, MA.: Harvard University Press.

Oliver A. 2005. The English National Health Service: 1979–2005. *Health Econ* 14:S75–S99.

Powell M. 2000. Analysing the 'new' British National Health Service. *Int J Health Plan M* 15:89–101.

Remington PL, Smith MY, Williamson DF, Anda RF, Gentry EM, and Hogelin GC. 1988. Design, characteristics and usefulness of state-based behavioral risk factor surveillance, 1981–87. *Public Health Rep* 103:366–75.

Robinson R. 2000. Managed care in the United States: A dilemma for evidence-based policy? *Health Econ* 9:1–7.

Saltman RB, Busse R, and Figueras J, eds. 2004. *Social Health Insurance Systems in Western Europe*. Berkshire, England: Open University Press.

Shekelle PG, Morton SC, and Keeler EB. 2006. *Costs and Benefits of Health Information Technology. Evidence Report/Technology Assessment No. 132*. AHRQ Publication No. 06-E006. Rockville, MD: Agency for Healthcare Research and Quality.

Singer PA and Bowman KW. 2002. Quality end-of-life care: A global perspective. *BMC Palliative Care* 1:4, http://www.biomedcentral.com/1472-684X/1/4 (accessed June 1, 2007).

Weisbrod BA. 1991. The health care quadrilemma: An essay on technological change, insurance, quality of care, and cost containment. *Journal of Economic Literature* 29:523–52.

Wheeler DL, Barrett T, Benson DA, Bryant SH, Canese K, Chetvernin V, *et al*. 2007. Database resources of the National Center for Biotechnology Information. *Nucleic Acids Res* 35:D5–D12.

Wilbur RL. 1932. The economics of public health and medical care. Address at the tenth annual dinner meeting of the Boards of Counsel of the Milbank Memorial Fund, March 17, 1932. Milbank Memorial Fund *Quarterly Bulletin* 10 (3): L169–90. Reprinted in 2005 *Milbank Quarterly* 83 (4): 523–36.

World Bank. 1993. *World Development Report 1993: Investing In Health*. New York: Oxford University Press.

All publications relating to the RAND experiment can be found at: http://www.rand.org/health/projects/hie/hiepubs.html.

Uncertainty and the Welfare Economics of Medical Care
(1963, Abridged)

by Kenneth J. Arrow*

I. Introduction: Scope and Method

This paper is an exploratory and tentative study of the specific differentia of medical care as the object of normative economics. It is contended here, on the basis of comparison of obvious characteristics of the medical-care industry with the norms of welfare economics, that the special economic problems of medical care can be explained as adaptations to the existence of uncertainty in the incidence of disease and in the efficacy of treatment.

It should be noted that the subject is the *medical-care industry*, not *health*. The causal factors in health are many, and the provision of medical care is only one. Particularly at low levels of income, other commodities such as nutrition, shelter, clothing, and sanitation may be much more significant. It is the complex of services that center about the physician, private and group practice, hospitals, and public health, which I propose to discuss.

The focus of discussion will be on the way the operation of the medical-care industry and the efficacy with which it satisfies the needs of society differ from a norm, if at all. The "norm" that the economist usually uses for the purposes of such comparisons is the operation of the competitive model, that is, the flows of services that would be offered and purchased and the prices that would be paid for them if each individual in the market offered or purchased services at the going prices as if his decisions had no influence over them, and the going prices were such that the amount of services which were available equalled [*sic*] the total amounts which other individuals were willing to purchase, with no imposed restrictions on supply or demand.

Note: Bracketed numbers throughout the text refer to references in the original journal article which can be found in the Notes section of this book.

*The author is professor of economics at Stanford University. He wishes to express his thanks for useful comments to F. Bator, R. Dorfman, V. Fuchs, Dr. S. Gilson, R. Kessel, S. Mushkin, and C. R. Rorem. This paper was prepared under the sponsorship of the Ford Foundation as part of a series of papers on the economics of health, education, and welfare.

The interest in the competitive model stems partly from its presumed descriptive power and partly from its implications for economic efficiency. In particular, we can state the following well-known proposition (First Optimality Theorem). If a competitive equilibrium exists at all, and if all commodities relevant to costs or utilities are in fact priced in the market, then the equilibrium is necessarily *optimal* in the following precise sense (due to V. Pareto): There is no other allocation of resources to services which will make all participants in the market better off.

Both the conditions of this optimality theorem and the definition of optimality call for comment. A definition is just a definition, but when the *definiendum* is a word already in common use with highly favorable connotations, it is clear that we are really trying to be persuasive; we are implicitly recommending the achievement of optimal states.[1] It is reasonable enough to assert that a change in allocation which makes all participants better off is one that certainly should be made; this is a value judgment, not a descriptive proposition, but it is a very weak one. From this it follows that it is not desirable to put up with a non-optimal allocation. But it does not follow that if we are at an allocation which is optimal in the Pareto sense, we should not change to any other. We cannot indeed make a change that does not hurt someone; but we can still desire to change to another allocation if the change makes enough participants better off and by so much that we feel that the injury to others is not enough to offset the benefits. Such interpersonal comparisons are, of course, value judgments. The change, however, by the previous argument ought to be an optimal state; of course there are many possible states, each of which is optimal in the sense here used.

However, a value judgment on the desirability of each possible new distribution of benefits and costs corresponding to each possible reallocation of resources is not, in general, necessary. Judgments about the distribution can be made separately, in one sense, from those about allocation if certain conditions are fulfilled. Before stating the relevant proposition, it is necessary to remark that the competitive equilibrium achieved depends in good measure on the initial distribution of purchasing power, which consists of ownership of assets and skills that command a price on the market. A transfer of assets among individuals will, in general, change the final supplies of goods and services and the prices paid for them. Thus, a transfer of purchasing power from the well to the ill will increase the demand for medical services. This will manifest itself in the short run in an increase in the price of medical services and in the long run in an increase in the amount supplied.

With this in mind, the following statement can be made (Second Optimality Theorem): If there are no increasing returns in production, and if certain other minor conditions are satisfied, then every optimal state is a competitive equilibrium corresponding to some initial distribution of purchasing power. Operationally, the significance of this proposition is that if the conditions of the two optimality theorems are satisfied, and if the allocation mechanism in the real world satisfies the conditions for a competitive model, then social policy can confine itself to steps taken to alter the distribution of purchasing power. For any given distribution of purchasing power, the market will, under the assumptions made, achieve a competitive equilibrium which is necessarily optimal; and any optimal state is a competitive equilibrium corresponding to some distribution of purchasing power, so that any desired optimal state can be achieved.

The redistribution of purchasing power among individuals most simply takes the form of money: taxes and subsidies. The implications of such a transfer for individual satisfactions are, in general, not known in advance. But we can assume that society can *ex post* judge the distribution of satisfactions and, if deemed unsatisfactory, take steps to correct it by subsequent transfers. Thus, by successive approximations, a most preferred social state can be achieved, with resource allocation being handled by the market and public policy confined to the redistribution of money income.[2]

If, on the contrary, the actual market differs significantly from the competitive model, or if the assumptions of the two optimality theorems are not fulfilled, the separation of allocative and distributional procedures becomes, in most cases, impossible.[3]

The first step then in the analysis of the medical-care market is the comparison between the actual market and the competitive model. The methodology of this comparison has been a recurrent subject of controversy in economics for over a century. Recently, M. Friedman [15] has vigorously argued that the competitive or any other model should be tested solely by its ability to predict. In the context of competition, he comes close to arguing that prices and quantities are the only relevant data. This point of view is valuable in stressing that a certain amount of lack of realism in the assumptions of a model is no argument against its value. But the price-quantity implications of the competitive model for pricing are not easy to derive without major—and, in many cases, impossible—econometric efforts.

In this paper, the institutional organization and the observable mores of the medical profession are included among the data to be used in assessing the competitiveness of the medical-care market. I shall also examine the presence or absence of the preconditions for the equivalence of competitive equilibria and optimal states. The major competitive preconditions, in the sense used here, are three: the *existence* of competitive equilibrium, the *marketability* of all goods and services relevant to costs and utilities, and *nonincreasing returns*. The first two, as we have seen, insure that competitive equilibrium is necessarily optimal; the third insures that every optimal state is the competitive equilibrium corresponding to some distribution of income.[4] The first and third conditions are interrelated; indeed, nonincreasing returns plus some additional conditions not restrictive in a modern economy imply the existence of a competitive equilibrium, i.e., imply that there will be some set of prices which will clear all markets.[5]

The concept of marketability is somewhat broader than the traditional divergence between private and social costs and benefits. The latter concept refers to cases in which the organization of the market does not require an individual to pay for costs that he imposes on others as the result of his actions or does not permit him to receive compensation for benefits he confers. In the medical field, the obvious example is the spread of communicable diseases. An individual who fails to be immunized not only risks his own health, a disutility which presumably he has weighed against the utility of avoiding the procedure, but also that of others. In an ideal price system, there would be a price which he would have to pay to anyone whose health is endangered, a price sufficiently high so that the others would feel compensated; or, alternatively, there would be a price which would be paid to him by others to induce him to undergo the immunization procedure. Either system would lead to an optimal state, though the distributional implications would be different. It is, of course, not hard to see that such price systems could not, in fact, be practical; to approximate an optimal state it would be necessary to have collective intervention in the form of subsidy or tax or compulsion.

By the absence of marketability for an action which is identifiable, technologically possible, and capable of influencing some individual's welfare, for better or for worse, is meant here the failure of the existing market to provide a means whereby the services can be both offered and demanded upon payment of a price. Nonmarketability may be due to intrinsic technological characteristics of the product which prevent a suitable price from being enforced, as in the case of communicable diseases, or it may be due to social or historical controls, such as those prohibiting an individual from selling himself into slavery. This distinction is, in fact, difficult to make precise, though it is obviously of importance for policy; for the present purposes, it will be sufficient to identify nonmarketability with the observed absence of markets.

The instance of nonmarketability with which we shall be most concerned is that of risk-bearing. The relevance of risk-bearing to medical care seems obvious; illness is to a considerable extent an unpredictable phenomenon. The ability to shift the risks of illness to others is worth a price which many are willing to pay. Because of pooling and of superior willingness and ability, others are willing to bear the risks. Nevertheless, as we shall see in greater detail, a great many risks are not covered, and indeed the markets for the services of risk-coverage are poorly developed or nonexistent. Why this should be so is explained in more detail in Section IV.C below; briefly, it is impossible to draw up insurance policies which will sufficiently distinguish among risks, particularly since observation of the results will be incapable of distinguishing between avoidable and unavoidable risks, so that incentives to avoid losses are diluted.

The optimality theorems discussed above are usually presented in the literature as referring only to conditions of certainty, but there is no difficulty in extending them to the case of risks, provided the additional services of risk-bearing are included with other commodities.[6]

However, the variety of possible risks in the world is really staggering. The relevant commodities include, in effect, bets on all possible occurrences in the world which impinge upon utilities. In fact, many of these "commodities," i.e., desired protection against many risks, are simply not available. Thus, a wide class of commodities is nonmarketable, and a basic competitive precondition is not satisfied.[7]

There is a still more subtle consequence of the introduction of risk-bearing considerations. When there is uncertainty, information or knowledge becomes a commodity. Like other commodities, it has a cost of production and a cost of transmission, and so it is naturally not spread out over the entire population but concentrated among those who can profit most from it. (These costs may be measured in time or disutility as well as money.) But the demand for information is difficult to discuss in the rational terms usually employed. The value of information is frequently not known in any meaningful sense to the buyer; if, indeed, he knew enough to measure the value of information, he would know the information itself. But information, in the form of skilled care, is precisely what is being bought from most physicians, and, indeed, from most professionals. The elusive character of information as a commodity suggests that it departs considerably from the usual marketability assumptions about commodities.[8]

That risk and uncertainty are, in fact, significant elements in medical care hardly need argument. I will hold that virtually all the special features of this industry, in fact, stem from the prevalence of uncertainty.

The nonexistence of markets for the bearing of some risks in the first instance reduces welfare for those who wish to transfer those risks to others for a certain price, as well as for those who would find it profitable to take on the risk at such prices. But it also reduces the desire to render or consume services which have risky consequences; in technical language, these commodities are complementary to risk-bearing. Conversely, the production and consumption of commodities and services with little risk attached act as substitutes for risk-bearing and are encouraged by market failure there with respect to risk-bearing. Thus the observed commodity pattern will be affected by the nonexistence of other markets.

The failure of one or more of the competitive preconditions has as its most immediate and obvious consequence a reduction in welfare below that obtainable from existing resources and technology, in the sense of a failure to reach an optimal state in the sense of Pareto. But more can be said. I propose here the view that, when the market fails to achieve an optimal state, society will, to some extent at least, recognize the gap, and nonmarket social institutions will arise attempting to bridge it.[9] Certainly this process is not necessarily conscious; nor is it uniformly successful in approaching more closely to optimality when the entire range of consequences is considered. It has always been a favorite activity of economists to point out that actions which on their face achieve a desirable goal may have less obvious consequences, particularly over time, which more than offset the original gains.

But it is contended here that the special structural characteristics of the medical-care market are largely attempts to overcome the lack of optimality due to the nonmarketability of the bearing of suitable risks and the imperfect marketability of information. These compensatory institutional changes, with some reinforcement from usual profit motives, largely explain the observed noncompetitive behavior of the medical-care market, behavior which, in itself, interferes with optimality. The social adjustment towards optimality thus puts obstacles in its own path.

The doctrine that society will seek to achieve optimality by nonmarket means if it cannot achieve them in the market is not novel. Certainly, the government, at least in its economic activities, is usually implicitly or explicitly held to function as the agency which substitutes for the market's failure.[10] I am arguing here that in some circumstances other social institutions will step into the optimality gap, and that the medical-care industry, with its variety of special institutions, some ancient, some modern, exemplifies this tendency.

It may be useful to remark here that a good part of the preference for redistribution expressed in government taxation and expenditure policies and private charity can be reinterpreted as desire for insurance. It is noteworthy that virtually nowhere is there a system of subsidies that has as its aim simply an equalization of income. The subsidies or other governmental help go to those who are disadvantaged in life by events the incidence of which is popularly regarded as unpredictable: the blind, dependent children, the medically indigent. Thus, optimality, in a context which includes risk-bearing, includes much that appears to be motivated by distributional value judgments when looked at in a narrower context.[11]

This methodological background gives rise to the following plan for this paper. Section II is a catalogue of stylized generalizations about the medical-care market which differentiate it from the usual commodity markets. In Section III the behavior of the market is compared with that of the competitive model which disregards the fact of uncertainty. In Section IV, the medical-care market is compared, both as to behavior and as to preconditions, with the ideal competitive market that takes account of uncertainty; an attempt will be made to demonstrate that the characteristics outlined in Section II can be explained either as the result of deviations from the competitive preconditions or as attempts to compensate by other institutions for these failures. The discussion is not designed to be definitive, but provocative. In particular, I have been chary about drawing policy inferences; to a considerable extent, they depend on further research, for which the present paper is intended to provide a framework.

II. A Survey of the Special Characteristics of the Medical-Care Market[12]

This section will list selectively some characteristics of medical care which distinguish it from the usual commodity of economics textbooks. The list is not exhaustive, and it is not claimed that the characteristics listed are individually unique to this market. But, taken together, they do establish a special place for medical care in economic analysis.

A. The Nature of Demand

The most obvious distinguishing characteristics of an individual's demand for medical services is that it is not steady in origin as, for example, for food or clothing, but irregular and unpredictable. Medical services, apart from preventive services, afford satisfaction only in the event of illness, a departure from the normal state of affairs. It is hard, indeed, to think of another commodity of significance in the average budget of which this is true. A portion of legal services, devoted to defense in criminal trials or to lawsuits, might fall in this category but the incidence is surely very much lower (and, of course, there are, in fact, strong institutional similarities between the legal and medical-care markets.)[13]

In addition, the demand for medical services is associated, with a considerable probability, with an assault on personal integrity. There is some risk of death and a more considerable risk of impairment of full functioning. In particular, there is a major potential for loss or reduction of earning ability. The risks are not by themselves unique; food is also a necessity, but avoidance of deprivation of food can be guaranteed with sufficient income, where the same cannot be said of avoidance of illness. Illness is, thus, not only risky but a costly risk in itself, apart from the cost of medical care.

B. Expected Behavior of the Physician

It is clear from everyday observation that the behavior expected of sellers of medical care is different from that of business men in general. These expectations are relevant because medical care belongs to the category of commodities for which the product and the activity of production are identical. In all such cases, the customer cannot test the product before consuming it, and there is an element of trust in the relation.[14] But the ethically understood restrictions on the activities of a physician are much more severe than on those of, say, a barber. His behavior is supposed to be governed by a concern for the customer's welfare which would not be expected of a salesman. In Talcott Parsons's terms, there is a "collectivity-orientation," which distinguishes medicine and other professions from business, where self-interest on the part of participants is the accepted norm.[15]

A few illustrations will indicate the degree of difference between the behavior expected of physicians and that expected of the typical businessman.[16] (1) Advertising and overt price competition are virtually eliminated among physicians. (2) Advice given by physicians as to further treatment by himself or others is supposed to be completely divorced from self-interest. (3) It is at least claimed that treatment is dictated by the objective needs of the case and not limited by financial considerations.[17] While the ethical compulsion is surely not as absolute in fact as it is in theory, we can hardly suppose that it has no influence over resource allocation in this area. Charity treatment in one form or another does exist because of this tradition about human rights to adequate medical care.[18] (4) The physician is relied on as an expert in certifying to the existence of illnesses and injuries for various legal and other purposes. It is socially expected that his concern for the correct conveying of information will, when appropriate, outweigh his desire to please his customers.[19]

Departure from the profit motive is strikingly manifested by the overwhelming predominance of nonprofit over proprietary hospitals.[20] The hospital per se offers services not too different from those of a hotel, and it is certainly not obvious that the profit motive will not lead to a more efficient supply. The explanation may lie either on the supply side or on that of demand. The simplest explanation is that public and private subsidies decrease the cost to the patient in nonprofit hospitals. A second possibility is that the association of profit-making with the supply of medical services arouses suspicion and antagonism on the part of patients and referring physicians, so they do prefer nonprofit institutions. Either explanation implies a preference on the part of some group, whether donors or patients, against the profit motive in the supply of hospital services.[21]

Conformity to collectivity-oriented behavior is especially important since it is a commonplace that the physician-patient relation affects the quality of the medical care product. A pure cash nexus would be inadequate; if nothing else, the patient expects that the same physician will normally treat him on successive occasions. This expectation is strong enough to persist even in the Soviet Union, where medical care is nominally removed from the market place [14, pp. 194–96]. That purely psychic interactions between physician and patient have effects which are objectively indistinguishable in kind from the effects of medication is evidenced by the use of the placebo as a control in medical experimentation; see Shapiro [25].

C. Product Uncertainty

Uncertainty as to the quality of the product is perhaps more intense here than in any other important commodity. Recovery from disease is as unpredictable as is its incidence. In most commodities, the possibility of learning from one's own experience or that of others is strong because there is an adequate number of trials. In the case of severe illness, that is, in general, not true; the uncertainty due to inexperience is added to the intrinsic difficulty of prediction. Further, the amount of uncertainty, measured in terms of utility variability, is certainly much greater for medical care in severe cases than for, say, houses or automobiles, even though these are also expenditures sufficiently infrequent so that there may be considerable residual uncertainty.

Further, there is a special quality to the uncertainty; it is very different on the two sides of the transaction. Because medical knowledge is so complicated, the information possessed by the physician as to the consequences and possibilities of treatment is necessarily very much greater than that of the patient, or at least so it is believed by both parties.[22] Further, both parties are aware of this informational inequality, and their relation is colored by this knowledge.

To avoid misunderstanding, observe that the difference in information relevant here is a difference in information as to the consequence of a purchase of medical care. There is always an inequality of information as to production methods between the producer and the purchaser of any commodity, but in most cases the customer may well have as good or nearly as good an understanding of the utility of the product as the producer.

D. Supply Conditions

In competitive theory, the supply of a commodity is governed by the net return from its production compared with the return derivable from the use of the same resources elsewhere. There are several significant departures from this theory in the case of medical care.

Most obviously, entry to the profession is restricted by licensing. Licensing, of course, restricts supply and therefore increases the cost of medical care. It is defended as guaranteeing a minimum of quality. Restriction of entry by licensing occurs in most professions, including barbering and undertaking.

A second feature is perhaps even more remarkable. The cost of medical education today is high and, according to the usual figures, is borne only to a minor extent by the student. Thus, the private benefits to the entering student considerably exceed the costs. (It is, however, possible that research costs, not properly chargeable to education, swell the apparent difference.) This subsidy should, in principle, cause a fall in the price of medical services, which, however, is offset by rationing through limited entry to schools and through elimination of students during the medical-school career. These restrictions basically render superfluous the licensing, except in regard to graduates of foreign schools.

The special role of educational institutions in simultaneously subsidizing and rationing entry is common to all professions requiring advanced training.[23] It is a striking and insufficiently remarked phenomenon that such an important part of resource allocation should be performed by nonprofit-oriented agencies.

Since this last phenomenon goes well beyond the purely medical aspect, we will not dwell on it longer here except to note that the anomaly is most striking in the medical field. Educational costs tend to be far higher there than in any other branch of professional training. While tuition is the same, or only slightly higher, so that the subsidy is much greater, at the same time the earnings of physicians rank highest among professional groups, so there would not at first blush seem to be any necessity for special inducements to enter the profession. Even if we grant that, for reasons unexamined here, there is a social interest in subsidized professional education, it is not clear why the rate of subsidization should differ among professions. One might expect that the tuition of medical students would be higher than that of other students.

The high cost of medical education in the United States is itself a reflection of the quality standards imposed by the American Medical Association since the Flexner Report, and it is, I believe, only since then that the subsidy element in medical education has become significant. Previously, many medical schools paid their way or even yielded a profit.

Another interesting feature of limitation on entry to subsidized education is the extent of individual preferences concerning the social welfare, as manifested by contributions to private universities. But whether support is public or private, the important point is that both the quality and the quantity of the supply of medical care are being strongly influenced by social nonmarket forces.[24, 25]

One striking consequence of the control of quality is the restriction on the range offered. If many qualities of a commodity are possible, it would usually happen in a competitive market that many qualities will be offered on the market, at suitably varying prices, to appeal to different tastes and incomes. Both the licensing laws and the standards of medical-school training have limited the possibilities of alternative qualities of medical care. The declining ratio of physicians to total employees in the medical-care industry shows that substitution of less trained personnel, technicians, and the like, is not prevented completely, but the central role of the highly trained physician is not affected at all.[26]

E. Pricing Practices

The unusual pricing practices and attitudes of the medical profession are well known: extensive price discrimination by income (with an extreme of zero prices for sufficiently indigent patients) and, formerly, a strong insistence on fee for services as against such alternatives as prepayment.

The opposition to prepayment is closely related to an even stronger opposition to closed-panel practice (contractual arrangements which bind the patient to a particular group of physicians). Again these attitudes seem to differentiate professions from business. Prepayment and closed-panel plans are virtually nonexistent in the legal profession. In ordinary business, on the other hand, there exists a wide variety of exclusive service contracts involving sharing of risks; it is assumed that competition will select those which satisfy needs best.[27]

The problems of implicit and explicit price-fixing should also be mentioned. Price competition is frowned on. Arrangements of this type are not uncommon in service industries, and they have not been subjected to antitrust action. How important this is is hard to assess. It has been pointed out many times that the apparent rigidity of so-called administered prices considerably understates the actual flexibility. Here, too, if physicians find themselves with unoccupied time, rates are likely to go down, openly or covertly; if there is insufficient time for the demand, rates will surely rise. The "ethics" of price competition may decrease the flexibility of price responses, but probably that is all.

III. Comparisons with the Competitive
Model under Certainty

A. Nonmarketable Commodities

As already noted, the diffusion of communicable diseases provides an obvious example of nonmarket interactions. But from a theoretical viewpoint, the issues are well understood, and there is little point in expanding on this theme. (This should not be interpreted as minimizing the contribution of public health to welfare; there is every reason to suppose that it is considerably more important than all other aspects of medical care.)

Beyond this special area there is a more general interdependence, the concern of individuals for the health of others. The economic manifestations of this taste are to be found in individual donations to hospitals and to medical education, as well as in the widely accepted responsibilities of government in this area. The taste for improving the health of others appears to be stronger than for improving other aspects of their welfare.[28]

In interdependencies generated by concern for the welfare of others there is always a theoretical case for collective action if each participant derives satisfaction from the contributions of all.

B. Increasing Returns

Problems associated with increasing returns play some role in allocation of resources in the medical field, particularly in areas of low density or low income. Hospitals show increasing returns up to a point; specialists and some medical equipment constitute significant indivisibilities. In many parts of the world the individual physician may be a large unit relative to demand. In such cases it can be socially desirable to subsidize the appropriate medical-care unit. The appropriate mode of analysis is much the same as for water-resource projects. Increasing returns are hardly apt to be a significant problem in general practice in large cities in the United States, and improved transportation to some extent reduces their importance elsewhere.

C. Entry

The most striking departure from competitive behavior is restriction on entry to the field, as discussed in II.D above. Friedman and Kuznets, in a detailed examination of the pre-World War II data, have argued that the higher income of physicians could be attributed to this restriction.[29]

There is some evidence that the demand for admission to medical school has dropped (as indicated by the number of applicants per place and the quality of those admitted), so that the number of medical-school places is not as significant a barrier to entry as in the early 1950's [28, pp. 14–15]. But it certainly has operated over the past and it is still operating to a considerable extent today. It has, of course, constituted a direct and unsubtle restriction on the supply of medical care.

There are several considerations that must be added to help evaluate the importance of entry restrictions: (1) Additional entrants would be, in general, of lower quality; hence, the addition to the supply of medical care, properly adjusted for quality, is less than purely quantitative calculations would show.[30] (2) To achieve genuinely competitive conditions, it would be necessary not only to remove numerical restrictions on entry but also to remove the subsidy in medical education. Like any other producer, the physician should bear all the costs of production, including, in this case, education.[31] It is not so clear that this change would not keep even unrestricted entry down below the present level. (3) To some extent, the effect of making tuition carry the full cost of education will be to create too few entrants, rather than too many. Given the imperfections of the capital market, loans for this purpose to those who do not have the cash are difficult to obtain. The lender really has no security. The obvious answer is some form of insured loans, as has frequently been argued; not too much ingenuity would be needed to create a credit system for medical (and other branches of higher) education. Under these conditions the cost would still constitute a deterrent, but one to be compared with the high future incomes to be obtained.

If entry were governed by ideal competitive conditions, it may be that the quantity on balance would be increased, though this conclusion is not obvious. The average quality would probably fall, even under an ideal credit system, since subsidy plus selected entry draw some highly qualified individuals who would otherwise get into other fields. The decline in quality is not an over-all social loss, since it is accompanied by increase in quality in other fields of endeavor; indeed, if demands accurately reflected utilities, there would be a net social gain through a switch to competitive entry.[32]

There is a second aspect of entry in which the contrast with competitive behavior is, in many respects, even sharper. It is the exclusion of many imperfect substitutes for physicians. The licensing laws, though they do not effectively limit the number of physicians, do exclude all others from engaging in any one of the activities known as medical practice. As a result, costly physician time may be employed at specific tasks for which only a small fraction of their training is needed, and which could be performed by others less well trained and therefore less expensive. One might expect immunization centers, privately operated, but not necessarily requiring the services of doctors.

In the competitive model without uncertainty, consumers are presumed to be able to distinguish qualities of the commodities they buy.

Under this hypothesis, licensing would be, at best, superfluous and exclude those from whom consumers would not buy anyway; but it might exclude too many.

D. Pricing

The pricing practices of the medical industry (see II.E above) depart sharply from the competitive norm. As Kessel [17] has pointed out with great vigor, not only is price discrimination incompatible with the competitive model, but its preservation in the face of the large number of physicians is equivalent to a collective monopoly. In the past, the opposition to prepayment plans has taken distinctly coercive forms, certainly transcending market pressures, to say the least.

Kessel has argued that price discrimination is designed to maximize profits along the classic lines of discriminating monopoly and that organized medical opposition to prepayment was motivated by the desire to protect these profits. In principle, prepayment schemes are compatible with discrimination, but in practice they do not usually discriminate. I do not believe the evidence that the actual scale of discrimination is profit-maximizing is convincing. In particular, note that for any monopoly, discriminating or otherwise, the elasticity of demand in each market at the point of maximum profits is greater than one. But it is almost surely true for medical care that the price elasticity of demand for all income levels is less than one. That price discrimination by income is not completely profit-maximizing is obvious in the extreme case of charity; Kessel argues that this represents an appeasement of public opinion. But this already shows the incompleteness of the model and suggests the relevance and importance of social and ethical factors.

Certainly one important part of the opposition to prepayment was its close relation to closed-panel plans. Prepayment is a form of insurance, and naturally the individual physician did not wish to assume the risks. Pooling was intrinsically involved, and this strongly motivates, as we shall discuss further in Section IV below, control over prices and benefits. The simplest administrative form is the closed panel; physicians involved are, in effect, the insuring agent. From this point of view, Blue Cross solved the prepayment problem by universalizing the closed panel.

The case that price discrimination by income is a form of profit maximization which was zealously defended by opposition to fees for service seems far from proven. But it remains true that this price discrimination, for whatever cause, is a source of nonoptimality. Hypothetically, it means everyone would be better off if prices were made equal for all, and the rich compensated the poor for the changes in the relative positions. The importance of this welfare loss depends on the actual amount of discrimination and on the elasticities of demand for medical services by the different income groups. If the discussion is simplified by considering only two income levels, rich and poor, and if the elasticity of demand by either one is zero, then no reallocation of medical services will take place and the initial situation is optimal. The only effect of a change in price will be the redistribution of income as between the medical profession and the group with the zero elasticity of demand. With low elasticities of demand, the gain will be small. To illustrate, suppose the price of medical care to the rich is double that to the poor, the medical expenditures by the rich are 20 per cent of those by the poor, and the elasticity of demand for both classes is .5; then the net social gain due to the abolition of discrimination is slightly over 1 per cent of previous medical expenditures.[33]

The issues involved in the opposition to prepayment, the other major anomaly in medical pricing, are not meaningful in the world of certainty and will be discussed below.

IV. Comparison with the Ideal Competitive Model under Uncertainty

A. Introduction

In this section we will compare the operations of the actual medical-care market with those of an ideal system in which not only the usual commodities and services but also insurance policies against all conceivable risks are available.[34] Departures consist for the most part of insurance policies that might conceivably be written, but are in fact not. Whether these potential commodities are nonmarketable, or, merely because of some imperfection in the market, are not actually marketed, is a somewhat fine point.

To recall what has already been said in Section I, there are two kinds of risks involved in medical care: the risk of becoming ill, and the risk of total or incomplete or delayed recovery. The loss due to illness is only partially the cost of medical care. It also consists of discomfort and loss of productive time during illness, and, in more serious cases, death or prolonged deprivation of normal function. From the point of view of the welfare economics of uncertainty, both losses are risks against which individuals would like to insure. The nonexistence of suitable insurance policies for either risk implies a loss of welfare.

B. The Theory of Ideal Insurance

In this section, the basic principles of an optimal regime for risk-bearing will be presented. For illustration, reference will usually be made to the case of insurance against cost in medical care. The principles are equally applicable to any of the risks. There is no single source to which the reader can be easily referred, though I think the principles are at least reasonably well understood.

As a basis for the analysis, the assumption is made that each individual acts so as to maximize the expected value of a utility function. If we think of utility as attached to income, then the costs of medical care act as a random deduction from this income, and it is the expected value of the utility of income after medical costs that we are concerned with. (Income after medical costs is the ability to spend money on other objects which give satisfaction. We presuppose that illness is not a source of satisfaction in itself; to the extent that it is a source of dissatisfaction, the illness should enter into the utility function as a separate variable.) The expected-utility hypothesis, due originally to Daniel Bernoulli (1738), is plausible and is the most analytically manageable of all hypotheses that have been proposed to explain behavior under uncertainty. In any case, the results to follow probably would not be significantly affected by moving to another mode of analysis.

It is further assumed that individuals are normally risk-averters. In utility terms, this means that they have a diminishing marginal utility of income. This assumption may reasonably be taken to hold for most of the significant affairs of life for a majority of people, but the presence of gambling provides some difficulty in the full application of this view. It follows from the assumption of risk aversion that if an individual is given a choice between a probability distribution of income, with a given mean m, and the certainty of the income m, he would prefer the latter. Suppose, therefore, an agency, a large insurance company plan, or the government, stands ready to offer insurance against medical costs on an actuarially fair basis; that is, if the costs of medical care are a random variable with mean m, the company will charge a premium m, and agree to indemnify the individual for all medical costs.

Under these circumstances, the individual will certainly prefer to take out a policy and will have a welfare gain thereby.

Will this be a social gain? Obviously yes, if the insurance agent is suffering no social loss. Under the assumption that medical risks on different individuals are basically independent, the pooling of them reduces the risk involved to the insurer to relatively small proportions. In the limit, the welfare loss, even assuming risk aversion on the part of the insurer, would vanish and there is a net social gain which may be of quite substantial magnitude. In fact, of course, the pooling of risks does not go to the limit; there are only a finite number of them and there may be some interdependence among the risks due to epidemics and the like. But then a premium, perhaps slightly above the actuarial level, would be sufficient to offset this welfare loss. From the point of view of the individual, since he has a strict preference for the actuarially fair policy over assuming the risks himself, he will still have a preference for an actuarially unfair policy, provided, of course, that it is not too unfair.

In addition to a residual degree of risk aversion by insurers, there are other reasons for the loading of the premium (i.e., an excess of premium over the actuarial value). Insurance involves administrative costs. Also, because of the irregularity of payments there is likely to be a cost of capital tied up. Suppose, to take a simple case, the insurance company is not willing to sell any insurance policy that a consumer wants but will charge a fixed-percentage loading above the actuarial value for its premium. Then it can be shown that the most preferred policy from the point of view of an individual is coverage with a deductible amount; that is, the insurance policy provides 100 per cent coverage for all medical costs in excess of some fixed-dollar limit. If, however, the insurance company has some degree of risk aversion, its loading may also depend on the degree of uncertainty of the risk. In that case, the Pareto optimal policy will involve some element of coinsurance, i.e., the coverage for costs over the minimum limit will be some fraction less than 100 per cent (for proofs of these statements, see Appendix) [Appendixes not included in this volume, Ed.].

These results can also be applied to the hypothetical concept of insurance against failure to recover from illness. For simplicity, let us assume that the cost of failure to recover is regarded purely as a money cost, either simply productive opportunities foregone or, more generally, the money equivalent of all dissatisfactions. Suppose further that, given that a person is ill, the expected value of medical care is greater than its cost; that is, the expected money value attributable to recovery with medical help is greater than resources devoted to medical help. However, the recovery, though on the average beneficial, is uncertain; in the absence of insurance a risk-averter may well prefer not to take a chance on further impoverishment by buying medical care. A suitable insurance policy would, however, mean that he paid nothing if he doesn't benefit; since the expected value is greater than the cost, there would be a net social gain.[35]

C. Problems of Insurance

1. THE MORAL HAZARD. The welfare case for insurance policies of all sorts is overwhelming. It follows that the government should undertake insurance in those cases where this market, for whatever reason, has failed to emerge. Nevertheless, there are a number of significant practical limitations on the use of insurance. It is important to understand them, though I do not believe that they alter the case for the creation of a much wider class of insurance policies than now exists.

One of the limits which has been much stressed in insurance literature is the effect of insurance on incentives. What is desired in the case of insurance is that the event against which insurance is taken be out of the control of the individual. Unfortunately, in real life this separation can never be made perfectly. The outbreak of fire in one's house or business may be largely uncontrollable by the individual, but the probability of fire is somewhat influenced by carelessness, and of course arson is a possibility, if an extreme one. Similarly, in medical polices the cost of medical care is not completely determined by the illness suffered by the individual but depends on the choice of a doctor and his willingness to use medical services. It is frequently observed that widespread medical insurance increases the demand for medical care. Coinsurance provisions have been introduced into many major medical policies to meet this contingency as well as the risk aversion of the insurance companies.

To some extent the professional relationship between physician and patient limits the normal hazard in various forms of medical insurance. By certifying to the necessity of given treatment or the lack thereof, the physician acts as a controlling agent on behalf of the insurance companies. Needless to say, it is a far from perfect check; the physicians themselves are not under any control and it may be convenient for them or pleasing to their patients to prescribe more expensive medication, private nurses, more frequent treatments, and other marginal variations of care. It is probably true that hospitalization and surgery are more under the casual inspection of others than is general practice and therefore less subject to moral hazard; this may be one reason why insurance policies in those fields have been more widespread.

2. ALTERNATIVE METHODS OF INSURANCE PAYMENT. It is interesting that no less than three different methods of coverage of the costs of medical care have arisen: prepayment, indemnities according to a fixed schedule, and insurance against costs, whatever they may be. In prepayment plans, insurance in effect is paid in kind—that is, directly in medical services. The other two forms both involve cash payments to the beneficiary, but in the one case the amounts to be paid involving a medical contingency are fixed in advance, while in the other the insurance carrier pays all the costs, whatever they may be, subject, of course, to provisions like deductibles and coinsurance.

In hypothetically perfect markets these three forms of insurance would be equivalent. The indemnities stipulated would, in fact, equal the market price of the services, so that value to the insured would be the same if he were to be paid the fixed sum or the market price or were given the services free. In fact, of course, insurance against full costs and prepayment plans both offer insurance against uncertainty as to the price of medical services, in addition to uncertainty about their needs. Further, by their mode of compensation to the physician, prepayment plans are inevitably bound up with closed panels so that the freedom of choice of the physician by the patient is less than it would be under a scheme more strictly confined to the provision of insurance. These remarks are tentative, and the question of coexistence of the different schemes should be a fruitful subject for investigation.

3. THIRD-PARTY CONTROL OVER PAYMENTS. The moral hazard in physicians' control noted in paragraph 1 above shows itself in those insurance schemes where the physician has the greatest control, namely, major medical insurance. Here there has been a marked rise in expenditures over time. In prepayment plans, where the insurance and medical service are supplied by the same group, the incentive to keep medical costs to a minimum is strongest. In plans of the Blue Cross group, there has developed a conflict of interest between the insurance carrier and the medical-service supplier, in this case particularly the hospital.

The need for third-party control is reinforced by another aspect of the moral hazard. Insurance removes the incentive on the part of individuals, patients, and physicians to shop around for better prices for hospitalization and surgical care. The market forces, therefore, tend to be replaced by direct institutional control.

4. ADMINISTRATIVE COSTS. The pure theory of insurance sketched in Section B above omits one very important consideration: the costs of operating an insurance company. There are several types of operating costs, but one of the most important categories includes commissions and acquisition costs, selling costs in usual economic terminology. Not only does this mean that insurance policies must be sold for considerably more than their actuarial value, but it also means there is a great differential among different types of insurance. It is very striking to observe that among health insurance policies of insurance companies in 1958, expenses of one sort or another constitute 51.6 per cent of total premium income for individual policies, and only 9.5 per cent for group policies [26, Table 14–1, p. 272]. This striking differential would seem to imply enormous economies of scale in the provision of insurance, quite apart from the coverage of the risks themselves. Obviously, this provides a very strong argument for widespread plans, including, in particular, compulsory ones.

5. PREDICTABILITY AND INSURANCE. Clearly, from the risk-aversion point of view, insurance is more valuable, the greater the uncertainty in the risk being insured against. This is usually used as an argument for putting greater emphasis on insurance against hospitalization and surgery than other forms of medical care. The empirical assumption has been challenged by O. W. Anderson and others [3, pp. 53–54], who asserted that

out-of-hospital expenses were equally as unpredictable as in-hospital costs. What was in fact shown was that the probability of costs exceeding $200 is about the same for the two categories, but this is not, of course, a correct measure of predictability, and a quick glance at the supporting evidence shows that in relation to the average cost the variability is much lower for ordinary medical expenses. Thus, for the city of Birmingham, the mean expenditure on surgery was $7, as opposed to $20 for other medical expenses, but of those who paid something for surgery the average bill was $99, as against $36 for those with some ordinary medical cost. Eighty-two per cent of those interviewed had no surgery, and only 20 per cent had no ordinary medical expenses [3, Tables A–13, A–18, and A–19 on pp. 72, 77, and 79, respectively].

The issue of predictability also has bearing on the merits of insurance against chronic illness or maternity. On a lifetime insurance basis, insurance against chronic illness makes sense, since this is both highly unpredictable and highly significant in costs. Among people who already have chronic illness, or symptoms which reliably indicate it, insurance in the strict sense is probably pointless.

6. POOLING OF UNEQUAL RISKS. Hypothetically, insurance requires for its full social benefit a maximum possible discrimination of risks. Those in groups of higher incidences of illness should pay higher premiums. In fact, however, there is a tendency to equalize, rather than to differentiate, premiums, especially in the Blue Cross and similar widespread schemes. This constitutes, in effect, a redistribution of income from those with a low propensity to illness to those with a high propensity. The equalization, of course, could not in fact be carried through if the market were genuinely competitive. Under those circumstances, insurance plans could arise which charged lower premiums to preferred risks and draw them off, leaving the plan which does not discriminate among risks with only an adverse selection of them.

As we have already seen in the case of income redistribution, some of this may be thought of as insurance with a longer time perspective. If a plan guarantees to everybody a premium that corresponds to total experience but not to experience as it might be segregated by smaller subgroups, everybody is, in effect, insured against a change in his basic state of health which would lead to a reclassification. This corresponds precisely to the use of a level premium in life insurance instead of a premium varying by age, as would be the case for term insurance.

7. GAPS AND COVERAGE. We may briefly note that, at any rate to date, insurances against the cost of medical care are far from universal. Certain groups—the unemployed, the institutionalized, and the aged—are almost completely uncovered. Of total expenditures, between one-fifth and one-

fourth are covered by insurance. It should be noted, however, that over half of all hospital expenses and about 35 per cent of the medical payments of those with bills of $1,000 a year and over, are included [26, p. 376]. Thus, the coverage on the more variable parts of medical expenditure is somewhat better than the over-all figures would indicate, but it must be assumed that the insurance mechanism is still very far from achieving the full coverage of which it is capable.

D. Uncertainty of Effects of Treatment

1. There are really two major aspects of uncertainty for an individual already suffering from an illness. He is uncertain about the effectiveness of medical treatment, and his uncertainty may be quite different from that of his physician, based on the presumably quite different medical knowledges.

2. IDEAL INSURANCE.This will necessarily involve insurance against a failure to benefit from medical care, whether through recovery, relief of pain, or arrest of further deterioration. One form would be a system in which the payment to the physician is made in accordance with the degree of benefit. Since this would involve transferring the risks from the patient to the physician, who might certainly have an aversion to bearing them, there is room for insurance carriers to pool the risks, either by contract with physicians or by contract with the potential patients. Under ideal insurance, medical care will always be undertaken in any case in which the expected utility, taking account of the probabilities, exceeds the expected medical cost. This prescription would lead to an economic optimum. If we think of the failure to recover mainly in terms of lost working time, then this policy would, in fact, maximize economic welfare as ordinarily measured.

3. THE CONCEPTS OF TRUST AND DELEGATION. In the absence of ideal insurance, there arise institutions which offer some sort of substitute guarantees. Under ideal insurance the patient would actually have no concern with the informational inequality between himself and the physician, since he would only be paying by results anyway, and his utility position would in fact be thoroughly guaranteed. In its absence he wants to have some guarantee that at least the physician is using his knowledge to the best advantage. This leads to the setting up of a relationship of trust and confidence, one which the physician has a social obligation to live up to. Since the patient does not, at least in his belief, know as much as the physician, he cannot completely enforce standards of care. In part, he replaces direct observation by generalized belief in the ability of the physician.[36] To put it another way, the social obligation for best

practice is part of the commodity the physician sells, even though it is a part that is not subject to thorough inspection by the buyer.

One consequence of such trust relations is that the physician cannot act, or at least appear to act, as if he is maximizing his income at every moment of time. As a signal to the buyer of his intentions to act as thoroughly in the buyer's behalf as possible, the physician avoids the obvious stigmata of profit-maximizing. Purely arms-length bargaining behavior would be incompatible, not logically, but surely psychologically, with the trust relations. From these special relations come the various forms of ethical behavior discussed above, and so also, I suggest, the relative unimportance of profit-making in hospitals. The very word, "profit," is a signal that denies the trust relations.

Price discrimination and its extreme, free treatment for the indigent, also follow. If the obligation of the physician is understood to be first of all to the welfare of the patient, then in particular it takes precedence over financial difficulties.

As a second consequence of informational inequality between physician and patient and the lack of insurance of a suitable type, the patient must delegate to the physician much of his freedom of choice. He does not have the knowledge to make decisions on treatment, referral, or hospitalization. To justify this delegation, the physician finds himself somewhat limited, just as any agent would in similar circumstances. The safest course to take to avoid not being a true agent is to give the socially prescribed "best" treatment of the day. Compromise in quality, even for the purpose of saving the patient money, is to risk an imputation of failure to live up to the social bond.

The special trust relation of physicians (and allied occupations, such as priests) extends to third parties so that the certifications of physicians as to illness and injury are accepted as especially reliable (see Section II.B above). The social value to all concerned of such presumptively reliable sources of information is obvious.

Notice the general principle here. Because there are barriers to the information flow and because there is no market in which the risks involved can be insured, coordination of purchase and sales must take place through convergent expectations, but these are greatly assisted by having clear and prominent signals, and these, in turn, force patterns of behavior which are not in themselves logical necessities for optimality.[37]

4. LICENSING AND EDUCATIONAL STANDARDS. Delegation and trust are the social institutions designed to obviate the problem of informational inequality. The general uncertainty about the prospects of medical treatment is socially handled by rigid entry requirements. These are designed to reduce the uncertainty in the mind of the consumer as to the

quality of product insofar as this is possible.[38] I think this explanation, which is perhaps the naive one, is much more tenable than any idea of a monopoly seeking to increase incomes. No doubt restriction on entry is desirable from the point of view of the existing physicians, but the public pressure needed to achieve the restriction must come from deeper causes.

The social demand for guaranteed quality can be met in more than one way, however. At least three attitudes can be taken by the state or other social institutions toward entry into an occupation or toward the production of commodities in general; examples of all three types exist. (1) The occupation can be licensed, nonqualified entrants being simply excluded. The licensing may be more complex than it is in medicine; individuals could be licensed for some, but not all, medical activities, for example. Indeed, the present all-or-none approach could be criticized as being insufficient with regard to complicated specialist treatment, as well as excessive with regard to minor medical skills. Graded licensing may, however, be much harder to enforce. Controls could be exercised analogous to those for foods; they can be excluded as being dangerous, or they can be permitted for animals but not for humans. (2) The state or other agency can certify or label, without compulsory exclusion. The category of Certified Psychologist is now under active discussion; canned goods are graded. Certification can be done by nongovernmental agencies, as in the medical-board examinations for specialists. (3) Nothing at all may be done; consumers make their own choices.

The choice among these alternatives in any given case depends on the degree of difficulty consumers have in making the choice unaided, and on the consequences of errors of judgment. It is the general social consensus, clearly, that the *laissez-faire* solution for medicine is intolerable. The certification proposal never seems to have been discussed seriously. It is beyond the scope of this paper to discuss these proposals in detail. I wish simply to point out that they should be judged in terms of the ability to relieve the uncertainty of the patient in regard to the quality of the commodity he is purchasing, and that entry restrictions are the consequences of an apparent inability to devise a system in which the risks of gaps in medical knowledge and skill are borne primarily by the patient, not the physician.

Postscript

I wish to repeat here what has been suggested above in several places: that the failure of the market to insure against uncertainties has created many social institutions in which the usual assumptions of the market are to some extent contradicted. The medical profession is only one example, though in many respects an extreme one. All professions share some of the same properties. The economic importance of personal and especially family relationships, though declining, is by no means trivial in the most advanced economies; it is based on nonmarket relations that create guarantees of behavior which would otherwise be afflicted with excessive uncertainty. Many other examples can be given. The logic and limitations of ideal competitive behavior under uncertainty force us to recognize the incomplete description of reality supplied by the impersonal price system.

Appendix [Five pages of theory and formulae appear in the original work. They are not included here to save space. Ed.]

SOURCE

Arrow KJ. 1963. Uncertainty and the welfare economics of medical care. *American Economic Review* 53 (5): 941–73. Copyright 1963 *American Economic Review*. Reprinted with permission of American Economic Association.

Small Area Variations in Health Care Delivery
(1973, Abridged)
A Population-based Health Information System Can Guide Planning and Regulatory Decision-Making

John Wennberg and Alan Gittelsohn

Recent regulation has extended planning and regulatory authority in the health field in a number of important areas. The 1972 amendments to the Social Security Act provide authority for regulating the construction of facilities and establish Professional Standard Review Organizations (PSRO's), which are accountable for setting standards and evaluating professional performance. Phase 3 of the Wage and Stabilization Act of 1970 and state insurance commissions provide authority for regulating dollar flow by controlling the price of services and the price of insurance.

Taken together, this legislation influences major factors determining how a specific health care organization performs—the expenditures it can incur, the facilities and manpower it can use, and the kind and amount of services it produces. While the immediate effects of these decisions are on an institution, there are important questions concerning their effects on the communities that receive the services: How much in the way of resources, money, manpower, and facilities is expended for the residents of the community? What cases are treated and what types of therapy employed? How do decisions made by the public sector change the situation? Answers to these questions depend on statistics that describe, on a per capita basis, the input of resources, and the production of services, and the effect of these on health status. If this information were available for the different communities of the region or state, it would be possible to appraise the impact of regulatory decisions on the equality of distribution of resources and dollars and the effectiveness of medical care services.

For technical and organizational reasons, documentation of the health care experience of populations has been restricted to large political jurisdictions such as counties, states, or nations. Studies at this level of aggregation have used indicators that support direct comparisons among areas. Relationships between the supply of manpower, facilities, and expenditures in the population on whose behalf these resources are expended are expressed as direct input rates—for example, the number of physicians or beds per thousand persons or per capita expenditures. The quantity of services produced or the kinds of cases treated are commonly expressed as "utilization rates." Examples of hospital utilization statistics include the number of days the residents of an area spent in hospital (called "patient days"), number of surgical procedures, and number of cases of a given diagnosis admitted—all expressed in terms of events per thousand persons at risk. These rates are commonly calculated on an annual basis and, for utilization, are often "age-adjusted" so as to remove the effect of age as an explanation of difference between regions.

With these indicators, a number of studies have shown population-based differences in use of health manpower and facilities and delivery of health services that are difficult to attribute to differences in illness rates. In Canada, hospital utilization rates tend to be as much as 50 percent higher than rates in the United States. Variations among states are large. Medicare expenditures per enrollee in 1970 were twice as high in California as in Arkansas. The number of physicians per thousand persons has been up to three times higher in some states than in others. International comparisons and studies of regions within states show that there are large differences in the rate of delivery of specific surgical procedures (1).

In 1969, there was implemented in the state of Vermont a data system to monitor aspects of health care delivery in each of the 251 towns of the state. When the population of the state is grouped into 13 geographically distinct hospital catchment, or service, areas, variations in health care are often more apparent than they are when the population is divided into fewer, larger areas. Population rates can be used to make direct statistical comparisons between each of the 13 hospital service areas. Since the medical care in each area is delivered predominantly by local physicians, variations tend to reflect differences in the way particular individuals and groups practice medicine. The specificity of the information in Vermont's data system makes it possible to appraise the impact that decisions controlling facility construction, the price of insurance, and the unit price of service have on the quality of distribution of facilities and dollars in a given population.

Our article examines the extent to which beds and manpower use, expenditures, and utilization vary among hospital service areas in Vermont. Variations in utilization appear to indicate that the effectiveness of a given level of delivery of service is uncertain. Observed variations in expenditure are evaluated in terms of lateral transfer of income among areas; these variations occur because in some areas the average price of insurance is consistently higher than the average per capita reimbursement. Past decisions of the Price Commission and the state Hill-Burton agency are reviewed. Evidence is presented that their decisions, based on institutional rather than population data, have served to increase rather than decrease inequalities among areas.

Concepts and Measures

Vermont, with a population in 1970 of 444,000, is largely rural; less than a third of its population lives in towns and villages of over 2,500 persons. The state is organized administratively into 251 towns, averaging 37 square miles (1 square mile=2.59 square kilometers) in area and ranging in population from 10 to 35,000 persons, with a median of 825. Relevant health data on these populations have been assembled from sources of data and published reports in order to develop files of hospital discharges, nursing home admissions, Medicare reimbursements, health manpower, facilities, expenditures, and mortality (2). Several special surveys were necessary to complete data sets. At least the following data on each patient are available: age, sex, residence, length of stay in the hospital, diagnoses, procedures, and referring in attending physician and surgeon. In this article, data describing the use of medical services are based on 1969 abstracts, hospital and nursing home discharges, and home health agency encounters—except for (i) Medicare Part B, which is an estimate for 1972 based on all billings processed by the third-party carrier during January and February 1972, and (ii) a 1963 patient origins study by the Vermont State Health Department that we used to estimate 1963 hospital expenditure rates. We believe that, for each set of data used in this article, the information includes nearly the total medical care experience of the populations under study.

To study particular health care systems, we have grouped towns into hospital service areas surrounding the hospital used most frequently by the town (Table 1 and Fig. 1). Residents of towns located near a hospital show a high percentage of use of the local facility. In the smaller, more rural towns located between hospitals, use tends to be divided. Service areas were set up to maintain geographic continuity (3). Three areas contain two hospitals in the same community, while the remainder contain a single facility. Three areas with populations under 5,000 have been excluded, leaving 13 available for analysis. Twelve of the 13 areas are served primarily by community hospitals, varying in bed size from 32 to 207. Area 12 contains a 100-bed community hospital and a 587-bed teaching hospital, which serves both as a community hospital and as the principal referral hospital for most of the state. A university hospital in New Hampshire is the principal referral hospital for three service areas located in the eastern portion of Vermont. [Fig. 1, Map of Vermont, deleted to save space, Ed.]

Measures of health care delivery include age-adjusted utilization rate and indices of manpower, facilities, and expenditures. Estimates of manpower and facilities in a geographically defined population present

Table 1 Admissions, by Area of Residence, and Admissions to Hospital in Area, by Residential Status, Vermont, 1969

Hospital service area	Population	Admissions, by area of residence				Admissions to hospital in area		
		Number	Local (%)	Referral (%)	Other (%)	Number	Residents	Non-residents
1	12,301	2,669	81	12	7	2,526	85	15
2	18,762	2,798	85	13	2	2,910	82	18
3	7,960	1,271	72	11	17	1,658	55	45
4	18,057	3,060	86	7	7	3,735	71	29
5	31,187	4,469	85	6	9	5,171	74	26
6	32,886	5,637	82	16	2	5,550	83	17
7	12,175	2,595	76	18	6	2,703	73	27
8	20,170	3,676	86	10	4	3,538	89	11
9	20,624	3,454	75	14	11	3,235	80	20
10	53,389	8,553	86	10	4	8,515	87	13
11	53,002	8,544	82	14	4	7,713	91	9
12	109,750	17,423	95*		5	24,400	67	33
13	13,200	1,760	63	31	5	1,862	60	40

*Includes referral hospital, which was located within the service area.

technical and conceptual difficulties. Patient mobility, regionalization of specialized services, and the absence of residential qualifications for admission to facilities contribute to these difficulties. While the number of hospital beds physically situated in an area provides a rough index of supply, it does not account for hospitalization of residents outside the area or for local use by nonresidents. We have estimated the rate of input of hospital beds based on total hospital utilization by the population of each service area. Estimates are made by allocating facilities to each service area of the state in proportion to the use of these facilities by residents. For example, if 10 percent of the hospital's admissions originate in a given service area, 10 percent of its beds are assigned to that area. The sum of all hospitals' contributions to the service area provides a measure of total input of beds to that service area (4). In effect, the procedure assigns an average cost and unit of effort to each admission (3, 4).

A similar allocation approach has been used to develop estimates of nursing home beds, hospital expenditures, medical manpower, and non-physician hospital staff. For each physician acting as an attending physician or surgeon in the hospital, one full-time equivalent (FTE) physician was allocated to the area, in proportion to the distribution of his patients' residences. The sums within specialty classes and overall physicians for a given service area have been used as estimates of physician labor input. Active physicians in the state who did not use hospitals (fewer than 10 percent) were assigned to the hospital service area in which their practices were located. Estimates of expenditures for hospitals and nursing homes by each hospital service area were based on allocations of total reported institutional expenditures, according to frequency of admission of area residents. Medicare Part B expenditures were obtained directly from reimbursement data on the unit record claims forms.

Variations among Service Areas

Tables 2 and 3 present the ranges of variation in expenditures, input of manpower and facilities, and production of health services, measured by utilization, for the 13 hospital service areas of Vermont.

VARIATIONS IN USE OF RESOURCES: We recorded variations of hospital bed rates and nonphysician manpower over the 13 service areas. The number of beds per 10,000 persons ranged from 34 to 59, and the number of hospital personnel per 10,000 persons from 68 to 128. Nursing home beds varied from 9 to 65, nursing home employees from 8 to 52. The input of physician efforts ranged between 8 and 12 FTE physicians per 10,000 persons, with individual specialties having wider variations. The input of internists and general surgeons was more than twice in some areas what

Table 2 Variation in Utilization, Facilities, Manpower, and Expenditure Rates among 13 Hospital Service Areas, Vermont, 1969

Resource input and utilization indicators	Lowest two areas		Entire state	Highest two areas	
Utilization rates per 1,000 persons					
Hospital days	1,015	1,027	1,250	1,380	1,495
Hospital discharges	122	124	144	195	197
All surgical procedures	36	49	55	61	69
Respiratory disease	10	13	16	29	36
Genitourinary disease	8	9	12	15	18
Circulatory disease	12	13	17	22	25
Digestive disease	15	16	19	24	26
Nursing home admissions, age 65 and over	14	22	52	81	81
Beds per 10,000 persons					
Hospital	34	36	42	51	59
Nursing home	9	26	42	62	65
Personnel per 10,000 persons					
Hospital	68	76	100	119	128
Nursing home	8	23	32	51	52
FTE physicians per 10,000 persons	7.9	8.4	10.3	11.9	12.4
General practice	1.5	1.7	2.5	3.8	4.4
Internal medicine	.9	.9	1.6	1.7	2.6
Pediatrics	.1	.2	.7	1.1	1.2
Obstetrics	.1	.2	.7	1.0	1.1
General surgery	.7	.9	1.1	1.5	1.7
Expenditures per capita ($)					
Hospitals	58	63	89	92	120
Nursing homes	5	13	17	25	26
Medicare Part B, age 65 and over (1972)	54	84	127	147	162

it was in others; pediatrician and obstetrician effort was more than 10 times greater in some areas than in others.

VARIATIONS IN EXPENDITURES: The estimated 1969 per capita expenditures for hospital services were more than twice as much in some areas as in others; for nursing home services, they were more than five times greater in one area than another. The range of reimbursement from Medicare Part B among Vermont communities is larger than that among the 50 states—and reimbursements can be up to twice as great in one state as another.

Estimated Part B expenditures in 1972, primarily reflecting physician services, ranged between $54 and $162 per capita. Greater variations are seen for specific types of Medicare services. Reimbursement for diagnostic x-ray services differed by 400 percent over service areas, electrocardiogram reimbursements by 600 percent, and total laboratory services by 700 percent.

Differences in expenditures among areas apparently are long-standing. Estimated expenditures for hospital services in 1963 correlated .82 with 1969 rates (5). Both 1963 and 1969 hospital expenditures related to 1972 Medicare reimbursements ($r=.79$ and .75, respectively). Of Medicare reimbursements to physicians, 52 percent were for services delivered in hospitals.

VARIATIONS IN UTILIZATION: Hospital discharge rates for all causes, adjusted for age composition, varied from a low of 122 to a high of 197 per 1,000 persons. The Vermont rate of 144 was similar to the rate for the New England region. Age-adjusted hospital patient days per 1,000 persons ranged between 1,015 and 1,495. Nursing home admissions rates varied from 1.3 to 10.0 and were not significantly correlated with hospital admissions or expenditures.

The variations in the use of hospitals for broad classes of diagnoses and in rate of performance of surgical procedures is shown in Table 2. The annual rate at which respiratory conditions were treated in hospitals showed marked differences among areas: the lowest rate was ten admissions per 1,000 persons, the highest 36. Defining surgery as procedures (excluding biopsies) generally requiring anesthesia and performed in operating rooms, the total surgery rate varied between 360 and 689 per 10,000 persons over the 13 service areas.

The age-adjusted rates of nine frequently performed surgical procedures are exhibited in Table 3. The rates vary tremendously over the 13 service areas, the most striking example being tonsillectomy, which varied from a low of 13 to a high of 151 cases per 10,000 persons. The neighbors of the highest tonsillectomy area recorded rates of 32, 35, 38, and 39. Primary appendectomy rates ranged from 10 to 32, with a state total of 18 per 10,000 persons. Similar variations were observed in the rate of removal

Table 3 Variations in Number of Surgical Procedures Performed per 10,000 Persons for the 13 Vermont Hospital Service Areas and Comparison Populations, Vermont, 1969 (rates adjusted to Vermont age composition)

Surgical procedure	Lowest two areas		Entire state	Highest two areas	
Tonsillectomy	13	32	43	85	151
Appendectomy	10	15	18	27	32
Hemorrhoidectomy	2	4	6	9	10
Males					
Hernioplasty	29	38	41	47	48
Prostatectomy	11	13	20	28	38
Females					
Cholecystectomy	17	19	27	46	57
Hysterectomy	20	22	30	34	60
Mastectomy	12	14	18	28	33
Dilation and curettage	30	42	55	108	141
Varicose veins	6	7	12	24	28

of prostates, gall bladders, and uteri. For each of the procedures, the differences in rates were statistically significant by chi-square tests.

The per capita number of days spent in a hospital, reflecting the combined effect of medical decisions about admissions and about length of stay, also varied widely over the Vermont service areas. Tonsillectomy days per 10,000 persons, adjusted for age, varied from 17 to a high of 314. Appendectomy days range from 42 to 204, prostatectomy from 65 to 524, hysterectomy from 64 to 616, and mastectomy from 21 to 198.

Evaluation of Variations

There are a number of indications that there is uncertainty concerning the value of a given level of health care delivery. This appears to apply to the aggregate of all services, as measured by expenditures, as well as to specific procedures. Expenditures for hospitalization and for physician services under Medicare Part B show no significant correlation with age-adjusted mortality ($r=05$ and .01) and perinatal mortality ($r=.08$ and .10). Hospitalization rates for specific admitting diagnoses and for surgical procedures are almost 10 times greater in some hospital service areas as in others. Neither the medical literature nor our data provides substantial clues as to whether spending six times more for electrocardiograms or seven times more for laboratory services results in greater improvement in health for persons age 65 and over than does a lesser expenditure. Tonsillectomy provides an example of variability. Assuming that age-specific rates remain stable, there is a 19 percent probability that a child living in Vermont will have his tonsils removed by age 20. The probability recorded in the highest service area is over 66 percent, as contrasted with probabilities ranging from 16 percent to 22 percent in the five neighboring communities, which are ostensibly similar in demographic characteristics. There are no data available that would allow us to relate these variations to the prevalence of tonsillitis, but it appears that the variations are more likely to be associated with differences in beliefs among physicians concerning the indications for, and efficacy of, the procedure.

Because of lack of data on the prevalence of disease in Vermont communities, the relationship between health needs and input of physician services cannot be measured directly. However, since a general association exists between serious illness and age, the age structure of the population should be an indicator of the relative health needs of the community. The percentage of the population 65 years of age and [older] varied among service areas from 8.9 to 13.4. Multiple regression analysis of the influence of community size, population structure, and income on supply of physicians shows that physicians concentrate their efforts in the more populous service areas and in those with higher per capita incomes. They tend to avoid areas with larger proportions of persons age 65 and above. The multiple correlation between rate of physician input and population size, income, and age structure was $r = .90$, a result significant at the .001 level. The simple correlations were .51, .60, and −.64, respectively. Hospital service areas with small populations have proportionately more persons age 65 and over. These data suggest a poor correspondence between physician input and population need.

Factors intrinsic to the operation of the health care system appear to be responsible for variations in performance. The results of most medical encounters are primarily dependent on medical decisions and the economic circumstances and behavior of patients in care. The wide variations in utilization rates between different Vermont populations suggests that provider and consumer behavior is rarely uniform, even when economic circumstances are more or less constant, as they are for Medicare enrollees. The observation that native Vermonters of similar age and income use physician services approximately one-half as often as nonnatives suggests the importance of consumer behavior (6). Further evidence suggests that once a patient is "in the system," the actual services he receives depend in part on provider characteristics.

Table 4 Simple Correlation between Medical Manpower Rates and Rates for Surgical and Diagnostic Procedures and 13 Vermont Hospital Service Areas, 1969

Procedure	Physicians performing surgery		Physicians not performing surgery
	General surgeon	General practitioner	
Surgical			
Most complex	.54	−.25	−.19
Intermediate A	.21	−.21	−.04
Intermediate B	.68	.12	−.42
Intermediate C	.55	.16	−.39
Least complex	.48	.40	−.27
Mastectomy	.48	−.20	−.24
Hysterectomy	.39	−.21	−.34
Cholecystectomy	.48	.24	−.04
Appendectomy	.31	.14	−.28
Tonsillectomy and adenoidectomy	.46	.42	−.28
Varicose veins	.07	.31	−.16
Dilation and curettage	.08	.38	−.42
Total	.54	.19	−.44
Diagnostic			
Electrocardiogram	−.12	−.36	.41
Laboratory	−.06	−.30	.30
X-ray	−.10	−.28	.35

The correlation between the total surgery rate and the input of physicians performing surgery is positive and significant, with $r = .64$. Table 4 presents simple correlation coefficients for three categories of physicians and selected surgical procedures ranked by complexity (7). The supply of general surgeons is positively related to the surgery rate at all levels of surgical complexity and for nearly all types of individual procedures. Populations served by proportionately higher numbers of general practitioners performing surgery tend to have lower surgery rates for the more complex procedures and higher rates for the less complex procedures. By contrast, a higher supply of physicians who did not perform surgery, particularly internists, tends to be either associated with lower surgery rates or unrelated altogether.

The ancillary, nonsurgical diagnostic procedures obtained through Medicare Part B exhibited opposite trends. Electrocardiogram, x-ray, and laboratory expenditure rates among persons age 65 and over tend to correlate positively with the supply of internists and other physicians who do not perform surgery and to be unrelated to the supply of surgeons. All three kinds of procedures are positively related to the input of hospital beds and non-surgeons, the multiple correlation being $r = .69$ for x-rays, .67 for electrocardiograms, and .82 for laboratory procedures.

Variations in the health care experience of different Vermont populations may be explained more by behavioral and distributional differences than by differences in illness patterns. We are, of course, unable to state which utilization rates are "normal" or which input rate represents a better allocation of resources. For example, for a given kind of surgery or diagnostic technique, it is not clear which rate indicates that medically unnecessary procedures are being performed or that not enough is being done. An important reason for uncertainty is that few prospective studies under controlled circumstances have been performed. Because the outcome of one type of service compared to another (or to none at all) is often not known, the variation in therapeutic and diagnostic procedures observed among different Vermont communities cannot be strictly evaluated (8). However, given the magnitude of these variations, the possibility of too much medical care and the attendant likelihood of iatrogenic illness is presumably as strong as the possibility of not enough service and unattended morbidity and mortality.

While interpretation of variations in utilization poses rather than answers questions concerning effectiveness, the data provide prima fascia evidence of inequality in the input of resources. Variations in expenditure, sustained in large part through third-party payment mechanisms, pose questions of equity, since the price of insurance is not adjusted to reflect these differences. Under Medicare Part B, the enrollee and the federal treasury each contribute $68 annually (1972). The lowest per capita reimbursement in the B areas of Vermont is $54, 20 percent less than the average amount contributed by the enrollee. In contrast, the highest reimbursement in the state was $164 per capita, representing a benefit recovery that exceeded combined patient and federal contributions by more than 20 percent. A similar situation obtains for private medical and hospital insurance. Under Blue Cross–Blue Shield, premiums are established on a Vermont- and a New Hampshire-wide "community rating" basis, with residents of low expenditure areas paying similar amounts or similar levels of coverage as residents of high expenditure areas.

Price Commission and Hill-Burton Decisions

A review of the decisions of the Hill-Burton and Price Commission agencies in Vermont reveals the difficulties of public regulation without the benefit of information about variations in per capita facility and manpower input, expenditures and service utilization. The information available to these agencies is based on indicators that do not describe the experience of the population receiving services from the regulated health care organizations. They cannot take into account the effect of their decision on lateral transfer of income nor appraise the value of increasing the rate of delivery of services.

The planning method used by the Hill-Burton agency in Vermont is similar to that used in most states. The formula for estimating hospital bed need is based on manifest demand, as measured by hospital patient days (without reference to the population), and an average daily patient census equal to 80 percent of a hospital's total beds. Population coverage enters the formula only through projected growth. No account is taken of the admissions of area residents to other hospitals or services delivered to nonresident patients (which in area 12, for example, comprise over one-third of all admissions). The single underlying premise is that demand, in terms of the total number of days the hospital bed is used, constitutes need.

Application of the Hill-Burton technique is illustrated by the recommendations for more hospital beds in the state contained in the 1971 Vermont State Plan (9) (Table 5). The recommended increase bore little relation to existing bed input and service utilization. The greatest increment (44 percent) was assigned to a hospital with a bed rate of 5.9 and a patient day rate of 1,495, both the highest in all 13 areas. The lowest increment (2 percent) was assigned to a hospital with a bed rate of 3.4 and a patient day rate of 1,015, both the lowest in all 13 areas. The second highest increase (27 percent) was assigned to a hospital of intermediate service utilization and bed rates, but with an average daily census approaching 100 percent and a mean length of stay exceeding the state average by 22 percent.

Since 1969, three hospitals in Vermont have undertaken construction projects financed under the Hill-Burton program. Assuming that the geographic distribution of patients using these facilities remains the same, the increased number of beds in two of the hospitals will move the bed input rates in the service areas to the second and third highest positions in the state. Examination of subsequent years' data will be required to

Table 5 Population-based Indicators of Bed Input and Patient Days, Compared to Bed Need as Determined by Hill-Burton Planning Formula (Vermont service areas, ranked by 1969 bed input rates)

Hospital service areas*	Bed input (per 1,000 persons)	Patient days (per 1,000 persons)	Percent increase in bed need
1	5.9	1,495	44
2	4.4	1,361	5
3	4.3	1,027	22
4	4.0	1,292	27
5	3.7	1,174	18
6	3.7	1,132	8
7	3.6	1,077	6
8	3.4	1,015	2

*Contains only hospital service areas that are coterminus with Hill-Burton areas.

ascertain whether the increase in bed input is associated with increase in service utilization or a general drop in average daily census.

The Federal Price Commission's control of expenditures on hospitals is indirect, since it is concerned with limiting increases in prices of routine, daily hospital services and ancillary services, including x-ray and laboratory procedures. Decisions are based on unit pricing structure and other institutional contingencies and do not take volume of services into consideration. Since the expenditure rate for a community represents the combined effects of volume and unit price, both factors must be considered. For hospital expenditures, the per capita rate may be expressed as a function of the patient day rate and the average cost per patient day. Over the 13 service areas, volume and the weighted average cost per day each accounted for nearly 40 percent of the variation in per capita hospital expenditures, with the rest attributed to differences in the amount of ancillary services. The implication is that the two factors are of about equal importance in the determination of expenditures.

Since the inception of phase II Price Commission guidelines limiting annual increases in unit service price to under 6 percent, three Vermont hospitals have initiated requests for exceptions. The first was withdrawn voluntarily before a public hearing was held, the second was denied, and the third was approved. The hospital receiving the exception was the principal institution serving an area that ranked first in the state in hospital manpower input rate and first in patient day rate. While the average patient day charges were relatively low, the high admission rate resulted in the per capita expenditure rate that ranked second highest in the state.

Both the Hill-Burton and the Price Commission decisions have served to *increase* variations in health care in Vermont. The decisions of the Price Commission to award a selective exception to a Vermont area with high hospital manpower use and expenditure rates will probably *increase* the disparities among areas and increase horizontal transfer of income. The building of additional facilities in high utilization areas presumably will lead to increased utilization. Both decisions probably will result in the delivery of additional health services without evidence that additional health services are of specific value for the receiving population.

For the Medicare and Medicaid populations, PSRO's are assigned broad responsibility for establishing the medical necessity of current health care patterns within their particular regions. This responsibility suggests that PSRO's are the appropriate agency to come to grips with the meaning of variations in population-based utilization rates among different medical care markets. However, rational inquiry into the meaning of variations in probability of surgical removal of organs, diagnostic procedures, hospital admission case mix, and so forth, will often require formal testing of an hypothesis concerning the relations between health care and outcome. This is a long-range proposition and requires a high level of organization and technical attainment, which will not be easily developed. However, specifically in those instances where public decisions received the implementation of new health care technology (for example, the installation of coronary intensive care units), it seems reasonable to tie implementation to the willingness of PSRO's to develop explicit clinical standards and perform prospective evaluations of the effect of the technology on medical outcome. This strategy could convert the essentially uncontrolled experiments in health care delivery that characterize the majority of health care efforts to a situation in which both the profession and the public can read some certainty concerning the value of the investment.

Short of engaging in extensive evaluation of alternative levels of service, PSRO's could provide a valuable service by reviewing medical necessity for more routine methods of peer review. Population-based indicators of resource input, utilization, and mortality are particularly useful in identifying communities whose health care experience deviates from regional averages. These profiles can aid in the selection of areas for further review, when the likelihood is high that medically unnecessary care is being delivered. Further, continuous monitoring of these communities will identify the successes and failures of PSRO's in dealing with performance that departs from regional norms.

Summary and Conclusions

Health information about total populations is a prerequisite for sound decision-making and planning in the health care field. Experience with a population-based health data system in Vermont reveals that there are wide variations in resource input, utilization of services, and expenditures among neighboring communities. Results show prima facie inequalities in the input of resources that are associated with income transfer from areas of lower expenditure to areas of higher expenditure. Variations in utilization indicate that there is considerable uncertainty about the effectiveness of different levels of aggregate, as well as specific kinds of, health services.

Informed choices in the public regulation of the health care sector require knowledge of the relation between medical care systems and the population groups being served, and they should take into account the effect of regulation on equality and effectiveness. When population-based data on small areas are available, decisions to expand hospitals, currently based on institutional pressures, can take into account any community's regional ranking in regard to bed input in utilization rates. Proposals by hospitals for unit price increases and the regulation of the actuarial rate of insurance programs can be evaluated in terms of per capita expenditures and income transfer between geographically defined populations. The PSRO's can evaluate the wide variations in level of services among residents of different communities. Coordinated exercise of the authority vested in these regulatory programs may lead to explicit strategies to deal directly with inequality and uncertainty concerning the effectiveness of health care delivery. Population-based health information systems, because they can provide information on the performance of health care systems and regulatory agencies, are an important step in the development of rational public policy for health.

Source

Wennberg J and Gittelsohn A. 1973. Small area variations in health care delivery. *Science*, New Series 182 (4117): 1102–08. Copyright 1973 *Science*. Reprinted with permission of American Association for the Advancement of Science.

Quantifying the Burden of Disease: The Technical Basis for Disability-adjusted Life Years
(1994)

C.J.L. Murray

Detailed assumptions used in constructing a new indicator of the burden of disease, the disability-adjusted life year (DALY), are presented. Four key social choices in any indicator of the burden of disease are carefully reviewed. First, the advantages and disadvantages of various methods of calculating the duration of life lost due to a death at each age are discussed. DALYs use a standard expected-life lost based on model life-table West Level 26. Second, the value of time lived at different ages is captured in DALYs using an exponential function which reflects the dependence of the young and the elderly on adults. Third, the time lived with a disability is made comparable with the time lost due to premature mortality by defining six classes of disability severity. Assigned to each class is a severity weight between 0 and 1. Finally, a three percent discount rate is used in the calculation of DALYs. The formula for calculating DALYs based on these assumptions is provided.

Introduction

This paper provides the technical basis for a new measure of the burden of disease: the disability-adjusted life year (DALY). It is one of four papers in this issue of the *Bulletin of the World Health Organization* on the Global Burden of Disease study (*1–3*); this first one details the conceptual basis for the indicator, the second examines the empirical basis for measuring time lost due to premature mortality by cause, the third describes the time lived with a disability by cause, and the fourth presents summary results and a sensitivity analysis. In this article, the rationale for measuring the burden of disease, the need for a single indicator of burden, some general concepts used in the design of an indicator of the burden of disease, a series of specific value choices, and some computational aspects are analysed in turn.

Why Measure the Burden of Disease?

The intended use of an indicator of the burden of disease is critical to its design. At least four objectives are important.

Note: Alphabetic superscript notations throughout the text refer to references in the original journal article which can be found in the Notes section of this book.

— to aid in setting health service (both curative and preventive) priorities;

— to aid in setting health research priorities;

— to aid in identifying disadvantaged groups and targeting of health interventions;

— to provide a comparable measure of output for intervention, programme and sector evaluation and planning.

Not everyone appreciates the ethical dimension of health status indicators (4). Nevertheless, the first two objectives listed for measuring the burden of disease could influence the allocation of resources among individuals, clearly establishing an ethical dimension to the construction of an indicator of the burden of disease.

Single and Multiple Indicators of Disease Burden

Since Sullivan's proposal of a composite index of health status incorporating information on morbidity and mortality (5, 6), there has been extensive debate on the utility of such single indicators of health status (7). For our purposes, this debate on the value of constructing single indicators can be reduced to a basic choice between explicit and implicit valuations. Decision-makers who allocate resources to competing health programmes must choose between the relative importance of different health outcomes such as mortality reduction or disability prevention. Because money is unidimensional, the allocation of resources between programmes defines a set of relative weights for different health outcomes. The only exception to this is in a completely free market for health care where such decisions between competing health programmes are not made by a central authority but by individuals, one health problem at a time.

Even in the USA, competitive resource allocation choices are still made for at least subsegments of the population such as Medicaid, Medicare and Veterans Administration beneficiaries. If the process of choosing relative weights of different types of health outcomes is left entirely to the political or bureaucratic process there is a high probability that similar health outcomes may be weighted inconsistently, perhaps reflecting the political voices of different constituencies. More importantly, there may be no open discussion or debate on key value choices or differential weightings. The wide variation in the implied value of saving a life in public safety legislation is but one example (8).

Alternatively, we can explicitly choose a set of relative values for different health outcomes and construct a single indicator of health. The black box of the decision-maker's relative values is then opened for public scrutiny and influence. Both this paper and the others in this series on the burden of disease are predicated on the desirability of making implicit values explicit. Development of a single indicator of the burden of disease for use in planning and evaluating the health sector is described below.

Some General Concepts

This paper is not intended to present a new paradigm for measuring health, nor to firmly identify one intellectual tradition such as utilitarianism, human rights, or Rawls' theory of justice (9) as the basis for the social preferences incorporated into DALYs. Rather, the majority of the paper is devoted to a discussion of several types of social preferences which must be incorporated into any indicator of health status. In order to derive a usable indicator, a particular stand is also taken on each of the social values described. The philosophical basis for this position will not be argued in detail. For the interested reader, an indicator very similar to DALYs has been developed based on Rawls' device of the "original position." That is a type of thought experiment where a group of individuals, ignorant of each other's social position, age, sex and other characteristics, are asked to choose the values and institutions to govern society. An "original position" could be invoked for a more specific task such as choosing the values to be incorporated in a health indicator.[a, b] Further philosophical treatment is excluded here.

However, four general concepts in the development of DALYs, which have enjoyed wide consensus with the groups involved in the study, are presented. These concepts are not derived from one particular conception of the good and may in fact be based on mutually inconsistent ethical frameworks. Nevertheless, the purpose of this paper is to explain the technical assumptions underlying DALYs and not to propose a unified ethical framework for all health sector analysis. In our discussion of the details of various social preferences incorporated into the indicator, we make reference to these concepts. The reader who finds these concepts intuitively plausible may feel comfortable with DALYs as a measurement tool.

(1) *To the extent possible, any health outcome that represents a loss of welfare should be included in an indicator of health status*

Any health outcome that affects social welfare should in some way be reflected in the indicator of the burden of disease. In other words, if society would be willing to devote some resources to avert or treat a health outcome, that outcome should be included in the total estimated burden. As will be seen later, this is at odds with one major stream of work on the measurement of disability which ignores all forms of disability below some thresholds of severity and duration. Note that by making reference to the concept of welfare we are not claiming that DALYs are the best measure of the health component of social welfare. Nor that maximizing DALYs gained from health interventions up to some cost per DALY would be consistent with an objective of maximizing social welfare, although this argument has been formally made (*10*). The link between health maximization, as measured by DALYs or any other measure, and welfare maximization would require another paper to adequately address the complexities of this issue.

(2) *The characteristics of the individual affected by a health outcome that should be considered in calculating the associated burden of disease should be restricted to age and sex*

Every health outcome such as the premature death of a 45-year-old man from a heart attack or permanent disability from blindness due to a road accident in a 19-year-old woman can be characterized by a set of variables. Some of these variables define the specific health outcome itself such as the etiology, type, severity or duration of the disability. Others are individual characteristics such as sex, age, income, educational attainment, religion, ethnicity, occupation, etc. In the most general terms, the task of constructing a burden of disease measure is to take an *n*-dimensional matrix of information on health outcomes and collapse this into a single number. To transform this complex array of information, what are the variables that should be included or indeed allowed to be considered? Some might argue that all the variables may be relevant and none should be excluded *a priori*. At the limit, this is a form of total relativism since every health outcome becomes unique and there is no meaning to an aggregate indicator.

Others might want to include variables that are unacceptable to the authors. The government of South Africa under apartheid implicitly put a higher relative weight on health outcomes in whites as compared to blacks. Nearly everyone would agree that attributes such as race, religion or political beliefs have no place in the construction of a health indicator. Some, however, might see a logic of including income or educational status such that the health of the wealthy counted more than the health of the poor. Estimations of the cost of disease (*11, 12*) use methods that value equivalent health outcomes in higher income groups as more costly than the same outcomes in the poor.

The set of variables that can be considered are restricted here to those defining the particular health outcome and individual characteristics that are general to all communities and households, namely age and sex. Daniels (*13*) has argued that differentiation by age should not be viewed as pitting the welfare of one age group against another, but rather as viewing an individual during different phases of the life-cycle. Variables defining subgroups such as income or education, which not all individuals or households can hope to belong to, are expressly excluded from consideration. This is a fundamental value choice founded on our notions of social justice. Some readers, with different values and conceptions of social justice, might conclude that other information should be included in assessing health status.

(3) *Treating like health outcomes as like*

We articulate a principle of treating like health outcomes as like. For example, the premature death of a 40-year-old woman should contribute equally to estimates of the global burden of disease irrespective of whether she lives in the slums of Bogota or a wealthy suburb of Boston. Treating like events equally also ensures comparability of the burden of disease across different communities and in the same community over a period of time. Community-specific characteristics such as local levels of mortality should not change the assumptions incorporated into the indicator design. The value of a person's health status is his or her own and does not depend on his or her neighbour's health status. A concrete example of this will be discussed in the section on the duration of time lost due to premature mortality. The approach presented means that occasionally we will sacrifice consistency with cost-effectiveness measures but retain comparability of burden across communities and a plausible treatment of equity.

(4) *Time is the unit of measure for the burden of disease*

Many health indicators measure the occurrence of events such as disease incidence or death per unit time and others measure these events per unit population. The units of measure are specific to the entity studied such as infant deaths for the infant mortality rate or measles cases in the measles attack rate. For a composite health indicator, a more general unit of measure is required. The best candidate for a general unit of measure is time itself, denominated in years or days. Using time as the unit of measure also provides a simple and intuitive method to combine the time lived with a disability with the time lost due to premature mortality. Measuring health status using time is not a new idea; the concept of years of life lost from dying young has been in use for nearly 45 years (*14*). The development of time-based measures and the myriad modifications of this approach are explored more fully below.

Incidence versus Prevalence Perspectives

With time as the chosen unit of measure, the burden of disease could still be an incidence- or prevalence-based indicator. Time lost due to premature mortality is a function of death rates and the duration of life lost due to a death at each age. Because death rates are incidence rates, there is no obvious alternative for mortality to using an incidence approach. There are no calculated measures of the prevalence of the dead. In contrast, for disability both incidence and prevalence measures are in routine use. There are at least two ways of measuring the aggregate time lived with a disability. One method is to take point prevalence measures of disability, adjusting for seasonal variation if present, and estimate the total time lived with the disability as prevalence × one year. The alternative is to measure the incidence of disabilities and the average duration of each disability. Incidence × duration will then provide an estimate of the total time lived with the disability.

If the incidence of disabilities is constant over time and the population age-structure is also constant, then the prevalence and incidence approaches yield exactly the same total amount of time lived with a disability. For nearly all populations the age structure is not constant and for many diseases such as lung cancer, cervical cancer, stomach cancer, HIV infection, and leprosy the incidence is changing over time. For the Global Burden of Disease study, we have chosen to use an incidence perspective for three reasons. First, with the method of calculating time lived with disabilities is more consistent with the method for calculating time lost due to premature mortality. Second, an incidence perspective is more sensitive to current epidemiological trend and will reflect the impact of health interventions more rapidly. The results of the Global Burden of Disease study, presented in Murray et al. (3) have also been calculated using a prevalence approach. These prevalence-based measures of the burden of disease will be published at a later date (15). Third, measuring the incidence or deriving it from prevalence data and information on case-fatality and remission rates imposes a level of internal consistency and discipline that would be missing if the prevalence data were used uncritically.

Specific Value Choices in Designing an Indicator of Burden

In the following sections, we address in detail the four key social preferences or values that must be incorporated into an indicator of the burden of disease. These are: the duration of time lost due to a death at each age, the value of time lived at different ages, non-fatal health outcomes (converting time lived with a disability to be comparable with time lost due to premature mortality), and time preference.

The Duration of Time Lost due to Premature Death

Since Dempsey (14) introduced the concept of measuring lost time due to mortality rather than crude or age-standardized death rates, a wide variety of methods for measuring years of life lost have been proposed (16–23).

Because the same terms have been used to describe quite different measures of lost time, there is substantial confusion on the precise method used in any particular study.

At least four different methods of estimating the duration of time lost due to premature death are possible. The following terminology is introduced in an attempt to clarify the discussion and comparison of methods: potential years of life lost, period expected years of life lost, cohort expected years of life lost, and standard expected years of life lost. Each measure is defined and its advantages and disadvantages are reviewed. In the earliest literature on measuring years of life lost, there was also considerable debate about the 'zero mortality assumption' (17–19). Using this assumption, calculating the years of life lost due to a particular disease entails recalculating a life-table in the absence of mortality from that cause at any age. Thus the number of years of life lost due to a tuberculosis death at age 40 would be different from a motor vehicle accident at age 40. Such methods violate the concept of treating like health outcomes identically and are not discussed further.

(1) *Potential years of life lost* are calculated by defining a potential limit to life and calculating the years lost due to each death as the potential limit minus the age at death. The formula for the number of years of potential life lost in a population is in notation:

$$x = L$$

$$\Sigma\, d_x\, (L - x)$$

$$x = 0$$

where d_x is deaths at age x, and L is the potential limit to life. A wide range of potential limits to life have been in [sic] used in practice, ranging from 60 to 85 (16–18, 22–25). The choice of the upper limit is arbitrary and the arguments are made on statistical grounds. Dempsey (14) proposed that the limit to life be selected as life expectancy at birth for a given population. Romeder & McWhinnie (16) have argued that the potential years of life lost should be calculated based only on deaths over age 1 to avoid being too heavily affected by infant mortality. This is a strange argument which has little intuitive appeal. If the indicator is to be used in informing resource allocation decisions, we would not want to ignore infant deaths. Proponents of the potential years of life lost approach, point to its ease of calculation and the egalitarian treatment of all deaths at a given age as equally important in contributing to the estimated total. If the potential limit to life is chosen as close to life expectancy, the results for the younger age groups are not substantially different from those for expected years of life lost (discussed below). The major disadvantage is in the treatment of deaths in the older population. Deaths over the arbitrary potential limit to life, for example 65 as calculated by the Centers for Disease Control (CDC) in the USA, do not contribute to the estimated burden of disease. This runs counter to our first principle because society clearly does care about the health of these groups and expends substantial resources in all countries on their health care. Even in high mortality populations, societies do appear to care about the health of the population over 60 or 70.

(2) An alternative is to calculate the *period expected years of life lost* (17–19, 21), using the local expectation of life at each age as the estimate of the duration of life lost at each age. Period expected years of life lost has become the standard method of estimating years of life lost in many cost-effectiveness studies (26, 27). This method is seen as a more 'realistic' estimate of the stream of life gained by averting a death, given competing risks of death in a particular population. More formally,

$$\sum_{x=0}^{x=l} d_x e_x$$

where l is the last age group and e_x is the expectation of life at each age. Because the expectation of life does not drop to zero at an arbitrary age, this method has the advantage of providing a more appealing estimate of the stream of lost life due to deaths in the older age groups. However, application of the period expectation method with locally different values of life expectancy would lead us to conclude that the death of a 40-year-old woman in Kigali contributes less to the global burden of disease than the death of a 40-year-old woman in Paris because the expectation of life at age 40 in Rwanda is lower than in France. Equivalent health outcomes would be a greater burden in richer communities than in poorer communities. As this runs counter to the principle of treating like events as like, this method is not used for estimating disability-adjusted life years.

The claim that period expected years of life lost are a more realistic estimate of the true duration of time lost due to premature mortality rests on three questionable assumptions. First, if a death is averted, that individual will then be exposed to the same mortality risks as the average individual in the population. In other words, the individual whose death is averted would not have a higher risk of subsequent death than the rest of the population. This may not be true for many chronic disabling conditions; likewise, because much mortality is concentrated in the chronically ill, averting a random death from injury may save more years than average expectation. For the population as a whole, the assumption of being exposed to the average mortality risk is reasonable. When evaluating specific interventions in a cost-effectiveness study, care must be taken to evaluate directly this question of interdependent mortality risks.

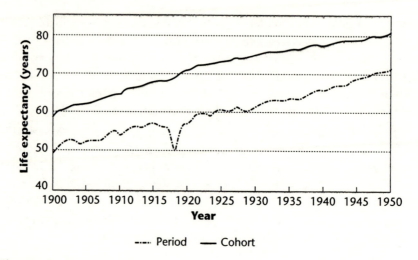

Figure 1 Period and cohort life expectancy at birth, 1900–1950, USA females. WHO 94082.

Second, period life expectancies are calculated based on the assumption that someone alive today will be exposed in the future to currently observed age-specific mortality rates at each age. Twentieth century mortality history demonstrates that this is a completely fallacious assumption, particularly in a population with moderate or high mortality (Fig. 1). Mortality has been declining at a steady pace throughout the last decades so that the life expectancy of a cohort, the real expectation of life based on the mortality experience of a group over time, is much higher than the period life expectancy based on currently observed rates. Fig. 1 shows how the cohort life expectancy at birth for US females has been 10–15 years higher than period life expectancy from 1900 to 1950.

Third, if we conceive of the burden of disease as the gap between current conditions and some ideal, why would one choose current mortality patterns to define that ideal and the existing gap? Such a standard would also have to be changed each year as life expectancy increases, leading to paradoxical situations where improvements in life expectancy could increase the expected years of life lost due to some large causes.[c]

(3) A third method for estimating the duration of time lost due to premature mortality is defined as *cohort expected years of life lost*:

$$\sum_{x=0}^{x=1} d_x \, e_x^c$$

where e^c is the estimated cohort life expectancy at each age. Clearly, cohort life expectancies must be estimated since we cannot know today the mortality experience a cohort will experience. However, the estimates based on past patterns of mortality decline are likely to be closer to the truth than period life expectancies. The difference in absolute terms between period and cohort expected years of life lost will be greatest for high mortality populations where substantial absolute mortality decline can be expected in the next decades. Despite the logical advantages of the cohort approach over the period approach, it still suffers from the criticism that it will not treat like events as like because cohort life expectancy will still differ from community to community. While inappropriate for measuring burden of disease, cohort life expectancy is the most attractive method of estimating the benefits of interventions for cost-effectiveness analysis.

(4) The advantages of the cohort expectation approach in the treatment of deaths at older ages and the egalitarian nature of the potential years of life lost methods can be combined. *Standard expected years of life lost can be defined as:*

$$\sum_{x=0}^{x=1} d_x e_x^*$$

where $e*$ is the expectation of life at each age based on some ideal standard. For DALYs, the standard has been chosen to match the highest national life expectancy observed; Japanese females have already achieved a period life expectancy at birth of close to 82 years. For a specific standard, the expectations are based on model life-table West Level 26 which has a life expectancy at birth for females of 82.5. Using a model life-table makes the standard expectations at each age easily available through publications and software distributed by the United Nations Population Division and eliminates some peculiarities of the Japanese age-specific mortality. Choosing one family of model life-tables over any other makes little or no difference to the results at such a low mortality level. With this indicator, deaths at all ages, even after age 82.5, contribute to the total estimated burden of disease while all deaths at the same age will contribute equally to the total estimated burden of disease.

Should the same standard expectation of life at each age be used for males as well as for females? One could argue on grounds of fostering equity that a male death at age 40 should count as the same duration of life lost as a female death at age 40. There appears, however, to be a biological difference in survival potential between males and females (*28, 29*).

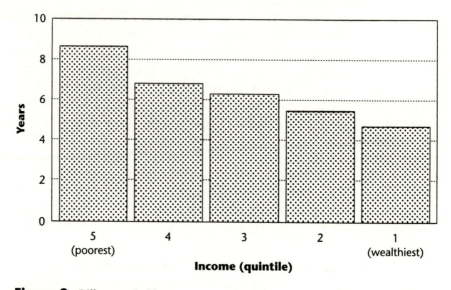

Figure 2 Differences in life expectancy at birth for males and females, by income quintile, in urban Canada, 1986.
WHO 94083.

The average sex differences in life expectancy at birth in low mortality populations is 7.2 years (*30*). Not all this difference is biological; a large share is due to injury deaths among young males and higher levels of risk factors such as smoking. If we examine high-income groups in low-mortality populations, the gap in life expectancy between males and females narrows considerably. Fig. 2 shows the differences in life expectancy by income groups in Canada (*31*). Where males are not exposed to high risks due to occupation, smoking, alcohol or injuries, the residual gap in life expectancy is narrowing dramatically. Projecting this forward, the ultimate gap in life expectancy at birth between the sexes is likely to approach 2 or 3 years. Independent estimates of the biological differences in survival potential have generated similar estimates (*33*). For the burden of disease study, we have chosen to use a life expectancy at birth of 80 for males and 82.5 for females from model life-table West. [Citation 32 is not in the original, Ed.]

In summary, the duration of time lost due to premature mortality can be measured by at least four different methods. Fig. 3 shows a comparison for a hypothetical population where period life expectancy at birth is 55. Four terms have been introduced to try and clarify the different methods of calculation, although this terminology is not yet in general usage. For the calculation of DALYs, we have chosen to use the standard expected years of life lost method with slight differences in the standard for males and females. To illustrate, the first two columns

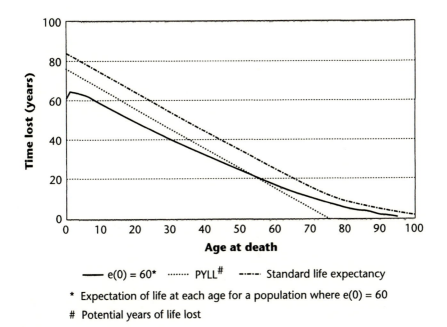

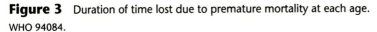

* Expectation of life at each age for a population where e(0) = 60
# Potential years of life lost

Figure 3 Duration of time lost due to premature mortality at each age.
WHO 94084.

of Table 1 provide an abridged listing of the standard male and female expectancies used.

Social Value of the Time Lived at Different Ages

In all societies social roles vary with age. The young, and often the elderly, depend on the rest of society for physical, emotional and financial support. Given different roles and changing levels of dependency with age, it may be appropriate to consider valuing the time lived at a particular age unequally. Higher weights for a year of time at a particular age does not mean that the time lived at that age is *per se* more important to the individual, but that because of social roles the social value of that time may be greater. Fig. 4 illustrates graphically two contrasting approaches to the value of the time lived at different ages: uniform value or unequal age weights with more importance given to time in the middle age group.

Unequal weights can be justified within two different conceptual frameworks. First, the theory of human capital views individuals as a type of machine with costs of maintenance and expected output. The value of time at each age for this human production machine should be proportionate to productivity. Several of the original proponents of measuring the years of life lost proposed measures of working years of life lost (17–19). Piot &

Table 1 Standard Life Expectancy and DALYs Lost Due to Premature Death at Each Age[a]

Age (years)	Life expectancy		Death DALYs	
	Females	Males	Female	Males
0	82.50	80.00	32.45	32.34
1	81.84	79.36	33.37	33.26
5	77.95	75.38	35.85	35.72
10	72.99	70.40	36.86	36.71
15	68.02	65.41	36.23	36.06
20	63.08	60.44	34.52	34.31
25	58.17	55.47	32.12	31.87
30	53.27	50.51	29.31	29.02
35	48.38	45.56	26.31	25.97
40	43.53	40.64	23.26	22.85
45	38.72	35.77	20.24	19.76
50	33.99	30.99	17.33	16.77
55	29.37	26.32	14.57	13.92
60	24.83	21.81	11.97	11.24
65	20.44	17.50	9.55	8.76
70	16.20	13.58	7.33	6.55
75	12.28	10.17	5.35	4.68
80	8.90	7.45	3.68	3.20

[a] Life expectancy is calculated for the age at the beginning of the interval.

Sundaresan calculated the years of healthy living in the productive age groups as a health sector outcome measure.[d] Several World Bank authors (33, 34) have used productivity weights in the calculation of years of life gained in cost-effectiveness studies. Barnum (34), in particular, suggests using average wage rates by age as the weighting factors. The logical extension of the human capital approach would be to weight time by other human attributes that correlate with productivity such as income, education, geographical location or even, in some economies, ethnicity. The obvious inequity is why no-one explicitly calls for this extension, even though it would only be logically consistent. Because of this apparent inconsis-

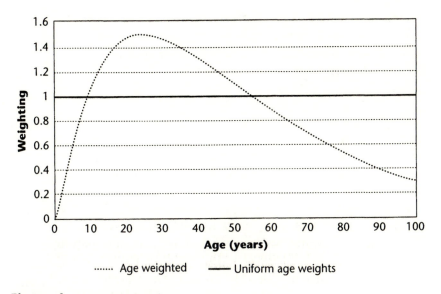

Figure 4 Age-weight function.

WHO 94085.

tency in the application of the human capital concept and because the human capital approach inadequately reflects human welfare, productivity weights are not used in the development of disability-adjusted life years.

Alternatively, we can view unequal age-weights as an attempt to capture different social roles at different ages. As all individuals can aspire to belong to each age group in his or her lifetime, Daniels argues that it is not unjust to discriminate by age (13). The concept of dependency and social role is broader than formal sector wage productivity and is not linked to total income levels. Unequal age-weights also has broad intuitive appeal. There has been little formal empirical work on measuring individual preferences for age-weights in the community; however, informal polling of tuberculosis programme managers by the author in an annual training course has revealed that everyone polled believes that the time lived in the middle age groups should be weighted as more important than the extremes. Not surprisingly there was no consensus on the precise weights to be used, only on the general functional form.

Having chosen to use unequal age-weights to capture different social roles through the life-cycle, how should specific weights be selected? With little empirical work on preferences for age-weights based on differing social roles as opposed to productivity, the only option was to use a modified Delphi method with a group of public health experts. One must also choose between establishing a set of discrete weights for each age or define a continuous mathematical function for the weights at each age.

Discrete age weights allow for great flexibility in the pattern chosen but require time-consuming iterative computations in their application.

For reasons of convenience, it is preferable to define a continuous age-weighting function. Functions of the form:

$$Cxe^{-\beta x}$$

where β is a constant having the general form shown in Fig. 4. This conforms to the basic age-weighting pattern desired. Only a narrow range of β provides reasonable age patterns, approximately between 0.03 and 0.05. Based on informal polling of the advisory board for this study, we chose a β of 0.04. As discussed by Murray et al. (3), the results are largely insensitive to the specific β chosen but are sensitive in certain qualitative ways to the difference between equal and unequal age-weights.

The constant C in the equation is chosen so that the introduction of unequal age-weights does not change the global estimated burden of disease from the total that would be estimated with uniform age-weights. Its value thus depends on the age and sex pattern of results of the global burden of disease in real populations detailed in Murray et al. (3). In another article on the global burden of disease published in this issue of the *Bulletin*, C equals 0.16243. If the age-weighting function were changed, for example by altering β, the constant would necessarily change as well.

Non-fatal Health Outcomes

Measuring non-fatal health outcomes in terms commensurate with time lost due to premature mortality has been the subject of extensive research for three decades (35). Disease-specific measures such as attack rates date from the nineteenth century, but more general measures of non-fatal health outcomes became a major issue in the 1960s. A series of authors formulated models for composite indicators of mortality and morbidity (5, 6, 36–39).[e] While each indicator had notable differences, they all defined a series of health states ranging from health to death, a series of weights reflecting the severity of these states and in some cases probabilities of movement from one state to another over time. Since these pioneering studies, intellectual efforts have evolved on three largely independent lines. Remarkably, for reasons of disciplinary focus, geographical and institutional locus, and types of health systems, the different strands of work on measuring non-fatal health outcomes have proceeded in relative isolation (40). The result is substantially different vocabulary, methods, and objectives and not surprisingly confusion. To provide the context for the disability-adjusted life year approach, the three domains of work will be briefly outlined.

Joint measures of non-fatal health outcomes and premature mortality were obviously of use in cost-effectiveness analyses of health projects (*41–43*). Consequently one line of development has been pursued by health economists interested in using the measures at the level of the individual or beneficiaries of a specific intervention. The now familiar term, the quality-adjusted life year (QALY), has become a standard tool in health programme evaluation in industrialized countries (*43–45*). In the work on QALYs, the focus has been on developing sophisticated methods for measuring individual preferences for time spent in different health states. For example, Nord (*46*) reviews five approaches developed to elicit utility weights for health states. Boyle & Torrance (*47*) have discussed a comprehensive system of health states, but this has yet to be applied. For most cost-effectiveness studies, health states have been defined *ad hoc* for a particular intervention such as coronary artery bypass grafting (*48*). The dimensions of physical, mental or social function within each state has received little attention in the QALY literature.

The second school of work has been the burgeoning field of health status indicators pursued largely in North America (see *49–51* for proceedings of three general conferences). Rather than the emphasis on choosing utility weights as in the estimation of QALYs field, the major thrust has been defining the precise dimensions of health status and practical survey instruments for measurement. Beginning initially with a narrow vision of disease, the measures have progressively incorporated variables related to physical function, mental function, and more recently social function (*52*). The term health-related quality of life has been used for this broader vision. The indicators themselves are weighted aggregates of a multitude of variables measuring specific functions or dimensions of physical, mental and social function. Research on new survey instruments has explored the differences between self-reported, proxy reported, independently observed, and objective functional tests. Reliability, various forms of validity (although rarely criterion validity), and feasibility of application are the basis for choice between indicators. The weights used in collapsing measurements of multiple variables into a single indicator have not been as much a topic for concern as in the QALY literature; frequently they are chosen on arbitrary grounds such as equal weighting.

The third cluster of work on measuring non-fatal health outcomes also dates from the early 1970s. A World Health Organization initiative in collaboration with the WHO Centre for the Classification of Diseases in Paris, and various nongovernmental organizations led to the publication of a draft classification of impairments, disabilities and handicaps in 1975[f] and the *International classification of impairments, disabilities and handicaps* (ICIDH) in 1980 (*53*). The conceptual framework that emerged from this process is substantially different from the QALY or health status index approaches.

In the manual of the ICIDH, a linear progression from disease to pathology to manifestation to impairment to disability to handicap is proposed. Impairment is defined at the level of the organ system, disability is the impact on the performance of the individual, and handicap is the overall consequences, which depend on the social environment. For example, a loss of a finger or an eye is an impairment. The consequent disability may be the loss of fine motor function or sight. Depending on the need in particular environments, the loss of function could lead to a handicap or disadvantage. The loss of fine motor function may be a greater handicap, in this terminology, for a concert violonist than for a bank-teller. Note the major difference between this approach which sees handicap as a completely different axis from disability and the health status field which adds social function as one more in a long list of variables incorporated in a measure of health-related quality of life.

Both the World Health Organization and the United Nations Statistical Division have adopted the ICIDH. Currently, other countries are adopting the ICIDH as the basis for measuring disability and handicap. Le Réseau d'Espérance de Vie en Santé (REVES) is an independent network of academics and government agencies that are concerned with quantifying healthy life (54). In line with the ICIDH, REVES has proposed three indicators: impairment-free life expectancy, disability-free life expectancy, and handicap-free life expectancy (55). Reflecting the concerns of some associations of people with disabilities and handicaps, some members of REVES are actively opposed to the use of weights for different health states in calculating composite health indicators. *De facto*, in any of the health expectancies, weights of 0 and 1 are used somewhat arbitrarily. These health expectancies, such as disability-free life expectancy, weight all the time spent with a moderate or severe disability as equal to the time lost due to premature mortality, a weight of one. Mild disability is given a weight of zero. The threshold below which disability is weighted with zero is not clearly defined in this literature. Often a threshold is justified by pointing out that nearly everyone has some mild impairment, disability or handicap so that if milder outcomes were included, health expectancies would approach zero in all environments. If weights between zero and one were chosen as in DALYs, this would not occur.

Given the diverse approaches to measuring nonfatal health outcomes, many possible strategies could have been used for measuring the burden of disease. Prior to the Global Burden of Disease study, the only effort to evaluate the burden of disease due to disability and premature mortality by cause for an entire population was the Ghana Health Assessment Project (25). While that study was path-breaking, it did not publish the methods or rationale used for defining, measuring and weighting disability. Learning from past experience, we chose to deal more directly with disability measurement issues and to develop a practical approach that could be applied to over 100 diseases and their sequelae. Four key issues had to be addressed: defining disability classes, separating duration and severity, mapping diseases through to disabling sequelae, and choosing weights for different classes.

In the terminology of the *International classification of impairments, disabilities, and handicaps,* we have chosen to measure disability, not handicap. Handicap or disadvantage is an attractive concept because it focuses on the impact, given a particular social context of the individual. In some cases, similar disabilities may lead to a greater handicap for an already disadvantaged person than for the more fortunate. In many cases, however, allocating resources to avert handicap, as opposed to disability, could exacerbate inequalities. The manual of the ICIDH itself gives the following example: "Subnormality of intelligence is an impairment, but it may not lead to appreciable activity restriction; factors other than the impairment may determine the handicap because the disadvantage may be minimal if the individual lives in a remote rural community, whereas it could be severe in the child of university graduates living in a large city, of whom more might be expected." (53, p. 31).

Pursuing handicap could and probably would lead us to invest in avoiding mental retardation in the rich and well-educated but not in the poor. On even the most minimal principles of equity, this is unacceptable. The principle of treating like events as like requires using disability instead of handicap.

Having decided to measure disability, the challenge is to develop a way of capturing the multiple dimensions of human function in a simple scheme. Six disability classes have been defined between perfect health and death. Each class represents a greater loss of welfare or increased severity than the class before. Disabilities in the same class may restrict different abilities or functional capacities but their impact on the individual is considered to be similar. Table 2 provides a definition of each of the six classes. Limited ability has been arbitrarily defined as a 50% or more decrease in ability.

The classes are also defined operationally. A class is defined by the set of disabling sequelae included in that class. For those who work with individuals with a disability, looking at the set of disabling sequelae included in that class may make it much clearer what a Class 3 disability is. Operational validation forces us to ask: are the disabling sequelae in each class approximately similar and does each class represent a group of sequelae more severe than the class before? As explained below, the final distribution of disabling sequelae by class was subject to the review of an independent group of experts.

The separation in the development of the disability-adjusted life year of duration of disability and severity must be emphasized. Severity of a

Table 2 Definitions of Disability Weighting

	Description	Weight
Class 1	Limited ability to perform at least one activity in one of the following areas: recreation, education, procreation or occupation.	0.096
Class 2	Limited ability to perform most activities in one of the following areas: recreation, education, procreation or occupation.	0.220
Class 3	Limited ability to perform activities in two or more of the following areas: recreation, education, procreation or occupation.	0.400
Class 4	Limited ability to perform most activities in all of the following areas: recreation, education, procreation or occupation.	0.600
Class 5	Needs assistance with instrumental activities of daily living such as meal preparation, shopping or housework.	0.810
Class 6	Needs assistance with activities of daily living such as eating, personal hygiene or toilet use.	0.920

disability could be a function of duration. A similar loss of function is argued to be worse per unit time if it is expected to be permanent [rather] than temporary. Man can endure suffering if the prospect of relief is near. In DALYs, severity or class weights are not a function of the time spent in each class but only of the class itself. This allows comparisons between the time lived with short- and long-term disabilities with the time lost due to premature mortality. A numerical example illustrates: 100 people each losing 0.1 of a DALY is a burden equal to 1 person losing 10 DALYs. We should note that experience in Oregon, with the application of cost-effectiveness to health resource allocation decisions, demonstrated that many individuals are against the separation of severity and duration (56). Through a series of town meetings, priorities for intervention based solely on cost-effectiveness criteria were modified. Analysis of these modifications demonstrated a concern for a larger quantum of benefits accruing to individuals as compared to the same number of QALYs accruing to more individuals (57). This concern would be captured better through a series of dispersion weights that adjusted for DALYs by the size of health gain affecting the individual because part of this effect relates to the duration of time lost due to mortality rather than just the severity of the disability. Because experience is limited only to Oregon, we have not introduced dispersion weights into the analysis and have maintained the separation of disability duration and severity.

A major obstacle between public health studies on particular diseases and work on disability has been the absence of a probability map from disease through to impairments and disabilities. On paper arrows may be drawn from disease all the way to handicap, but even those who work on disability can rarely provide concrete information on the probability that someone with a particular disease will go on to suffer disabilities of differing severity. For the Global Burden of Disease study, such a mapping from disease through impairment to disability was developed. The details of the map and specific problems encountered are discussed in Murray & Lopez (2).

To compare the time lived in six disability classes with the time lost due to premature mortality, a weight for each class is required. At least five types of methods have been proposed to elicit preferences for health states from individuals (45, 46): rating scales, magnitude estimation, standard gamble, time trade-off, and person trade-off. In brief,

(a) rating scales ask individuals to place different states on a scale from 0 to 100;

(b) magnitude estimation asks direct questions about the relative value of the time spent in one state compared to another;

(c) standard gambles ask individuals to choose between the certainty of living in a health state versus a chance of getting well at a probability p and dying at probability $1 - p$;

(d) time trade-offs elicit how much time an individual would exchange living in one state versus being healthy, such as 0.4 years of healthy life versus 1 year in a particular health state; and

(e) in person trade-offs, individuals are asked to choose between curing a certain number of individuals in one disability class versus another number in a different class.

Time trade-off questions differ from the other methods because they confound questions of the utility of time spent in disability classes and the time preference rate discussed below. The last three methods all try to elicit the point at which the individual is indifferent between the two choices being offered. When the individual is indifferent the two outcomes are then equivalent and a weight is derived. Specific weights depend not only on the type of question used but on the group of respondents. Health care providers, patients, families of patients, and the general public may give different results to a specific question (46). The specific weights may depend on the question and respondent type but the ordinal ranking of health states is often less sensitive to the specific formulation.

Weights for the six classes have been chosen by a group of independent experts who had not been involved in the estimation of the incidence, duration or mortality of any disease, convened at the Centers for Disease Control. They chose weights based on both the word definitions and the set of disabling sequelae in each class. *De facto*, they used a magnitude estimation method to choose a number between 0 and 1 for each of the six classes. Their votes were averaged to generate the final class weights provided in Table 2. How much do the specific weights matter? For classes 3 through 6, even if the weight is changed up or down by 0.1 it will have only a minor effect on the estimated burden of disease by cause. For Classes 1 and 2, however, the incidence times duration of disability is much higher and a change of weight from 0.05 to 0.1, for example, could have a significant effect on the results. Future work at the country level and at the global and regional level will benefit from a broader exercise to elicit weights for the six disability classes.

Time Preference

At the simplest level, time preference is the economic concept that individuals prefer benefits now rather than in the future. The value of goods or services today is greater than in one or ten years. If offered the choice between 100 dollars from a completely reliable source today or 100 dollars in 1 year, most will prefer their money today. If offered 110 in one year versus 100 today, some may choose the 110 dollars. The bank interest rate on a savings account is the rate at which individuals are willing to forego consumption today for consumption in the future. The market rate of interest is the aggregate rate at which individuals in society as a whole discount future consumption. It is standard practice in economic appraisal of projects to use the discount rate to discount benefits in the future (58). The process of discounting future benefits converts them into present-value terms which can then be compared with project costs also discounted if they are spread over more than one year to determine cost-effectiveness.

However, despite the uniform use of discounting in cost-benefit and cost-effectiveness analysis, there is no consensus on the conceptual justification for discounting or on the appropriate discount rate (59, 60). Simplifying, there are two approaches to choosing the discount rate. One can use the social opportunity cost of capital as captured by the market rate of return on investment. Distortions of the market caused by corporate taxation and other interventions can complicate determining the social opportunity cost of capital. In practice, discount rates based on the social opportunity cost of capital are high (between 8% and 15%). The World Bank and the U.S. Congressional Budget Office have used a 10% discount rate for many years in project appraisal (61). Studies of long-term return on investments, however, suggest a lower discount rate of 1–3%. The alternative concept is that society, like individuals, has a social time preference which should be used for discounting future benefits to society. This rate is thought to be lower than the market rate of interest (closer to 1–3%) (59).

Discounting years of health life or their equivalent has been used since Piot & Sundaresan in 1967 in many cost-effectiveness analyses.[g] However, as health policy researchers have become more familiar with time preference, discounting health benefits has become highly controversial (62–75). While a detailed discussion of arguments for and against discounting is beyond the scope of this paper, a brief review of some arguments for social time preference may put discounting in a sharper perspective.

- First, individuals may have a pure time preference for no clear reason except myopia. Myopia is not a persuasive basis for social time preference. There is no reason to value welfare *per se* today more than welfare *per se* of the same individuals. Nor is there a reason for society to value the welfare *per se* of those alive today more than the welfare *per se* of those who are yet to be born.

- Second, if consumption is expected to grow in the future and there is decreasing marginal utility of consumption, then a marginal unit of consumption in the future will lead to less utility in the future and should be discounted. This logic for a positive discount rate may be reversed for health benefits. Disability-adjusted life years represent a measure of time gained or lost in the future. Time gives the potential to consume and derive utility; it is not equivalent to a fixed number of units of consumption. In fact, in the face of growing consumption a future DALY may yield more utility than a current DALY.

- Third, there is uncertainty correlating with time so that future outcomes need to be discounted to reflect the finite but non-zero risk that society will not exist at that time. Or in a less extreme form, it may be reasonable to expect an individual to incorporate his or her future risk of death each year into individual time preference, on average about 1% per year. For society, the equivalent risk of extinction will be much lower. Defining a plausible risk of social extinction is difficult, but attempts have been made to use certain probability distributions for estimates of uncertainty correlating with time.

- Fourth, Keeler & Cretin (75) have formalized a commonly appreciated problem known as the time paradox. If one argues that health benefits should not be discounted or should be discounted at a rate lower than monetary costs, one will always choose to put off investing in a health project until the future. Benefits will be the same in present-value terms because they are not discounted. But the costs in present-value terms will be lower if the project is deferred to the future. Costs are lower because the budget could be invested and yield a positive return. A thousand dollars today will turn into $1,100 or $1,050 in a year. Only when costs and benefits are discounted at the same rate do we become indifferent to the time when a project is implemented. The time paradox depends on three critical assumptions: (a) the opportunity for health intervention will be the same in the future with similar costs and benefits, (b) it is politically feasible for society to receive more resources for health in the future in exchange for putting off current expenditure, and (c) the rate of return in other sectors or in financial markets is higher than in the health sector. If any of these do not hold, the time paradox is no longer relevant.

- Fifth, if health benefits are not discounted, then we may conclude that 100% of resources should be invested in any disease eradication plans with finite costs as this will eliminate infinite streams of DALYs which will outweigh all other health investments that do not result in eradication.

Recognizing that the debate on discounting health benefits will not be resolved in the near future, we have chosen a low positive rate of 3 percent for the calculation of DALYs. This is consistent with the long-term yield on investments. There is also a precedent in the World Bank Disease Control Priorities Study (27) that used a 3 percent rate. It avoids the difficulty of the time paradox and of overvaluing eradication programmes when no discount rate is used. Murray et al. (3) provide the sensitivity of the Global Burden of Disease results to varying the discount rate between zero and ten percent.

Introducing discounting into the computation of DALYs raises a number of technical questions. It complicates the choice between incidence and prevalence perspectives. With discounting, even with constant incidence rates, the number of DALYs computed using an incidence perspective for disability will be lower than using a prevalence perspective, because the stream of disability into the future will be discounted so that the last years in the stream will count much less than the first. Second, years of life lost due to premature mortality and years lived with a disability must be compared carefully. If we calculated the time lost from premature mortality which will occur in the future from current disease incidence, we get a different result than if we calculate the time lost due to premature mortality occurring this year. Even if death rates were constant over time, discounting would introduce a difference. The only practical solution, however, is to assess the time lived with a disability by using current incidence and the time lost due to premature mortality by using current death rates.

Third, we can calculate the discounted stream of lost life due to premature mortality at age a by discounting the number of years as estimated from the standard.

$$\frac{1}{r} - \frac{e^{-rL}}{r}$$

where r is the discount rate and L is the standard expectation of life at age a. An expectation of life is the average number of years expected, but expected deaths will be distributed over many ages. Because discounting is a nonlinear function, the average of a discounted distribution is not equal to the discounted value of the average of a distribution. A more precise estimate of the discounted life expectation would take into account the distribution of the ages of death. Discounting the survivorship function, however, yields results that are only marginally different.

The discounted duration of time lost due to premature death at each age, calculated using the survivorship function method, for females ranges from 0.8% to 2.3% (from 1% to 3% for males) less than the direct method. Because of the minor differences and the tremendous advantages of defining a single formula for calculating DALYs, the direct method for discounting has been chosen.

DALY Formula

In summary, the disability-adjusted life year is an indicator of the time lived with a disability and the time lost due to premature mortality. The duration of time lost due to premature mortality is calculated using standard expected years of life lost where model life-table West with an expectation of life at birth of 82.5 for females and 80 for males has been used. Time lived at different ages has been valued using an exponential function of the form $Cxe^{-\beta x}$. Streams of time have been discounted at 3%. A continuous discounting function of the form $e^{-r(x-a)}$ has been used where r is the discount rate and a is the age of onset.[h] Disability is divided into six classes, with each class having a severity weight between 0 and 1. Time lived in each class is multiplied by the disability weight to make it comparable with the years lost due to premature mortality.

A general formula for the number of DALYs lost by one individual can be developed:

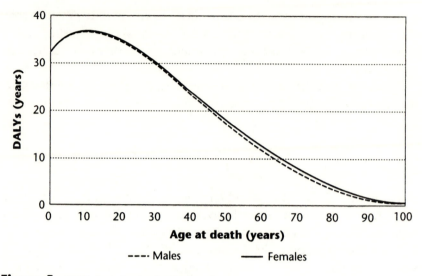

Figure 5 DALYs lost due to death at each age.
WHO 94086.

$$x = a + L$$
$$\int DCxe^{-\beta x} e^{-r(x-a)} \, dx$$
$$x = a$$

The solution of the definite integral from the age of onset a to $a+L$ where L is the duration of disability or time lost due to premature mortality gives us the DALY formula for an individual:

$$-\left[\frac{DCe^{-\beta a}}{(\beta + r)^2} \left[e^{-(\beta + r)(L)} (1 + (\beta + r)(L + a)) - (1 + (\beta + r)a) \right] \right]$$

where D is the disability weight (or 1 for premature mortality), r is the discount rate, C is the age-weighting correction constant, β is the parameter from the age-weighting function, a is the age of onset, and L is the duration of disability or time lost due to premature mortality. This formula can be conveniently written in a spreadsheet cell to facilitate calculation of DALYs. In the specific form used for calculating DALYs, r equals 0.03, β equals 0.04, and C equals 0.16243. The general form of the DALY formula facilitates the sensitivity testing presented in Murray et al. (3). Fig. 5 presents the number of DALYs lost due to a death at each age for a male and a female. This pattern is the aggregate results of the duration of time lost due to premature mortality, age-weighting and discounting but the figure does not reflect any disability.

Conclusion

Disability-adjusted life years as an indicator is consistent with a long line of work on composite indicators of non-fatal health outcomes and premature mortality. While DALYs must be viewed as only one more step in a long development process, there are several aspects about them that are worth noting when comparing DALYs by cause, age, sex, and region with other indicators.

- The particular set of value choices—the duration of life lost, the value of life lived at different ages, comparison of the time lived with a disability with the time lost due to mortality, and the time preference—all differ from past indicators. They have been selected in such a way that the indicator is comparable across a wide range of environments. We also believe that value choices reflect a broad consensus among those practising international public health. However, as the sensitivity analysis shows (3), many of the conclusions of the Global Burden of Disease study are unaffected by changes in those parameters.

- Apart from the specific value choices, the major difference between DALYs and more widely available measures such as potential years of life lost is, of course, the inclusion of the time lived with a disability. As demonstrated elsewhere (3), 34% of the global burden of disease is due to disability; some causes such as neuropsychiatric diseases appear as major problems using DALYs but not using potential years of life lost.

- Estimates of the burden of disease denominated in DALYs can easily be used in conjunction with the literature on cost-effectiveness of health interventions. For example, the largest compendium of international health interventions has reported results in terms of cost per DALY (27). This facilitates using estimates of the burden of disease in determining health resource allocations.

- The more original aspect of DALYs is not their design but the successful application of the indicator to measure the burden of disease for over 100 diseases in eight regions for five age groups among males and females. While details such as the distribution of disabling sequelae by class are bound to be changed in the future as more information is obtained, it is already established as a feasible alternative for assessing the burden of disability and premature mortality.

Acknowledgments

This work would not have been possible without the tremendous efforts of Caroline Cook. Extensive comments from P. Musgrove, M. Reich and A. Lopez were very helpful. J.-L. Bobadilla, D. Jamison, J. Zeitlin, W. Whang, J. Kim, S. Anand, J. Koplan, K. Hill, J.-M. Robine, R. Wilkins and R. Rannan-Eliya provided constructive comments and suggestions for improvement.

SOURCE

Murray, C. J. L. 1994. Quantifying the burden of disease: The technical basis for disability-adjusted life years. *Bulletin of the World Health Organization* 72 (3): 429–45. English version reprinted with permission of WHO Press.

CHAPTER 14

MEDICAL ETHICS AND HUMAN RESEARCH

We live in a time when the words "impossible" and "unsolvable" are no longer part of the scientific community's vocabulary. Each day we move closer to trials that will not just minimize the symptoms of disease and injury but eliminate them.
—Christopher Reeve (1952–2004), American actor

PROFESSIONALS INVOLVED IN MEDICAL and preventive care often cite the Hippocratic Oath with the dictum "Do no harm" (see Volume I, Chapter 1) as the beginning of medical ethics, but the evolution of the field usually gets little attention. It was the rise of scientifically focused clinical practice in the late nineteenth century that brought medical ethics, specifically informed consent, to the attention of the medical community as a pressing matter. For example, in 1891 Prussia, TB among people in prison was rampant. Concerned that forcing medical interventions on prisoners was a breach of medical ethics, the Prussian interior minister issued a decree that tuberculin, an antigen that could determine whether an inmate had been exposed to TB, "must in no case be used against the patient's will."

The rise of scientific medicine brought with it a need for experimentation, and some researchers did not hesitate to use human subjects without their consent. In 1898, for instance, German professor and physician Alfred Neisser infected a cohort of prostitutes with syphilis to examine the potential for a vaccine to protect against the disease. None of the subjects was asked about participating in the study prior to being infected. When controversy about the study arose, Neisser contended the subjects had become infected as a result of their work, not his administration of sera from syphilitic patients. Neisser also contended that no informed consent was needed, a stance backed by the Royal Disciplinary Court. The court's decision had no standing with the public, however, and the resulting uproar led the minister for religious, educational, and medical affairs to issue a directive banning such experiments unless consent was clearly given by the subject. Unfortunately, the directive lacked the force of law.

The advancement of medical ethics as a response to torture under the guise of "medical experimentation" by the National Socialists (Nazis) cannot be overstated. Under the Nazis, a wide assortment of groups (Jews, gays and lesbians, Roma, and the mentally retarded, among others) were considered subhuman and therefore sent to concentration camps for extermination or to provide forced labor. Some concentration camp prisoners were selected to serve as subjects in experiments designed to address a wide variety of questions. Most of these questions were of dubious scientific importance, and others constituted human response to outright torture. The subjects could not refuse to participate, and few survived the experiments. Some Nazi experiments included conjoining twins by sewing them together, changing eye color by intraocular injections, exposing subjects to extreme temperatures, or denying them food and water (except for salt water) to assess the physiological consequences. Subjects were also purposefully infected with malaria and injected with experimental treatments, such as those for gangrene and other varieties of battlefield infection. They were also subjected to mustard gas and other chemical weapon exposures to test the effectiveness of possible treatments. Nazi efforts at forced sterilization were particularly noteworthy; they began with chemicals (which were not considered rapid enough to have the desired effects) and progressed to radiation (which quickly rendered the subjects sterile).

The Allied capture of 23 individuals responsible for many of these experiments led to the "Doctors' Trial" (*USA vs. Karl Brandt, et al.*) in Nuremberg, where 20 physicians and 3 Nazi Party officials were tried for war crimes. One of the defenses offered by the defendants was the lack of international law on human experimentation. Seven of the defendants were convicted and received death sentences, seven were acquitted, and the rest received prison terms of ten years to life. One consequence of the Doctors' Trial was the creation of the "Nuremberg Code," a document that provides a basis for assessing whether a given medical study constitutes "research" and defines key concepts such as informed consent, coercion, beneficence, and equipoise (See Appendix A). Despite its importance, the Nuremberg Code was not incorporated into any American law, and during the latter half of the twentieth century some medical research in clear violation of these principles became public. For example, the Tuskegee Syphilis Study was conducted in the absence of informed consent from the subjects studied, and during Project MK-ULTRA, the United States Central Intelligence Agency surreptitiously studied the effects of lysergic acid diethylamide (LSD) and other drugs in subjects who never consented to participate in such research.

In 1964, during its meeting in Helsinki, the General Assembly of the World Medical Organization adopted a set of principles governing human experimentation. The Declaration of Helsinki builds upon the Nuremberg Code in providing a basis for physician behavior regarding clinical research. During the last third of the twentieth century, it was revised four times. Not all revisions have been accepted by national regulatory authorities; for instance, the U.S. Food and Drug Administration will not recognize any revision of the document past the third revision in 1989 (See Appendix B).

Among the major triggers for developing means to protect research subjects after World War II was the Tuskegee Syphilis Study. Begun in 1932 when treatments for the disease were noxious and often toxic, the study sought to determine whether patients with syphilis were better off if not exposed to the prevailing modalities of treating the disease. In association with the Tuskegee Institute, the U.S. Public Health Service identified 399 African American men with syphilis as part of an effort to create treatment programs for impoverished blacks. Initially, the men were to be followed for under a year and then offered treatment for the disease. However, leadership of the study changed with the retirement of the study's creator, Taliaferro Clark. Clark's successor, Raymond H. Vonderlehr, changed the study into a long-term observational investigation of the natural history of syphilis. Within 15 years, however, penicillin emerged as a standard of care for syphilis; significantly, penicillin lacked the toxicity of prior treatments. None of the 399 subjects in the study were offered penicillin or any other treatment for their disease. In 1972, a spirited PHS investigator in San Francisco, Peter Buxtun, who had been trying to bring the questionable ethical basis for the study to the attention of the CDC for six years, went to the *Washington Star* newspaper to bring public attention to the study. During the resulting public uproar, a commission was established to investigate the ethical lapses present in the Tuskegee Study. Its report, the Belmont Report (See Appendix C), established three principles as the basis for ethical clinical research: respect for persons, including the voluntary provision of informed consent by all research subjects; beneficence; and justice, insofar as all study procedures are administered fairly.

In the United States, legislation required that Institutional Review Boards (IRBs) be created at all institutions receiving federal funds. IRBs were charged with assuring that all research undertaken at their institutions constituted bona fide medical research and ensured that subjects were provided with an appropriate informed consent process. In the European Union, similar regulations were legislated and led to the creation of Ethics Committees at each institution undertaking research. Ethics committees function as IRBs, assuring that basic ethical principals are followed in clinical research undertaken at individual institutions.

CLINICAL TRIALS

Implicit in the provisioning of informed consent is the monitoring of clinical studies to assure that untoward or adverse events are not increased among those receiving a drug or other modality being investigated. The development of the randomized trial after World War II allowed for large-scale human experimentation. A monitoring committee otherwise divorced from the trial was needed to assure that safety, equipoise, and beneficence remained present in the trial. In the absence of any of these three components, the trial would lose its ethical basis and would need to be halted. By the 1960s in the United States, the NIH had become a major patron of large-scale clinical research studies. The National Heart Institute, in particular, assembled a committee to review the means by which clinical trials were conducted. The committee's report, known as the *Greenberg Report* (after its chair, Professor Bernard Greenberg, an eminent statistician), detailed the general approach to multicenter randomized trials and was explicit in the need for a data monitoring committee (often referred to as a data and safety monitoring board or committee) to assure that the safety of the subjects was preserved within the contexts of a randomized clinical study. Since then, data monitoring committees are mandatory for all clinical research evaluations in which comparisons with either placebo or some other comparator is undertaken.

The issue of whether a given clinical study is representative of the population to which the results are to be generalized followed the disclosure of the Tuskegee study in the 1970s and controversy regarding the role of hormone replacement therapy (HRT) during the 1980s. HRT was a modification of estrogen replacement therapy designed to mitigate the effects of menopause on cardiovascular disease risk while minimizing the risk of endometrial cancer. In the wake of feminism concurrent with the development of this controversy, attention focused on the degree to which government-supported research included all members of society, especially minorities and women. Regulations to assure that such representation was present in all U.S. government-supported clinical research studies were implemented during the 1980s. However, controversy about the lack of data regarding the efficacy of HRT persisted, and it led to the creation of the Women's Health Initiative (WHI) together with the Office on Women's Health at the NIH. The WHI sought to address the issue of whether HRT was indeed warranted as a therapeutic modality in postmenopausal women. As the century drew to a close, the WHI randomized trials had subjects enrolled and follow-up had begun.

Although the NIH crafted and funded a direct effort to specifically answer questions about women's health, it did not do the same for other minorities.

Instead, the agency chose to require that all clinical studies include minorities. Indeed, the United States was not the only country that chose to redress an imbalance in the clinical research arena. Australia, for example, began the Australian Aboriginal Birth Cohort Study in 1987 to focus on aboriginal health issues. Whether such efforts will succeed in meaningfully incorporating minorities into clinical research on a global scale remains unclear.

SELECTED READINGS

Anesthesiologist Henry K. Beecher provides our first reading. In 1941, Beecher was selected as the world's first endowed professor of anesthesia by Harvard University. During the course of his career he became concerned with the lax ethical practices surrounding human experimentation. Some claim Beecher's concern was rooted in trying to protect the reputation of solid scientific research; others claim he was motivated by deep religious convictions. Yet others believe Beecher may have been haunted by guilt because he participated in some less than ethical clinical studies. Regardless of his motivation, Beecher began writing on medical ethics in 1959. As his career progressed, he grew steadily agitated with the ethically questionable behaviors he witnessed in medical research. At the Brook Lodge Conference Center in Michigan in 1965, Beecher spoke to journalists and shocked them by stating that ". . . breaches of ethical conduct in experimentation are by no means rare, but are almost, one fears, universal." He then set out to document his claims, putting together a manuscript damning the nation's leading hospitals, medical schools, and industry. The *New England Journal of Medicine* accepted Beecher's manuscript, and it is reproduced here. The paper made an impact, sowing the seeds that led to federal legislation governing the rules of human experimentation in the United States.

The second reading, by George J. Annas and Sherman Elias, reminds us that risks and benefits need to be balanced when bringing a new drug or medical technology to market. Thalidomide is the focus of this piece, but the larger point is that technological advances, especially pharmaceutical ones, are not unbridled cures for all ills. However, these technologies are not so inherently dangerous that they should not be used if they have been proven efficacious for specific therapies. The risk–benefit proposition that attends any therapeutic decision is neither black nor white but rather a spectrum of grays. If an established set of side effects is demonstrated, it may be possible to develop systems that will mitigate those risks. For example, the manufacturer of thalidomide has since implemented a risk-mitigation system that has been used with success so that patients in need of thalidomide can now access the drug. Annas and Elias note that trust in technology alone is not sufficient to assure public safety in health care. Risk-taking judgments must be made by humans and should not be based on an assumption that technology alone can render the risk–benefit proposition moot.

Our third reading, by Arthur L. Caplan, discusses the fallout of government mandating payment for treatments for a given disease, specifically the 1972 decision that Medicare will cover all treatments for end-stage renal disease (ESRD). At the time Medicare coverage for ESRD began, the major therapeutic modality, renal dialysis, was still in the process of winning acceptance in the medical community. Funding for the program was small compared with overall Medicare expenses. With the recent epidemic increase in diabetes, however, the number of persons with ESRD has grown considerably, and the expenditures required to deal with the mandate far exceed what was expected. Caplan uses the example of ESRD as a straw man with which to examine many of the contentions raised against a national health insurance plan in the United States. He raises the two major ethical queries: 1) Who bears the burden of cost for new medical technologies? If the burden falls to the federal government, who will make the decision on which technologies are developed and deployed? 2) Do we, as a society, want decisions regarding allocation of a given therapeutic technology to be influenced and informed by ethical and biomedical scientific considerations? This question will need to be addressed if expenditures for ESRD, and future technologies, are not to overwhelm the resources of third-party payers.

BIBLIOGRAPHY

Angell M. 1997. The ethics of clinical research in the third world. *N Engl J Med* 337 (12): 847–49.

Armitage P. 1982. The role of randomization in clinical trials. *Stat Med* 1:345–52.

Bartlett EE. 2001. Did medical research routinely exclude women? An examination of the evidence. *Epidemiology* 12 (5): 584–86.

Bendek TG. 1978. The 'Tuskegee Syphilis' study: Analysis of moral versus methodological aspects. *J Chron Dis* 31:35–50.

Bull JP. 1959. The historical development of clinical therapeutic trials. *J Chron Dis* 10:218–48.

Bush JK. 1994. The industry perspective on the inclusion of women in clinical trials. *Acad Med* 69 (9): 708–15.

Cairns J, Cohen L, Colton T, DeMets DL, Deykin D, Friedman L, Greenwald P, Hutchison GB, and Rosner B. 1991. Issues in the early termination of the aspirin component of the Physicians' Health Study: Data Monitoring Board of the Physicians' Health Study. *Ann Epidemiol* 41(5): 395–405.

Cochrane AL. 1972. *Effectiveness and Efficiency: Random Reflections on Health Services.* London: Nuffield Provincial Hospital Trust.

Coleman CH, Bouësseau M-C, and Reis A. 2008. The contribution of ethics to public health. *Bull WHO* 86 (8): 1578–79.

Comstock GW. 1978. Uncontrolled ruminations on modern controlled trials. *Am J Epidemiol* 108 (2): 81–84.

Chavkin W. 1994. Women and clinical research. *J Am Med Women's Assoc* 49 (4): 99–100.

Doll R. 1982. Clinical trials: Retrospect and prospect. *Stat Med* 1:337–44.

Dubois MY and Burris JF. 1994. Inclusion of women in clinical research. *Acad Med* 69 (9): 693–94.

Fuchs FD, Klag MJ, and Whelton PK. 2000. The classics: A tribute to the fiftieth anniversary of randomized clinical trial. J Clin Epidemiol 53:335–42.

Harrison RW 3rd. 2001. Impact of biomedical research on African Americans. *J Natl Med Assoc* 93 (3 Suppl.): 6S–7S.

Jones JH. 1993. *Bad Blood: The Tuskegee Syphilis Experiment.* New York: The Free Press.

Kampmeier RH. 1974. Final report on the "Tuskegee Syphilis Study." *Southern Med J* 67 (11): 1349–53.

Katz RV, Kegeles SS, Kressin NR, Green BL, Wang MQ, James SA, Russell SL, and Claudio C. 2006. The Tuskegee Legacy Project: Willingness of minorities to participate in biomedical research. *Journal of Health Care for the Poor and Underserved* 17:698–715.

Keitt SK. 2003. Sex and gender: The politics, policy, and practice of medical research. *Yale J Health Policy Law Ethics* 3 (2): 253–78.

Killen J, Grady C, Folkers GK, and Fauci AS. 2002. Ethics of clinical research in the developing world. *Nature Reviews* 2:210–15.

Krebs J. 2008. The importance of public-health ethics. *Bull WHO* 86 (8): 579.

McCarthy CR. 1994. Historical background of clinical trials involving women and minorities. *Acad Med* 69 (9): 695–98.

Merkatz RB and Junod SW. 1994. Historical background of changes in FDA policy on the study and evaluation of drugs in women. *Acad Med* 69 (9): 703–7.

Merton V. 1993. The exclusion of pregnant, pregnable, and once-pregnable people (a.k.a. women) from biomedical research. *Am J Law Med* 19 (4): 369–451.

Miller FG, Caplan AL, and Fletcher JC. 1998. Dealing with Dolly: Inside the national bioethics advisory commission. *Health Affairs* 17 (3): 264–67.

Nowak R. 1994. Problems in clinical trials go far beyond misconduct (in Special News Report). *Science,* New Series 264 (5165): 1538–41.

Organization, review and administration of cooperative studies (Greenberg Report): A report from the Heart Special Project Committee to the National Advisory Heart Council, May 1967. 1988. *Control Clin Trials* 9 (2): 137–48.

Page AK. 2002. Prior agreements in international clinical trials: Ensuring the benefits of research to developing countries. *Yale J Health Policy Law Ethics* 3 (1): 35–66.

Pendergast P and Hirsch HL. 1986. The Dalkon Shield in perspective. *Med Law* 5:35–44.

Pinn VW. 1994. The role of the NIH's Office of Research on Women's Health. *Acad Med* 69 (9): 698–702.

Sackett D, Rosenberg W, Muir Gray J, Haynes RB, and Richardson W. 1996. Evidence based medicine: What it is and what it isn't. *BMJ* 312:71–72.

The controlled therapeutic trial [editorial]. 1948. *BMJ* 2:791–92.

Thomas SB and Quinn SC. 1991. The Tuskegee Syphilis Study, 1932 to 1972: Implications for HIV education and AIDS risk education programs in the black community. *AJPH* 81 (11): 1498–1505.

Tunis SR, Stryer DB, and Clancy CM. 2003. Practical clinical trials: Increasing the value of clinical research for decision making for clinical and health policy. *JAMA* 290 (12): 1623–32.

Vandenbroucke JP. 1987. A short note on the history of the randomized controlled trial. *J Chronic Dis* 40:985–86.

Vandenbroucke JP. 1998. Clinical investigation in the 20th century: The ascendency of numerical reasoning. *Lancet* 352 (Suppl. 2): 12–16.

Vollmann J and Winau R. 1996. Informed consent in human experimentation before the Nuremberg code. *BMJ* 313 (7070): 1445–49.

Weijer C and Fuchs A. 1994. The duty to exclude: Excluding people at undue risk from research. Review. *Clin Invest Med* 17 (2): 115–22.

Ethics and Clinical Research
(1966)

Henry K. Beecher, M.D.
Boston

Human experimentation since World War II has created some difficult problems with the increasing employment of patients as experimental subjects when it must be apparent that they would not have been available if they had been truly aware of the uses that would be made of them. Evidence is at hand that many of the patients in the examples to follow never had the risk satisfactorily explained to them, and it seems obvious that further hundreds have not known that they were subjects of an experiment although grave consequences have been suffered as a direct result of experiments described here. There is a belief prevalent in some sophisticated circles that attention to these matters would "block progress." But, according to Pope Pius XII,[1] ". . . science is not the highest value to which all other orders of values . . . should be subordinated."

I am aware that these are troubling charges. They have grown out of troubling practices. They can be documented, as I propose to do, by examples from leading medical schools, university hospitals, private hospitals, government military departments (the Army, the Navy and the Air Force), governmental institutes (the National Institute of Health), Veterans Administration hospitals and industry. The basis for the charges is broad.*

I should like to affirm that American medicine is sound, and most progress in it soundly attained. There is, however, a reason for concern in certain areas, and I believe the type of activities to be mentioned will do great harm to medicine unless soon corrected. It will certainly be charged that any mention of these matters does a disservice to medicine, but not one so great, I believe, as a continuation of the practices to be cited.

Experimentation in man takes place in several areas: in self-experimentation; in patient volunteers and normal subjects; in therapy; and in the different areas of *experimentation on a patient not for his benefit but*

---

*At the Brook Lodge Conference on "Problems and Complexities of Clinical Research" I commented that "what seem to be breaches of ethical conduct in experimentation are by no means rare, but are almost, one fears, universal." I thought it was obvious that I was by "universal" referring to the fact that examples could easily be found in *all* categories where research in man takes place to any significant extent. Judging by press comments, that was not obvious: hence, this note.

for that, at least in theory, of patients in general. The present study is limited to this last category.

Reasons for Urgency of Study

Ethical errors are increasing not only in numbers but in variety—for example, in the recently added problems arising in transplantation of organs.

There are a number of reasons why serious attention to the general problem is urgent.

Of transcendent importance is the enormous and continuing increase in available funds, as shown below.

Since World War II the annual expenditure for research (in large part in man) in the Massachusetts General Hospital has increased a remarkable 17-fold. At the National Institutes of Health, the increase has been a gigantic 624-fold. This "national" rate of increase is over 36 times that of the Massachusetts General Hospital. These data, rough as they are, illustrate the vast opportunities and concomitantly extended responsibilities.

Taking into account the sound and increasing emphasis of recent years that experimentation in man must precede general application of new procedures in therapy, plus the great sums of money available, there is reason to fear that these requirements in these resources may be greater than the supply of responsible investigators. All this heightens the problems under discussion.

Medical schools and university hospitals are increasingly dominated by investigators. Every young man knows that he will never be promoted to a tenured post, to a professorship in a major medical school, unless he has proved himself as an investigator. If the ready availability of money for conducting research is added to this fact, one can see how great the pressures are on ambitious young physicians.

Money Available for Research Each Year

	Massachusetts General Hospital	**National Institutes of Health***
1945	$ 500,000†	$ 701,800
1955	2,222,816	36,063,200
1965	8,384,342	436,600,000

*National Institutes of Health figures based upon decade averages, including funds for construction, kindly supplied by Dr. John Sherman of National Institutes of Health.

† Approximation, supplied by Mr. David C. Crockett, of Massachusetts General Hospital.

Implementation of the recommendations of the President's Commission on Heart Disease, Cancer and Stroke means that further astronomical sums of money will become available for research in man.

In addition to the foregoing three practical points there are others that Sir Robert Platt[2] has pointed out: a general awakening of social conscience; greater power for good or harm in new remedies, new operations and new investigative procedures than was formerly the case; new methods for preventive treatment with their advantages and dangers that are now applied to communities as a whole as well as to individuals, with multiplication of the possibilities for injury; medical science has shown how valuable human experimentation can be in solving problems of disease and its treatment; one can therefore anticipate an increase in experimentation; and the newly developed concept of clinical research as the profession (for example, clinical pharmacology)—and this, of course, could lead to unfortunate separation between the interests of science and the interests of the patient.

Frequency of Unethical or Questionably Ethical Procedures

Nearly everyone agrees that ethical violations do occur. A preliminary examination of the matter was based on 17 examples, which were easily increased to 50. These 50 studies contained references to 186 further likely examples, on the average 3.7 leads per study; they at times overlapped from paper to paper, but this figure indicates how conveniently one can proceed in a search for such material. The data are suggestive of widespread problems, but there is need for another kind of information, which was obtained by examination of 100 consecutive human studies published in 1964, in an excellent journal; 12 of these seemed to be unethical. If only one quarter of them is truly unethical, this still indicates the existence of a serious situation. Pappworth,[3] in England, has collected, he says, more than 500 papers based upon unethical experimentation. It is evident from such observations that unethical or questionably ethical procedures are not uncommon.

The Problem of Consent

All so-called codes are based on the bland assumption that meaningful or informed consent is readily available for the asking. As pointed out elsewhere,[4] this is very often not the case. Consent in any fully informed sense may not be obtainable. Nevertheless, except, possibly, in the most trivial situations, it remains a goal toward which one must strive for sociological, ethical and clear-cut legal reasons. There is no choice in the matter.

If suitably approached, patients will accede, on the basis of trust, to about any request their physician may make. At the same time, every experienced clinician investigator knows that patients will often submit to inconvenience and some discomfort, if they do not last very long, but the usual patient will never agree to jeopardize seriously his health or his life for the sake of "science."

In only 2 of the 50* examples originally compiled for this study was consent mentioned. Actually, it should be emphasized in all cases for obvious moral and legal reasons, but it would be unrealistic to place much dependence on it. In any precise sense statements regarding consent are meaningless unless one knows how fully the patient was informed of all risks, and if these are not known, that fact should also be made clear. A far more dependable safeguard than consent is the presence of a truly *responsible* investigator.

Examples of Unethical or Questionably Ethical Studies

These examples are not cited for the condemnation of individuals; they are recorded to call attention to a variety of ethical problems found in experimental medicine, for it is hoped that calling attention to them will help to correct abuses present. During ten years of study of these matters it has become apparent that thoughtlessness and carelessness, not a willful disregard of the patient's rights, account for most of the cases encountered. Nonetheless, it is evident that in many of the examples presented, the investigators have risked the health or the life of their subjects. No attempt has been made to present the "worst" possible examples; rather, the aim has been to show the variety of problems encountered.

References to the examples presented are not given, for there is no intention of pointing to individuals, but rather, a wish to call attention to widespread practices. All, however, are documented to the satisfaction of the editors of the *Journal*.

Known Effective Treatment Withheld

EXAMPLE 1. It is known that rheumatic fever can usually be prevented by adequate treatment of streptococcal respiratory infections by the parenteral administration of penicillin. Nevertheless, definitive treatment was withheld, and placebos were given to a group of 109 men in service, while benzathine penicillin G was given to others.

---

*Reduced here to 22 for reasons of space.

The therapy that each patient received was determined automatically by his military serial number arranged so that more men received penicillin than received placebo. In a small group of patients studied 2 cases of acute rheumatic fever and 1 of acute nephritis developed in the control patients, whereas these complications did not occur among those who received the benzathine penicillin G.

EXAMPLE 2. The sulfonamides were for many years the only antibacterial drugs effective in shortening the duration of acute streptococcal pharyngitis and in reducing its suppurative complications. The investigators in this study undertook to determine if the occurrence of the serious nonsupperative complications, rheumatic fever and acute glomerulonephritis, would be reduced by this treatment. This study was made despite the general experience that certain antibiotics, including penicillin, will prevent the development of rheumatic fever.

The subjects were a large group of hospital patients; a control group of approximately the same size, also with exudative Group A streptococcus, was included. The latter group received only nonspecific therapy (no sulfadiazine). The total group denied the effective penicillin comprised over 500 men.

Rheumatic fever was diagnosed in 5.4 per cent of those treated with sulfadiazine. In the control group rheumatic fever developed in 4.2 per cent.

In reference to this study a medical officer stated in writing that the subjects were not informed, did not consent and were not aware that they had been involved in the experiment, and yet admittedly 25 acquired rheumatic fever. According to this same medical officer *more than 70* who had known definitive treatment withheld were on the wards with rheumatic fever when he was there.

EXAMPLE 3. This involved the study of the relapse rate in typhoid fever treated in two ways. In an earlier study by the present investigators chloramphenicol had been recognized as an effective treatment for typhoid fever, being attended by half the mortality that was experienced when this agent was not used. Others had made the same observations, indicating that to withhold this effective remedy would be a life-or- death decision. The present study was carried out to determine the relapse rate under the two methods of treatment; of 408 charity patients, 251 were treated with chloramphenicol, of whom 20, or 7.97 per cent, died. Symptomatic treatment was given, but chloramphenicol was withheld in 157, of whom 36, or 22.9 per cent, died. According to the data presented, 23 patients died in the course of this study who would not have been expected to succumb if they had received specific therapy.

Study of Therapy

EXAMPLE 4. TriA (triacetyloleandomycin) was originally introduced for the treatment of infection with gram-positive organisms. Spotty evidence of hepatic dysfunction emerged, especially in children, and so the present study was undertaken on 50 patients, including mental defectives or juvenile delinquents who were inmates of a children's center. No disease other than acne was present; the drug was given for treatment of this. The ages of the subjects ranged from thirteen to thirty-nine years. "By the time half of the patients had received the drug for four weeks, the high incidence of significant hepatic dysfunction . . . led to the discontinuation of administration for the remainder of the group at three weeks." (However, only two weeks after the start of the administration of the drug, 54 per cent of the patients showed abnormal excretion of bromsulfalein.) Eight patients with marked hepatic dysfunction were transferred to the hospital "for more intensive study." Liver biopsy was carried out in these 8 patients and repeated in 4 of them. Liver damage was evident. Four of these hospitalized patients, after their liver-function tests returned to normal limits, received a "challenge" dose of the drug. Within two days hepatic dysfunction was evident in 3 of the 4 patients. In 1 patient a second challenge dose was given after the first challenge and again led to evidence of abnormal liver function. Flocculation tests remained abnormal in some patients as long as five weeks after discontinuance of the drug.

Physiologic Studies

EXAMPLE 5. In this controlled, double-blind study of the hematologic toxicity of chloramphenicol, it was recognized that chloramphenicol is "well known as the cause of aplastic anemia" and that there is a "prolonged morbidity and high mortality of aplastic anemia" and that ". . . chloramphenicol-induced aplastic anemia can be related to dose . . ." The aim of this study was "further definition of the toxicology of the drug . . ."

Forty-one randomly chosen patients were given either 2 or 6 gm. of chloramphenicol per day; 12 control patients were used. "Toxic bone-marrow depression, predominantly affecting erythropoiesis, developed in 2 of 20 patients given 2.0 gm. and in 18 of 21 given 6 gm. of chloramphenicol daily." The smaller dose is recommended for routine use.

EXAMPLE 6. In a study of the effect of thymectomy on the survival of skin homografts 18 children, 3 and a half months to eighteen years of age, about to undergo surgery for congenital heart disease, were selected. Eleven were to have total thymectomy as part of the operation, and 7 were to serve as controls. As part of the experiment, full-thickness skin homografts from an unrelated adult donor were secured to the chest wall in each case. (Total thymectomy is occasionally, although not usually part of the primary cardiovascular surgery involved, and whereas it may not greatly add to the hazards of the necessary operation, its eventual effects in children are not known.) This work was proposed as part of a long-range study of "the growth and development of these children over the years." No difference in the survival of the skin homograft was observed in the 2 groups.

EXAMPLE 7. This study of cyclopropane anesthesia and cardiac arrhythmias consisted of 31 patients. The average duration of this study was three hours, ranging from two to four and a half hours. "Minor surgical procedures" were carried out in all but 1 subject. Moderate to deep anesthesia, with endotracheal intubation and controlled respiration, was used. Carbon dioxide was injected into the closed respiratory system until cardiac arrhythmias appeared. Toxic levels of carbon dioxide were achieved and maintained for considerable periods. During the cyclopropane anesthesia a variety of pathologic cardiac arrhythmias occurred. When the carbon dioxide tension was elevated above normal, ventricular extrasystoles were more numerous than when the carbon dioxide tension was normal, ventricular arrhythmias being continuous in 1 subject for ninety minutes. (This can lead to fatal fibrillation.)

EXAMPLE 8. Since the minimum blood-flow requirements of the cerebral circulation are not accurately known, this study was carried out to determine "cerebral hemodynamic and metabolic changes . . . before and during acute reductions in arterial pressure induced by drug administration and/or postural adjustments." Forty-four patients whose ages varied from the second to the tenth decade were involved. They included normotensive subjects, those with essential hypertension and finally a group with malignant hypertension. Fifteen have abnormal electrocardiogram. Few details about the reasons for hospitalization are given.

Signs of cerebral circulatory insufficiency, which were easily recognized, included confusion and in some cases a nonresponsive state. By alteration in the tilt of the patient "the clinical state of the subject could be changed in a matter of seconds from one of alertness to confusion, and for the remainder of the flow, the subject was maintained in the latter state." The femoral arteries were cannulated in all subjects, and the internal jugular veins in 14.

The mean arterial pressure fell in 37 subjects from 109 to 48 mm. of mercury, with signs of cerebral ischemia. "With the onset of collapse, cardiac output and right ventricular pressures decreased sharply."

Since signs of cerebral insufficiency developed without evidence of coronary insufficiency the authors concluded that "the brain may be more sensitive to acute hypotension than is the heart."

EXAMPLE 9. This is a study of the adverse circulatory responses elicited by intra-abdominal maneuvers:

> When the peritoneal cavity was entered, a deliberate series of maneuvers was carried out [in 68 patients] to ascertain the effect of stimuli and the areas responsible for development of the expected circulatory changes. Accordingly, the surgeon rubbed localized areas of the parietal and visceral peritoneum with a small ball sponge as discretely as possible. Traction on the mesenteries, pressure in the area of the celiac plexus, traction on the gallbladder and stomach, and occlusion of the portal and caval veins were the other stimuli applied.

Thirty-four of the patients were sixty years of age or older; 11 were seventy or older. In 44 patients the hypotension produced by the deliberate stimulation was "moderate to marked." The maximum fall produced by manipulation was from 200 systolic, 105 diastolic, to 42 systolic, 20 diastolic; the average fall in mean pressure in 26 patients was 53 mm. of mercury.

Of the 50 patient studied, 17 showed either atrioventricular dissociation with nodal rhythm or nodal rhythm alone. A decrease in the amplitude of the T wave and elevation or depression of the ST segment were noted in 25 cases in association with manipulation and hypotension or, at other times, in the course of anesthesia and operation. In only 1 case was the change pronounced enough to suggest myocardial ischemia. No case of myocardial infarction was noted in the group studied although routine electrocardiograms were not taken after operation to detect silent infarcts. Two cases in which electrocardiograms were taken after operation showed T-wave and ST-segment changes that had not been present before.

These authors refer to a similar study in which more alarming electrocardiographic changes were observed. Four patients in the series sustained silent myocardial infarctions; most of their patients were undergoing gallbladder surgery because of associated heart disease. It can be added further that in the 34 patients referred to above as being sixty years of age or older, some doubtless had heart diseases that could have made risky the maneuvers carried out. In any event, this possibility might have been a deterrent.

EXAMPLE 10. Starling's law—"that the heart output per beat is directly proportional to the diastolic filling"—was studied in 30 adult patients with atrial fibrillation and mitral stenosis sufficiently severe to require valvulotomy. "Continuous alterations of the length of the segment of left ventricular muscle were recorded simultaneously in 13 of these patients by means of a mercury-filled resistance gauge sutured to the surface of the left ventricle." Pressures of the left ventricle were determined by direct puncture simultaneously with the segment length in 13 patients and without the segment length in an additional 13 patients. Four similar unanesthetized patients were studied through catheterization on the left side of the heart transeptally. In all 30 patients arterial pressure was measured through the catheterized brachial artery.

EXAMPLE 11. To study the sequence of ventricular contraction in human bundle-branch block, simultaneous catheterization of both ventricles was performed in 22 subjects; catheterization of the right side of the heart is carried out in the usual manner; the left side was catheterized transbronchially. Extrasystoles were produced by tapping on the epicardium in subjects with normal myocardium while they were undergoing thoracotomy. Simultaneous pressures were measured in both ventricles through needle puncture in this group.

The purpose of this study was to gain increased insight into the physiology involved.

EXAMPLE 12. This investigation was carried out to examine the possible effect of vagal stimulation on cardiac arrest. The authors had in recent years transected the homolateral vagus nerve immediately below the origin of the recurrent laryngeal nerve as palliation against cough and pain in bronchogenic carcinoma. Having been impressed with the number of reports of cardiac arrest that seem to follow vagal stimulation, they tested the effects of intrathoracic vagal stimulation during 30 of their surgical procedures, concluding, from these observations in patients under satisfactory anesthesia, that cardiac irregularities in cardiac arrest due to vagovagal reflex were less common than had previously been supposed.

EXAMPLE 13. This study presented a technic for determining portal circulation time in hepatic blood flow. It involved the transcutaneous injection of the spleen and catheterization of the hepatic vein. This was carried out in 42 subjects, of whom 14 were normal; 16 had cirrhosis (varying degrees), 9 acute hepatitis, and 4 hemolytic anemia.

No mention is made of what information was divulged to the subjects, some of whom were seriously ill. This study consisted in the development of a technic, not of therapy, in the 14 normal subjects.

Studies to Improve the Understanding of Disease

EXAMPLE 14. In this study of the syndrome of impending hepatic coma in patients with cirrhosis of the liver certain nitrogenous substances were administered to 9 patients with chronic alcoholism and advanced cirrhosis: ammonium chloride, di-ammonium citrate, urea or dietary protein. In all patients a reaction that included mental disturbances, a "flapping tremor" and electroencephalographic changes developed. Similar signs had occurred in only 1 of the patients before these substances were administered:

> The first sign noted was usually clouding of the consciousness. Three patients had a second or third course of administration of a nitrogenous substance with the same results. It was concluded that marked resemblance between this reaction and impending hepatic coma, implied that the administration of these [nitrogenous] substances to patients with cirrhosis may be hazardous.

EXAMPLE 15. The relation of the effects of ingested ammonia to liver disease was investigated in 11 normal subjects, 6 with acute virus hepatitis, 26 with cirrhosis, and 8 miscellaneous patients. Ten of these patients had neurologic changes associated with either hepatitis or cirrhosis.

The hepatic and renal veins were cannulated. Ammonium chloride was administered by mouth. After this, a tremor that lasted for three days developed in 1 patient. When ammonium chloride was ingested by 4 cirrhotic patients with tremor and mental confusion the symptoms were exaggerated during the test. The same thing was true of the fifth patient in another group.

EXAMPLE 16. This study was directed toward determining the period and activity of infectious hepatitis. Artificial induction of hepatitis was carried out in an institution for mentally defective children in which a mild form of hepatitis was endemic. The parents gave consent for the intramuscular injection or oral administration of the virus, but nothing is said regarding what was told them concerning the appreciable hazards involved.

A resolution adopted by the World Medical Association states explicitly: "Under no circumstances is a doctor permitted to do anything which would weaken the physical or mental resistance of a human being except from strictly therapeutic or prophylactic indications imposed in the interest of the patient." There is no right to risk an injury to 1 person for the benefit of others.

EXAMPLE 17. Live cancer cells were injected into 22 human subjects as part of this study of immunity to cancer. According to a recent review, the subjects (hospitalized patients) were "merely told they would be receiving 'some cells'"—". . . the word cancer was entirely omitted. . . ."

EXAMPLE 18. Melanoma was transplanted from a daughter to her volunteering and informed mother, "in the hope of gaining a better understanding of cancer immunity and in the hope that the production of tumor antibodies might be helpful in the treatment of the cancer patient." Since the daughter died on the day after the transplantation of the tumor into her mother, the hope expressed seems to have been more theoretical than practical, and the daughter's condition was described as "terminal" at the time the mother volunteered to be a recipient. The primary implant was widely excised on the twenty-fourth day after it had been placed in the mother. She died from metastatic melanoma on the four hundred and fifty-first day after transplantation. The evidence that this patient died of diffuse melanoma that metastasized from a small piece of transplanted tumor was considered conclusive.

Technical Study of Disease

EXAMPLE 19. During bronchoscopy a special needle was inserted through a bronchus into the left atrium of the heart. This was done in an unspecified number of subjects, both with cardiac disease and with normal hearts.

The technic was a new approach whose hazards were at the beginning quite unknown. The subjects with normal hearts were used, not for their possible benefit but for that of patients in general.

EXAMPLE 20. The percutaneous method of catheterization of the left side of the heart has, it is reported, led to 8 deaths (1.09 per cent death rate) and other serious accidents in 732 cases. There was, therefore, need for another method, the transbronchial approach, which was carried out in the present study in more than 500 cases, with no deaths.

Granted that a delicate problem arises regarding how much should be discussed with the patients involved in the use of the new method, nevertheless where the method is employed in a given patient for *his* benefit, the ethical problems are far less than when the potentially extremely dangerous method is used "in 15 patients with normal hearts, undergoing bronchoscopy for other reasons." Nothing was said about what was told any of the subjects, and nothing was said about the granting of permission, which was certainly indicated in the 15 normal subjects used.

EXAMPLE 21. This was a study of the effect of exercise on cardiac output and pulmonary-artery pressure in 8 "normal" persons (that is, patients whose diseases were not related to the cardiovascular system), in 8 with congestive heart failure severe enough to have recently required complete bed rest, in 6 with hypertension, in 2 with aortic insufficiency, in 7 with mitral stenosis and in 5 with pulmonary emphysema.

Intracardiac catheterization was carried out, and the catheter then inserted into the right or left main branch of the pulmonary artery. The brachial artery was usually catheterized; sometimes, the radial or femoral arteries were catheterized. The subjects exercised in a supine position by pushing their feet against weighted pedals. "The ability of these patients to carry on sustained work was severely limited by weakness and dyspnea." Several were in severe failure. This was not a therapeutic attempt but rather a physiologic study.

Bizarre Study

EXAMPLE 22. There is a question whether ureteral reflux can occur in the normal bladder. With this in mind, vesicourethrography was carried out on 26 normal babies less than forty-eight hours old. The infants were exposed to x-rays while the bladder was filling and during voiding. Multiple spot films were made to record the presence or absence of ureteral reflux. None was found in this group, and fortunately no infection followed the catheterization. What the results of the expensive x-ray exposure may be, no one can yet say.

Comment on Death Rates

In the foregoing examples a number of procedures, some with their own demonstrated death rates, were carried out. The following data were provided by 3 distinguished investigators in the field and represent widely held views.

CARDIAC CATHETERIZATION: right side of the heart, about 1 death per 1,000 cases; left side, 5 deaths per 1,000 cases. "Probably considerably higher in some places, depending on the portal of entry." (One investigator had 15 deaths in his first 150 cases.) It is possible that catheterization of a hepatic vein or renal vein would have a lower death rate than that of catheterization of the right side of the heart, for if it is properly carried out, only the atrium is entered en route to the liver or the kidney, not the right ventricle, which can lead to serious cardiac irregularities. There is always the possibility, however, that the ventricle will be entered inadvertently. This occurs in at least half of the cases, according to 1 expert— "but if properly done is too transient to be of importance."

LIVER BIOPSY: the death rate here is estimated at 2 to 3 per 1,000, depending in considerable part of the condition of the subject.

ANESTHESIA: the anesthesia death rate can be placed in general at about 1 death per 2,000 cases. The hazard is doubtless higher when certain practices such as deliberate evocation of ventricular extrasystoles under cyclopropane are involved.

Publication

In the view of the British Medical Research Council[5] it is not enough to ensure that all investigation is carried out in an ethical manner: it must be made unmistakably clear in the publications that the proprieties have been observed. This implies editorial responsibility in addition to the investigator's. The question rises, then, about valuable data that have been improperly obtained.* It is my view that such material should not be published.[5] There is a practical aspect to the matter: failure to obtain publication would discourage unethical experimentation. How many would carry out such experimentation if they *knew* its results would never be published? Even the suppression of such data (by not publishing it) would constitute a loss to medicine, in a specific localized sense, this loss, it seems, would be less important than the far-reaching moral loss to medicine if the data thus obtained were to be published. Admittedly, there is room for debate. Others believe that such data, because of their intrinsic value, obtained at a cost of great risk or damage to the subjects, should not be wasted but should be published with stern editorial comment. This would have to be done with exceptional skill, to avoid an odor of hypocrisy.

Summary and Conclusions

The ethical approach to experimentation and man has several components: two are more important than the others, the first being informed consent. The difficulty of obtaining this is discussed in detail. But it is absolutely essential to *strive* for it for moral, physiologic and legal reasons. The statement that consent has been obtained has little meaning unless the subject or his guardian is capable of understanding what is to be undertaken and unless all hazards are made clear. If these are not known this, too, should be stated. In such a situation the subject at least knows that he is to be a participant in an experiment. Secondly, there is the more reliable safeguard provided by the presence of an intelligent, informed, conscientious, compassionate, responsible investigator.

Ordinary patients will not knowingly risk their health or their life for the sake of "science." Every experienced clinician investigator knows this. When such risks are taken and a considerable number of patients are involved, it may be assumed that informed consent has not been obtained in all cases.

The gain anticipated from an experiment must be commensurate with the risk involved.

An experiment is ethical or not at its inception; it does not become ethical *post hoc*—ends do not justify means. There is no ethical distinction between ends and means.

In the publication of experimental results it must be made unmistakably clear that the proprieties have been observed. It is debatable whether

---

*As far as principle goes, a parallel can be seen in the recent Mapp decision by the United States Supreme Court. It was stated there that evidence unconstitutionally obtained cannot be used in any judicial decision, no matter how important the evidences to the ends of justice.

data obtained unethically should be published even with stern editorial comment.

SOURCE

Beecher HK. 1966. Ethics and clinical research. *N Engl J Med* 274 (24): 1354–60. Copyright 2006 *New England Journal of Medicine*. Reprinted with permission of the Massachusetts Medical Society.

Thalidomide and the Titanic: Reconstructing the Technology Tragedies of the Twentieth Century
(1999)

George J. Annas, JD, MPH, and Sherman Elias, MD

Abstract

The *Titanic* has become a metaphor for the disastrous consequences of an unqualified belief in the safety and invincibility of new technology. Similarly, the thalidomide tragedy stands for all of the "monsters" that can be inadvertently or negligently created by modern medicine. Thalidomide, once banned, has returned to the center of controversy with the Food and Drug Administration's (FDA's) announcement that thalidomide will be placed on the market for the treatment of erythema nodosum leprosum, a severe dermatological complication of Hansen's disease. Although this indication is very restricted, thalidomide will be available for off-label uses once it is on the market.

New laws regarding abortion and a new technology, ultrasound, make reasonable the approval of thalidomide for patients who suffer from serious conditions it can alleviate. In addition, the FDA and the manufacturer have proposed the most stringent postmarketing monitoring ever used for a prescription drug, including counseling, contraception, and ultra-sonography in the event of pregnancy.

The *Titanic*/thalidomide lesson for the FDA and public health is that rules and guidelines alone are not sufficient to guarantee safety. Continuous vigilance will be required to ensure that all reasonable postmarketing monitoring steps are actually taken to avoid predictable and preventable teratogenic disasters.

At the close of the 20th century, there seems to be a longing to make some sense of the century's most celebrated technological tragedies. The tragedies of the *Titanic* and thalidomide rank at or near the top in our pro-progress culture's consciousness of technological disasters. Each has had a much wider impact on the world than is reflected in the loss of life and limb, and each has come to stand for disaster caused by a combination of greed and overconfidence in technology.

The *Titanic*, of course, has become a metaphor for the disastrous consequences of an unqualified belief in the safety and invincibility of new technology.[1] Although only 1,500 people lost their lives when the ship went down, it was the total surprise the world felt at the sinking of this "unsinkable" ship that presaged the collapse of the old order of British invincibility and technological superiority. The *Titanic* probably was the safest passenger ship of its time, but human mistakes and overreliance on technology magnified the loss of life when the ship sank. Survivor Lawrence Beesley noted, reflecting on the tragedy and how similar tragedies might be avoided in the future, "The range of the wireless apparatus might be extended, but the principal defect is the lack of an operator for night duty on some ships. The awful fact that the *California* lay a few miles away, able to save every soul on board, and could not catch the message because the operator was asleep, seems too cruel to dwell upon."[2] The *Titanic* has, of course, been symbolically raised at century's end by its celebration in the most commercially successful film in history, *Titanic*, in which the story of the ship's sinking is reconstructed for our technological age. Even when the story is reconstructed with a "love conquers all" theme, we remain fascinated with the idea that nature, whether in the form of an iceberg, a tornado, a volcano, or an asteroid, can cause harm uncontrollable by technology.

The thalidomide tragedy of midcentury is much more recent than the *Titanic* tragedy, but it already stands for all of the deformities and "monsters" that can be inadvertently or negligently created by modem medicine.[3,4] Thalidomide's harm cannot be totally controlled. Nonetheless, through a combination of careful medical postmarketing monitoring and new laws, today thalidomide can be thought of as doing more good than harm. Thalidomide also holds wider postmarketing lessons for all drugs that carry potentially devastating dangers.

Thalidomide as Teratogen

The popular medical belief that the human fetus was protected from maternal drug exposures in the *sanctum sanctorum* of the uterus[5] was shattered in 1961 when Lenz[6] in Germany and McBride[7] in Australia independently suggested that prenatal exposure to thalidomide was the cause of serious birth defects. These abnormalities came to be known as thalidomide embryopathy, which includes amelia or phocomelia, cranial nerve palsies, microtia, choanal atresia, congenital heart defects (e.g., ductus, conotruncal defects), bowel atresias, gallbladder aplasia, and urogenital abnormalities.[8] Thalidomide was first introduced in Germany in 1958 as an anticonvulsive agent but was soon found unsuitable for this indication. Nonetheless, clinicians recognized that this drug was useful for a variety of other ailments, including morning sickness caused by pregnancy, hypertension, and migraines.[9] In the United States, Richardson-Merrill hoped ultimately to have thalidomide approved as an over-the-counter drug and planned to recommend it as treatment for myriad problems including alcoholism, anorexia, asthma, cancer, poor schoolwork, premature ejaculation, psychasthenia, and tuberculosis.[4]

By 1961, thalidomide was widely prescribed in Europe. Pregnant women in 48 countries took thalidomide, resulting in the live births of more than 8,000 affected infants.[4] Of infants exposed between days 35 and 48 after the last menstrual period, 20% to 30% had severe limb defects and other organ defects.[10,11] In the United States, the drug had failed to receive Food and Drug Administration (FDA) approval, not because of potential teratogenicity but because of concerns about peripheral neuropathy.[4] Even though Richardson-Merrill distributed more than 2.5 million thalidomide tablets to 1,267 physicians who gave them to some 20,000 patients in "clinical trials," only 17 affected infants were reported in the United States.[4] Once thalidomide was withdrawn from the market worldwide, affected infants continued to be born up to about May 1963 and very exceptionally beyond this date.[4,8] The drug's legalization in Brazil and use in South America, may, however, have resulted in at least 34 cases of thalidomide embryopathy since 1965.[12] The next chapter in history's most notorious human teratogen is about to be written.

New Indications for Thalidomide

Thalidomide has returned to the center of an emotionally charged controversy. On July 16, 1998, the FDA cleared thalidomide for marketing by a New Jersey-based pharmaceutical company, Celgene, Inc, for erythema nodosum leprosum, a severe dermatological complication of Hansen's disease (formerly known as leprosy).[13] Hansen's disease affects about 7,000 people in the United States, and approximately 50 of them are affected by erythema nodosum leprosum. The FDA has announced that thalidomide will be among the most tightly restricted drugs ever to be marketed in the United States.[14] The drug policy question is how strict these postmarketing approval controls should be.

Celgene, in cooperation with the FDA, has developed the System for Thalidomide Education and Prescribing Safety (STEPS) program. This program includes mandatory registration of all physicians who prescribe the medication and all patients who take it, as well as mandatory contraceptive measures for both males and females.[14] Women who take thalidomide must have a negative pregnancy test result, show proof that they are using 2 forms of contraception, and submit to monthly pregnancy tests (weekly in the first month).[14] Drawings of deformed infants must appear on every package of the drug. Both the patient and the physician must sign a document signifying that the patient understands the risks and is using contraception.[13,14] Prescriptions are limited to a 1-month supply. Whether thalidomide use in males affects sperm or fetal development is unknown, but males taking the drug will be counseled to use condoms when having intercourse with women of childbearing age.[14] Thalidomide causes not only birth defects but also peripheral neuropathy, and patients must be monitored to determine "how dose and use of the drug affects onset of this side effect and irreversibility."[14] These controls put thalidomide among the most stringently regulated drugs in the United States, but this may not be saying much.

Although thalidomide would be marketed for use in erythema nodosum leprosum, physicians would be able to prescribe it for so-called off-label uses (i.e., for other than erythema nodosum leprosum). For example, thalidomide has been shown to be effective in the treatment of oral aphthous ulcers of the mouth and oropharynx in patients with HIV infection.[15] Such ulcers can be extensive and debilitating, and thalidomide appears effective for pain relief and allows patients to eat and in some cases avoid a cachectic death. More than half of the patients with these ulcers are completely healed by 4 weeks of drug therapy, and almost 90% are at least partially healed.[15] Indeed, thalidomide appears to be so successful in oral aphthous ulcer treatment that within the last few years buyer's clubs have been purchasing the drug in Brazil, where it is legally available, and distributing it illegally to AIDS patients in the United States. Just as in the early 1960s, claims have also been made for the beneficial effects of thalidomide in many conditions, including macular degeneration, rheumatoid arthritis, diabetes mellitus, graft-vs-host disease following bone marrow transplants, autoimmune diseases, and some cancers. Thus, the off-label use of thalidomide may inevitably lead to exposure of many fetuses.

Risk-Benefit Analysis

Did the FDA properly weigh the risks and benefits of introducing thalidomide to the US market? The major risk is the inevitable tragedy that infants will again be born with the thalidomide embryopathy. Extensive regulations will be helpful but do not guarantee prevention of such births. The closest analogy is Accutane, an antiacne medication that can also cause severe birth defects.[16] The FDA tightly regulates its use. Nonetheless, up to 8 infants with isotretinoin-related malformations are born each year in the United States (A. A. Mitchell, oral communication, April 29, 1998).

Since the 1960s, a legal change and a technological development—*Roe v Wade*[17] and ultrasonography—have made thalidomide a "different" drug today. These 2 changes make it reasonable to treat thalidomide in a similar way to the other approximately 30 drugs that carry a serious risk to the fetus.[11] Since 1973 and the US Supreme Court's decision in *Roe v Wade*, American women have had a constitutional right to terminate their pregnancies prior to fetal viability. At the time that thalidomide failed to obtain FDA approval in the United States, abortion, with a few exceptions, was a crime. The thalidomide tragedy itself had a direct role in helping to change the public's attitude toward abortion. In late 1962, Sherri Chessen Finkbine read a newspaper article linking thalidomide to birth defects and later discovered that the "headache pills" her husband had obtained on a trip to England contained thalidomide.[18] Unable to have an abortion in Arizona, she ultimately flew to Sweden for the abortion of what turned out to be an affected fetus. Her story was widely publicized, and a Gallup poll conducted soon thereafter showed that 52% of Americans thought she had done the right thing.[18] Also, the major potential effect of thalidomide on the fetus is limb deformity, which can now be observed relatively early in pregnancy by ultrasound, a technology not available in the 1960s.

Any reasonable attempt to prevent the birth of infants with physical disabilities requires counseling patients who are taking thalidomide not to become pregnant and urging those in whom contraception fails either to discontinue the drug or to agree to have their fetuses evaluated for severe structural anomalies by high-resolution ultrasonography. Most major fetal malformations can be detected by ultrasonography, at least by 18 to 20 weeks' gestation. The final abortion decision, nonetheless, must be the woman's. Women, not the government, their employers, or their physicians, must make the final decisions about continuing or not continuing their pregnancies.[19]

The most compelling benefit of FDA approval of thalidomide is that it makes thalidomide available to patients who have conditions it can alleviate. In cases in which the suffering is great, no reasonable medical alternatives are available, and thalidomide is effective, the FDA is correct to conclude that its teratogenicity alone should not preclude its use. Women should not be denied effective therapy for severe existing disease solely because the therapy poses potentially severe risks to their fetuses. Because of thalidomide's teratogenicity, however, physicians have a responsibility not to prescribe it to fertile women unless no reasonable medical alternative exists, the condition being treated is serious, reliable contraception is used, and the woman is fully informed of the drug's risks and benefits. The American College of Obstetricians and Gynecologists (ACOG) also concluded that neither thalidomide nor any drug should be prevented from being introduced or withdrawn from the market solely because it is teratogenic. Instead, ACOG strongly supports efforts to prevent exposure to known teratogenic agents in women who are pregnant or contemplating pregnancy.[20]

Thalidomide's resurrection provides an opportunity to determine whether some drugs are potentially so dangerous that their use should be restricted to the conditions for which the drug is FDA approved. So far this opportunity has been missed, but the birth of even one affected infant from off-label use will undoubtedly provoke this debate. As long as off-label uses are permitted, the FDA should insist not only that prescriptions for such uses be subject to the FDA's safeguards for approved uses but also that patients be informed that thalidomide has not been approved for the off-label use contemplated.

Approval of thalidomide is consistent with other FDA drug approvals. Many valuable drugs have potential teratogenicity, including warfarin, lithium, angiotensin-converting enzyme inhibitors, nonsteroidal antiinflammatory drugs, aminoglycosides, immunosuppressants, and antineoplastic drugs.[10,11] Even the Thalidomide Victims Association of Canada agreed to help Celgene obtain FDA approval for thalidomide, so long as steps are taken to fully inform physicians and patients and to try to prevent harm to fetuses. The organization successfully resisted thalidomide's being given a totally new name (Celgene wanted to call it Synovir; it will be marketed as Thalomid) and got the labeling changed from "Avoid pregnancy" to "Do not get pregnant."[21]

Learning from Tragedies

Not all tragedies can be redeemed, but we can learn from all tragedies. The FDA has the responsibility to ensure that thalidomide is safely introduced in the United States. But physicians and their patients must share responsibility for its proper use. Only if everyone meets these responsibilities is there a realistic opportunity to obtain the benefits of thalidomide and to minimize the risks by preventing birth defects. The FDA, for example, has recently been severely criticized for its performance in postmarketing monitoring of drug safety.[22, 23] As more and more powerful drugs are approved for marketing, it has become apparent that much more careful postmarketing monitoring is needed than has been tolerated to date. In the absence of careful monitoring, many powerful drugs—such as the new diabetes drug troglitazone, which can cause severe liver toxicity—would have to be banned as unsafe.[24] Physicians have a central role in postmarketing monitoring and should prescribe thalidomide only after determining that it is the best drug for a serious condition and counseling fertile women patients to avoid pregnancy. And fertile women should take all reasonable steps to avoid pregnancy while taking thalidomide.

The *Titanic* can be reconstructed as myth but not raised intact (it is in 2 pieces). Thalidomide, because of changes in both law and medical technology, can be raised from its mythical monster drug status and reintroduced as a therapeutic component of modern medicine. Like preventing death at sea, preventing thalidomide-affected births will require not only medical technology but also human alertness. The decision to use thalidomide should be based on a realistic assessment of risks and benefits, as well as specific FDA, physician, and patient action to minimize predictable harm to fetuses.

The major lesson that the *Titanic* disaster holds regarding thalidomide is that wrapping a tragedy in the myth of a love story can obscure its horror and transform a tragic lesson into entertainment. FDA approval of thalidomide itself comes packaged as a mythical, although somewhat more complex, love story. Randy Warren, an affected child of a mother who took the drug, has dramatically argued in support of FDA approval: "Our hearts tell us this [thalidomide] did horrible things to our mothers and to ourselves, but our heads tell us 'How can we deny it to people who are suffering?'" [21] The myth, of course, is that society and the FDA have ever cared deeply about the suffering of people with Hansen's disease, when historically the United States has isolated "lepers" in "leper colonies" and left them to fend for themselves with the help of private charity.[25] Similarly, women with AIDS in the United States were denied zidovudine for years because of the fear that it was teratogenic.

Society is perfectly capable of being indifferent to human suffering and would continue to be in this instance if a private corporation, Celgene, had not thought it could profit from manufacturing and selling thalidomide. Ignoring commercial and profit motives here could lead to complacency in monitoring and result in the same type of disaster as the sinking of the *Titanic*. The *Titanic*'s owners reduced the number of lifeboats to save money, and the crew was unfamiliar with their operation.[1] The *Titanic*/thalidomide lesson for the FDA and public health is that continuous vigilance is required to ensure that all reasonable steps are taken to avoid predictable and preventable disasters. For the safety of the public's health, this broad lesson should be applied by the FDA, physicians, and drug companies to require rigorous postmarketing monitoring of all new and potentially dangerous drugs.

SOURCE

Annas GJ and Elias S. 1999. Thalidomide and the Titanic: Reconstructing the technology tragedies of the twentieth century. *Am J Public Health* 89:98–101. Copyright 1999 *American Journal of Public Health*. Reprinted with permission of American Public Health Association.

Kidneys, Ethics, and Politics: Policy Lessons of the ESRD Experience
(1981)

Arthur L. Caplan, The Hastings Center

Abstract

This article examines the policy lessons to be learned from the American experience with the End-Stage Renal Disease program. This program was instituted in 1972 as an amendment to the Social Security Act to provide reimbursement for the costs of therapy to those persons suffering from renal failure. The article tries to debunk certain common myths that have arisen concerning the ESRD program, by examining the history and evolution of renal dialysis technology as well as the social policies concerning dialysis pursued in England and Sweden. It argues that while the ESRD program is not a genuine instance of a 'mini' national health insurance program, there are important moral, social, and policy lessons to be learned from this unique effort to provide renal therapies to those Americans in need.

The Medical Treatment of End-stage Renal Disease— What Are the Policy Issues?

In 1972 Congress passed Public Law 92-603 as an amendment to the Medicare and Medicaid provisions of the Social Security Act. Under the bill persons suffering from end-stage renal disease (ESRD) were guaranteed special federal coverage for the costs of their treatment. The ESRD program now covers approximately 50,000 patients at a cost of over one billion dollars per year for various forms of renal therapy, primarily dialysis and kidney transplantation.[1] While ESRD patients currently constitute about 0.2 percent of the total Medicare population, they account for 5 percent of all Medicare expenditures.[2]

The ESRD program was viewed by many of its proponents and opponents at the time of its inception as a first step toward a national health insurance program for all Americans. As former Secretary of Health, Education, and Welfare, Joseph Califano noted in Congressional hearing on the ESRD program in 1977:[3]

> While there have been and continue to be problems in the administration and evaluation of the ESRD program, we have gained

valuable experience that will help us as we consider options for a National Health Insurance proposal. For the ESRD program is, in fact, a miniature National Health Insurance program for those with a specific life-threatening illness.

The policy dispute over the feasibility of some form of national health insurance for all Americans has been greatly influenced by the "experience" of the ESRD program. Critics of such proposals use the ESRD experience to argue that federal reimbursement for health care services would be much too expensive and too inefficient to be affordable or desirable. Proponents of national health insurance argue that the ESRD program delivers necessary services to those who could not afford to purchase them from their personal income, and that thousands of lives have been saved as the direct result of government intervention in the financing of health care, both in America and in other countries.

A good deal of philosophical attention has focused on the issues of resource allocation that surrounded the provision of renal dialysis and renal transplants prior to 1972. Proposed criteria for deciding who should get the scarce kidney or kidney machine abound in the ethics literature.[4] Yet, despite all the analytical attention that has been given to establishing criteria for micro-allocation of therapies for renal failure, little attention has been paid in the existing philosophical literature to the ethical and policy implications at the macro-allocative level of ESRD. Moreover, the analysis of the history and evolution of renal therapy in the United States and other countries raises serious questions as to the legitimacy and relevance of many of the discussions concerning allocating scarce medical sources.[5] There are solid grounds for skepticism concerning many of the discussions of the ethics of resource allocation in health care, since these presume that renal dialysis and kidney transplantation were, in the late 1960s, accurately characterized as both the established and sole forms of therapy available to individuals afflicted with renal failure.[6]

This paper will try to show that during the late 1960s and early 1970s, when ethical discussion of the allocation of renal therapies flourished in the popular press and in professional journals, renal dialysis and kidney transplantation occupied an ambiguous status somewhere between experiment and therapy in the minds of many health professionals. This ambiguity had much more influence over micro-allocation decisions than did any specific normative theory of micro-allocation. To ignore the conceptual and empirical ambiguities surrounding the evolution of both renal therapies and the ESRD reimbursement program is to run the risk of providing an ethical and policy analysis that simply misses the mark in terms of correctly framing the moral issues surrounding the care of those suffering from renal failure.

An exclusive focus on the morality of micro-allocation with regard to renal dialysis and transplantation also ignores the crucial role played by the ESRD experience in influencing the current policy debate over national health insurance.[7] While no one would deny that the ESRD program provides medically necessary services to people in dire need, the enormous costs associated with this program leave open the policy questions of how others with either equally pressing medical needs, or more ambiguous needs, can hope to have them fulfilled by any possible form of governmentally-backed insurance.[8]

Four questions loom especially large in assessing the moral and policy implications of the ESRD experience in the past twenty years:

1. Is the ESRD program a 'good' prototype of a National Health Insurance program? 'Good' here meaning the degree to which the ESRD program represents:
   (a) the expected costs of a more comprehensive national health program of some type;
   (b) the expected costs of therapies for noncontroversial health care needs.

2. Can useful inferences be drawn from the history of ESRD treatment and funding for future planning in other areas of health treatment and funding?

3. Is the experience of other countries with ESRD treatment and funding similar or dissimilar to the American experience, and is this experience properly understood by American health planners?

4. What does the case of ESRD reveal about the difficulties surrounding the normative analysis of issues in health policy?

A Set of Myths and Misapprehensions about Renal Dialysis and Renal Transplant

It is important to realize that a significant mythology has somehow arisen about the history, costs, and funding of ESRD.[9] Some of the most common myths are:

1. The increase in the number of persons in America now receiving renal dialysis therapy is attributable *solely* to the availability of funding.[10]

2. The allocation of the supply of renal dialysis and transplants is contingent upon the availability of funds to reimburse medical professionals for these services.[11] Countries with socialized systems of

medical care never did and do not now exclude persons in need from the supply of treatments for renal failure.[12]

3. The needs of persons determine the nature of the health care supply that is available.

4. The current cost of treatment for renal failure is simply a result of the need for treatment rising to meet the availability of federal funds.[13]

The easiest way to debunk these elements of the mythology surrounding ESRD is to review the history of the technology and its funding. If some headway can be made in this enterprise, a more realistic and reasonable assessment can then be made of the ESRD program and the lessons of this program for health policy in general.

A Brief History of Renal Dialysis Technology

One of the most puzzling gaps in the current normative analyses of the ESRD program is the lack of attention to the key role of technological evolution in micro- and macro-allocative decisions. As new technologies appear and evolve in medicine, the criteria for allocating these technologies shift and evolve as well. The history of chronic renal dialysis therapy contains at least four stages of development: invention, advertising, acceptance, and mastery. Allocation policies cannot be understood or analyzed without being placed in the context of this sequence.

Invention

Artificial kidney machines capable of removing waste materials from blood existed in the years following the Second World War. By 1950 several American medical centers had functioning artificial kidney machines.[14] These machines were used to "rest" the kidneys of diseased patients in the hope that the rest would allow malfunctioning kidneys to regain their normal function.

The major technological problem confronting patients interested in a mechanical kidney was access to their circulatory systems rather than access to the machine itself. The use of the artificial kidney machine required the insertion of tubes or cannulas into an artery and a vein. Since each treatment destroyed an accessible artery and vein, physicians using the artificial kidney quickly ran out of usable sites for gaining access to a patient's circulation. Thus, artificial kidneys could only be used as therapies to treat acute cases of renal failure. Chronic filtration of the blood was impossible.

The problem of circulatory access remained unsolved until the invention of the arterio-venous shunt by Belding Scribner of the University of Washington in 1959. As Richard Rettig has correctly noted, "This was the critical technological invention that ushered in the use of the artificial kidney to maintain the lives of those suffering from chronic kidney failure."[15]

Scribner realized[16] that by placing a permanent tube or shunt between an accessible artery and vein, blood circulation to these vessels could be maintained while permitting continuous access to the general circulation. The subcutaneous shunt could simply be removed for short periods of time and replaced by a shunt leading to the kidney machine. By permanently "short-circuiting" the circulation in an artery and vein through a shunt, a permanent access site could be maintained in place in a chronically ill person.

Scribner's shunt entirely changed the nature of medical intervention for renal failure. What had formerly been only an acute therapy for both acute and chronic renal failure now became a potential chronic therapy for cases of chronic[17] disability.

Advertising

Scribner spent the next three years, from 1959 to 1962, disseminating his new invention to the medical community. He made presentations at various medical society meetings and brought samples of his shunt with him to demonstrate to interested colleagues.[18] A steady procession of young physicians came to Seattle from around the country to study Scribner's technique.[19]

One of the most active participants in this form of advertising the new shunt technology was the hospital system of the Veterans Administration (VA). In 1963 the VA announced a program for establishing dialysis centers in thirty VA hospitals around the country.[20] This was a critical step in the course of disseminating renal dialysis treatment for chronic renal failure, for many physicians in renal medicine received training in VA hospitals and learned to perform dialytic therapy in the setting of chronic care institutions. Since the VA population is primarily institution-based, it was reasonable for the VA to ask for funds for the construction of renal dialysis units in VA hospitals.

By 1968 about 1,000 people were receiving long-term renal dialysis in the United States,[21] and thousands of other persons could have benefitted from it. A number of persons were trained or in training to learn to administer chronic dialysis.

Acceptance

By 1968 the first of what eventually became a torrent of articles was published on the normative issues of allocating renal dialysis machines.[22] Only nine years had passed since Scribner's invention of the arterio-venous shunt and only six years had passed since the shunt was advertised among health professionals. The short time from Scribner's invention to the first article on the ethics of micro-allocation is significant since this entire period was one in which renal dialysis (and transplantation) held a rather ambiguous status in the eyes of the medical profession.

Some physicians were convinced that dialysis for chronic renal failure was a legitimate medical therapy. Scribner's initial success had made dialysis appear to some funding agencies to be more a proven therapy than an experimental procedure. Research grants were difficult to obtain for a procedure that seemed to require only the provision of treatment to persons in need.[23]

But other physicians remained unconvinced and adopted the attitude that dialysis (and transplantation) were better understood as experimental procedures.[24] Scribner had obtained good results using his shunt with his own patients during this period, but physicians at other centers had encountered problems in matching his favorable morbidity and mortality rates. And the art of carrying out renal dialysis was slow to evolve, partly due to the small number of persons capable of carrying out dialysis, and partly because of insufficient research funds.

One other factor that played a key role in the medical profession's skeptical attitude toward dialysis during the 1960s was that dialysis was in direct competition with other techniques for treating renal failure.[25] Renal transplantation, from living and cadaver donors, held out great promise as a less costly[26] and less disruptive treatment. While immuno-logical rejection posed great difficulties for transplant proponents, many believed that this problem could be solved, and that a transplant would be far more attractive to potential patients than a long course of weekly dialysis sessions.

The debate over the experimental status of renal dialysis was not" officially"[27] settled until 1967, when the influential government commission, The Committee on Chronic Kidney Disease, headed by Dr. C. W. Gottschalk, issued a report that stated:[28]

> The Committee believes that transplantation and dialysis techniques are sufficiently perfected at present to warrant launching a national treatment program and urges this course of action. . . . Approximately 5,000 patients with chronic uremia died in fiscal year 1967 because of a lack of adequate treatment facilities and by 1973, when

treatment capabilities may meet demand, a minimum of 24,000 additional medically suitable patients will have died without the opportunity for treatment . . .

Mastery

The fourth and last stage in the evolution and development of renal dialysis took place from 1968 to about 1977. During this period the iatrogenic effects of chronic renal dialysis were observed and techniques were developed to avoid them. While dialysis had been employed as a temporary procedure for persons in acute renal failure since the early 1950s, the technique had not been used as a treatment for *chronic* renal failure. From 1968 to 1977 enough patient-hours were accumulated on dialysis machines to detect a number of complications and side effects of chronic treatment. Imbalances in metabolites, anemia, hepatitis, cardiovascular anomalies, neuropathy, hypertension, psychiatric problems, and osteodystrophy all emerged as problems directly attributable to chronic renal dialysis.[29] Various techniques evolved for coping with these problems, ranging from alternating the length and frequency of dialysis to providing supplementary salts and metabolites to those receiving dialysis.[30]

The differences between the acceptance and mastery stages in the evolution of renal dialysis are worth emphasizing. At the end of the third stage, in 1968, Scribner's shunt had gained acceptance among the medical community. A sizable number of trained medical personnel and a fair number of dialysis centers, in the VA hospitals and elsewhere, existed to provide dialysis, but only about 1,000 persons were receiving dialysis, and few had been in dialysis for more than five years. By 1977, however, 35,000 persons were receiving dialysis in the United States, and many had been on dialysis for ten years or more.[31]

A significant amount of time was needed to move from the stage where chronic dialysis was accepted as a legitimate therapy by the medical profession, to the stage at which the medical profession could legitimately be said to have mastered the technique. These stages are crucial for understanding the normative criteria that influenced patient selection during the history of renal dialysis therapy.

Who Got the Kidney Machine?

From 1959 to 1977 the pool of persons receiving dialysis for chronic renal failure expanded rapidly. So did the number of personnel prepared to offer dialysis and the number of sites at which dialysis could be obtained.

Perhaps the most marked shift in the composition of the recipient pool for chronic dialysis in the United States took place between the period of acceptance of the technique in the late 1960s and mastery of the technique in the late 1970s. In the late 1960s, the majority of dialysis recipients were young (25 to 45), middle-class persons with no other illnesses. In the words of a physician, "We had what was in many ways an idealized population. A large fraction of the patients were living in a productive period of their lives. They were young and had little else wrong with them."[32]

By the late 1970s, however, the patient pool had shifted considerably. Recipients were often either much older or much younger than in the 1960s. Age and complicating diseases, such as diabetes or alcoholism, were rarely invoked as contraindications for chronic dialysis. Many more poor and minority persons received dialysis.[33]

The shift in the composition of the patient population for dialysis is usually attributed to the ethical biases of physicians in the selection of dialysis recipients, and to the availability of funds for chronic dialysis after 1972.[34] But the history of renal dialysis therapy clearly reveals a number of other factors at work in influencing the composition of the patient pool over the years. Fewer centers and trained personnel existed in the 1960s. Physicians in the 1960s had not fully mastered the technique of chronic dialysis, having had no experience with its possible side effects. And chronic renal dialysis was a treatment in competition with other treatments for renal failure during much of the 1960s. In such circumstances, the desires of dialysis specialists, both for success as compared to alternative therapies, and for mastery over complications, greatly influenced the type of patients they selected. In 1967 physicians wanted "healthy" patients, since a good track record and a "clean" data sample were essential to both competitive success and technical mastery. In 1977 neither of these concerns carried as much weight.

A Short History of Federal Funding for ESRD

In 1972 Congress passed Public Law 92-603 as an amendment to the Social Security Act. Under this law Medicare coverage was extended to those under 65 suffering from end-stage renal disease.

The portion of the law concerning ESRD was passed with little debate or analysis. Few cost estimates were obtained and no study of possible supply options was undertaken. The highlight of the legislative process prior to the passage of the law was the dialysis of the vice-president of the National Association of Patients on Hemodialysis and Transplantation before the House Ways and Means Committee in November of 1971. The actual amendment was passed after thirty minutes of debate in the Senate and ten minutes in the House in October of 1972.[35]

The need for therapy for ESRD seemed clear to the legislators. All that stood between the 24,000 untreated persons cited in the Gottschalk Report and life was money.[36] Renal patients and physicians wanted the law passed and lobbied for it. In addition, the ESRD program was only an amendment to much larger Medicare/Medicaid program.

The bill provided reimbursement for renal therapy to "kidney disease centers" which met minimal standards for utilization and admission. Physicians were paid a fixed fee per month for a kidney patient seen in a center, a lower fee for patients treated at home. Reimbursement fees were also set for overhead center costs. No limits were set on total reimbursement expenditures for the ESRD programs.[37]

One immediate effect of the bill was to encourage the creation of dialysis centers, both in and out of medical centers. With reimbursement available at maximum rates for center dialysis, efforts to encourage home dialysis and self-dialysis waned. In 1972, 40 percent of all patients were being dialyzed in their homes. This percentage fell to 15 percent by 1978.[38]

Extracts from the European Experience with ESRD: Britain and Sweden

The British experience with ESRD has differed to some extent from the American. Britain has had a national health insurance scheme in place since 1946. However, confronted by the large costs of renal therapy, the Department of Health and Social Security took the unusual step of getting a cap on the total amount of money available for renal failure. In the words of their 1971 report:[39]

> We actually set aside a sum of money which we told the Hospitals Boards should be spent on dialysis and we determined where it should be spent and how much should be spent. At this time this was a great change from our normal method of control and indeed we have hardly repeated it since.
>
> This cap on total expenditures had the effect of increasing the percentage of patients in Britain on home as opposed to center dialysis. In 1976, 66 percent of all patients in the United Kingdom were receiving home dialysis.[40]

A most interesting aspect of the British experience with ESRD is that despite the availability of government funds for ESRD, the number and composition of the population of patients receiving dialysis and transplants closely parallels the American experience. In the invention and advertising stages, British physicians were as selective as their American counterparts in placing patients in renal failure on dialysis. Four out of five candidates were rejected. The average patient was middle-aged, male, married, working, and owned his own home.[41] As in America, the small number of trained personnel and the scarcity of dialysis equipment undoubtedly caused the rationing of treatment.

The acceptance stage of renal technology showed many parallels as well. Victor Parsons, chief nephrologist at King's College Hospital in London, in commenting about dialysis in the late 1960s writes:[42]

> Individual desire to go on living or the desire to be treated [for renal failure] was not considered. . . . Very often the patients were unaware they were up for selection. This enabled the renal units to achieve high survival rates, and quite rightly since in the early stages it was important that the treatment should be seen in its best possible light. To have adopted a totally non-selective policy at the outset would have led the technique into disrepute as being nothing but a technical exercise in the prolongation of a very poor quality of life.

Technological and scientific concerns with demonstrating the superiority, efficacy, and safety of dialysis were as much on the minds of British physicians operating under a socialized system of health care as they were on the minds of American physicians under a fee-for-service system.

As the technology of dialysis passed from the stage of acceptance to that of mastery during the 1970s, the pool of dialysis patients in Britain quickly expanded. More centers were built and professional staff trained. The tacitly agreed-upon maximum age for dialysis treatment rose from 45 in 1963 to 60 in 1978.[43] The financial limits imposed by the cap on overall funding for dialysis continues to discourage British physicians from dialyzing those over 60.[44]

The patterns of dialysis allocation manifested in the British experience strongly highlight the role of technological evolution in determining the composition of the patient pool. Technological and scientific considerations play just as central a role in understanding micro-allocation decisions in the socialized health care system of Britain as they did in the fee-for-service system in the United States.

Further evidence for the role of technology evolution in allocation is provided by the Swedish experience with dialysis. The number and nature of persons receiving treatment over the past twenty years parallels that in the United States despite the availability of public funds. In the 1960s, Swedish physicians were highly selective in admitting persons for dialysis. As a recent review of the state of renal therapy in Sweden notes:[45]

... it became a question for nephrologists who had commenced or planned to start long-term dialysis treatment, not only to show that the therapy can prolong life but also that these patients can be rehabilitated, i.e., care for their families and be able to work and pay their taxes. This is in itself remarkable as previously no such criteria had been established to justify the treatment of chronically ill patients.

And, as in the United States and United Kingdom, the shift of renal dialysis from the stage of acceptance in the 1960s to mastery in the 1970s[46]

has led to a slackening of the previously strict requirements for complete rehabilitation. Nowadays even patients who do not measure up to these requirements—such as the elderly and patients with severe complicating illnesses—are considered for active treatment.

Popular Mythology Revisited

Before returning to the general issues raised at the beginning of this article, the five popular myths underlying many discussions of the implications of ESRD for health policy deserve some comment. The history of funding and technology in the area of ESRD is in conflict with all of them.

1. *The increase in the number of persons receiving renal dialysis is attributable solely to the availability of funds.* This statement is false for a number of reasons. The increase in patient numbers is attributable to shifts in the status of renal dialysis, from invention to acceptance as a therapy, and from acceptance to mastery of the therapy by the medical profession. The British and Swedish experiences with ESRD plainly reveal that factors other than government funding have been at work in expanding the pool of persons receiving dialysis.

2. *The allocation of the supply of renal dialysis (and transplants) is contingent upon the availability of funds to reimburse medical professionals for these services.* This claim is false since the supply available for meeting health needs is contingent on much more than money. Scientific and technological concerns affect both the nature of the supply (home dialysis, center dialysis, or transplants) and who gets the supply (young, old, healthy, etc.). The mode of funding may affect the degree to which some patients receive treatment (spending caps in Britain produce a mode of supply that excludes persons over 60).

3. *Countries with socialized systems of medical care never did and do not now exclude patients from treatment for renal failure.* While this claim is be-

lieved by many health planners and critics of the American health care system, it is quite false. Rationing existed in Britain and Sweden in a form similar to that which existed in the United States and which continues to exist in Britain today.[47]

4. *The needs of persons determine the nature of the health care supply that is available.* This statement is false because it overlooks the role played by technological evolution in determining the nature and kind of available health care. Technological competition plays a key role in determining the nature of the health care supply. The mode of health care funding also determines supply. Incentives for center dialysis in America have produced a very different supply for renal therapy than that available in Britain.

5. *The current cost of the supply for those in need due to renal failure is simply a result of need rising to meet the availability of federal funds to pay the costs.* While many health policy analysts appear to believe this statement,[48] the ESRD experience shows that it is simply not true. The rise in the cost of renal dialysis was not due solely to supply rising to meet the windfall of federal dollars.

The high costs of treatment of ESRD can also be attributed to the nature and timing of the availability of federal funds. By funding the ESRD program in 1972, the government paid for a technology that was still midway between acceptance and mastery. The cost of "working the bugs out" of dialysis was paid by Medicare. The cost of expanding the number of centers and the numbers of trained personnel to staff them was also borne by the United States taxpayer in the form of amortized costs included in treatment fees. The real policy issue arising from the ESRD program, which the fifth myth overlooks, is at what point (if ever) should the federal government pay for new technologies in medicine—at the time of invention, acceptance, or mastery?

Finally, it is not true that the need for dialysis simply expanded. What happened was that the mastery of renal dialysis technology allowed the medical profession to accept a wider pool of candidates for dialysis. Today, as medicine tries to deal with renal failure in poorer nations, the cost of the supply for persons in these areas has actually begun to drop![49]

The Lessons of the ESRD Experience

The ESRD program is not a good prototype for or mini-experiment in national health insurance. Most forms of medical services available today reached the stage of mastery by the medical profession decades ago. Unlike renal dialysis, one would not have to include the high costs of advertising or mastery in covering standard medical regimens under a national health insurance program. In the case of renal dialysis the technology and the funding for it evolved simultaneously. But one would not have to anxiously await the development of costly new technologies in most areas of medicine. Nor would it be necessary to build buildings, train personnel, and perfect techniques—happily, we do not have to start from near scratch in planning the reimbursement of most medical therapies.

The British experience with dialysis funding cannot be overlooked in thinking about the costs of national health insurance. Open-ended funding produces much higher costs in the form of more costly modes of supply. Yet capping the total amount of funds available for any given evolving therapy runs the very real risk that no mode of therapy will emerge that can meet the needs of all patients.

The issue facing any national health insurance program is the stance it will adopt toward new and evolving medical therapies. The problem is that our knowledge of technological evolution is so poor that it is hard to classify or analyze the state of particular treatments. Since need and demand are not the sole determinants of cost, our ignorance about the way in which various modes of medical therapy evolve is a major stumbling block for anticipating the ultimate cost of any national health insurance program.[50] It is hard to anticipate the cost of treating medical needs when the evolutionary status of various treatments is controversial and the possibility exists that treatments not possible today could be possible in five or ten years.

There is also an important lesson in the ESRD experience for those concerned with the ethics of health care. Much of the literature on the ethics of micro-allocation in the area of dialysis and transplant simply misses the mark. By ignoring the history of renal technology and funding, philosophers and theologians have managed to give some very convincing answers to the wrong question.[51] The question is not who should get the kidney machine. In thinking about the normative issues surrounding ESRD, the questions are: who should pay for developing and disseminating new medical therapies, and how should ethical and scientific considerations influence the allocation of newly evolved technologies?

Serious problems surround the history of decision-making and public policy regarding ESRD. The government bought a still-developing treatment when it thought it had purchased a mastered therapy. This error has been a very expensive one, not only in terms of the large costs of paying for center dialysis for a tiny percentage of the population, but in terms of the damage done to the prospects for discussing *some* form of national health insurance. There may be nothing that can be done about the former cost. But this need not be true of the latter, if we really can learn from the experience of ESRD.

The author gratefully acknowledges the support of the Education Division of the National Endowment for the Humanities and the Henry J. Kaiser Family Foundation in the writing of this article.

SOURCE

Caplan AL. 1981. Kidneys, Ethics, and Politics: Policy Lessons of the ESRD Experience. *Journal of Health Politics, Policy and Law* 6 (3): 488–501. Copyright 1981 Department of Health Administration, Duke University. Reproduced with permission of Duke University Press.

CHAPTER 15

GLOBAL HEALTH

The landscape of public health is complex and rapidly changing. The challenges are unprecedented. But this landscape also reveals a spirit of global solidarity and a strong desire for fairness in health. And this gives us an occasion for unprecedented optimism as well.

> —Dr. Margaret Chan (b. 1947), Director General of the World Health Organization
> Singapore, April 3, 2007

ALTHOUGH THE GREEKS WERE KNOWN for hygiene and the Romans for their public works, modern man had a much harder time learning not to foul his nest. The economic engine of the Industrial Revolution needed the balance of the Sanitary Revolution to bring both hygiene and public works back as respectable concepts to maintain the public's health (see Volume I, Part II). Twentieth-century man's devotion to technology sometimes blinded him to simple solutions and in some instances made problems worse. For example, the Green Revolution of the mid twentieth century expanded marginal lands for agriculture and introduced new seed stocks for high yields. Although some geographic areas benefited in terms of increased agricultural production, others were ecologically devastated, and the gap between the developed and developing worlds widened. Another example is that of the Bacteriologic Revolution, which led many in the early twentieth century to believe mankind could finally control or eliminate infectious diseases. Although one disease was successfully eradicated (smallpox) and others were significantly reduced (polio and measles), new diseases such as HIV became pandemic and antibiotic-resistant organisms such as MDR TB began to cast their shadows.

It was not until the second half of the twentieth century that the developed world accepted that technology was not always the answer. For instance, the seventh cholera pandemic (El Tor) began in Indonesia in 1961 and continued for at least 40 years. The case fatality rate at the beginning of the pandemic was about 50 percent, and the technologic answer at the time was to treat cholera victims with intravenous (IV) electrolyte solution therapy, a technique developed for battlefield conditions during the two world wars. IV therapy supplies are expensive and often difficult to transport to areas that lack infrastructure or that suffer from political unrest. A simpler alternative, oral rehydration therapy (ORT), was tested in Pakistan and India in the 1960s and found to be as effective as IV therapy. Experts, however, rejected the simple replacement. They warned that only trained medical personnel should be allowed to administer ORT and recommended that IV therapy remain the treatment of choice.

The medical experts were challenged in 1971 as the Bangladesh War of Independence caused 10 million refugees to flee into the border area of West Bengal, India. Dr. Dilip Mahalanabis from the Johns Hopkins Center for Medical Research and Training in Calcutta was assigned to one of the refugee camps. When he arrived, he found 350,000 refugees already encamped and another 6,000 arriving daily. It was not long before his 16-bed hospital was overwhelmed with cholera cases. Mahalanabis defied the experts and began training paramedical personnel and family members in the use of ORT solution. The case fatality rate at his camp fell to 3.6 percent, leading *The Lancet* in 1978 to call ORT "the most important medical discovery of the twentieth century."[1]

Another major development affecting global public health during the twentieth century was the creation of the WHO as an operating arm of the UN. Formed during World War II, the WHO serves as a coordinator among national public health agencies and as an initiator of health activity in response to emerging global health crises, such as HIV or global influenza pandemics. It provides a nexus for the orderly collection and dissemination of global public health information, often gleaned from its own surveillance systems or assembled from those of national health authorities. At the time the agency was created, WHO defined health as "a state of complete physical, mental, and social well-being and not merely the absence of disease or infirmity." This definition and the agency's prestige allow it to sometimes cajole governments into accepting public health realities they may prefer not to acknowledge.

Multiple efforts at improving national and global public health occurred over the course of the twentieth century. In Canada, the Lalonde Report[2] was presented in the House of Commons in 1974. This report is widely recognized for being the first governmental document to challenge the biomedical health care system, identifying the need to look beyond care of the sick in order to improve public health. In 1977, the World Health Assembly (composed of representatives from WHO member states) highlighted the need to promote health so that all global citizens could be "economically productive" by the year 2000. In 1978, the International Conference on Primary Health Care met in Alma-Ata, USSR (now Almaty, Kazakhstan), and issued a declaration calling for access to primary health care for all populations (see Appendix D). In 1986, the first International Conference on Health Promotion met in Ottawa, Canada, and called for a focus on health promotion, including building healthy public policy. The *Ottawa Charter* noted the need for creating supportive environments, strengthening community action, developing personal skills, and reorienting health care services toward prevention of illness and promotion of health in order to achieve "Health for All" by 2000 (Appendix E). The WHO launched its Healthy Cities project for 34 European cities in 1988. In 1990, mayors and political representatives from participating European cities met in Milan, Italy, to issue their commitment to the initiative for health and sustainable development (Appendix 5).

In contrast to the WHO and European approaches to public health, the United States put the responsibility for personal health—and as an extension, public health—on individuals rather than government. The groundwork for the Healthy People initiative was set by the 1979 surgeon general's report and two additional documents: the 1980 *Promoting Health/Preventing Disease: Objectives for the Nation* and the 1990 *Healthy People 2000: National Health Promotion and Disease Prevention Objectives*. The focus on individual responsibility for health continued in the United States, but the scope expanded in 1993 when the nation hosted the International Healthy Cities and Communities Conference. That conference spawned a US-based Healthy Communities movement that recognizes, as does the *Ottawa Charter*, the interaction of health with quality of life at the community level. Rather than seeking a national agenda or focusing only on individual responsibility, the Healthy Communities movement encourages local collaborations for improving the health and well-being of community residents. In 1998, 10 years after it began in the United States, Surgeon General David Sacher endorsed the Healthy Communities agenda. The CDC followed by creating its own Healthy Communities initiatives shortly thereafter.

As the century ended, the United Nations held a global summit and issued the United Nations Millennium Declaration on September 18, 2000 (see Appendix G). The Millennium Development Goals covered economic, environmental, health, and social justice issues designed to create a better world with better global health. The goals were:

1. Eradicate extreme poverty and hunger

2. Achieve universal primary education

3. Promote gender equality and empower women

4. Reduce child mortality

5. Improve maternal health

6. Combat HIV/AIDS, malaria, and other diseases

7. Ensure environmental sustainability

8. Develop a global partnership for development

More than 60 indicators were created to track progress toward achieving the goals. The indicators were monitored by an interagency group of experts led by the Department of Economic and Social Affairs of the United Nations. Annual progress reports on the goals are available on the UN website. These reports generally state that although fewer people are dying of AIDS and the world is edging slowly toward universal primary education and safe drinking water, the remaining targets for development are unlikely to be met. Conversely, a demographic shift (epidemiologic transition) occurred during the course of the twentieth century. This shift changed the disease profiles of developed nations so that conditions associated with aging, such as cancer and heart disease, emerged as major public health challenges. Alzheimer's disease, for instance, did not present much public health interest until sufficient numbers of elderly were living long enough to develop the disease. With continued population aging, it seems likely that new problems, such as worn-out organ systems, will become significant public health concerns in the twenty-first century.

CURRENT PANDEMICS

In 2000, between 1.0 and 1.3 billion people globally were estimated to smoke cigarettes. Smokers and people exposed to ETS carry a known risk of premature death. The impact of cigarette smoking on such a massive scale will generate a global pandemic of cardiovascular disease, cerebrovascular disease, chronic obstructive lung disease, and cancers of the lung, buccal cavity, lips, cervix, larynx, and bladder during the next few decades. Moreover, as discretionary incomes increase globally, the opportunity to "light up" will also increase as the tobacco industry targets its advertising toward these as yet untapped customers. The impact of smoking initiation will likely be greatest in rapidly industrializing countries, such as China, where disposable income is rapidly increasing. On the other hand, the negative effects of ETS on public health can be curbed. For instance, a number of U.S. cities and states have conclusively demonstrated that banning smoking in public places reduces the number of acute cardiac events in the population by as much as 20 percent. Despite these results, governments across the globe face a difficult choice; continue their dependence on lucrative tobacco taxes or face increasing health care costs as a result of the effects of smoking. The choice is not an easy one.

As the twenty-first century began, waistlines expanded as countries industrialized and adopted a Western lifestyle. High-fat diets as well as sedentary occupations and avocations yielded higher body mass indices (BMIs), increases in insulin resistance, and an increased prevalence of diabetes. The complications of diabetes are significant: cardiovascular disease, peripheral neuropathies, cerebrovascular disease, wound infections, peripheral vascular disease, diabetic liver disease (nonalcoholic fatty liver disease or nonalcoholic steatohepatitis), and malignancies. The resources needed to address the complications of diabetes have the potential to overwhelm many nations. In terms of public health, considerable attention needs to be focused on the increased occurrence of obesity.

The HIV pandemic continues in Africa, its principal epicenter; among a new generation of gay and bisexual men; and among intravenous drug users not residing in countries with free needle exchange programs. In Africa, denial regarding the etiology and means of spread of HIV precluded the deployment of early and effective preventive measures to contain the epidemic. Botswana and other African nations suffered disastrous impacts of HIV in terms of family disruption as well as labor force and economic losses. Although HAART therapy promises to convert HIV infection from a death sentence into a chronic disease, such therapy has considerable costs and creates an expanding pool of people who can continue to pass on the disease. This is true for countries that have denied the epidemic (Botswana), for those with active sex industries (Thailand), and for those that have diverted public health resources from HIV to bioterrorism (United States). Hopes persist for the development of a vaccine or genetic therapy that can prevent HIV infection though efforts to date have not yielded positive results.

EMERGING ISSUES

Bioterrorism, as well as new and emerging infectious agents, pose serious public health threats insofar as their control is predicated upon the operation of national public health systems. During the latter part of the twentieth century, resources to maintain such systems were constrained in the United States by a lack of political will, in the crumbling Soviet Union (and Eastern Europe) by economic strife, and in nations not yet having the infrastructure or wealth necessary to run a public health system. New infectious agents are increasingly challenging public health efforts. Some of these agents are man-made, such as MDR TB, while others come from novel interfaces between humans and animals, such as Ebola virus. Increased wealth feeds an increasing demand for exotic animals, whether for entertainment or as a food source, and new man–animal interactions make cross-species transmission of infectious agents likely to occur, especially in the African savannah and the rain forests and markets of Africa,

South America, and Southeast Asia. Advances in international commerce, particularly passenger aviation, hold the potential for the explosive spread of new pathogens before health authorities even become aware of their existence. Real-time surveillance for such outbreaks has begun, but it is not yet clear that those efforts will be able to identify new epidemics early enough to prevent their transition to regional or global pandemics.

Advances in information technology hold great potential for advancing public health. For example, data mining and new computational capacities allowed scientists to map the human genome. This was the first step in finding insights into the propensity of some people to develop specific diseases, understanding disease pathophysiology, and developing effective prevention and treatment regimens. However, the same information is also subject to potential abuse, whether in the workplace, in commercialization of screening tests, or in the identification of new therapies. The challenge is how to make bioinformatics readily available to researchers while protecting the health information of individual subjects. This arena remains a challenging frontier.

Defining and containing the costs of health care has been an evolving area since the establishment of health economics as a discipline in the early 1960s. The growth of health care spending in the United States and the constraints imposed by national health care systems elsewhere made the study of health care from an economic perspective inevitable. Aging populations with chronic comorbidities, rising incomes, access to information, and new technologies all raised expectations for health care services in the second half of the twentieth century. In response to rising costs, insurance companies restricted access to expensive treatments and those not demonstrated as cost-effective by outcomes research. Pharmaceutical companies focused their business interests on developing drugs that reduce health care utilization and on those with high demand, especially lifestyle drugs. This shift in production had profound effects on vaccine development and production as well as on the development of "orphan" drugs, those designed to address rare diseases.

Globalization was a reality by the time Millennium Island in Kiribati, Micronesia (pronounced Keer-ee-bas and located on the International Date Line in the South Pacific), welcomed the new millennium at midnight on January 1, 2000. Television cameras captured the ceremony and broadcast it around the world in real time. Audiences on every continent watched as 70 traditional dancers set the backdrop for President Teburoro Tito to raise and pass a torch to a boy who then passed it to an old man in a canoe. President Tito said, "Let us put aside all divisions. Let us unite in love and peace." Television cameras then followed the progress of celebrations around the world for 23 more hours.

The ability of real-time information to be broadcast around the globe clearly demonstrates how the communities and nations of the world have become intertwined, in terms of economic development, information sharing, maintenance of a habitable environment, and public health. Raising populations out of poverty is important for improving public health, as are providing public education and clean water for all. Infectious diseases know no borders; preventing and containing them is important for global public health. Finally, reducing the effects of chronic disease and disability are important, not only for humanitarian purposes, but also for reducing the economic burden on nations. For public health and surveillance systems to best serve us all, they require considerable care and maintenance so they can function effectively.

In the face of the constraints placed on the public health infrastructure by governments at all levels, several foundations stepped forward with innovative social investment models. The pioneer in this area was the Robert Wood Johnson Foundation, which began with a program focused on the health status of those lacking access to care. Over time, this organization has broadened its focus to include the health status of minorities and cost-of-care issues. During the 1990s, the William and Melinda Gates Foundation began operations with a focus on global health issues, particularly the development of affordable treatments and preventive strategies for developing countries. It has recently partnered with the Institute for One World Health, a not-for-profit pharmaceutical company with interests in addressing neglected diseases in developing countries. Other foundations, such as the Soros Foundation and the Buffet Foundation, are also concerned, in part, with health issues facing developing countries, especially population control. The financial support of these nongovernmental organizations has been key to the creation of some form of public health infrastructure in areas where either no or insufficient governmental financial support exists.

With the backdrop of private foundation support and the rise of the Internet, the question arises as to what systems will evolve to address emerging public health issues on a global scale. Although the overhead costs for the use of the Internet are small and data systems continue to gather, process, and transmit information at ever-increasing speeds, there remain large areas of the globe without the ability to receive, much less respond, to such information. In other areas, the infrastructure to receive and respond to information exists, but the political will to cooperate to solve global public health issues remains problematic. How these issues are resolved has yet to be determined. They will likely require not only financial resources, but also creativity, persistence, and perhaps technologies yet to be developed.

SELECTED READINGS

The first reading, by Linda Irvine and colleagues, reviews the major global efforts at public health that emerged primarily in the second half of the twentieth century. Beginning with the creation of the World Health Organization in 1948, the authors methodically review the international conferences and their consensus documents addressing global public health, culminating with Health For All in the 21st Century.

In the second reading, Christopher Murray and Alan Lopez describe the Global Burden of Disease (GBD) Study commissioned by the World Bank in 1991. A massive undertaking, the GBD project was designed to provide a comprehensive assessment of the burden of 107 diseases and injuries and 10 selected risk factors for the world and 8 major regions within it. The authors tell us that by century's end, one-third of children in the developing world did not live past age five. This unfortunate statistic is remarkably similar to that determined by John Graunt for Greater London in 1662 (See Vol I, Chap 2). We learn from the GBD study that regional differences, as well as differences between the developed and developing world, are stark; that the rise of China and the fall of the Soviet Union significantly affected the public health of those nations; and that epidemiologic transition brings with it some interesting paradoxes. Primarily, however, we learn of the difficulties in putting together disparate data sets to bring together a picture of global health.

Our final reading, by Susan Okie, describes the Gates–Buffet effect, that is, the recognition by philanthropic organizations that in a shrinking world facing global economic challenges, many individual nations cannot serve their own populations, much less provide resources for others. For example, when the WHO could not adequately provide for antimalaria research and prevention campaigns, the Gates Foundation heavily invested in those ventures. Other philanthropies, such as the Robert Wood Johnson and the Clinton Foundations, also seek to improve public and global health, respectively. We can only hope that this interest in global health by philanthropic foundations will continue to grow and help to improve public health for all.

BIBLIOGRAPHY

Alyward RB, Hull HF, Cochi SL, Sutter RW, Olivé J-M, and Melgaard B. 2000. Disease eradication as a public health strategy: A case study of poliomyelitis eradication. *Bull WHO* 78 (3): 285–97.

Barrett R, Kuzawa CW, McDade T, and Armelagos GJ. 1998. Emerging and re-emerging infectious diseases: The third epidemiologic transition. *Annual Review of Anthropology* 27:247–71.

Barua D. 1993. Application of science in practice by the World Health Organization in diarrhoeal diseases control. *J Diarrhoeal Dis Res* 11:193–96.

Brown TM, Cueto M, and Fee E. 2006. The World Health Organization and the transition from "international" to "global" public health. *Am J Public Health* 96 (1): 62–72.

Davies JK, Kelly MP, eds. 1993. *Healthy Cities: Research and Practice.* New York: Routledge.

de Onis M, Onyango AW, Borghi E, Garza C, Yang H, and the WHO Multicentre Growth Reference Study Group. 2006. Comparison of the World Health Organization (WHO) child growth standards and the National Center for Health Statistics/WHO international growth reference: Implications for child health programmes. *Public Health Nutr* 9 (7), doi:10.1017/PHN20062005.

Ezzati M, Lopez AD, Rodgers A, Vander Hoorn S, Murray CJL, and the Comparative Risk Assessment Collaborating Group. 2002. Selected major risk factors and global and regional burden of disease. *Lancet* 360:1347–60.

Fontaine O and Newton C. 2001. Public Health Classics: A revolution in the management of diarrhoea. *Bull World Health Organ* 79 (5): 471–72. [Commentary on Mahalanabis, *et al.*]

Gostin LO. 2005. World health law: Toward a new conception of world health governance for the 21st century. *Yale J Health Policy Law Ethics* 1:413–24.

Guest G, ed. 2005. *Globalization, Health, and the Environment: An Integrated Perspective.* Lanham, MD: AltaMira Press.

Hirschhorn N. 1968. Decrease in net stool output in cholera during intestinal perfusion with glucose containing solutions. *N Eng J Med* 279:176–80.

Kaplan WA. 2006. Can the ubiquitous power of mobile phones be used to improve health outcomes in developing countries? Globalization and Health 2:9, doi:10.1186/1744-8603-2-9,. http://www.globalizationandhealth.com/content/2/1/9 (accessed June 1, 2007).

Lalonde M. 1981. *A New Perspective on the Health of Canadians: A Working Document.* Ottawa: Minister of Supply and Services Canada Cat. No. H32- 1374, http://www.hc-sc.gc.ca/hcs -sss/com/lalonde/index_e.html (accessed May 16, 2007).

Lindblade KA, Eisele TP, Gimnig JE, Alaii JA, Odhiambo F, O. ter Kuile F, Hawley WA, Wannemuehler KA, Phillips-Howard PA, Rosen DH, Nahlen BL, Terlouw DJ, Kubaje Adazu K, Vulule JM, and Slutsker L. 2004. Sustainability of reductions in malaria transmission and infant mortality in western Kenya with use of insecticide-treated bednets: 4 to 6 years of follow-up. *JAMA* 291:2571–80.

Mahalanabis D, Choudhuri AB, Bagchi NG, Bhattacharya AK, and Simpson TW. 1973. Oral fluid therapy of cholera among Bangladesh refugees. *The Johns Hopkins Medical Journal* 132:197–205.

Newman RD and Mercer MA. 2000. Environmental health consequences of land mines. Review. Int *J Occup Environ Health* 6 (3): 243–48.

Phillips DR. 1994. Epidemiological transition: Implications for health and health care provision. *Geografiska Annaler.* Series B, Human Geography 76 (2): 71–89.

Phillips RA. 1964. Water and electrolyte losses in cholera. *Fed Proc* 23:705–12. Reprinted in 1982 *Nutr Rev* 40 (4): 113–15.

Pierce NF, Sack RB, Mitra RC, Banwell JG, Brigham KL, Fedson DS, and Mondal A. 1969. Replacement of water and electrolyte losses in cholera by an oral glucose-electrolyte solution. *Ann Intern Med* 70 (6): 1173–81.

Report of a field trial by an international working group. 1977. A positive effect on the nutrition of Philippine children of an oral glucose electrolyte solution given at home for the treatment of diarrhoea. *Bull WHO* 55:87–94.

Ruxin JN. 1994. Magic bullet: The history of oral rehydration therapy. Med Hist 38 (4): 363–97.

Samadi AR, Islam R, and Huq MI. 1983. Replacement of intravenous therapy by oral rehydration solution in a large treatment centre for diarrhoea with dehydration. *Bull WHO* 61:471–76.

Santosham M, Keenan EM, Broun D, and Glass R. 1997. Oral rehydration therapy for diarrhea: An example of reverse transfer of technology. *Pediatrics* 100 (5): e10, http://www .pediatrics.org/cgi/content/full/100/5/e10 (accessed June 1, 2009).

Stoto MA, Abel C, and Dievler A, eds. 1996. *Healthy Communities: New Partnerships for the Future of Public Health*. Washington, DC: National Academy Press.

Strong K, Mathers C, Leeder S, and Beaglehole R. 2005. Preventing chronic diseases: How many lives can we save? *Lancet* 366 (9496): 1578–82. Review.

Takano T, ed. 2003. *Healthy Cities & Urban Policy Research*. USA and London: Spon Press.

The Health Committee of the League of Nations. 1933. Editorial. *Canadian Med Assoc J*, (March): 309–11.

Tilson H and Berkowitz B. 2006. The public health enterprise: Examining our twenty-first-century challenges. *Health Affairs* 25 (4): 900–910.

Wagstaff A and Claeson M. 2004. *The Millenium Development Goals for Health: Rising to the Challenges*. Washington, DC: The International Bank for Reconstruction and Development / The World Bank Pub. No. 29673. http://www-wds.worldbank.org/servlet/WDSCon tentServer/WDSP/IB/2004/07/15/000009486_20040715130626/Rendered/PDF/ 296730PAPER0Mi1ent0goals0for0health.pdf (accessed June 1, 2009).

Walsh JA and Warren KS. 1979. Selective primary health care: An interim strategy for disease control in developing countries. *N Engl J Med* 301:967–74.

World Health Organization. 1998. *The World Health Report 1998—Life in the 21st Century: A Vision for All*. Geneva: World Health Organization.

A Review of Major Influences on Current Public Health Policy in Developed Countries in the Second Half of the 20th Century
(2006)

Linda Irvine, Lawrie Elliott, Hilary Wallace, Iain K Crombie

Abstract

Public health policy underwent substantial transformation during the latter half of the 20th century. The landmark statement was the 1948 World Health Organization (WHO) constitution, which identified good health as a fundamental right and gave the responsibility to governments to achieve it for all the people. However, following World War II, developed countries made substantial investment in health care with less attention paid to public health.

The importance of public health was slowly recognised over the period from 1970 to 2000 with the publication of several reports from different organisations. The first authoritative policy statement that the important determinants of health lay outside health care was in the Lalonde Report from Canada. These ideas were subsequently expressed in the WHO Alma-Ata declaration and were emphasised a year later by the US Surgeon General. The idea of setting goals for health improvement also began in the 1970s. The Lalonde Report and the United Kingdom Black Report recommended that targets be used, but the first explicitly stated health targets were set by the US in 1979. WHO also identified the need for such targets at this time, but did not introduce them until 1984. Since then health targets have become a central feature of public health policy in developed countries.

The Ottawa Conference on Health Promotion in 1986 championed the view that health promotion was central to achieving health goals internationally. It helped clarify the types of actions needed: that individuals need to be provided with a supportive environment and economic resources to be able to lead healthy lives. In a further development, the Healthy Cities Project was launched with the specific aim of involving political decision-makers in building a strong lobby for public health at the local level. The Healthy Cities Project illustrates how to provide means and opportunity for interventions to be implemented in communities.

Concerns with inequalities in health were emphasized in the WHO declaration of Alma-Ata, and were the focus of the United Kingdom

Black Report. The Jakarta Conference on Health Promotion in 1997 urged international action on poverty, as it is the major threat to health. International acceptance of the need to tackle inequalities took longer than the acceptance of health targets, but it is now an important feature of public health policy.

The advent for the 21st century marked the coming of age of public health. The renewed version of 'Health for All,' 'Health for All in the 21st Century,' emphasized the one constant goal of WHO that all individuals should achieve their full health potential. Public health is now regarded internationally as being a priority with this WHO goal being adopted as the overarching goal of policy. The challenges it faces in tackling problems such as obesity, inequalities in health, smoking, alcohol and substance abuse are great and will require policies which tackle the economic, social and environmental determinants of health.

Introduction

Public health policy in developing countries underwent substantial transformation during the latter half of the 20th century. Preventive health care and health promotion became established, following the realisation that good health could not be achieved within the existing health care systems. The massive investment in curative medicine, which developed countries made following World War II, had not led to a corresponding improvement in the health of the people.[1] The main causes of mortality at that time were coronary heart disease, stroke, cancer and accidents, while the role of life-threatening infectious and communicable diseases had diminished. The 1950s and 1960s witnessed major advances in the understanding of the causes and risk factors of these chronic diseases.[2] The widespread recognition that good health is dependent upon many individual, social and internal factors led experts in the field of public health to outline a new vision of public health policy.

This paper reviews the key events and reports that have influenced the development of public health policy in many industrialised countries during the second half of the 20th century. The development of current public health resulted from the actions of groups of individuals, of countries and international organisations. By far the most influential organisation was the World Health Organization (WHO), although actions taken in Canada and the US, and subsequently in Europe, also contributed to the creation of public health policy internationally. These developments really began with the inaugural constitution of WHO[3] that established the principles within which public health would develop.

The Origins of the World Health Organization

The United Nations (UN) was established in 1945 and 51 countries signed the UN Charter. With the formation of the UN came the decision to establish an independent health organisation. During the following year, at the International Health Conference in New York, the participating countries approved the name and the Constitution of the World Health Organization.[3] The World Health Assembly and the Executive Board were established as the governing bodies of WHO. The WHO constitution came into effect in April 1948 and WHO became fully operational following the First World Health Assembly in June 1948. The Constitution provided the widely quoted definition of health: "health is a state of complete physical, mental and social well-being and not merely the absence of disease or infirmity." The constitution also states that: "the enjoyment of the highest attainable standard of health is one of the fundamental rights of every human being without distinction of race, religion, political beliefs, economic or social condition." Further it gives responsibility to individual countries stating that: "Governments have a responsibility for the health of their peoples which can be fulfilled only by the provision of adequate health and social measures."

Japan took responsibility to facilitate an environment in which people can lead a healthy life at an early stage. This is reflected in the 1946 constitution of Japan.[4] Article 25 of the constitution states that: "All people shall have the right to maintain the minimum standards of wholesome and cultured living." It goes on to say: "In all spheres of life, the State shall use its endeavours for the promotion and expansion of social welfare and security, and of public health." During the following year the Public Centre Law was amended and public health services were separated from curative services.[5] Other developed countries did not take this type of action at that time, instead focusing their intention on improving health care delivery.

The Lalonde Report

More than 20 years after the formation of WHO, several events changed the way health was perceived and the ways in which it could be improved. The first of these was the publication in 1974 of the internationally acclaimed document 'A New Perspective on the Health of Canadians,'[6] or the Lalonde Report, as it is generally known. This was the first government document to suggest factors other than health care contribute to the health of the population. The Lalonde Report draws on the work of Thomas McKeown, a Scottish doctor and epidemiologist.[7] McKeown suggested that the growth in world population of the industrial world during the period from the late 18th century to the middle of the 20th century owed less to the advances in medicine than to improved living standards.[8] In particular, he emphasised the role of diet and nutritional status, resulting from better economic conditions.

The Lalonde Report reviewed the major causes of early death and years of life lost, and identified the 'grizzly litany of destructive life-style habits' as well as the environmental factors which contributed to these. Based on these assessments, the report proposed the 'health field concept.' This suggested that human biology, lifestyle, the environment and health care services were all critical factors in determining health status. Further, the report stated that any major improvements in health would mainly come from improvements in life-style and the environment and from a better understanding of human biology.[9] The report stated two broad objectives: a) to reduce mental and physical health hazard for those at high risk; and b) to improve the accessibility of good mental and physical health care. To achieve these, five distinct strategies were proposed, covering: a) health promotion; b) a regulatory strategy; c) a research strategy; d) health care efficiency; and e) goal setting. Within these strategies a total of 74 courses of action were identified. The goal-setting strategy identified the need to set specific targets for reductions in morbidity and mortality together with specific dates for their achievement. Although initially the report was received sympathetically within Canada it had little significant impact.[9] However, the report was widely circulated both in Canada and abroad and is now seen as a landmark document.

The Concept of 'Health for All'

The Lalonde Report was shortly followed by an even more influential document from WHO. The 30th World Health Assembly in 1977 revealed that large numbers of people, and in some cases entire countries, were not experiencing the level of help that was intended under the WHO constitution. The World Health Assembly therefore proposed actions to make substantial improvements in health by the end of the century. Resolution WHA30.43 stated that the main social targets of governments and the WHO in the coming decades should be the "attainment by citizens of the world by the year 2000 of a level of health that will permit them to lead a socially and economically productive life." This became popularly known as 'Health for All by the Year 2000.'[10] Since its introduction, Health for All has provided a framework for health improvement and has had a major influence on public health policy development.

The Alma-Ata Conference

Health for All was launched as a global movement in the 1978 International Conference on Primary Care. This was held at Alma-Ata in Kazakhstan, then part of the USSR. The health status of hundreds of millions of people in the world was deemed to be unacceptable.[11] The conference established that the attainment of health required the action of social and economic sectors as well as the health sector. The conference declaration, the 'Alma-Ata Declaration,'[11] outlined the role of primary health care in addressing this. The declaration was an important milestone in the promotion of world health. The conference objectives were to promote the concept of primary health care in all countries, to begin to develop it and devise principles for it, outlining the role of governments and other organisations and to formulate recommendations for the development of primary care.

The declaration highlighted two main areas for action. The first was to re-orient health care away from expensive urban hospitals and advanced technology and towards primary care and the establishment of community health centres and community health workers. The declaration went further, stating that health services went beyond medical care to include agriculture, food, industry, education and housing.

The second area for action was to improve the delivery of services. The principles covered four topics: a) equity of care which stresses the need to target vulnerable populations and achieve equal access to health; b) empowerment and respect which could be enhanced by designing interventions to enable communities to increase their control over their own health; c) participation with communities and planning care was also seen as important; and d) the need to address intra-sectoral activity, i.e. promoting and providing services where people live. These essentials of primary care were adopted at the conference at Alma-Ata and were endorsed by the World Health Assembly in resolution WA32.30 in the following year.[10]

Healthy People

Similar innovations were occurring in the 1970s in the USA.[12] Concern with the avoidance of preventable causes of disease, including smoking, alcohol and diet, featured in the 'Forward Plan for Health' in 1974.[13] Subsequently Congress passed the Health Information and Promotion Act which created what was finally called the Office of Disease Prevention and Health Promotion. This led to the publication, in 1979, of the Surgeon General's report 'Healthy People: The Surgeon General's Report on Health Promotion and Disease Prevention.'[1] It explicitly recognised the contribution of the Lalonde Report. It also noted that although the health of the American people had never been better, international data confirmed that health status in America lagged behind many developed countries. Life expectancy, infant mortality and mortality from cancer and cardiovascular disease were worse than in many other industrialised countries. This occurred despite massive investment in health care in the previous two decades. The report acknowledged that a 700% increase in health spending from 1960 to 1978 (from $27 billion to $192 billion) had failed to show a corresponding improvement in health. The report also clarified that expenditure had been mainly for the treatment of disease and disability with little directed towards prevention of disease. The report, therefore, stressed that "the renewed national commitment efforts designed to prevent disease and to promote health" was the way to ensure improved health and quality of life.

'Healthy People' acted on the recommendations of the Lalonde Report and pioneered the introduction of national health targets. The document set goals to reduce mortality among infants, children, adolescents and young adults and to increase independence among older people. This formal setting of targets is thought to have given credibility to the aims and methods of health promotion in the US.[12]

The Black Report

A further influential document was 'Inequalities in Health,' or the Black Report,[14] which was published in 1980 in the UK. In 1977 the Labour government commissioned an expert committee to investigate why the NHS in the UK had apparently failed to reduce social inequalities in health. The concept that deprivation and ill health were linked was not new, but the Black Report produced convincing evidence that poverty and ill health were inextricably linked in that material deprivation was a major determinant of ill health and death. It also concluded that people's behaviour is constrained by structural and environmental factors over which they have no control. The report made 37 recommendations for tackling inequalities, among them that national health goals should be set. It also suggested that, following discussion among all relevant agencies, measures be put in place to tackle diet, smoking, alcohol and physical inactivity. The report was explicitly rejected by the incoming Conservative government, but it had a substantial impact on political thought in countries such as Sweden and Ireland.

Health Targets

The developments in the 1970s in WHO led to the publication of 'Health Targets for Europe'[15] in 1984. The 32 member states of the WHO European Region adopted the European Health for All policy with its 38 targets.

This represented an act of solidarity and unity on health among the European countries. Health for All was not imposed on countries by law and regulations; nevertheless it began to influence health policy-makers across the region. The strategy was based on five key principles: a) equity, a reduction in inequalities in health; b) empowerment, enabling individuals to reach their full physical and mental ability; c) participation by communities in health policy decision-making; d) co-operation between agencies involved in health; and e) local primary care providing preventive care at the local level. The first target was to achieve equity in health. Eleven targets sought to improve the quality of life, reduce mortality and morbidity from chronic diseases, and improve the health of certain groups. Promoting a healthy life-style was the theme for five targets, while improving the environment was the topic for another eight. Six targets sought to improve health systems, and seven targets encouraged individual countries to establish their own Health for All policies to support health promotion.

The targets were very ambitious and were criticised for being political rather than scientific in nature; nonetheless most countries adopted the Health for All concept. The use of targets, however, varied greatly between countries. A recent review of the use of the targets concluded that while most countries initially attempted to use the 38 targets, by the end of the 1990s, no European country had formally incorporated the full scope of the strategy into its health policy.[16] The European countries also agreed [on] a process for monitoring progress towards the targets, both individually and collectively. Over 200 indicators, both quantitative and qualitative were agreed.[17] Regular monitoring exercises have been carried out and published in WHO health reports.

The First WHO Conference on Health Promotion

Over this period there were substantial developments in the field of health promotion. The first WHO conference on health promotion in 1986 produced the 'Ottawa Charter.'[18] The Charter builds on the declaration of Alma-Ata[11] and provided the basis for the development of health promotion policy. Five action areas were identified in the Charter: a) to build healthy public policy by making healthy choices easy for the community; b) to create supportive environments including the provision of affordable housing and effective transportation policy; c) to strengthen community action by empowering communities to be involved in health promotion activities; d) to develop personal skills through education, information and life-skills training; and e) to achieve the reorientation of the health care services. The aims were to achieve a greater balance between curative and preventive services, and to ensure that health professionals fully appreciate the social and environmental causes of ill health.

Healthy Cities Project

The Healthy Cities Project is a worldwide effort promoted by the WHO.[19] The term 'healthy cities' was introduced in the mid 1980s at a conference in Canada. The concept was quickly adopted by the European Office of WHO and the WHO Healthy Cities Project was launched in 11 European countries in 1987. Following its success and rapid expansion within Europe, it was later adopted by WHO offices of the African, American, Eastern Mediterranean, South East and Western Pacific regions. The Healthy Cities Project seeks to enhance the physical, mental, social and environmental well-being of the people who live and work in cities. It incorporates a broad definition of health that emphasizes the prevention of community problems. This approach encompasses all aspects of people's lives, including housing, education, religion, employment, nutrition, leisure and recreation, health and medical care, good transportation, a clean and green environment, friendly people, and safe streets and parks.

Subsequent Conferences on Health Promotion

The second International Conference on Health Promotion was held in Adelaide in 1988. The Conference statement[20] reiterated the principles outlined in the Ottawa Charter. It stressed the need to develop strategies for healthy public policy action and the need to address the issues of equity, access and development. It called upon governments to set explicit health goals that emphasise health promotion. Crucially it recommended that government be accountable for the health consequences of their policies or lack of policies, and that they should measure and report the health impact of their policies. The conference also identified four key areas as priorities for health public policy for immediate action: a) supporting the health of women; b) food and nutrition; c) tobacco and alcohol; and d) creating supportive environments. Finally, it stressed the importance of developing new health alliances and the need for strong advocacy to put health high on the agenda of policy members.

The fourth Conference, held in Jakarta in July 1997[21] focused on developing effective health promotion strategies for the 21st century. Poverty was acknowledged as the greatest threat to health, but the conference recognised that global challenges were leading to new challenges. The declaration stated that the creation of new partnerships for health between different sectors at all levels of society and government were required.

The Acheson Report

Health inequalities became even more apparent in most countries during the 1990s. Soon after the UK elections in 1997, the new Labour government invited Sir Donald Acheson, former Chief Medical Officer in England, to undertake an independent review of inequalities of health in England. The report 'Independent Inquiry into Inequalities in Health Report'[22] was published in 1998. The report found that, despite increasing prosperity, the health gap between social classes had widened since the 1980s. The scientific evidence showed that the roots of ill health were determined by factors such as income, employment and education as well as the material environment and life-style. The report's key recommendations were that: a) all policies likely to affect health should be evaluated in terms of their impact on health inequalities; b) a high priority should be given to the health of families and children; and c) further steps should be taken to reduce inequalities and improve the living standards of poor households.

Renewal of Health for All

Health For All in the 21st century represents a reinvigoration of the original WHO Health for All programme. The Health for All 21 renewal process started in 1995. The World Health Assembly held in Geneva in May 1998 then adopted the new global Health for All policy 'Health for All in the 21st Century.'[23] The new policy follows the 'Health for All by the Year 2000.' The strategy sets global priorities and targets for 2020. The targets aim to make it possible for people throughout the world to reach the highest possible level of health.[24]

The European region's response to the global Health for All policy is the document Health 21. It sets 21 targets which cover health outcomes, the determinants of health, and health policies and sustainable health systems. Member states are expected to use this as a framework within which they will set their own targets, based on national priorities.[25] Further, within the European Union political developments such as the Treaty of Maastricht[26] and the Treaty of Amsterdam[27] have given legislative support to public health initiatives. In essence, these treaties enshrine the principles first laid out in the WHO's 1946 constitution.

Conclusions

This paper has reviewed some of the major influences and key events which led to the development of current public health policy internationally. However these may not have been the sole factors. It is likely that

---

Box 1

PRINCIPLES OF PUBLIC HEALTH
- Individuals have the right to the highest attainable standard of health
- Governments have a duty to ensure the health of their people
- Inequalities in health are unacceptable
- Improvements in health will mainly come from improvements in life-style and the environment
- Health targets are an important feature of policy
- The social and physical environment is the major determinant of health behaviour
- Government should act to empower individuals enabling them to improve their health

---

there were a host of factors and individuals which created the culture and intellectual climate in which the major and very public events could occur. Thus, the signal events identified in this paper could be better interpreted as the culmination of the effects of a myriad of factors. However, because of their prominence the signal events will have reinforced the effects of the individual factors.

The events and reports together identify a set of fundamental principles upon which current public health policy is based (see Box 1). The right of each individual to good health and the duty of governments to ensure this were clearly stated in the inaugural WHO constitution. Japan appears to be unique in recognising immediately the principles espoused by WHO and acted to separate preventive services from curative ones. In other countries public health continued to focus for many years on disease surveillance, infectious disease control, screening and ensuring effective delivery of health care.

Concerns with inequalities in health reached national and international consciousness in the 1970s. They were emphasised in the 1978 WHO declaration of Alma-Ata, and were the focus of the Black Report which, although commissioned in the 1970s, was published in 1980. Although Sweden issued a report on inequalities in 1984, international acceptance of the need to tackle inequalities took longer but it is now an important feature of public health policy.

Recognition that the important determinants of health lay outside health care, Japan apart, only began influencing public health policy in developed countries in the 1970s. The first authoritative statement of this was in the Lalonde Report. However, these ideas were mentioned in the Alma-Ata declaration in 1978 and were emphasised by the US Surgeon General in 1979. The speed of the international recognition suggests these ideas may have been developing independently in several countries.

What is important about them is that they set the direction for future public health endeavour.

The setting of goals for health improvement occurred almost at the same time. The Lalonde Report in 1974 and the Black Report in 1980 recommended that targets be set. The first explicitly stated health targets were produced by the US in 1978. WHO identified the need for such targets in 1978, but did not produce an explicit list until 1984. Since then health targets have become a central feature of public health policy in developed countries, providing more detailed instruction for the direction of public health policy.

The idea that the social and physical environment is the major determinant of health behaviour was clearly stated in the Black Report. It gained international prominence in the Ottawa Charter, which emphasised that individuals need to be provided with a supportive environment and economic resources to be able to lead healthy lives. The Adelaide Recommendations reiterated the Ottawa goals, but extended them by placing responsibility directly on governments for achieving these goals.

Public health is regarded internationally as being a priority. One question that could be asked is why it was so slow to develop despite the publication of the landmark documents which mapped out the way forward. The explanation could lie in the political and economic context of the second half of the 20th century, where the focus for health was on the increased provision of health services. Now, there is considerable political will in individual countries to deliver the public health agenda. The expectations being placed on public health are high: that it deliver major increases in both length and quality of life. The challenges it faces in tackling problems such as obesity, inequalities in health, smoking, alcohol misuse and substance abuse are great and will require policies which are truly based on the principles outlined in this paper.

SOURCE

Irvine L, Elliott L, Wallace H, and Crombie IK. 2006. A review of major influences on current public health policy in developed countries in the second half of the 20th century. *J R Soc Health* 126 (2): 73–8. Copyright 2006 *Journal of the Royal Society of Health*. Reprinted with permission of Sage Publications.

Mortality by Cause for Eight Regions of the World: Global Burden of Disease Study
(1997)

Christopher J. L. Murray and Alan D. Lopez

Summary

BACKGROUND Reliable information on causes of death is essential to the development of national and international health policies for prevention and control of disease and injury. Medically certified information is available for less than 30% of the estimated 50.5 million deaths that occur each year worldwide. However, other data sources can be used to develop cause-of-death estimates for populations. To be useful, estimates must be internally consistent, plausible, and reflect epidemiological characteristics suggested by community-level data. The Global Burden of Disease Study (GBD) used various data sources and made corrections for miscoding of important diseases (e.g., ischaemic heart disease) to estimate worldwide and regional cause-of-death patterns in 1990 for 14 age-sex groups in eight regions, for 107 causes.

METHODS Preliminary estimates were developed with available vital-registration data, sample-registration data for India and China, and small-scale population-study data sources. Registration data were corrected for miscoding, and Lorenz-curve analysis was used to estimate cause-of-death patterns in areas without registration. Preliminary estimates were modified to reflect the epidemiology of selected diseases and injuries. Final estimates were checked to ensure that numbers of deaths in specific age-sex groups did not exceed estimates suggested by independent demographic methods.

FINDINGS 98% of all deaths in children younger than 15 years are in the developing world. 83% and 59% of deaths at 15–59 and 70 years, respectively, are in the developing world. The probability of death between birth and 15 years ranges from 22.0% in sub-Saharan Africa to 1.1% in the established market economies. Probabilities of death between 15 and 60 years range from 7.2% for women in established market economies to 39.1% for men in sub-Saharan Africa. The probability of a man or woman dying from a non-communicable disease is higher in sub-Saharan Africa and other developing regions than in established market economies. Worldwide in 1990, communicable, maternal, perinatal, and nutritional disorders accounted for 17.2 million deaths, non-communicable diseases for 28.1 million deaths and injuries for 5.1 million deaths. The leading causes of death in 1990 were ischaemic heart disease (6.3 million deaths), cerebrovascular accidents (4.4 million deaths), lower respiratory infections (4.3 million), diarrhoeal diseases (2.9 million), perinatal disorders (2.4 million), chronic obstructive pulmonary disease (2.2 million), tuberculosis (2.0 million), measles (1.1 million), road-traffic accidents (1.0 million), and lung cancer (0.9 million).

INTERPRETATION Five of the ten leading killers are communicable, perinatal, and nutritional disorders largely affecting children. Non-communicable diseases are, however, already major public health challenges in all regions. Injuries, which account for 10% of global mortality, are often ignored as a major cause of death and may require innovative strategies to reduce their toll. The estimates by cause have wide CIs, but provide a foundation for a more informed debate on public-health priorities.

Introduction

This paper, the first of a series of four, reports on the 5-year Global Burden of Disease Study (GBD). (The other three papers will follow in the next three issues of *The Lancet*.) The study was initiated in 1992 at the request of the World Bank and was done in collaboration with WHO. Preliminary results were used by the World Bank[1] and published by WHO.[2] The GBD was designed to address three primary goals: to provide information on non-fatal health outcomes for debates on international health policy, which are generally focused on mortality; to develop unbiased epidemiological assessments for major disorders; and to quantify the burden of disease with a measure that could also be used for cost-effectiveness analysis. There were four specific objectives:

- To develop internally consistent estimates of mortality for 107 causes of death by age, sex, and geographic region.

- To develop internally consistent estimates of incidence, prevalence, duration, and case-fatality for 483 disabling sequelae of the 107 causes.

- To estimate the fraction of mortality and disability attributable to ten major risk factors.

- To develop various projection scenarios of mortality and disability estimates by cause, age, sex, and region.

Final results, including chapters on each major condition by the investigators who contributed to this study are available.[3,4] The results published here supersede the preliminary results.[2,3] This paper reports on regional and global patterns of mortality by cause.

Methods

Design

The GBD can be divided into five components, which were all studied simultaneously and are interlinked: causes of death, descriptive epidemiology of disabling sequelae, burden attributable to selected risk factors, projections of burden from 1990 to 2020, and sensitivity analysis. In the cause-of-death component, data from vital registration and sample registration systems were combined with the results of population-monitoring laboratories and disease-specific epidemiological studies and models to develop regional estimates of mortality for different age-sex groups according to a clear set of algorithms.

For each of the 107 disorders, the number of disabling sequelae selected to be investigated in depth was limited. For example, diabetes mellitus was restricted to five sequelae—diabetes itself, retinopathy, neuropathy, diabetic foot, and amputation. In total, 483 sequelae were selected for direct assessment. For each sequela, average age at onset, duration, incidence, prevalence, and case-fatality rates by age, sex, and region were estimated by an iterative process. In 1992, disease specialists for each condition were identified. Based on a review of published and unpublished studies and surveys, the specialists developed first-round estimates of duration, incidence, remission, case-fatality, prevalence, and death rates. Estimates were critically reviewed, and their internal consistency was ascertained with a computer program (DisMod) that modelled disease or injury process. Major inconsistencies were identified and epidemiological estimates revised to correct them. Throughout the study, four complete cycles of international review, revision, and internal-consistency analysis were done to generate the final set of estimates.[4]

To assist identification and modification of inconsistent estimates of incidence, prevalence, duration, and case-fatality, a simple model that formalised the relation between incidence, remission, case-fatality, and prevalence was developed. Susceptible people in the population were assumed to be at risk of incurring a disease or disability at rate i, from which they could die at general mortality rate m. Patients' diseases remit at rate r, or they die from general causes at the same rate as the susceptibles (m) or die from cause-specific mortality at rate f. If these rates can be assumed to be constant in the short term, for example for a year, a set of ordinary differential equations can be defined to characterise movement between

susceptible, diseased, recovered, and dead. DisMod uses the finite difference method to solve these equations.[3]

We assessed the burden of disease and injury attributable to ten major
risk factors—malnutrition, poor water, sanitation and hygiene, unsafe
sex, alcohol, occupation, tobacco use, hypertension, physical inactivity,
illicit use of drugs, and air pollution. For most risk factors, estimates of
attributable death and disability were made from estimates for prevalence
of exposure by age, sex, and region, relative risks for the exposed from
several previously published studies, and the regional pattern of burden.

Three alternative projection scenarios of the burden of disease were
developed for each region. Simple models related causes-specific mortality and disability to a limited set of major socioeconomic factors. The
methods, which included several steps to incorporate other information,
such as the spread of HIV, are detailed in the fourth paper of this series.

Indicators of Burden of Disease

The results of the GBD were analysed by means of various epidemiological
and demographic indicators, including incidence and prevalence rates,
life expectancy, probabilities of death in different age-groups, disability-
adjusted life expectancy, years of life lost because of premature death,
years of life lived with disability (adjusted for the severity of disability),
and disability-adjusted life years (DALYs), calculated as the sum of years
of life lost and years of life lived with disability. DALYs, which were developed specifically for the GBD, are time-based health-outcome measures,
similar to quality-adjusted life years, that include weights for time spent
in less-than-perfect health. Such composite measures of the burden of
disease allowed us to compare the burden of premature mortality with
non-fatal health outcomes, such as disability. All measures of health outcome implicitly or explicitly include social values. Four key areas in which
social values were important in the construction of a health-outcome indicator were years of life lost because of death in each age group; time lost
because of premature death compared with time lives in a health state
worse than perfect health; the discounting of future health; and the value
of a year of life lived in the different age-groups. The choice of values incorporated into DALYs and their selection have been extensively debated
and discussed.[3,5-7] Severity weights on a scale of 0 (perfect health) to 1
(death) were assigned to each of the 483 disabling sequelae. How these
disability severity weights were developed is described in more detail in
the second paper of this series. An extensive sensitivity analysis of the GBD
results to changes in various social values showed that the main findings
are largely unaffected by changes in the discount rate, age weights, or health-
state preferences.[3]

GBD Regions

We made assessments for eight geographic regions that were delineated by the World Bank.[1] These regions were: the established market economies, mainly consisting of high-income Organisation for Economic Cooperation and Development members; the formerly socialist economies of Europe, which stretched from Czechoslovakia to Siberia; Latin America and the Caribbean; China; India; the middle eastern crescent, which included North Africa, the Middle East, Pakistan, and the Central Asian Republics of the former Soviet Union; other Asia and islands, which covered the rest of Asia and the Pacific; and sub-Saharan Africa.

GBD Classification System

For the GBD we used a tree structure to show rankings of causes of death and disability.[8] At the first level were three groups of causes of mortality.

Group 1 consisted of communicable diseases, maternal, perinatal, and nutritional disorders.

Group 2 consisted of non-communicable diseases.

Group 3 consisted of all intentional or unintentional injuries.

Group 1 causes of death included disorders, the specific mortality of which typically declines faster than all-cause mortality during epidemiological transition. In the theory of the epidemiological transition, as total mortality decreases, the cause-of-death structure should shift from group 1 to group 2 causes.[9] As a result, group 1 causes account for only a small proportion of deaths in low-mortality populations (and, conversely, dominate the cause-of-death pattern in high-mortality populations). The non-communicable diseases in group 2 are, therefore, the most important health problems for populations that have undergone the epidemiological transition.

Each of the three groups contained several major subcategories that were mutually exclusive and exhaustive. Specifically, group 1 was divided into infectious and parasitic causes, respiratory infections, maternal causes, perinatal disorders, and nutritional deficiencies. Group 2 contained 14 categories of non-communicable diseases. Group 3 was subdivided into unintentional and intentional injuries. Third and fourth levels of branching were used to identify all the 107 specific causes of death.

Regional Demographic Estimates

Many sources provide much information about the basic demography of each region in the world. The database for estimating rates of child mortality in all regions is more developed than that for adult mortality.[10,11] Indeed, demographers disagree about rates of adult mortality in some developing regions without good vital registration systems, where mortality is estimated indirectly from census and survey data.[12] For example, estimates of adult mortality by age and sex from the World Bank and the United Nations Population Division can differ by as much as 50%; but, in general, the discrepancies are less extreme. Demographic estimates of deaths and population in 1990 by age and sex[1] form the basis of the GBD.

Detailed Methods for Estimation of Causes of Death

Mortality rates specific for age, sex, and cause for each region were estimated in four steps: preparation of preliminary estimates, largely from vital registration and sample registration data; correction of estimates for selected causes by specific methods; adjustment of cause-specific mortality rates for selected causes based on epidemiological analyses; and final adjustments to ensure that the sum of cause-specific mortality rates was identical to total age-specific mortality rates estimated from demographic methods.

Table 1 Sources and Methods Used to Estimate Mortality by Cause for Each Region in 1990

	Vital registration (% coverage)		
	Under 5	≥ 5	Total
EME	99	99	99
FSE	99	99	99
IND*	–	–	–
CHN*	–	–	–
OAI	2.1	13.6	10.2
SSA	0.4	1.7	1.1
LAC	27.6	47.2	42.6
MEC	12.3	27.1	21.8

*See text.

EME=established market economies; FSE=formerly socialist economies of Europe; IND=India; CHN=China; OAI=other Asia and islands; SSA=sub-Saharan Africa; LAC=Latin America and the Caribbean; MEC=middle eastern crescent.

Correction of ICD-9 Miscoding in Areas with Good
Vital Registration Data

For those study areas with good vital registration data available, adjustments were made to correct for problems related to the coding of causes of death. The rules of the International Classification of Diseases (ICD) specify that the underlying cause of death should be given as the primary cause of death. The various ICD conventions are arbitrary methods to deal with the multicausal nature of mortality. For example, liver cancer, in a patient known to have hepatitis B, is coded as the cause of death. By contrast, in ICD-10, deaths from lymphoma among HIV patients are coded to HIV and not to lymphoma. In our study we followed the principles of the ICD to give only a single cause of death for the primary tabulations. We estimated the proportion of deaths associated with each cause. In some cases, in which ambiguous ICD-9 rules and conventions were followed, we used an arbitrary convention to estimate rates for the underlying cause of death for the primary tabulations.[3]

Although medically certified causes of death are generally a reliable source of information on the broad causes-of-death pattern in a community, correction algorithms were necessary for three specific situations. First, based on statistical evidence[8,13] ICD-9 Chapter XVI deaths in the age-group 0–4 years were proportionately distributed across all group 1 causes within that age-sex group. For each age-group older than 5 years, chapter XVI deaths were proportionately distributed across group 2 causes. Second, for deaths from injuries that could not be classified as intentional or unintentional, deaths were proportionately redistributed across all other (known) injuries. Third, deaths from unspecified environmental and accidental causes (E928, including E929.9) were redistributed across all causes of unintentional injury.

Coding of cardiovascular disease across communities and within the same community over time has been notoriously variable.[14–16] Large proportions of deaths from heart failure (ICD-9 428), ventricular arrhythmias (ICD-9 427.1, 427.4, 427.5), general atherosclerosis (ICD-9 440.9), and ill-defined descriptions and complications of heart disease (ICD-9 429.0, 429.1, 429.2 and 429.9) are likely to be actually deaths from ischaemic heart disease. We developed a correction algorithm to redistribute a proportion of these deaths to ischaemic heart disease.[17] Before correction, the ratio of the highest ischaemic heart disease mortality rate in people over 30 years of age (Finland) to the lowest (Japan) was 6.3 to 1.0 (figure 1). After correction, the ratio was 2.3 to 1.0.

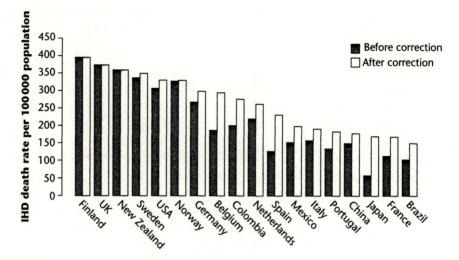

Figure 1 Mortality rates by country for ischaemic heart disease (IHD) before and after adjustment for miscoding

Age-standardised rates for men and women aged ≥30, about 1990.

Preliminary Estimates for Each Region

For the established market economies and formerly socialist economies of Europe, preliminary estimates were derived solely from vital registration data (which covered virtually all deaths in both regions) after correction for miscoding (table 1). For China, preliminary estimates (rural and urban) were calculated from data from the 1991 disease surveillance points—a sample registration system that covered a representative sample of 10 million people, and included 52,734 deaths adjusted to match the total deaths in each age-group and sex-group in China. For India, cause-of-death patterns in urban areas were based on the nearly complete urban registration system in Maharashtra State.[18] Estimates of mortality by cause for rural areas were based on the survey of causes of death (rural), a system that currently includes over 1,300 primary-health centres[19] and provides useful information on causes of mortality in rural areas. However, since the cause of death is assigned by non-medical personnel, the returns from this system are likely to be useful only for estimating broad cause-of-death patterns and not for specific causes. Detailed rates of specific causes were based on the extensive analysis and follow-up studies done as part of the Andhra Pradesh Burden of Disease Study (P Mahapatra and G N V Ramana, personal communication).

In Latin America and the Caribbean, other Asia and islands, the middle eastern crescent, and sub-Saharan Africa, some vital registration data are available, but most deaths are not recorded on the existing systems (table 1). Moreover, the deaths that are recorded are not representative of mortality for the entire region. Therefore, we divided each of these regions into a registration area, for which vital registration data were available, and a residual area. To develop plausible estimates of mortality by cause in the residual areas, we used a new method based on the geographical inequality of death distribution to estimate mortality rates specific for age and sex from all causes combined.[3] For both registration areas we then compared the percentage distribution of recorded deaths in each age-group assigned to groups 1, 2, and 3 with the percentage predicted by cause-of-death models. Building on substantial previous experience with cause-of-death models,[8,13,20–22] we developed a new set from a dataset of 103 observations from 67 countries, from the years 1950 to 1991. Separate models were developed for both sexes in each of the seven GBD age-groups: 0–4, 5–14, 15–29, 30–44, 45–59, 60–69, and 70 years or older. The number of SD above or below the predicted value for each group showed how much the registration areas in the region deviated from the cause-of-death patterns reflected in the models. To estimate the division of all-cause mortality into groups 1, 2, and 3 in the residual areas, the pattern of deviation of the cause-of-death structure as compared with the cause-of-death models was assumed to be similar to that of the registration areas.

In sub-Saharan Africa, a slightly different method was used because registration data were available only for South Africa. The region was divided into southern Africa (South Africa, Botswana, Namibia, Mozambique, Zimbabwe, Swaziland, Zambia, and Malawe) and Northern Africa (all other countries in sub-Saharan Africa). The inequality-of-death distribution method was then used to estimate the all-cause mortality for Southern Africa, based on the vital registration data from South Africa. The distribution of deaths across groups 1, 2, and 3 for registered deaths in South Africa was within one SD of that predicted by the models. For Northern Africa, we applied the same pattern of deviation as suggested by the registration areas of South Africa because the observed patterns were consistent with evidence from various population-monitoring laboratories (e.g., Senegal,[23] The Gambia,[24] Ghana,[25] Kenya,[26] and Tanzania[27]).

For preliminary estimates for the more detailed causes within each group in the developing regions, the proportionate distribution for a given age-sex group was assumed to be the same as in the registration areas.

Specific Corrections

For a number of disease categories specific corrections were also applied. To estimate the total cancer-death rates for each age-sex group, the preliminary estimates described earlier were used. For regions with vital registration data (table 1), those were used to estimate the distribution of total cancer deaths by site. In India, the distribution by site of cancer in the urban areas was based on the vital registration data from Maharashtra, and in the rural areas, based on the Andhra Pradesh Burden of Disease Study (P Mahapatra and G N V Ramana, personal communication). For other regions and the population in Latin America and the Caribbean, site-specific distributions were estimated from a set of published estimates of site-specific mortality based on the International Agency for Cancer Research network of registries for 1985.[28] However, in these estimates, the proportion of total cancer deaths that were attributed to "other and unknown" primary sites, was very small compared with areas that have better vital registration. The site distribution of cancer deaths in these estimates was based on the assumption that the low proportion of cancer deaths estimated for other and unknown cancers by Parkin and colleagues[31] is due to misdiagnosis of metastatic cancers or other coding errors.

Epidemiological Estimates

Epidemiological assessments were used to adjust preliminary-round mortality estimates for selected causes. Because of the greater emphasis on study of infectious-disease epidemiology in most developing countries, there are epidemiologically based estimates of mortality for many more diseases in group 1 than group 2. Since epidemiological assessments tend to yield monitoring rates that are higher than those based on vital registration, the final results are often biased towards group 1 diseases and away from group 2 diseases.

Epidemiological estimates of war deaths, because of their sporadic but intense nature, were incorporated in a slightly different way. We chose to classify war deaths as additional to deaths estimated from the basic demographic analyses used to calculate the number of deaths in each age-sex group in each region. The epidemiological estimates of war deaths were not, therefore, subject to the internal consistency algorithm.

Internal Consistency Algorithms

To ensure that the sum of cause-specific deaths equalled the number of deaths from all causes in any given age-sex group, two additional adjustment algorithms were applied separately, one for neonatal causes[6] and one for all other age-groups. To assess the extent of overestimation of mortality in each of the age-sex groups and in each region we compared the number of SD above or below the proportionate mortality for a group, as predicted by the cause-of-death models, with the number of SD above or below the preliminary estimates. If preliminary estimates for group 1 or group 2 based on vital registration or sample registration data were already more than 2.5 SD above or below the expected value, we did not allow epidemiological assessments to increase the degree of deviation. If the preliminary assessment for group 1 was less than 2.5 SD greater than expected, or if that for group 2 was less than 2.5 SD below the expected value, the results from epidemiological assessments were permitted to change the proportion in either group by 2.0 SD. If a change of 2.0 SD would increase the percentage of deaths due to group 1 to be more than 2.5 SD above the mean, or decrease the percentage of deaths due to group 2 to be more than 2.5 SD below the mean, the percentage of deaths due to group 1 was set equal to a value 2.5 SD above the mean and the percentage of deaths due to group 2 was set equal to 2.5 SD below the mean.

Results

Figure 2 illustrates the distribution of all deaths worldwide by age and region. Because of a much younger population age distribution and higher mortality rates in children, 98% of deaths in children were in the developing world (all study regions except established market economies and formerly socialist economies of Europe). 32% of all deaths in the developing world occurred in children younger than 5 years, and 63% occurred

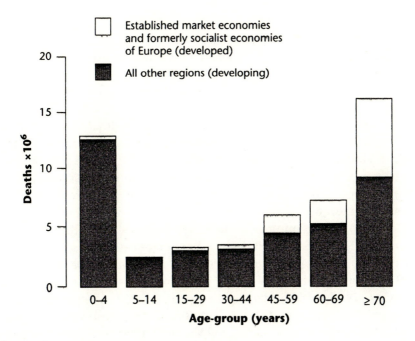

Figure 2 Distribution by age-group in study regions.

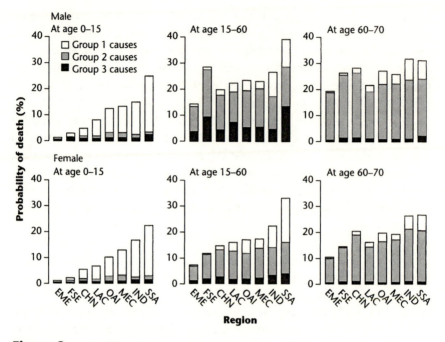

Figure 3 Probability of dying during three periods of life by broad-cause, group, sex, and region, 1990.

Abbreviations for regions given as footnote to table 1.

by the age of 60 years. Within developing regions, the age structure of death varied widely: 53% of all deaths in sub-Saharan Africa occurred between ages 0 and 4 years, compared with 11% in China. Interestingly, 83% of all adult deaths between 15 and 59 years occurred in developing countries. Even at 70 years or older, 59% of deaths worldwide were in the developing world. In established market economies, 4.6 million deaths occur each year at 70 years or older, as do 3.6 million in China alone. This emphasises that by 1990 the demographic transition was sufficiently advanced that only a handful of causes led to more deaths in established market economies and formerly socialist economies of Europe than in the developing world—several sites of cancer, dementias, Parkinson's disease, and a few others.

A useful way to summarise the results of this study is in probabilities of death (figure 3). Probabilities are shown for death from group 1, group 2, or group 3 causes. As expected, for girls the highest probability of death between birth and age 14 (22.0%) was in sub-Saharan Africa and the lowest (1.1%) in established market economies. At these ages, most of the regional difference was due to differences in the probability of a group 1 death. The regional rankings of probabilities for women aged 14–60 were the same as for child and adolescent death. For adult women, however, a large part of the regional difference was the higher probability of group 1 death, but the probability of non-communicable disease (group 2) death was higher in developing regions than in established market or formerly socialist economies of Europe. Figure 3 shows the unusually high probability of injury death among adult women in China, which is due mainly to high suicide rates in rural areas.

The regional rankings and prominence of group 1 causes in explaining regional differences in the probability of death between birth and 14 years are the same for boys and girls. Regional differences in the probability of death for men between 15 and 60 years are surprisingly different from that for children and women. Formerly socialist economies of Europe had a higher probability of death (28.4%) than any other region except sub-Saharan Africa (39.1%). Differences in adult risks of death were due to substantial variation in the probability of death from all three groups. Sub-Saharan Africa and India had higher risks of death among men, largely because of group 1 causes, such as tuberculosis and HIV. The remarkable excess mortality in men from the formerly socialist economies of Europe region was attributable to much higher risks of group 2 death and higher probabilities of group 3 death than in established market economies. The probability of death from group 3 injuries varied widely among regions from 3.4% in established market economies to 13.3% in sub-Saharan Africa.

50,467,000 people died in 1990; 53% of them were male. Worldwide, one death in three is from a group 1 cause (Table 2). One death in ten was from an injury, and slightly more than one death in two was from group 2 causes. Because of differences in population-age structure, mortality rates, and epidemiological patterns, there was a dramatic difference between established market and formerly socialist economies of Europe and the developing regions in the distribution of deaths. For the developing regions as a whole, group 1 conditions accounted for four of ten deaths, group 2 causes one death in two, and injuries one death in ten. For countries in the established market economies and formerly socialist economies of Europe, only one in 16 was due to group 1 causes, whereas group 2 accounted for more than 85% of all deaths. In sub-Saharan Africa, group 1 disorders accounted for 65% of all deaths, whereas in China these causes accounted for only 16% of deaths.

Table 3 gives the 30 leading causes of global mortality in 1990. Ischaemic heart disease was the leading cause of death worldwide, accounting for 6.26 million deaths (2.7 million in established market economies and formerly socialist economies of Europe; 3.6 million in the developing regions). Stroke was the next most common cause of death (4.38 million deaths, almost 3 million in developing countries), closely followed by acute respiratory infections (4.3 million, 3·. million in developing countries).

Table 2 Distribution of Deaths for Specific Causes (level-two categories) in 1990

	Deaths in region ($\times 10^3$)										
	EME	FSE	IND	CHN	OAI	SSA	LAC	MEC	Developed	Developing	World
All causes	7,121	3,791	9,371	8,885	5,534	8,202	3,009	4,553	10,912	39,554	50,467
Group 1											
Total group 1	453	214	4,775	1,405	2,190	5,316	943	1,945	667	16,573	17,241
Infectious and parasitic diseases	111	52	2,647	544	1,176	3,456	473	871	163	9,166	9,329
Respiratory infections	275	114	1,229	474	552	1,023	180	534	389	3,992	4,380
Maternal disorders	1	2	115	30	52	186	19	48	3	451	454
Perinatal disorders	46	36	660	276	331	503	96	395	82	2,361	2,443
Nutritional deficiencies	21	9	124	80	79	148	76	96	30	604	634
Group 2											
Total group 2	6,223	3,188	3,788	6,460	2,785	1,864	1,676	2,156	9,411	18,730	28,141
Malignant neoplasms	1,762	650	505	1,464	640	429	345	228	2,413	3,611	6,024
Other neoplasms	36	8	5	21	10	10	9	6	44	62	106
Diabetes mellitus	149	30	104	60	59	23	89	61	176	396	571
Endocrine disorders	46	4	2	14	9	23	27	17	50	93	143

Neuropsychiatric disorders	205	70	106	98	69	41	50	61	274	426	700
Sense-organ disorders	0	0	0	18	0	0	1	0	0	19	20
Cardiovascular disorders	3,175	2,071	2,266	2,568	1,349	815	789	1,295	5,245	9,082	14,327
Respiratory disorders	343	158	267	1,530	148	210	116	163	500	2,435	2,935
Digestive disorders	305	120	255	411	315	153	140	152	424	1,426	1,851
Genitourinary disorders	123	45	104	124	98	96	53	92	167	568	735
Skin disorders	12	2	2	12	2	7	3	2	14	29	43
Musculoskeletal disorders	32	5	3	36	9	1	9	2	37	60	97
Congenital anomalies	39	27	170	105	75	55	43	76	66	523	589
Oral disorders	0	0	0	0	0	0	0	0	0	2	2
Group 3											
Total group 3	445	389	808	1,020	559	1,022	389	452	834	4,251	5,084
Unintentional injuries	303	249	650	626	426	534	248	198	552	2,682	3,233
Intentional injuries	143	140	158	394	133	488	41	254	282	1,569	1,851

Abbreviations for regions as in table 1; developed=EME+FSE; developing=all other regions.

Table 3 30 Leading Causes of Death Worldwide in 1990

Rank	Cause of deaths	Number of deaths (×10³)
	All causes	50,467
1	Ischaemic heart disease	6,260
2	Cerebrovascular disease	4,381
3	Lower respiratory infections	4,299
4	Diarrhoeal diseases	2,946
5	Perinatal disorders	2,443
6	Chronic obstructive pulmonary disease	2,211
7	Tuberculosis (HIV seropositive excluded)	1,960
8	Measles	1,058
9	Road-traffic accidents	999
10	Trachea, bronchus, and lung cancers	945
11	Malaria	856
12	Self-inflicted injuries	786
13	Cirrhosis of the liver	779
14	Stomach cancer	752
15	Congenital anomalies	589
16	Diabetes mellitus	571
17	Violence	563
18	Tetanus	542
19	Nephritis and nephrosis	536
20	Drowning	504
21	War injuries	502
22	Liver cancer	501
23	Inflammatory heart diseases	495
24	Colon and rectum cancers	472
25	Protein-energy malnutrition	372
26	Oesophagus cancer	358
27	Pertussis	347
28	Rheumatic heart disease	340
29	Breast cancer	322
30	HIV	312

Other leading causes include diarrhoeal diseases (virtually all in developing countries), chronic obstructive pulmonary disease, tuberculosis, measles, low birthweight, road-traffic accidents, and lung cancer. Worldwide these top ten causes account for 52% of all deaths.

The leading causes of death for women and men in the age-group 15–44 are of great interest. In 1990, an estimated 2.7 million women in this age-group died. Maternal disorders were the leading causes of death, accounting for about 433,000 deaths (15.8% of deaths in this age-group). Tuberculosis remains a major cause of death among women in this age-group and causes about 10% of deaths. Suicide (7.0%), war (4.4%), road-traffic accidents (3.7%), HIV (3.4%), and stroke (2.7%) are also significant causes of death, more so in some regions than in others (e.g., in China, suicide is estimated to be the cause of almost one in four deaths for women in this age-group).

Cancer caused about 6 million deaths in 1990, 3.4 million in men. About 2.4 million cancer deaths occurred in established market economies and formerly socialist economies of Europe. By 1990, therefore, there were already 50% more cancer deaths in less developed countries than in developed countries. Lung cancer, trachea, bronchus, and lung) [*sic*] is the leading site of worldwide cancer deaths (table 3). Stomach cancer is the next most important site of cancer mortality, followed by liver, colon and rectum, oesophagus, and breast. Lung cancer caused almost twice as many male deaths in 1990 as the next most important site for men (stomach cancer). Other leading sites of male cancer mortality worldwide included liver (357,000 deaths), oesophagus (240,000), colon and rectum (237,000), prostate (193,000), and mouth and oropharynx (186,000). Breast cancer was the leading site of female cancer deaths in 1990, claiming about 50,000 more victims than the next most important site for mortality (stomach, with 282,000 deaths). Interestingly, lung cancer was already the third leading site of mortality from cancer in women in 1990, accounting for an estimated 237,000 deaths, slightly more than cervical cancer at 200,000.

Injuries, whether intentional or otherwise, were a major cause of death worldwide. In 1990, an estimated 5 million people died from group 3 causes (injuries). The risk of death from injury varied strongly by region, age, and sex. Worldwide, there were about two male deaths from violence for every female death (3.3 million compared with 1.7 million). Injuries accounted for about 12.5% of all male deaths, compared with 7.4% of female deaths. Equally striking was the regional variation in mortality from violent causes. In established market economies, for example, injuries from violence caused about 6% of all deaths in 1990, compared with 9–11% in other regions, rising to 12–13% in sub-Saharan Africa and Latin America and the Caribbean, where violence is a major cause of male deaths, accounting for about one in six deaths. Remarkably, 56% of all female suicides in the world occurred in China, whereas 40% of male homicides were in sub-Saharan Africa and a further 20% were in Latin America and the Caribbean.

For some diseases, the numbers of deaths estimated in the primary tabulations according to the rule of underlying cause greatly underestimated the real public-health importance of the disorder. For example, diabetes mellitus not only causes direct mortality but also increases an individual's risk of death from cardiovascular diseases. As part of the GBD, the burden attributable to diabetes, hepatitis B, Chagas' disease, tuberculosis, unipolar major depression, sexually transmitted diseases, and disorders causing blindness were calculated by a standard attributable risk method. In the primary tabulations diabetes mellitus accounted for 580,000 deaths in 1990, with adjustment for the heightened risk of death from other causes, 2.8 million deaths in 1990 were attributable to diabetes. Similarly, deaths directly attributable to hepatitis B and C in 1990 (about 105,000) represent only a fraction of the larger number of deaths attributable to cirrhosis and liver cancer, probably caused by hepatitis B. In total, hepatitis B and C caused about 820,000 deaths. Analyses of disorders such as trachoma, onchocerciasis, cataract, and glaucoma also suggest that large numbers of deaths are attributable to these disorders.

Discussion

Despite decades of sustained progress through development and targeted health interventions in all regions of the world in the reduction of child mortality due to group 1 causes, five of the ten leading causes of death are still communicable or perinatal disorders. With the exception of tuberculosis, these major causes largely affect children younger than 5 years. Seven disorders (lower respiratory infections, diarrhoeal diseases, perinatal disorders, tuberculosis, measles, malaria, and hepatitis B and C, including deaths from cirrhosis and liver cancer attributable to hepatitis C) accounted for 14.4 million deaths per year or 28.5% of worldwide mortality. Further reduction of mortality from these and other communicable diseases must remain one of the principal priorities for global public-health action.

One major finding from this study is the importance of non-communicable diseases in worldwide and regional patterns of death in all regions of the world. The probability of death from a non-communicable disease is higher in low-income regions such as sub-Saharan Africa than in high-income regions such as established market economies. This finding is at odds with the popular perception that many risk factors for non-communicable diseases are more prevalent in high-income than low-income populations, and that, consequently, the rates of these "diseases of affluence" must also be higher in the better-off populations. The apparent paradox of higher non-communicable death rates in the adults of the developing world must be attributable to the other major determinants of non-communicable disease mortality that are more common in these regions. Leading possibilities include the possible role of group 1 conditions in children as determinants of subsequent non-communicable diseases as adults.[29] There is clear evidence that, in aggregate, non-communicable disease rates drop as an area develops but the proportion of deaths due to non-communicable diseases is higher in established market economies and formerly socialist economies of Europe than in sub-Saharan Africa. Because of declines in fertility that accompany mortality decline, the populations of the developed regions have higher proportions of older people, and, therefore, the proportion of deaths due to non-communicable diseases is increased. The ratio of group 2 deaths to group 1 deaths has been proposed as a crude but useful indicator of the epidemiological transition.[30] These ratios range from more than 13 in established market economies and formerly socialist economies of Europe to 0.4 in sub-Saharan Africa. According to this criterion, China, followed distantly by Latin America and the Caribbean and other Asia and islands, are all further along the path of the combined demographic and epidemiological transitions than was thought to be the case, which may affect the potential demand for health services in these countries.

Injuries account for 10% of worldwide mortality, but they are often ignored. Five of the 25 leading causes of mortality (road-traffic accidents, self-inflicted injuries, violence, drownings, and war) are injuries. The regional patterns raise important epidemiological questions, such as: why suicide rates among women in China, other Asia and islands, and South India are so high; why women in India are 2.3 times more likely to die from a burn, whereas in all other regions combined, men are more likely to die from burns; and why is homicide so common? Much new descriptive epidemiology is urgently needed to reveal further the patterns and determinants of mortality from injury in different countries and regions of the world.

Many of our estimates are likely to have wide CIs. Since we integrated various estimation processes, used by several sources, into an internally consistent epidemiological profile, a precise 95% CI cannot be defined. The degree of uncertainty of the estimates does, however, vary from disease to disease, across age-groups, and between regions. For example, the estimates that are most uncertain are those for sub-Saharan Africa, particularly for the exact composition of group 2 and group 3 mortality. How should the degree of uncertainty associated with an estimate alter the way in which decision-makers interpret results? According to economic theory, when making decisions about programmes and policies, decision-makers should treat estimates that are certain or uncertain all in the same way. If there are wide CIs, decision-makers may invest resources to acquire more information to narrow the uncertainty. Disorders for which further information is gathered should be those that are major public-health concerns (e.g., tobacco-related disease in developing countries).

Much more research is required on the application and adaptation of promising methods for epidemiological surveillance in poorer populations. The disease surveillance points system in China seems to be the most useful alternative to complete vital registration, but much more research is required on how this approach might be adapted for different sociopolitical environments. Applied research on the cost-effectiveness of different systems for data collection is also needed. The system of collecting cause of death data via "verbal autopsies" needs to be assessed and improved to provide reliable data on broad categories of causes of death at low cost. What is also clear from this attempt at appraisal of worldwide mortality patterns is that even the levels of mortality rates among adults are not well known, especially in large parts of sub-Saharan Africa. As more and more regions undergo the epidemiological transition, death, particularly premature death, among adults will increasingly become a major public-health concern. Surveillance systems and research methods to reliably measure and monitor adult mortality must anticipate this trend.

This work was supported by the Edna McConnell Clark Foundation, the Rockefeller Foundation, the World Bank, and WHO. The views expressed are entirely those of the authors and do not reflect the opinions, policies, or standards of WHO. WHO considers that DALYs and the burden of disease approach discussed in these papers are potentially useful for health situation assessment but require further research.

SOURCE

Murray CJL and Lopez AD. 1997. Mortality by cause for eight regions of the world: Global Burden of Disease Study. *Lancet* 349 (9061): 1269–76. Copyright 1997 *The Lancet*. Reprinted with permission of *The Lancet*.

Global Health—The Gates–Buffett Effect
(2006)

Susan Okie, M.D.

Standing before a giant AIDS ribbon, Bill and Melinda Gates greeted some 26,000 researchers and public health workers on the opening night of last month's conference hosted by the International AIDS Society in Toronto. Bill Gates's voice echoed through the stadium as he assured the conference delegates, "Melinda and I have made stopping AIDS the top priority of our foundation. The Gateses spoke in turn, revealing both their passion and their clear-eyed intellectual engagement. Bill Gates talked of the new optimism he senses in Africa with the increased availability of antiretroviral drugs, but he warned that without increased prevention efforts, the provision of long-term treatment for infected persons is "simply unsustainable." Melinda Gates spoke of the stigmas that limit efforts to control AIDS, noting that government officials in many countries refused to accompany them when they meet with sex workers. The philanthropists promised to increase their foundation's funding for research on new prevention tools for women and called for expanded access to proven measures such as condoms, clean needles, and HIV testing. The demonstrators who had heckled previous speakers were silent; the Gateses were interrupted only by cheers.

In a world with many celebrities but few heroes, Bill Gates has attained heroic status by committing much of his enormous fortune to the advancement of global equity. He and his wife have targeted the causes of health disparities between rich and poor, and their foundation has become a driving force in international aid and in research on AIDS and other diseases. In June, the Bill and Melinda Gates Foundation's likely impact on global health was amplified when Warren Buffett, the world's second-richest man, announced plans to give most of his fortune to the foundation established by the richest one.

Buffett's gift, worth about $37 billion, will double the foundation's endowment from $29 billion to approximately $60 billion, making it by far the world's largest charitable foundation. The gift will also increase the foundation's annual giving from $1.36 billion last year to about $3 billion, or approximately $1 per year for every person in the poorer half of the world's population. By comparison, the World Bank estimates that the total health-related aid to developing countries in 2004 (from governments, international organizations, and private sources) was about $12.7 billion (see graph) [Graph not included to save space, Ed.].

If Gates donates more of his own fortune and if the value of Buffett's donated Berkshire Hathaway stock rises, the Gates Foundation's annual giving will increase further. Yet the projected cost of solving major health problems in the developing world is far higher than even the most optimistic projections for giving by Gates. In 2000, the United Nations adopted Millennium Development Goals to be achieved by 2015; they included substantially reducing child and maternal mortality, reversing the spread of HIV–AIDS and malaria, and reducing the prevalence of tuberculosis and associated mortality. It is estimated that to meet these health goals, international aid would have to increase by a factor of three to seven.[1]

Shortly after their marriage in 1994, Bill and Melinda Gates designated global health as the primary focus for their charitable giving and established the William H. Gates Foundation. By the end of 2005, the foundation (renamed in 1999) had awarded $10.2 billion in grants, about $6 billion of it for health-related projects. The mission of these grants can be summarized in three words: global health equity. The foundation holds that all human lives are of equal value, and the goal is to conquer diseases that disproportionately afflict the world's poor, preventing them from reaching their full potential. "Until we reduce the burden on the poor so that there is no real gap between us and them," Gates said in 2005, "[global health] will always be our priority."[2]

Some of the earliest major grants of this foundation aimed to increase access to life-saving vaccines in developing countries. Other key targets have included HIV–AIDS, malaria, tuberculosis, malnutrition, acute diarrheal and respiratory infections, tropical parasitic diseases, and maternal and child health. The foundation also mobilizes the resources for global health by promoting innovative financing mechanisms and product development and makes "focused investments . . . to achieve fundamental scientific breakthroughs," as exemplified by $450 billion in grants awarded last year to tackle 14 "grand challenges" in infectious disease, nutrition, and other fields. Recently, the foundation has begun to work on development issues that strongly influence health, such as clean water, sanitation, and girls' education.

The foundation has had several notable health-related achievements to date (see box), and some claim that the example set by Bill and Melinda Gates has been as important as the money they've donated. By calling attention to global inequities, they have attracted funding from others and made it fashionable for the rich or famous to become involved in solving global problems. Buffett's move reflects that trend—and seems likely to intensify it. "The golden age of global health started when Bill and Melinda Gates put $27 billion into their foundation," says Jim Yong

---

Key Health-Related Achievements of the Gates Foundation

An estimated 1.7 million deaths have been prevented through the work of the Global Alliance for Vaccines and Immunization (GAVI), which was formed in 2000 with the help of Gates funding and has received grants totaling $1.5 billion. About 90 million children have received hepatitis B vaccine, about 14 million have received *Haemophilus influenzae* type B and yellow fever vaccines, and about 21 million have benefited from expanded coverage with basic childhood vaccines. As a partnership of public and private organizations, governments, and pharmaceutical companies, GAVI also represents a successful model for alliances that the Gates Foundation is promoting in other areas.

An HIV-AIDS prevention initiative in India ($200 million) provides education, treatment for sexually transmitted diseases, condoms, and clean needles and syringes in six states with high rates of HIV infection. The national HIV–AIDS treatment program in Botswana ($50 million) is currently treating about 56,000 patients and has provided valuable lessons about scaling up HIV treatment. The foundation has also given $528 million for AIDS-vaccine research and $124 million for research on a microbicide to prevent sexual transmission of HIV. In August, it announced a 5-year, $500 million grant to the Global Fund to Fight AIDS, Tuberculosis, and Malaria, bringing its total contribution to the Global Fund to $650 million and its total funding for HIV–AIDS programs to about $2 billion.

Ten projects in malaria-vaccine development are being supported ($250 million) through the Malaria Vaccine Initiative of the international, nonprofit Program for Appropriate Technology in Health; one vaccine will soon be tested in a large phase 3 clinical trial in Africa. The first comprehensive national effort by a sub-Saharan African country to control malaria with the use of drugs, insecticide-treated bed nets, and other methods is being supported in Zambia ($35 million). The foundation is also supporting the development of better tuberculosis vaccines, including a genetically engineered, more immunologic version of the bacille Calmette-Guérin (BCG) vaccine, which researchers hope to test soon in large clinical trials in Africa and India.

More than 20 million mothers and infants have received basic health services through $110 million in grants for Saving Newborn Lives (a Save the Children initiative).

Kim, chief of the Division of Social Medicine and Health Inequalities at Brigham and Women's Hospital in Boston. "They completely changed the sense of scale. It was the Gateses who really got us dreaming."

"I think people watch what the Gateses do and assume that if they're doing it, it's not only a smart humanitarian move, but a smart business move," said Helene Gayle, a former official at the Centers for Disease Control and Prevention (CDC) who spent 5 years at the Gates Foundation and now heads CARE. "They've put global health on the front burner like never before."

According to Gayle, a trip to Africa in the early 1990s opened the couple's eyes to the vast health disparities between rich and poor countries. Gates has credited William Foege, a former director of the CDC, with awakening him to the potential social impact of his money—particularly by suggesting that he read the 1993 World Development Report, which starkly quantified the toll of disease in developing countries. From infectious disease experts, the couple learned that an amazing number of lives could be saved for what seemed to them relatively small investments. "We really did think it was too shocking to be true," Bill Gates has said.[2]

Buffett, for his part, has long intended to give away most of his $44 billion fortune, but he only recently decided to do so while he is still alive. He also changed his mind about where to donate it, choosing the foundation established by Gates, his friend and bridge partner, rather than the Susan Thompson Buffett Foundation, named for his late wife. That shift reflects his business philosophy of investing in companies that have a track record, rather than reinventing the wheel. By serving on the board of the Gates Foundation, he will have some say in how the funds are spent, and he made his gift contingent on Bill and Melinda's remaining at the helm.

The doubling of the foundation's budget comes at a time of change in the leadership of its health program. Earlier this year, Tadataka (Tachi) Yamada was named president of the foundation's Global Health Program, replacing Richard Klausner. Yamada, a gastroenterologist and former chairman of internal medicine at the University of Michigan Medical School, previously headed research and development at GlaxoSmithKline, where he oversaw a budget of more than $4 billion and more than 15,000 employees. Although his staff at the foundation is much smaller—just over 100 employees—the Buffett gift offers unique opportunities both for tackling the health problems that are already being addressed and for broadening the foundation's mandate. Yamada, who had been on the job for only 10 weeks when I spoke to him, had been traveling to field sites and listening to ideas about how to spend the additional money.

"I project that we're going to be spending a little bit more than half [the foundation's annual awards] on global health," Yamada said. "My initial reaction is to do more of what we're doing—to do it more completely or better." The foundation had invested in the development of new vaccines, drugs, and diagnostic tests for malaria, tuberculosis, HIV, and other infections, he noted, and some of these products will soon be ready for manufacture, large-scale testing, or distribution, requiring additional resources.

Yamada mentioned two new areas that are likely to become foci of giving: health information and human-resource development. The improvement of health information systems could enable developing countries to quantify health problems, helping them to set spending priorities, improve health care delivery, and measure the effects of interventions. Yamada recently saw an impressive model program in Manhica, Mozambique, created in cooperation with Spanish epidemiologists. In the area of human resources, he said, the foundation is interested in worker-training projects that will improve health care delivery. "I'm not just talking about nurses and doctors; I'm talking about a broader array of health care workers with varying levels of education—down to community workers with very little," he said.

Some have urged the foundation to broaden its focus to include deadly noncommunicable diseases. Yamada said his program would like to become involved in efforts to reduce smoking and tobacco use in developing countries, perhaps by reinforcing initiatives for countries to sign the World Health Organization's Framework Convention on Tobacco Control, a treaty that will require signatories to increase taxes on tobacco products, ban sales to minors, regulate advertising, and take other measures.

When the Buffett gift was announced, some observers expressed concern that aid from other sources would decline because the Gates Foundation would be perceived as rich enough to solve the developing world's health problems. But experts say that the foundation's actions have consistently led to increased funding from others. "Without Bill Gates, we would never have had the Global Fund," said Kim. "And for sure, there would be no PEPFAR," the President's Emergency Plan for AIDS Relief.

In the area of malaria control, the size of the foundation's grants has enabled it to energize research and forge partnerships among academia, government, and industry much more effectively than other institutions have, said Brian Greenwood, a professor at the London School of Hygiene and Tropical Medicine. Companies have been induced to develop drugs or vaccines for use in poor countries, because the foundation helps to pay the cost of development. "They have the potential to direct the overall pattern of what happens" in a field, Greenwood said. Critics have argued that such power to set the agenda has a downside. The foundation's grant making may not always reflect the priorities of recipients in developing countries, and its choices may influence the decisions of other funding agencies, potentially steering money away from basic science and toward product development. However, the Gates Foundation's wealth and independence allow it to take risks that could yield big payoffs. "Governments cannot afford to fail in the same way," noted Harvey V. Feinberg, president of the Institute of Medicine.

The history of the Global Alliance for Vaccines and Immunization (GAVI) illustrates both the dramatic progress that has been made and the continuing challenges. In the 1990s, childhood immunization rates with basic vaccines stopped increasing in developing countries, and newer vaccines against diseases such as hepatitis B and *Haemophilus influenza* type B were unavailable. Bill and Melinda Gates were attracted to a problem that might be attacked with money and technology; a $750 million Gates grant jump-started the alliance, and the foundation received a seat on GAVI's governing board. "Its intellectual input was critical," said Julian Lob-Levyt, president of GAVI. "I think the results-based nature of GAVI, which comes from Gates, is new in the development community."

GAVI now has almost $3.5 billion in commitments from governments and private sources, as well as $4 billion in long-term commitments to a new sister institution, the International Finance Facility for Immunization. In a financing innovation, pledges of future donations will be used to issue bonds on the financial market, allowing money to be spent up front to improve delivery systems, purchase vaccines in larger quantities, and assure manufacturers of the stable long-term market. Although Lob-Levyt predicts that financial incentives will attract new manufacturers and increase competition, lowering prices, the high cost of some vaccines remains problematic. In many countries, a weak health care infrastructure also represents a formidable barrier, so GAVI and the Gates Foundation have shifted course to address the underlying problem.

The Gates Foundation is still evolving, and its leaders acknowledged having made mistakes. For example, some early grants did not cover operating expenses for grantees; now they are included. The foundation staff underestimated the complexity of tasks such as delivering childhood vaccines in developing countries and found that in some cases, 5 years of funding for projects was not long enough to deliver results. Although the foundation is known for its "lean" structure, some grantees said the current staff levels are barely adequate to handle the existing workload, and Yamada said that it will have to grow in order to double its spending. Choosing worthy recipients, monitoring projects, and measuring their effects will be especially challenging. "For our largest grants, GAVI and the Global Fund, we know the results that they've produced and they are pretty substantial," said Yamada. "For others, it's harder to measure . . . [but] we're beginning to get some evidence." In Botswana, for example, where the foundation supports a national HIV–AIDS testing and treatment program, the prevalence of HIV infection among girls 15 to 19 years of age decreased by 22% between 2003 and 2005.

Perhaps the Gates Foundation's greatest influence derives from its assumption that intractable problems can be solved, given enough money and international cooperation. For example, as a condition of receiving $287 million in grants for AIDS-vaccine research that were announced in July, 165 scientists in 19 countries will have to share their data in a central repository. Yamada predicted that such collaboration will become more common in the future, even in industry.

"We're trying to deal with very difficult problems that people are suffering from in the developing world," he said. "The more information sharing there is, the more patients will benefit."

SOURCE

Okie S. 2006. Global health—The Gates–Buffet effect. *N Engl J Med* 55 (11): 1084–88. Copyright 2006 *New England Journal of Medicine*. Reprinted with permission of the Massachusetts Medical Society.

NUREMBERG CODE

Directives for Human Experimentation

1. The voluntary consent of the human subject is absolutely essential. This means that the person involved should have legal capacity to give consent; should be so situated as to be able to exercise free power of choice, without the intervention of any element of force, fraud, deceit, duress, over-reaching, or other ulterior form of constraint or coercion; and should have sufficient knowledge and comprehension of the elements of the subject matter involved as to enable him to make an understanding and enlightened decision. This latter element requires that before the acceptance of an affirmative decision by the experimental subject there should be made known to him the nature, duration, and purpose of the experiment; the method and means by which it is to be conducted; all inconveniences and hazards reasonable to be expected; and the effects upon his health or person which may possibly come from his participation in the experiment. The duty and responsibility for ascertaining the quality of the consent rests upon each individual who initiates, directs or engages in the experiment. It is a personal duty and responsibility which may not be delegated to another with impunity.

2. The experiment should be such as to yield fruitful results for the good of society, unprocurable by other methods or means of study, and not random and unnecessary in nature.

3. The experiment should be so designed and based on the results of animal experimentation and a knowledge of the natural history of the disease or other problem under study that the anticipated results will justify the performance of the experiment.

4. The experiment should be so conducted as to avoid all unnecessary physical and mental suffering and injury.

5. No experiment should be conducted where there is an a priori reason to believe that death or disabling injury will occur; except, perhaps, in those experiments where the experimental physicians also serve as subjects.

6. The degree of risk to be taken should never exceed that determined by the humanitarian importance of the problem to be solved by the experiment.

7. Proper preparations should be made and adequate facilities provided to protect the experimental subject against even remote possibilities of injury, disability, or death.

8. The experiment should be conducted only by scientifically qualified persons. The highest degree of skill and care should be required through all stages of the experiment of those who conduct or engage in the experiment.

9. During the course of the experiment the human subject should be at liberty to bring the experiment to an end if he has reached the physical or

mental state where continuation of the experiment seems to him to be impossible.

10. During the course of the experiment the scientist in charge must be prepared to terminate the experiment at any stage, if he has probable cause to believe, in the exercise of the good faith, superior skill and careful judgment required of him that a continuation of the experiment is likely to result in injury, disability, or death to the experimental subject.

SOURCE

Trials of War Criminals before the Nuremberg Military Tribunals under Control Council Law No. 10, Vol. 2, pp. 181–182. Washington, D.C.: U.S. Government Printing Office, 1949.

DECLARATION OF HELSINKI

Recommendations Guiding Doctors in Clinical Research
Adopted by the 18th World Medical Assembly, Helsinki, Finland, June 1964

INTRODUCTION

It is the mission of the doctor to safeguard the health of the people. His knowledge and conscience are dedicated to the fulfillment of this mission.

The Declaration of Geneva of the World Medical Association binds the doctor with the words, "The health of my patient will be my first consideration"; and the International Code of Medical Ethics declares that "Any act or advice which could weaken physical or mental resistance of a human being may be used only in his interest."

Because it is essential that the results of laboratory experiments be applied to human beings to further scientific knowledge and to help suffering humanity, the World Medical Association has prepared the following recommendations as a guide to each doctor in clinical research. It must be stressed that the standards as drafted are only a guide to physicians all over the world. Doctors are not relieved from criminal, civil and ethical responsibilities under the laws of their own countries.

In the field of clinical research a fundamental distinction must be recognized between clinical research in which the aim is essentially therapeutic for a patient, and clinical research the essential object of which is purely scientific and without therapeutic value to the person subjected to the research.

I. BASIC PRINCIPLES

1. Clinical research must conform to the moral and scientific principles that justify medical research, and should be based on laboratory and animal experiments or other scientifically established facts.
2. Clinical research should be conducted only by scientifically qualified persons and under the supervision of a qualified medical man.
3. Clinical research cannot legitimately be carried out unless the importance of the objective is in proportion to the inherent risk to the subject.
4. Every clinical research project should be preceded by careful assessment of inherent risks in comparison to foreseeable benefits to the subject or to others.

5. Special caution should be exercised by the doctor in performing clinical research in which the personality of the subject is liable to be altered by drugs or experimental procedure.

II. CLINICAL RESEARCH COMBINED WITH PROFESSIONAL CARE

1. In the treatment of the sick person, the doctor must be free to use a new therapeutic measure, if in his judgment it offers hope of saving life, re-establishing health, or alleviating suffering.

   If at all possible, consistent with patient psychology, the doctor should obtain the patient's freely given consent after the patient has been given a full explanation. In case of legal incapacity, consent should also be procured from the legal guardian; in case of physical incapacity the permission of the legal guardian replaces that of the patient.

2. The doctor can combine clinical research with professional care, the objective being the acquisition of new medical knowledge, only to the extent that clinical research is justified by its therapeutic value for the patient.

III. NON-THERAPEUTIC CLINICAL RESEARCH

1. In the purely scientific application of clinical research carried out on a human being it is the duty of the doctor to remain the protector of the life and health of that person on whom clinical research is being carried out.

2. The nature, the purpose, and the risk of clinical research must be explained to the subject by the doctor.

3a. Clinical research on a human being cannot be undertaken without his free consent, after he has been fully informed; if he is legally incompetent, the consent of the legal guardian should be procured.

3b. The subject of clinical research should be in such a mental, physical and legal state as to be able to exercise fully his power of choice.

3c. Consent should as a rule be obtained in writing. However, the responsibility for clinical research always remains with the research worker; it never falls on the subject even after consent is obtained.

4a. The investigator must respect the right of each individual to safeguard his personal integrity, especially if the subject is in a dependent relationship to the investigator.

4b. At any time during the course of clinical research the subject or his guardian should be free to withdraw permission for research to be continued. The investigator or the investigating team should discontinue the research if in his or their judgment, it may, if continued, be harmful to the individual.

SOURCE

THE BELMONT REPORT

Office of the Secretary
Ethical Principles and Guidelines for the Protection of Human Subjects of Research
The National Commission for the Protection of Human Subjects of Biomedical and
Behavioral Research
April 18, 1979

AGENCY: Department of Health, Education, and Welfare.

ACTION: Notice of Report for Public Comment.

SUMMARY: On July 12, 1974, the National Research Act (Pub. L. 93–348) was signed into law, there-by creating the National Commission for the Protection of Human Subjects of Biomedical and Behavioral Research. One of the charges to the Commission was to identify the basic ethical principles that should underlie the conduct of biomedical and behavioral research involving human subjects and to develop guidelines which should be followed to assure that such research is conducted in accordance with those principles. In carrying out the above, the Commission was directed to consider: (i) the boundaries between biomedical and behavioral research and the accepted and routine practice of medicine, (ii) the role of assessment of risk-benefit criteria in the determination of the appropriateness of research involving human subjects, (iii) appropriate guidelines for the selection of human subjects for participation in such research and (iv) the nature and definition of informed consent in various research settings.

The Belmont Report attempts to summarize the basic ethical principles identified by the Commission in the course of its deliberations. It is the outgrowth of an intensive four-day period of discussions that were held in February 1976 at the Smithsonian Institution's Belmont Conference Center supplemented by the monthly deliberations of the Commission that were held over a period of nearly four years. It is a statement of basic ethical principles and guidelines that should assist in resolving the ethical problems that surround the conduct of research with human subjects. By publishing the Report in the Federal Register, and providing reprints upon request, the Secretary intends that it may be made readily available to scientists, members of Institutional Review Boards, and Federal employees. The two-volume Appendix, containing the lengthy reports of experts and specialists who assisted the Commission in fulfilling this part of its charge, is available as DHEW Publication No. (OS) 78–0013 and No. (OS) 78–0014, for sale by the Superintendent of Documents, U.S. Government Printing Office, Washington, D.C. 20402.

Unlike most other reports of the Commission, the Belmont Report does not make specific recommendations for administrative action by the Secretary of Health, Education, and Welfare. Rather, the Commission recommended that the Belmont Report be adopted in its entirety, as a statement of the Department's policy. The Department requests public comment on this recommendation.

NATIONAL COMMISSION FOR THE PROTECTION OF HUMAN
SUBJECTS OF BIOMEDICAL AND BEHAVIORAL RESEARCH
MEMBERS OF THE COMMISSION

Kenneth John Ryan, M.D., Chairman, Chief of Staff, Boston
Hospital for Women.
Joseph V. Brady, Ph.D., Professor of Behavioral Biology, Johns
Hopkins University.
Robert E. Cooke, M.D., President, Medical College
of Pennsylvania.
Dorothy I. Height, President, National Council of Negro
Women, Inc.
Albert R. Jonsen, Ph.D., Associate Professor of Bioethics,
University of California at San Francisco.
Patricia King, J.D., Associate Professor of Law, Georgetown
University Law Center.
Karen Lebacqz, Ph.D., Associate Professor of Christian Ethics,
Pacific School of Religion.
*** David W. Louisell, J.D., Professor of Law, University
of California at Berkeley.
Donald W. Seldin, M.D., Professor and Chairman, Department
of Internal Medicine, University of Texas at Dallas.
***Eliot Stellar, Ph.D., Provost of the University and Professor
of Physiological Psychology, University of Pennsylvania.

*** Robert H. Turtle, LL.B., Attorney, VomBaur, Coburn,
Simmons & Turtle, Washington, D.C.

*** Deceased.

TABLE OF CONTENTS

ETHICAL PRINCIPLES & GUIDELINES FOR RESEARCH
INVOLVING HUMAN SUBJECTS

Scientific research has produced substantial social benefits. It has also
posed some troubling ethical questions. Public attention was drawn to
these questions by reported abuses of human subjects in biomedical experiments, especially during the Second World War. During the Nuremberg War Crime Trials, the Nuremberg code was drafted as a set of standards for judging physicians and scientists who had conducted biomedical
experiments on concentration camp prisoners. This code became the
prototype of many later codes (1) intended to assure that research involving human subjects would be carried out in an ethical manner.

The codes consist of rules, some general, others specific, that guide
the investigators or the reviewers of research in their work. Such rules
often are inadequate to cover complex situations; at times they come
into conflict, and they are frequently difficult to interpret or apply.
Broader ethical principles will provide a basis on which specific rules
may be formulated, criticized and interpreted.

Three principles, or general prescriptive judgments, that are relevant
to research involving human subjects are identified in this statement.

Other principles may also be relevant. These three are comprehensive, however, and are stated at a level of generalization that should assist scientists, subjects, reviewers and interested citizens to understand the ethical issues inherent in research involving human subjects. These principles cannot always be applied so as to resolve beyond dispute particular ethical problems. The objective is to provide an analytical framework that will guide the resolution of ethical problems arising from research involving human subjects.

This statement consists of a distinction between research and practice, a discussion of the three basic ethical principles, and remarks about the application of these principles.

PART A. BOUNDARIES BETWEEN PRACTICE & RESEARCH

A. Boundaries between Practice and Research

It is important to distinguish between biomedical and behavioral research, on the one hand, and the practice of accepted therapy on the other, in order to know what activities ought to undergo review for the protection of human subjects of research. The distinction between research and practice is blurred partly because both often occur together (as in research designed to evaluate a therapy) and partly because notable departures from standard practice are often called "experimental" when the terms "experimental" and "research" are not carefully defined.

For the most part, the term "practice" refers to interventions that are designed solely to enhance the well-being of an individual patient or client and that have a reasonable expectation of success. The purpose of medical or behavioral practice is to provide diagnosis, preventive treatment or therapy to particular individuals.(2) By contrast, the term "research' designates an activity designed to test an hypothesis, permit conclusions to be drawn, and thereby to develop or contribute to generalizable knowledge (expressed, for example, in theories, principles, and statements of relationships). Research is usually described in a formal protocol that sets forth an objective and a set of procedures designed to reach that objective.

When a clinician departs in a significant way from standard or accepted practice, the innovation does not, in and of itself, constitute research. The fact that a procedure is "experimental," in the sense of new, untested or different, does not automatically place it in the category of research. Radically new procedures of this description should, however, be made the object of formal research at an early stage in order to determine whether they are safe and effective. Thus, it is the responsibility of medical practice committees, for example, to insist that a major innovation be incorporated into a formal research project. (3)

Research and practice may be carried on together when research is designed to evaluate the safety and efficacy of a therapy. This need not cause any confusion regarding whether or not the activity requires review; the general rule is that if there is any element of research in an activity, that activity should undergo review for the protection of human subjects.

Part B. Basic Ethical Principles

B. Basic Ethical Principles

The expression "basic ethical principles" refers to those general judgments that serve as a basic justification for the many particular ethical prescriptions and evaluations of human actions. Three basic principles, among those generally accepted in our cultural tradition, are particularly relevant to the ethics of research involving human subjects: the principles of respect of persons, beneficence and justice.

1. RESPECT FOR PERSONS.—Respect for persons incorporates at least two ethical convictions: first, that individuals should be treated as autonomous agents, and second, that persons with diminished autonomy are entitled to protection. The principle of respect for persons thus divides into two separate moral requirements: the requirement to acknowledge autonomy and the requirement to protect those with diminished autonomy.

An autonomous person is an individual capable of deliberation about personal goals and of acting under the direction of such deliberation. To respect autonomy is to give weight to autonomous persons' considered opinions and choices while refraining from obstructing their actions unless they are clearly detrimental to others. To show lack of respect for an autonomous agent is to repudiate that person's considered judgments, to deny an individual the freedom to act on those considered judgments, or to withhold information necessary to make a considered judgment, when there are no compelling reasons to do so.

However, not every human being is capable of self-determination. The capacity for self-determination matures during an individual's life, and some individuals lose this capacity wholly or in part because of illness, mental disability, or circumstances that severely restrict liberty. Respect for the immature and the incapacitated may require protecting them as they mature or while they are incapacitated.

Some persons are in need of extensive protection, even to the point of excluding them from activities which may harm them; other persons require little protection beyond making sure they undertake activities freely and with awareness of possible adverse consequence. The extent of protection afforded should depend upon the risk of harm and the likelihood of benefit. The judgment that any individual lacks autonomy should be periodically reevaluated and will vary in different situations.

In most cases of research involving human subjects, respect for persons demands that subjects enter into the research voluntarily and with adequate information. In some situations, however, application of the principle is not obvious. The involvement of prisoners as subjects of research provides an instructive example. On the one hand, it would seem that the principle of respect for persons requires that prisoners not be deprived of the opportunity to volunteer for research. On the other hand, under prison conditions they may be subtly coerced or unduly influenced to engage in research activities for which they would not otherwise volunteer. Respect for persons would then dictate that prisoners be protected. Whether to allow prisoners to "volunteer" or to "protect" them presents a dilemma. Respecting persons, in most hard cases, is often a matter of balancing competing claims urged by the principle of respect itself.

2. BENEFICENCE.—Persons are treated in an ethical manner not only by respecting their decisions and protecting them from harm, but also by making efforts to secure their well-being. Such treatment falls under the principle of beneficence. The term "beneficence" is often understood to cover acts of kindness or charity that go beyond strict obligation. In this document, beneficence is understood in a stronger sense, as an obligation. Two general rules have been formulated as complementary expressions of beneficent actions in this sense: (1) do not harm and (2) maximize possible benefits and minimize possible harms.

The Hippocratic maxim "do no harm" has long been a fundamental principle of medical ethics. Claude Bernard extended it to the realm of research, saying that one should not injure one person regardless of the benefits that might come to others. However, even avoiding harm requires learning what is harmful; and, in the process of obtaining this information, persons may be exposed to risk of harm. Further, the Hippocratic Oath requires physicians to benefit their patients "according to their best judgment." Learning what will in fact benefit may require exposing persons to risk. The problem posed by these imperatives is to decide when it is justifiable to seek certain benefits despite the risks involved, and when the benefits should be foregone because of the risks.

The obligations of beneficence affect both individual investigators and society at large, because they extend both to particular research projects and to the entire enterprise of research. In the case of particular projects, investigators and members of their institutions are obliged to give forethought to the maximization of benefits and the reduction of risk that might occur from the research investigation. In the case of scientific research in general, members of the larger society are obliged to recognize the longer term benefits and risks that may result from the improvement of knowledge and from the development of novel medical, psychotherapeutic, and social procedures.

The principle of beneficence often occupies a well-defined justifying role in many areas of research involving human subjects. An example is found in research involving children. Effective ways of treating childhood diseases and fostering healthy development are benefits that serve to justify research involving children—even when individual research subjects are not direct beneficiaries. Research also makes it possible to avoid the harm that may result from the application of previously accepted routine practices that on closer investigation turn out to be dangerous. But the role of the principle of beneficence is not always so unambiguous. A difficult ethical problem remains, for example, about research that presents more than minimal risk without immediate prospect of direct benefit to the children involved. Some have argued that such research is inadmissible, while others have pointed out that this limit would rule out much research promising great benefit to children in the future. Here again, as with all hard cases, the different claims covered by the principle of beneficence may come into conflict and force difficult choices.

3. JUSTICE.—Who ought to receive the benefits of research and bear its burdens? This is a question of justice, in the sense of "fairness in distribution" or "what is deserved." An injustice occurs when some benefit to which a person is entitled is denied without good reason or when some burden is imposed unduly. Another way of conceiving the principle of justice is that equals ought to be treated equally. However, this statement requires explication. Who is equal and who is unequal? What considerations justify departure from equal distribution? Almost all commentators allow that distinctions based on experience, age, deprivation, competence, merit and position do sometimes constitute criteria justifying differential treatment for certain purposes. It is necessary, then, to explain in what respects people should be treated equally.

There are several widely accepted formulations of just ways to distribute burdens and benefits. Each formulation mentions some relevant property on the basis of which burdens and benefits should be distributed. These formulations are (1) to each person an equal share, (2) to each person according to individual need, (3) to each person according to individual effort, (4) to each person according to societal contribution, and (5) to each person according to merit.

Questions of justice have long been associated with social practices such as punishment, taxation and political representation. Until recently these questions have not generally been associated with scientific research. However, they are foreshadowed even in the earliest reflections on the ethics of research involving human subjects. For example, during the 19th and early 20th centuries the burdens of serving as research subjects fell largely upon poor ward patients, while the benefits of improved medical care flowed primarily to private patients. Subsequently, the exploitation of unwilling prisoners as research subjects in Nazi concentration camps was condemned as a particularly flagrant injustice. In this country, in the 1940's, the Tuskegee syphilis study used disadvantaged, rural black men to study the untreated course of a disease that is by no means confined to that population. These subjects were deprived of demonstrably effective treatment in order not to interrupt the project, long after such treatment became generally available.

Against this historical background, it can be seen how conceptions of justice are relevant to research involving human subjects. For example, the selection of research subjects needs to be scrutinized in order to determine whether some classes (e.g., welfare patients, particular racial and ethnic minorities, or persons confined to institutions) are being systematically selected simply because of their easy availability, their compromised position, or their manipulability, rather than for reasons directly related to the problem being studied. Finally, whenever research supported by public funds leads to the development of therapeutic devices and procedures, justice demands both that these not provide advantages only to those who can afford them and that such research should not unduly involve persons from groups unlikely to be among the beneficiaries of subsequent applications of the research.

Part C. Applications

C. Applications

Applications of the general principles to the conduct of research leads to consideration of the following requirements: informed consent, risk/benefit assessment, and the selection of subjects of research.

1. INFORMED CONSENT.—Respect for persons requires that subjects, to the degree that they are capable, be given the opportunity to choose what shall or shall not happen to them. This opportunity is provided when adequate standards for informed consent are satisfied. While the importance of informed consent is unquestioned, controversy prevails over the nature and possibility of an informed consent. Nonetheless, there is widespread agreement that the consent process can be analyzed as containing three elements: information, comprehension and voluntariness.

INFORMATION. Most codes of research establish specific items for disclosure intended to assure that subjects are given sufficient information. These items generally include: the research procedure, their purposes, risks and anticipated benefits, alternative procedures (where therapy is involved), and a statement offering the subject the opportunity to ask questions and to withdraw at any time from the research. Additional items have been proposed, including how subjects are selected, the person responsible for the research, etc.

However, a simple listing of items does not answer the question of what the standard should be for judging how much and what sort of information should be provided. One standard frequently invoked in medical practice, namely the information commonly provided by practitioners in the field or in the locale, is inadequate since research takes place precisely when a common understanding does not exist. Another standard, currently popular in malpractice law, requires the practitioner to reveal the information that reasonable persons would wish to know in order to make a decision regarding their care. This, too, seems insufficient since the research subject, being in essence a volunteer, may wish to know considerably more about risks gratuitously undertaken than do patients who deliver themselves into the hand of a clinician for needed care. It may be that a standard of "the reasonable volunteer" should be proposed: the extent and nature of information should be such that persons, knowing that the procedure is neither necessary for their care nor perhaps fully understood, can decide whether they wish to participate in the furthering of knowledge. Even when some direct benefit to them is anticipated, the subjects should understand clearly the range of risk and the voluntary nature of participation.

A special problem of consent arises where informing subjects of some pertinent aspect of the research is likely to impair the validity of the research. In many cases, it is sufficient to indicate to subjects that they are being invited to participate in research of which some features will not be revealed until the research is concluded. In all cases of research involving incomplete disclosure, such research is justified only if it is clear that (1) incomplete disclosure is truly necessary to accomplish the goals of the research, (2) there are no undisclosed risks to subjects that are more than minimal, and (3) there is an adequate plan for debriefing subjects, when appropriate, and for dissemination of research results to them. Information about risks should never be withheld for the purpose of eliciting the cooperation of subjects, and truthful answers should always be given to direct questions about the research. Care should be taken to distinguish cases in which disclosure would destroy or invalidate the research from cases in which disclosure would simply inconvenience the investigator.

COMPREHENSION. The manner and context in which information is conveyed is as important as the information itself. For example, presenting information in a disorganized and rapid fashion, allowing too little time for consideration or curtailing opportunities for questioning, all may adversely affect a subject's ability to make an informed choice.

Because the subject's ability to understand is a function of intelligence, rationality, maturity and language, it is necessary to adapt the presentation of the information to the subject's capacities. Investigators are responsible for ascertaining that the subject has comprehended the information. While there is always an obligation to ascertain that the information about risk to subjects is complete and adequately comprehended, when the risks are more serious, that obligation increases. On occasion, it may be suitable to give some oral or written tests of comprehension. Special provision may need to be made when comprehension is severely limited—for example, by conditions of immaturity or mental disability. Each class of subjects that one might consider as incompetent (e.g., infants and young children, mentally disabled patients, the terminally ill and the comatose) should be considered on its own terms. Even for these persons, however, respect requires giving them the opportunity to choose to the extent they are able, whether or not to participate in research. The objections of these subjects to involvement should be honored, unless the research entails providing them a therapy unavailable elsewhere. Respect for persons also requires seeking the permission of other parties in order to protect the subjects from harm. Such persons are thus respected both by acknowledging their own wishes and by the use of third parties to protect them from harm.

The third parties chosen should be those who are most likely to understand the incompetent subject's situation and to act in that person's best interest. The person authorized to act on behalf of the subject should be given an opportunity to observe the research as it proceeds in order to be able to withdraw the subject from the research, if such action appears in the subject's best interest.

VOLUNTARINESS. An agreement to participate in research constitutes a valid consent only if voluntarily given. This element of informed consent requires conditions free of coercion and undue influence. Coercion occurs when an overt threat of harm is intentionally presented by one person to another in order to obtain compliance. Undue influence, by contrast, occurs through an offer of an excessive, unwarranted, inappropriate or improper reward or other overture in order to obtain compliance. Also, inducements that would ordinarily be acceptable may become undue influences if the subject is especially vulnerable.

Unjustifiable pressures usually occur when persons in positions of authority or commanding influence—especially where possible sanctions are involved—urge a course of action for a subject. A continuum of such influencing factors exists, however, and it is impossible to state precisely where justifiable persuasion ends and undue influence begins. But undue influence would include actions such as manipulating a person's choice through the controlling influence of a close relative and threatening to withdraw health services to which an individual would otherwise be entitle.

2. ASSESSMENT OF RISKS AND BENEFITS.—The assessment of risks and benefits requires a careful arrayal of relevant data, including, in some cases, alternative ways of obtaining the benefits sought in the research. Thus, the assessment presents both an opportunity and a responsibility to gather systematic and comprehensive information about proposed research. For the investigator, it is a means to examine whether the proposed research is properly designed. For a review committee, it is a method for determining whether the risks that will be presented to subjects are justified. For prospective subjects, the assessment will assist the determination whether or not to participate.

THE NATURE AND SCOPE OF RISKS AND BENEFITS. The requirement that research be justified on the basis of a favorable risk/benefit assessment bears a close relation to the principle of beneficence, just as the moral requirement that informed consent be obtained is derived primarily from the principle of respect for persons. The term "risk" refers to a possibility that harm may occur. However, when expressions such as "small risk" or "high risk" are used, they usually refer (often ambiguously) both to the chance (probability) of experiencing a harm and the severity (magnitude) of the envisioned harm.

The term "benefit" is used in the research context to refer to something of positive value related to health or welfare. Unlike, "risk," "benefit" is not a term that expresses probabilities. Risk is properly contrasted to probability of benefits, and benefits are properly contrasted with harms rather than risks of harm. Accordingly, so-called risk/benefit assessments are concerned with the probabilities and magnitudes of possible harm and anticipated benefits. Many kinds of possible harms and benefits need to be taken into account. There are, for example, risks of psychological harm, physical harm, legal harm, social harm and economic harm and the corresponding benefits. While the most likely types of harms to research subjects are those of psychological or physical pain or injury, other possible kinds should not be overlooked.

Risks and benefits of research may affect the individual subjects, the families of the individual subjects, and society at large (or special groups of subjects in society). Previous codes and Federal regulations have required that risks to subjects be outweighed by the sum of both the anticipated benefit to the subject, if any, and the anticipated benefit to society in the form of knowledge to be gained from the research. In balancing these different elements, the risks and benefits affecting the immediate research subject will normally carry special weight. On the other hand, interests other than those of the subject may on some occasions be sufficient by themselves to justify the risks involved in the research, so long as the subjects' rights have been protected. Beneficence thus requires that we protect against risk of harm to subjects and also that we be concerned about the loss of the substantial benefits that might be gained from research.

THE SYSTEMATIC ASSESSMENT OF RISKS AND BENEFITS. It is commonly said that benefits and risks must be "balanced" and shown to be "in a favorable ratio." The metaphorical character of these terms draws attention to the difficulty of making precise judgments. Only on rare occasions will quantitative techniques be available for the scrutiny of research protocols. However, the idea of systematic, nonarbitrary analysis of risks and benefits should be emulated insofar as possible. This ideal requires those making decisions about the justifiability of research to be thorough in the accumulation and assessment of information about all aspects of the research, and to consider alternatives systematically. This procedure renders the assessment of research more rigorous and precise, while making communication between review board members and investigators less subject to misinterpretation, misinformation and conflicting judgments. Thus, there should first be a determination of the validity of the presuppositions of the research; then the nature, probability and magnitude of risk should be distinguished with as much clarity as possible. The method of ascertaining risks should be explicit, especially where there is no alternative to the use of such vague categories as small or slight risk. It should also be determined whether an investigator's estimates of the probability of harm or benefits are reasonable, as judged by known facts or other available studies.

Finally, assessment of the justifiability of research should reflect at least the following considerations: (i) Brutal or inhumane treatment of human subjects is never morally justified. (ii) Risks should be reduced to those necessary to achieve the research objective. It should be determined whether it is in fact necessary to use human subjects at all. Risk can perhaps never be entirely eliminated, but it can often be reduced by careful attention to alternative procedures. (iii) When research involves significant risk of serious impairment, review committees should be extraordinarily insistent on the justification of the risk (looking usually to the likelihood of benefit to the subject—or, in some rare cases, to the manifest voluntariness of the participation). (iv) When vulnerable populations are involved in research, the appropriateness of involving them should itself be demonstrated. A number of variables go into such judgments, including the nature and degree of risk, the condition of the particular population involved, and the nature and level of the anticipated benefits. (v) Relevant risks and benefits must be thoroughly arrayed in documents and procedures used in the informed consent process.

3. SELECTION OF SUBJECTS.—Just as the principle of respect for persons finds expression in the requirements for consent, and the principle of beneficence in risk/benefit assessment, the principle of justice gives rise to moral requirements that there be fair procedures and outcomes in the selection of research subjects.

Justice is relevant to the selection of subjects of research at two levels: the social and the individual. Individual justice in the selection of subjects would require that researchers exhibit fairness: thus, they should not offer potentially beneficial research only to some patients who are in their favor or select only "undesirable" persons for risky research. Social justice requires that distinction be drawn between classes of subjects that ought, and ought not, to participate in any particular kind of research, based on the ability of members of that class to bear burdens and on the appropriateness of placing further burdens on already burdened persons. Thus, it can be considered a matter of social justice that there is an order of preference in the selection of classes of subjects (e.g., adults before children) and that some classes of potential subjects (e.g., the institutionalized mentally infirm or prisoners) may be involved as research subjects, if at all, only on certain conditions.

Injustice may appear in the selection of subjects, even if individual subjects are selected fairly by investigators and treated fairly in the course of research. Thus injustice arises from social, racial, sexual and cultural biases institutionalized in society. Thus, even if individual researchers are treating their research subjects fairly, and even if IRBs are taking care to assure that subjects are selected fairly within a particular institution, unjust social patterns may nevertheless appear in the overall distribution of the burdens and benefits of research. Although individual institutions or investigators may not be able to resolve a problem that is pervasive in their social setting, they can consider distributive justice in selecting research subjects.

Some populations, especially institutionalized ones, are already burdened in many ways by their infirmities and environments. When research is proposed that involves risks and does not include a therapeutic component, other less burdened classes of persons should be called upon first to accept these risks of research, except where the research is directly related to the specific conditions of the class involved. Also, even though public funds for research may often flow in the same directions as public funds for health care, it seems unfair that populations dependent on public health care constitute a pool of preferred research subjects if more advantaged populations are likely to be the recipients of the benefits.

One special instance of injustice results from the involvement of vulnerable subjects. Certain groups, such as racial minorities, the economically disadvantaged, the very sick, and the institutionalized may continually be sought as research subjects, owing to their ready availability in settings where research is conducted. Given their dependent status and their frequently compromised capacity for free consent, they should be protected against the danger of being involved in research solely for administrative convenience, or because they are easy to manipulate as a result of their illness or socioeconomic condition.

(1) Since 1945, various codes for the proper and responsible conduct of human experimentation in medical research have been adopted by different organizations. The best known of these codes are the Nuremberg Code of 1947, the Helsinki Declaration of 1964 (revised in 1975), and the 1971 Guidelines (codified into Federal Regulations in 1974) issued by the U.S. Department of Health, Education, and Welfare Codes for the conduct of social and behavioral research have also been adopted, the best known being that of the American Psychological Association, published in 1973.

(2) Although practice usually involves interventions designed solely to enhance the well-being of a particular individual, interventions are sometimes applied to one individual for the enhancement of the well-being of another (e.g., blood donation, skin grafts, organ transplants) or an intervention may have the dual purpose of enhancing the well-being of a particular individual, and, at the same time, providing some benefit to others (e.g., vaccination, which protects both the person who is vaccinated and society generally). The fact that some forms of practice have elements other than immediate benefit to the individual receiving an intervention, however, should not confuse the general distinction between research and practice. Even when a procedure applied in practice may benefit some other person, it remains an intervention designed to enhance the well-being of a particular individual or groups of individuals; thus, it is practice and need not be reviewed as research.

(3) Because the problems related to social experimentation may differ substantially from those of biomedical and behavioral research, the Commission specifically declines to make any policy determination regarding such research at this time. Rather, the Commission believes that the problem ought to be addressed by one of its successor bodies.

SOURCE

U.S. Department of Health and Human Services. http://www.hhs.gov/ohrp/humansubjects/guidance/belmont.htm

DECLARATION OF ALMA-ATA

International Conference on Primary Health Care, Alma-Ata,
USSR, 6–12 September 1978

The International Conference on Primary Health Care, meeting in Alma-Ata this twelfth day of September in the year Nineteen hundred and seventy-eight, expressing the need for urgent action by all governments, all health and development workers, and the world community to protect and promote the health of all the people of the world, hereby makes the following

DECLARATION:

I

The Conference strongly reaffirms that health, which is a state of complete physical, mental and social wellbeing, and not merely the absence of disease or infirmity, is a fundamental human right and that the attainment of the highest possible level of health is a most important worldwide social goal whose realization requires the action of many other social and economic sectors in addition to the health sector.

II

The existing gross inequality in the health status of the people particularly between developed and developing countries as well as within countries is politically, socially and economically unacceptable and is, therefore, of common concern to all countries.

III

Economic and social development, based on a New International Economic Order, is of basic importance to the fullest attainment of health for all and to the reduction of the gap between the health status of the developing and developed countries. The promotion and protection of the health of the people is essential to sustained economic and social development and contributes to a better quality of life and to world peace.

IV

The people have the right and duty to participate individually and collectively in the planning and implementation of their health care.

V

Governments have a responsibility for the health of their people which can be fulfilled only by the provision of adequate health and social measures. A main social target of governments, international organizations and the whole world community in the coming decades should be the attainment by all peoples of the world by the year 2000 of a level of health that will permit them to lead a socially and economically productive life. Primary health care is the key to attaining this target as part of development in the spirit of social justice.

VI

Primary health care is essential health care based on practical, scientifically sound and socially acceptable methods and technology made universally accessible to individuals and families in the community through their full participation and at a cost that the community and country can afford to maintain at every stage of their development in the spirit of self-reliance and self-determination. It forms an integral part both of the country's health system, of which it is the central function and main focus, and of the overall social and economic development of the community. It is the first level of contact of individuals, the family and community with the national health system bringing health care as close as possible to where people live and work, and constitutes the first element of a continuing health care process.

VII

Primary Health Care:
1. reflects and evolves from the economic conditions and sociocultural and political characteristics of the country and its communities and is based on the application of the relevant results of social, biomedical and health services research and public health experience;
2. addresses the main health problems in the community, providing promotive, preventive, curative and rehabilitative services accordingly;
3. includes at least: education concerning prevailing health problems and the methods of preventing and controlling them; promotion of food supply and proper nutrition; an adequate supply of safe water and basic sanitation; maternal and child health care, including family planning; immunization against

the major infectious diseases; prevention and control of locally endemic diseases; appropriate treatment of common diseases and injuries; and provision of essential drugs;

4. involves, in addition to the health sector, all related sectors and aspects of national and community development, in particular agriculture, animal husbandry, food, industry, education, housing, public works, communications and other sectors; and demands the coordinated efforts of all those sectors;

5. requires and promotes maximum community and individual self-reliance and participation in the planning, organization, operation and control of primary health care, making fullest use of local, national and other available resources; and to this end develops through appropriate education the ability of communities to participate;

6. should be sustained by integrated, functional and mutually supportive referral systems, leading to the progressive improvement of comprehensive health care for all, and giving priority to those most in need;

7. relies, at local and referral levels, on health workers, including physicians, nurses, midwives, auxiliaries and community workers as applicable, as well as traditional practitioners as needed, suitably trained socially and technically to work as a health team and to respond to the expressed health needs of the community.

VIII

All governments should formulate national policies, strategies and plans of action to launch and sustain primary health care as part of a comprehensive national health system and in coordination with other sectors. To this end, it will be necessary to exercise political will, to mobilize the country's resources and to use available external resources rationally.

IX

All countries should cooperate in a spirit of partnership and service to ensure primary health care for all people since the attainment of health by people in any one country directly concerns and benefits every other country. In this context the joint WHO/UNICEF report on primary health care constitutes a solid basis for the further development and operation of primary health care throughout the world.

X

An acceptable level of health for all the people of the world by the year 2000 can be attained through a fuller and better use of the world's resources, a considerable part of which is now spent on armaments and military conflicts. A genuine policy of independence, peace, détente and disarmament could and should release additional resources that could well be devoted to peaceful aims and in particular to the acceleration of social and economic development of which primary health care, as an essential part, should be allotted its proper share.

The International Conference on Primary Health Care calls for urgent and effective national and international action to develop and implement primary health care throughout the world and particularly in developing countries in a spirit of technical cooperation and in keeping with a New International Economic Order. It urges governments, WHO and UNICEF, and other international organizations, as well as multilateral and bilateral agencies, nongovernmental organizations, funding agencies, all health workers and the whole world community to support national and international commitment to primary health care and to channel increased technical and financial support to it, particularly in developing countries. The Conference calls on all the aforementioned to collaborate in introducing, developing and maintaining primary health care in accordance with the spirit and content of this Declaration.

Source

Reproduced with permission of the World Health Organization. http://www.who .int/hpr/NPH/docs/declaration_almaata.pdf

OTTAWA CHARTER FOR HEALTH PROMOTION

First International Conference on Health Promotion
Ottawa, 21 November 1986—WHO/HPR/HEP/95.1

The first International Conference on Health Promotion, meeting in Ottawa this 21st day of November 1986, hereby presents this CHARTER for action to achieve Health for All by the year 2000 and beyond.

This conference was primarily a response to growing expectations for a new public health movement around the world. Discussions focused on the needs in industrialized countries, but took into account similar concerns in all other regions. It built on the progress made through the Declaration on Primary Health Care at Alma-Ata, the World Health Organization's Targets for Health for All document, and the recent debate at the World Health Assembly on intersectoral action for health.

HEALTH PROMOTION

Health promotion is the process of enabling people to increase control over, and to improve, their health. To reach a state of complete physical, mental and social well-being, an individual or group must be able to identify and to realize aspirations, to satisfy needs, and to change or cope with the environment. Health is, therefore, seen as a resource for everyday life, not the objective of living. Health is a positive concept emphasizing social and personal resources, as well as physical capacities. Therefore, health promotion is not just the responsibility of the health sector, but goes beyond healthy life-styles to well-being.

PREREQUISITES FOR HEALTH

The fundamental conditions and resources for health are:

- peace,
- shelter,
- education,
- food,
- income,

- a stable eco-system,
- sustainable resources,
- social justice, and equity.

Improvement in health requires a secure foundation in these basic prerequisites.

ADVOCATE

Good health is a major resource for social, economic and personal development and an important dimension of quality of life. Political, economic, social, cultural, environmental, behavioural and biological factors can all favour health or be harmful to it. Health promotion action aims at making these conditions favourable through advocacy for health.

ENABLE

Health promotion focuses on achieving equity in health. Health promotion action aims at reducing differences in current health status and ensuring equal opportunities and resources to enable all people to achieve their fullest health potential. This includes a secure foundation in a supportive environment, access to information, life skills and opportunities for making healthy choices. People cannot achieve their fullest health potential unless they are able to take control of those things which determine their health. This must apply equally to women and men.

MEDIATE

The prerequisites and prospects for health cannot be ensured by the health sector alone. More importantly, health promotion demands coordinated action by all concerned: by governments, by health and other social and economic sectors, by nongovernmental and voluntary organization, by local authorities, by industry and by the media. People in all walks of life are involved as individuals, families and communities. Professional and social groups and health personnel have a major responsibility to mediate between differing interests in society for the pursuit of health.

Health promotion strategies and programmes should be adapted to the local needs and possibilities of individual countries and regions to take into account differing social, cultural and economic systems.

HEALTH PROMOTION ACTION MEANS:

Build Healthy Public Policy

Health promotion goes beyond health care. It puts health on the agenda of policy makers in all sectors and at all levels, directing them to be aware of the health consequences of their decisions and to accept their responsibilities for health.

Health promotion policy combines diverse but complementary approaches including legislation, fiscal measures, taxation and organizational change. It is coordinated action that leads to health, income and social policies that foster greater equity. Joint action contributes to ensuring safer and healthier goods and services, healthier public services, and cleaner, more enjoyable environments.

Health promotion policy requires the identification of obstacles to the adoption of healthy public policies in non-health sectors, and ways of removing them. The aim must be to make the healthier choice the easier choice for policy makers as well.

Create Supportive Environments

Our societies are complex and interrelated. Health cannot be separated from other goals. The inextricable links between people and their environment constitutes the basis for a socioecological approach to health. The overall guiding principle for the world, nations, regions and communities alike, is the need to encourage reciprocal maintenance—to take care of each other, our communities and our natural environment. The conservation of natural resources throughout the world should be emphasized as a global responsibility.

Changing patterns of life, work and leisure have a significant impact on health. Work and leisure should be a source of health for people. The way society organizes work should help create a healthy society. Health promotion generates living and working conditions that are safe, stimulating, satisfying and enjoyable.

Systematic assessment of the health impact of a rapidly changing environment—particularly in areas of technology, work, energy production and urbanization—is essential and must be followed by action to ensure positive benefit to the health of the public. The protection of the natural and built environments and the conservation of natural resources must be addressed in any health promotion strategy.

Strengthen Community Actions

Health promotion works through concrete and effective community action in setting priorities, making decisions, planning strategies and implementing them to achieve better health. At the heart of this process is the empowerment of communities—their ownership and control of their own endeavours and destinies.

Community development draws on existing human and material resources in the community to enhance self-help and social support, and to develop flexible systems for strengthening public participation in and direction of health matters. This requires full and continuous access to information, learning opportunities for health, as well as funding support.

Develop Personal Skills

Health promotion supports personal and social development through providing information, education for health, and enhancing life skills. By so doing, it increases the options available to people to exercise more control over their own health and over their environments, and to make choices conducive to health.

Enabling people to learn, throughout life, to prepare themselves for all of its stages and to cope with chronic illness and injuries is essential. This has to be facilitated in school, home, work and community settings. Action is required through educational, professional, commercial and voluntary bodies, and within the institutions themselves.

Reorient Health Services

The responsibility for health promotion in health services is shared among individuals, community groups, health professionals, health service institutions and governments. Theym must work together towards a health care system which contributes to the pursuit of health.

The role of the health sector must move increasingly in a health promotion direction, beyond its responsibility for providing clinical and curative services. Health services need to embrace an expanded mandate which is sensitive and respects cultural needs. This mandate should support the needs of individuals and communities for a healthier life, and open channels between the health sector and broader social, political, economic and physical environmental components.

Reorienting health services also requires stronger attention to health research as well as changes in professional education and training. This must lead to a change of attitude and organization of health services which refocuses on the total needs of the individual as a whole person.

Moving into the Future

Health is created and lived by people within the settings of their everyday life; where they learn, work, play and love. Health is created by caring for oneself and others, by being able to take decisions and have control over one's life circumstances, and by ensuring that the society one lives in creates conditions that allow the attainment of health by all its members.

Caring, holism and ecology are essential issues in developing strategies for health promotion. Therefore, those involved should take as a guiding principle that, in each phase of planning, implementation and evaluation of health promotion activities, women and men should become equal partners.

COMMITMENT TO HEALTH PROMOTION

The participants in this Conference pledge:

- to move into the arena of healthy public policy, and to advocate a clear political commitment to health and equity in all sectors;
- to counteract the pressures towards harmful products, resource depletion, unhealthy living conditions and environments, and bad nutrition; and to focus attention on public health issues such as pollution, occupational hazards, housing and settlements;
- to respond to the health gap within and between societies, and to tackle the inequities in health produced by the rules and practices of these societies;
- to acknowledge people as the main health resource; to support and enable them to keep themselves, their families and friends healthy through financial and other means, and to accept the community as the essential voice in matters of its health, living conditions and well-being;
- to reorient health services and their resources towards the promotion of health; and to share power with other sectors, other disciplines and, most importantly, with people themselves;
- to recognize health and its maintenance as a major social investment and challenge; and to address the overall ecological issue of our ways of living.

The Conference urges all concerned to join them in their commitment to a strong public health alliance.

CALL FOR INTERNATIONAL ACTION

The Conference calls on the World Health Organization and other international organizations to advocate the promotion of health in all appropriate forums and to support countries in setting up strategies and programmes for health promotion.

The Conference is firmly convinced that if people in all walks of life, nongovernmental and voluntary organizations, governments, the World Health Organization and all other bodies concerned join forces in introducing strategies for health promotion, in line with the moral and social values that form the basis of this CHARTER, Health For All by the year 2000 will become a reality.

CHARTER ADOPTED AT AN INTERNATIONAL CONFERENCE ON HEALTH PROMOTION*
The move towards a new public health, November 17–21, 1986 Ottawa, Ontario, Canada

* Co-sponsored by the Canadian Public Health Association, Health and Welfare Canada, and the World Health Organization

SOURCE

Reproduced with permission of the World Health Organization. http://www.who .int/hpr/NPH/docs/ottawa_charter_hp.pdf

THE MILAN DECLARATION ON HEALTHY CITIES, 1990

We, the mayors and senior political representatives from the WHO Healthy Cities network, gathered in Milan on 5 and 6 April 1990, affirm our commitment to the principles of the Healthy City project and declare that:

1. CITIES' ROLE IN PROMOTING HEALTH

Health

Health is a positive concept emphasizing social and personal resources as well as physical capacities. Health is created and lived by people in the settings of their everyday lives.

We pledge our political support for healthy public policies and the creation of supportive environments in our cities that develop and sustain the health of all our citizens.

Health for All Policy

Cities are key partners in the WHO health for all movement.

We pledge our political support for the health for all policy and the attainment of its targets in our cities. This requires community participation, including, where appropriate, the decentralization of decision-making and resources to the local level.

Sustainability

Health depends on sustaining the world's natural resources, as well as the quality of the natural and built environments.

We pledge our political support for the protection of the health of citizens and the quality of their environment by ensuring that urban development is environmentally sustainable.

In particular, we recognize the adverse effects of traffic on health and the environment, and the need for comprehensive urban transport planning that takes account of these effects.

Equity

Harmful effects on people's health arise not only from poverty but also from other kinds of social and educational disadvantage.

We pledge our political support for programmes that promote equity and reduce inequalities in health within our cities.

In particular, in this United Nations International Year of Literacy, we recognize the vital contribution that our city educational systems play in creating and promoting health.

Intersectorality and Accountability

Health is mainly the result of society's combined action (or lack of action) on the physical and social environment. Improvements in health are due only in part to the advances of *medical care systems*.

We pledge our political support for the strengthening of intersectoral action on the broader determinants of health and for exploring with our city councils or other city authorities ways to make health and environmental impact assessment part of all urban planning decisions, policies and programmes.

International Dimensions

Peace is an essential prerequisite for health. In this context, we welcome the new openness in Europe and affirm our belief that cities play an essential role in building bridges of understanding within and between countries of Europe and the world.

We pledge our political support for the WHO Healthy Cities project within the national and international networks and organizations to which we belong, and will encourage the national and international development of the new public health movement.

2. ACTION FOR HEALTHY CITIES

We hereby confirm our commitment to the WHO Healthy Cities project, and specifically reconfirm our commitment to take what measures we can to ensure the effective operation of the project in our cities, namely:

- establishing effective intersectoral mechanisms for developing healthy public policies;
- developing a city health plan that identifies the major health challenges and proposes a comprehensive, citywide intersectoral strategy to address them;
- establishing an adequately staffed Healthy City organization;

- creating mechanisms for public accountability for the effects of decisionmaking on health;
- ensuring effective community participation in all decisions and actions affecting health.

To ensure the longterm success of the Healthy Cities movement, we seek to match the recent commitment of the WHO Regional Office for Europe by continuing our involvement at least until 1995. In addition, we will explore, with councils, participation in EXPO 1992 to be held in Seville, and EXPO 1995 to be held in Vienna and Budapest, as part the Healthy Cities exhibit/programme intended to give high visibility to successes of the Healthy Cities project.

We hereby pledge that, to promote the health of our cities and citizens, we will explore with our city councils other city authorities actions that can contribute to recent WHO policy initiatives, including:

- the European Charter on Environment and Health;
- the European Action Plan on Tobacco or Health;
- the WHO air quality guidelines;
- the WHO policy on the prevention [of] AIDS and the care of people with AIDS.

We recognize the need for additional resources, beyond those that can [be] provided by our own cities and WHO, to support the further growth and development of the project. Accordingly, we call on WHO:

- to take the lead in the European Region, with other partners, in establishing joint action in urban health that will provide funding and resources with particular emphasis on the cities in Europe with greatest problems and the fewest resources;
- to explore the establishment of increased financial support to the Healthy Cities project such as a European health fund;
- to explore and facilitate the establishment of a Healthy Cities institute [to] support the Healthy Cities movement;
- to facilitate the creation of a European Healthy Cities association;
- to broaden the Healthy Cities project to cities in the developing countries.

We will provide political support to WHO in its efforts to expand the resources available to the project. We undertake to report on our progress in implementing the action here described in our cities at the next Meeting of Mayors, which will take place at the 1992 Healthy Cities Symposium in Copenhagen.

3. CONCLUSIONS

- We recognize health and its maintenance as major social investments.
- We reiterate our commitment to the concepts and principles of health promotion as defined in the Ottawa Charter for Health Promotion.
- We challenge and support the WHO Healthy Cities project in its approach to address the overall ecological issues of our ways of living.
- We urge cities throughout Europe and beyond to participate in the Healthy Cities movement and to join us in our commitment to a strong public health alliance.

Updated 01 April 2006

SOURCE

Reproduced with permission of the WHO Regional Office for Europe, Copenhagen. http://www.euro.who.int/AboutWHO/Policy/20010927_8

UNITED NATIONS MILLENNIUM
DECLARATION

The General Assembly
Adopts the following Declaration:

United Nations Millennium Declaration

I. Values and Principles

1. We, heads of State and Government, have gathered at United Nations Headquarters in New York from 6 to 8 September 2000, at the dawn of a new millennium, to reaffirm our faith in the Organization and its Charter as indispensable foundations of a more peaceful, prosperous and just world.

2. We recognize that, in addition to our separate responsibilities to our individual societies, we have a collective responsibility to uphold the principles of human dignity, equality and equity at the global level. As leaders we have a duty therefore to all the world's people, especially the most vulnerable and, in particular, the children of the world, to whom the future belongs.

3. We reaffirm our commitment to the purposes and principles of the Charter of the United Nations, which have proved timeless and universal. Indeed, their relevance and capacity to inspire have increased, as nations and peoples have become increasingly interconnected and interdependent.

4. We are determined to establish a just and lasting peace all over the world in accordance with the purposes and principles of the Charter. We rededicate ourselves to support all efforts to uphold the sovereign equality of all States, respect for their territorial integrity and political independence, resolution of disputes by peaceful means and in conformity with the principles of justice and international law, the right to self-determination of peoples which remain under colonial domination and foreign occupation, non-interference in the internal affairs of States, respect for human rights and fundamental freedoms, respect for the equal rights of all without distinction as to race, sex, language or religion and international cooperation in solving international problems of an economic, social, cultural or humanitarian character.

5. We believe that the central challenge we face today is to ensure that globalization becomes a positive force for all the world's people. For while globalization offers great opportunities, at present its benefits are very unevenly shared, while its costs are unevenly distributed. We recognize that developing countries and countries with economies in transition face special difficulties in responding to this central challenge. Thus, only through broad and sustained efforts to create a shared future, based upon our common humanity in

all its diversity, can globalization be made fully inclusive and equitable. These efforts must include policies and measures, at the global level, which correspond to the needs of developing countries and economies in transition and are formulated and implemented with their effective participation.

6. We consider certain fundamental values to be essential to international relations in the twenty-first century. These include:

- **Freedom.** Men and women have the right to live their lives and raise their children in dignity, free from hunger and from the fear of violence, oppression or injustice. Democratic and participatory governance based on the will of the people best assures these rights.

- **Equality.** No individual and no nation must be denied the opportunity to benefit from development. The equal rights and opportunities of women and men must be assured.

- **Solidarity.** Global challenges must be managed in a way that distributes the costs and burdens fairly in accordance with basic principles of equity and social justice. Those who suffer or who benefit least deserve help from those who benefit most.

- **Tolerance.** Human beings must respect one other, in all their diversity of belief, culture and language. Differences within and between societies should be neither feared nor repressed, but cherished as a precious asset of humanity. A culture of peace and dialogue among all civilizations should be actively promoted.

- **Respect for nature.** Prudence must be shown in the management of all living species and natural resources, in accordance with the precepts of sustainable development. Only in this way can the immeasurable riches provided to us by nature be preserved and passed on to our descendants. The current unsustainable patterns of production and consumption must be changed in the interest of our future welfare and that of our descendants.

- **Shared responsibility.** Responsibility for managing worldwide economic and social development, as well as threats to international peace and security, must be shared among the nations of the world and should be exercised multilaterally. As the most universal and most representative organization in the world, the United Nations must play the central role.

7. In order to translate these shared values into actions, we have identified key objectives to which we assign special significance.

II. Peace, Security and Disarmament

8. We will spare no effort to free our peoples from the scourge of war, whether within or between States, which has claimed more than 5 million lives in the past decade. We will also seek to eliminate the dangers posed by weapons of mass destruction.

9. We resolve therefore:

- To strengthen respect for the rule of law in international as in national affairs and, in particular, to ensure compliance by Member States with the decisions of the International Court of Justice, in compliance with the Charter of the United Nations, in cases to which they are parties.

- To make the United Nations more effective in maintaining peace and security by giving it the resources and tools it needs for conflict prevention, peaceful resolution of disputes, peacekeeping, post-conflict peace-building and reconstruction. In this context, we take note of the report of the Panel on United Nations Peace Operations and request the General Assembly to consider its recommendations expeditiously.
- To strengthen cooperation between the United Nations and regional organizations, in accordance with the provisions of Chapter VIII of the Charter.
- To ensure the implementation, by States Parties, of treaties in areas such as arms control and disarmament and of international humanitarian law and human rights law, and call upon all States to consider signing and ratifying the Rome Statute of the International Criminal Court.
- To take concerted action against international terrorism, and to accede as soon as possible to all the relevant international conventions.
- To redouble our efforts to implement our commitment to counter the world drug problem.
- To intensify our efforts to fight transnational crime in all its dimensions, including trafficking as well as smuggling in human beings and money laundering.
- To minimize the adverse effects of United Nations economic sanctions on innocent populations, to subject such sanctions regimes to regular reviews and to eliminate the adverse effects of sanctions on third parties.
- To strive for the elimination of weapons of mass destruction, particularly nuclear weapons, and to keep all options open for achieving this aim, including the possibility of convening an international conference to identify ways of eliminating nuclear dangers.
- To take concerted action to end illicit traffic in small arms and light weapons, especially by making arms transfers more transparent and supporting regional disarmament measures, taking account of all the recommendations of the forthcoming United Nations Conference on Illicit Trade in Small Arms and Light Weapons.
- To call on all States to consider acceding to the Convention on the Prohibition of the Use, Stockpiling, Production and Transfer of Anti-personnel Mines and on Their Destruction, as well as the amended mines protocol to the Convention on conventional weapons.

10. We urge Member States to observe the Olympic Truce, individually and collectively, now and in the future, and to support the International Olympic Committee in its efforts to promote peace and human understanding through sport and the Olympic Ideal.

III. Development and Poverty Eradication

11. We will spare no effort to free our fellow men, women and children from the abject and dehumanizing conditions of extreme poverty, to which more than a billion of them are currently subjected. We are committed to making the right to development a reality for everyone and to freeing the entire human race from want.

12. We resolve therefore to create an environment—at the national and global levels alike—which is conducive to development and to the elimination of poverty.

13. Success in meeting these objectives depends, *inter alia*, on good governance within each country. It also depends on good governance at the international level and on transparency in the financial, monetary and trading systems. We are committed to an open, equitable, rule-based, predictable and non-discriminatory multilateral trading and financial system.

14. We are concerned about the obstacles developing countries face in mobilizing the resources needed to finance their sustained development. We will therefore make every effort to ensure the success of the High-level International and Intergovernmental Event on Financing for Development, to be held in 2001.

15. We also undertake to address the special needs of the least developed countries. In this context, we welcome the Third United Nations Conference on the Least Developed Countries to be held in May 2001 and will endeavour to ensure its success. We call on the industrialized countries:

   • To adopt, preferably by the time of that Conference, a policy of duty- and quota-free access for essentially all exports from the least developed countries;

   • To implement the enhanced programme of debt relief for the heavily indebted poor countries without further delay and to agree to cancel all official bilateral debts of those countries in return for their making demonstrable commitments to poverty reduction; and

   • To grant more generous development assistance, especially to countries that are genuinely making an effort to apply their resources to poverty reduction.

16. We are also determined to deal comprehensively and effectively with the debt problems of low- and middle-income developing countries, through various national and international measures designed to make their debt sustainable in the long term.

17. We also resolve to address the special needs of small island developing States, by implementing the Barbados Programme of Action and the outcome of the twenty-second special session of the General Assembly rapidly and in full. We urge the international community to ensure that, in the development of a vulnerability index, the special needs of small island developing States are taken into account.

18. We recognize the special needs and problems of the landlocked developing countries, and urge both bilateral and multilateral donors to increase financial and technical assistance to this group of countries to meet their special development needs and to help them overcome the impediments of geography by improving their transit transport systems.

19. We resolve further:

   • To halve, by the year 2015, the proportion of the world's people whose income is less than one dollar a day and the proportion of people who suffer from hunger and, by the same date, to halve the proportion of people who are unable to reach or to afford safe drinking water.

- To ensure that, by the same date, children everywhere, boys and girls alike, will be able to complete a full course of primary schooling and that girls and boys will have equal access to all levels of education.
- By the same date, to have reduced maternal mortality by three quarters, and under-five child mortality by two thirds, of their current rates.
- To have, by then, halted, and begun to reverse, the spread of HIV/AIDS, the scourge of malaria and other major diseases that afflict humanity.
- To provide special assistance to children orphaned by HIV/AIDS.
- By 2020, to have achieved a significant improvement in the lives of at least 100 million slum dwellers as proposed in the "Cities Without Slums" initiative.

20. We also resolve:
- To promote gender equality and the empowerment of women as effective ways to combat poverty, hunger and disease and to stimulate development that is truly sustainable.
- To develop and implement strategies that give young people everywhere a real chance to find decent and productive work.
- To encourage the pharmaceutical industry to make essential drugs more widely available and affordable by all who need them in developing countries.
- To develop strong partnerships with the private sector and with civil society organizations in pursuit of development and poverty eradication.
- To ensure that the benefits of new technologies, especially information and communication technologies, in conformity with recommendations contained in the ECOSOC 2000 Ministerial Declaration, are available to all.

IV. Protecting Our Common Environment

21. We must spare no effort to free all of humanity, and above all our children and grandchildren, from the threat of living on a planet irredeemably spoilt by human activities, and whose resources would no longer be sufficient for their needs.
22. We reaffirm our support for the principles of sustainable development, including those set out in Agenda 21, agreed upon at the United Nations Conference on Environment and Development.
23. We resolve therefore to adopt in all our environmental actions a new ethic of conservation and stewardship and, as first steps, we resolve:
- To make every effort to ensure the entry into force of the Kyoto Protocol, preferably by the tenth anniversary of the United Nations Conference on Environment and Development in 2002, and to embark on the required reduction in emissions of greenhouse gases.
- To intensify our collective efforts for the management, conservation and sustainable development of all types of forests.
- To press for the full implementation of the Convention on Biological Diversity and the Convention to Combat Desertification in those Countries Experiencing Serious Drought and/or Desertification, particularly in Africa.

- To stop the unsustainable exploitation of water resources by developing water management strategies at the regional, national and local levels, which promote both equitable access and adequate supplies.
- To intensify cooperation to reduce the number and effects of natural and man-made disasters.
- To ensure free access to information on the human genome sequence.

V. Human Rights, Democracy and Good Governance

24. We will spare no effort to promote democracy and strengthen the rule of law, as well as respect for all internationally recognized human rights and fundamental freedoms, including the right to development.
25. We resolve therefore:
    - To respect fully and uphold the Universal Declaration of Human Rights.
    - To strive for the full protection and promotion in all our countries of civil, political, economic, social and cultural rights for all.
    - To strengthen the capacity of all our countries to implement the principles and practices of democracy and respect for human rights, including minority rights.
    - To combat all forms of violence against women and to implement the Convention on the Elimination of All Forms of Discrimination against Women.
    - To take measures to ensure respect for and protection of the human rights of migrants, migrant workers and their families, to eliminate the increasing acts of racism and xenophobia in many societies and to promote greater harmony and tolerance in all societies.
    - To work collectively for more inclusive political processes, allowing genuine participation by all citizens in all our countries.
    - To ensure the freedom of the media to perform their essential role and the right of the public to have access to information.

VI. Protecting the Vulnerable

26. We will spare no effort to ensure that children and all civilian populations that suffer disproportionately the consequences of natural disasters, genocide, armed conflicts and other humanitarian emergencies are given every assistance and protection so that they can resume normal life as soon as possible.
    We resolve therefore:
    - To expand and strengthen the protection of civilians in complex emergencies, in conformity with international humanitarian law.
    - To strengthen international cooperation, including burden sharing in, and the coordination of humanitarian assistance to, countries hosting refugees and to help all refugees and displaced persons to return voluntarily to their homes, in safety and dignity and to be smoothly reintegrated into their societies.
    - To encourage the ratification and full implementation of the Convention on the Rights of the Child[12] and its optional protocols on the involvement

of children in armed conflict and on the sale of children, child prostitution and child pornography.

VII. MEETING THE SPECIAL NEEDS OF AFRICA

27. We will support the consolidation of democracy in Africa and assist Africans in their struggle for lasting peace, poverty eradication and sustainable development, thereby bringing Africa into the mainstream of the world economy.

28. We resolve therefore:
   - To give full support to the political and institutional structures of emerging democracies in Africa.
   - To encourage and sustain regional and subregional mechanisms for preventing conflict and promoting political stability, and to ensure a reliable flow of resources for peacekeeping operations on the continent.
   - To take special measures to address the challenges of poverty eradication and sustainable development in Africa, including debt cancellation, improved market access, enhanced Official Development Assistance and increased flows of Foreign Direct Investment, as well as transfers of technology.
   - To help Africa build up its capacity to tackle the spread of the HIV/AIDS pandemic and other infectious diseases.

VIII. STRENGTHENING THE UNITED NATIONS

29. We will spare no effort to make the United Nations a more effective instrument for pursuing all of these priorities: the fight for development for all the peoples of the world, the fight against poverty, ignorance and disease; the fight against injustice; the fight against violence, terror and crime; and the fight against the degradation and destruction of our common home.

30. We resolve therefore:
   - To reaffirm the central position of the General Assembly as the chief deliberative, policy-making and representative organ of the United Nations, and to enable it to play that role effectively.
   - To intensify our efforts to achieve a comprehensive reform of the Security Council in all its aspects.
   - To strengthen further the Economic and Social Council, building on its recent achievements, to help it fulfil the role ascribed to it in the Charter.
   - To strengthen the International Court of Justice, in order to ensure justice and the rule of law in international affairs.
   - To encourage regular consultations and coordination among the principal organs of the United Nations in pursuit of their functions.
   - To ensure that the Organization is provided on a timely and predictable basis with the resources it needs to carry out its mandates.
   - To urge the Secretariat to make the best use of those resources, in accordance with clear rules and procedures agreed by the General Assembly, in the interests of all Member States, by adopting the best management practices and

technologies available and by concentrating on those tasks that reflect the agreed priorities of Member States.

- To promote adherence to the Convention on the Safety of United Nations and Associated Personnel.
- To ensure greater policy coherence and better cooperation between the United Nations, its agencies, the Bretton Woods Institutions and the World Trade Organization, as well as other multilateral bodies, with a view to achieving a fully coordinated approach to the problems of peace and development.
- To strengthen further cooperation between the United Nations and national parliaments through their world organization, the Inter-Parliamentary Union, in various fields, including peace and security, economic and social development, international law and human rights and democracy and gender issues.
- To give greater opportunities to the private sector, non-governmental organizations and civil society, in general, to contribute to the realization of the Organization's goals and programmes.

31. We request the General Assembly to review on a regular basis the progress made in implementing the provisions of this Declaration, and ask the Secretary-General to issue periodic reports for consideration by the General Assembly and as a basis for further action.
32. We solemnly reaffirm, on this historic occasion, that the United Nations is the indispensable common house of the entire human family, through which we will seek to realize our universal aspirations for peace, cooperation and development. We therefore pledge our unstinting support for these common objectives and our determination to achieve them.

8th plenary meeting

8 September 2000

SOURCE

From the resolution adopted by the General Assembly, 8th plenary meeting, 8 September 2000. United Nations Millennium Declaration 2000. Reproduced with permission of the United Nations. http://www.un.org/millennium/declaration/ares552e.htm

NOTES*

PART I

Chapter 1   FOOD AND NUTRITION

Impact of Vitamin A Supplementation on Childhood Mortality

1. Sommer A, Tarwotjo I, Hussaini G. Susanto D. Increased mortality in mild vitamin A deficiency. *Lancet* 1983; ii: 585–88.
2. Sommer A. Mortality associated with mild, untreated xerophthalmia. *Trans Am Ophthalmol Soc* 1983; 81: 825–53.
3. Sommer A, Katz J, Tarwotjo I. Increased risk of respiratory disease and diarrhea in children with preexisting mild vitamin A deficiency. *Am J Clin Nutr* 1984; 40: 1090–95.
4. Sommer A, Tarwotjo I, Hussaini G. Incidence, prevalence and scale of blinding malnutrition. *Lancet* 1981; i: 1407–08.
5. Sommer A. Nutritional blindness: Xerophthalmia and keratomalacia. New York. Oxford University Press, 1982.
6. Sommer A. Field guide to the detection and control of xerophthalmia, 2nd ed. Geneva: World Health Organization, 1982.
7. Sommer A, Hussaini G, Muhilal, Tarwotjo I, Susanto J, Sarosa JS. History of night blindness: a simple tool for xerophthalmia screening. *Am J Clin Nutr* 1980; 33: 867–91.
8. McCullagh P, Nelder JA. Generalized linear models. New York: Chapman and Hall, 1983.
9. Breslow NE. Extra Poisson variation in log-linear models. *Appl Stats* 1984; 33: 38–44.
10. Hamill PVV. NCHS growth curves for children. Birth–16 years. United States. DHEW publication no (PHS) 76·1650. Washington: US Department of Health, Education and Welfare, 1977.
11. McLaren DS, Shirajian E, Tchalian M, Khoury G. Xerophthalmia in Jordan. *Am J Clin Nutr* 1965; 17: 117–10.
12. Pereira SM, Begum A, Duram ME. Vitamin deficiency in kwashiorkor. *Am J Clin Nutr* 1966; 19: 162–66.
13. Handayani T, Mujiani, Hull V, Rohde JE. Child mortality in a rural Javanese village. *Int J Epidemiol* 1961; 12: 66–92.
14. United Nations Childrens Fund. The State of the Worlds Children. New York: Oxford University Press, 1985: 140–41.
15. West KP Jr, Sommer A. Delivery of oral doses of vitamin A to prevent vitamin A deficiency and nutritional blindness. *Food Rev Intern* 1985; 1: 351–41S.

*Notes are in their original formats to comply with copyright.

16. Sinha DP, Bang FB. The effect of massive doses of vitamin A on the signs of vitamin A deficiency in preschool children. *Am J Clin Nutr* 1976; 29: 110–15.

17. Solon F, Fernandez TL, Lathom MC, Popkin BM. An evaluation of strategies to control vitamin A deficiencies in the Philippines. *Am J Clin Nutr* 1979; 32: 1445–53.

18. Cohen N, Rahman H, Matin MA, et al. Prevalence and determinants of nutritional blindness in Bangladeshi children. *Wld Hlth Statist Quart* 1985; 38: 317–30.

19. Brilliant LB, Pokhrel RP. Grassel NC, et al. Epidemiology of blindness in Nepal. *Bull WHO* 1965; 63: 375–66.

20. Brink EW, Perera WDA, Broske SP, et al. Vitamin A status of children in Sri Lanka. *Am J Clin Nutr* 1979; 32: 84–91.

21. Helen Keller International. Bangladesh blindness study: key results. Dhaka. HKI and Institute of Public Health, 1985.

22. Pereira SM, Begum A. Failure of a massive single oral dose of vitamin A to prevent deficiency. *Arch Dis Child* 1971; 46: 525–27.

23. Sommer A, Green WR, Kenyon KR. Clinical-histopatholologic correlations of vitamin A responsive and nonresponsive Bitot's spots. *Arch Ophthalmol* 1981; 99: 2014–27.

24. Brown KH, Gaffar A, Alamgir SM. Xerophthalmia, protein-calorie malnutrition, and infections in children. *J Pediatr* 1979; 95: 651–56.

25. Kochanowski BA, Ross AC. Stimulation of humoral immunity by vitamin A during suckling and postweaning in the rat. *J Nutr* (in press).

26. Nauss KM, Mark DA, Suskind RM. The effect of vitamin A deficiency on the in vitro cellular immune response of rats. *J Nutr* 1979; 109: 1815–23.

27. Mark DA, Nauss KM. Baliga BS, Suskind RM. Depressed transformation response by splenic lymphocytes from vitamin A-deficient rats. *Nutr Res* 1981; 1: 489–97.

28. Bhaskaram C, Reddy V. Cell-mediated immunity in iron- and vitamin-deficient children. *Br Med J* 1975; iii: 522.

29. Cohen BE, Elin RJ. Vitamin A-induced nonspecific resistance to infection. *J Infect Dis* 1974; 129: 597–600.

30. Sommer A, Muhilal, Tarwotjo I, Djunaedi E, Glover J. Oral versus intramuscular vitamin A in the treatment of xerophthalmia. *Lancet* 1980; i: 557–59.

31. Sommer A, Muhilal, Tarwotjo I. Protein deficiency and treatment of xerophthalmia. *Arch Ophthalmol* 1982; 100: 785–87.

The Nutrition Transition in Low-Income Countries: An Emerging Crisis

1. National Research Council, Committee on Diet and Health. Diet and health: Implications for reducing chronic disease risk. [Committee on Diet and, Food and Nutrition Board, Commission on Life Sciences] Washington, DC: National Academy Press, 1989

2. U.S. Dept. of Health and Human Services. The surgeon general's report on nutrition and health. Washington, DC: US DHHS, 1988

3. Harper AE. Transitions and health status: Implications for dietary recommendations. Am J Clin Nutr 1987; 45:1094–107

4. Omran AR. The epidemiologic transition: a theory of the epidemiology of population change. Milbank Mem Fund Q 1971; 49:509–8

5. Olshansky SJ, Ault AB. The fourth stage of the epidemiologic transition: the age of delayed degenerative diseases. Milbank Mem Fund Q 1986; 64:355–91

6. Harris DR. The prehistory of human subsistence: a speculative outline. In: Walcher DN, Kretchmer N, eds. *Food, nutrition, and evolution: food as an environmental factor in the genesis of human variability.* New York: Masson, 1981:15–37

7. Truswell AS. Diet and nutrition of hunter-gatherers. In: CIBA Foundation Symposium 49, *Health and disease in tribal societies.* Amsterdam: Elsevier/Excerpta Medica, 1977:213–26

8. Eaton SB, Shostak M, Konner M. *The Paleolithic prescription: a program of diet and exercise and a design for living.* New York, New York: Harper and Row; 1988

9. Eaton SB, Konner M. Paleolithic nutrition: a consideration of its nature and current implications. NEJM 1985; 312:283–9

10. Vargas LA. Old and new transitions and nutrition in Mexico. In: Swedlund AC, Armelagos GJ, eds. *Disease and populations in transition: anthropological and epidemiological perspectives.* New York, New York: Bergen and Carvey, 1990

11. Gordon KD. Evolutionary perspectives on human diet. In: Johnson FE, ed. *Nutritional Anthropology.* New York, New York: Liss, 1987:3–39

12. Brown PJ, Konner M. An anthropological perspective on obesity. In: Wurtman RJ, Wurtman JJ, eds. *Human Obesity.* Ann NY Acad Sci 1987; 499:29–46

13. Newman LF, ed. *Hunger in history: food shortage, poverty, and deprivation.* Cambridge, MA: Blackwell, 1990

14. Millo N. *Nutrition policy for food-rich countries: a strategic analysis.* Baltimore, MD: The Johns Hopkins University Press, 1990

15. Popkin BM, Haines PS, Reidy KC. Food consumption trends of U.S. women: patterns and determinants between 1977 and 1985. Am J Clin Nutr 1989; 49:1307–19

16. Popkin BM, Haines PS, Patterson R. Dietary changes in older Americans, 1977–87. Am J Clin Nutr 1992; 55:823–30

17. Crimmins EM, Saito Y, Ingegneri D. Changes in life expectancy and disability-free life expectancy in the United States. Popul Dev Rev 1989; 15:235–67

18. Menton KG, Soldo BJ. Dynamics of health changes in the oldest old: new perspectives and evidence. Milbank Mem Fund Q 1985; 63:206–85

19. Slattery ML, Randall DE. Trends and coronary heart disease mortality and food consumption in the United States between 1909 and 1980. Am J Clin Nutr 1988; 47:1060–7

20. Stephen AM, Wald NJ. Trends in individual consumption of dietary fat in the United States, 1920–1987. Am J Clin Nutr 1990; 52:457–69

21. Kuczmarski RJ. Prevalence of overweight and weight gain in the United States. Am J Clin Nutr 1992; 55 (suppl):495s–502s

22. Popkin BM, Paeratukul S, Ge K. Dietary and environmental correlates of obesity in a population study in China. Obesity Res, in press

23. Sobal J, Stunkard AJ. Socioeconomic status and obesity: a review of the literature. Psychol Bull 1989; 105:260–75

24. Byers T, Wold R, Williamson DF. Worldwide increases in body size during the 20th century: global fattening. In: Proceedings of XV International Congress of Nutrition. New York, New York: Gordon and Breech, in press

25. Helmert U, Shea S, Herman B, Griser E. Relationship with social class characteristics and risk factors for coronary heart disease in West Germany. Public Health 1990; 104:399–416

26. Hulshof KF, Lowik MR, Kok FJ, Wedel M, Brants HA, Hermus RJ, ten Hoor F. Diet another life-style factors in high and low socio-economic groups (Dutch Nutrition Surveillance System). Eur J Clin Nutr 1991; 45:441–50

27. Millo N. Toward healthy longevity. Scan J Soc Med 1991; 19:209–17

28. Oshaug A. Towards nutrition security. Presented at the International Conference on Nutrition, Oslo, Norway, 1991:1–99

29. Yamaguchi K. Changes in nutritional and health status in Japan after the Second World War. In: Proceedings of the International Symposium on Food, Nutrition, and Social Economic Development. Beijing: Chinese Academy of Preventive Medicine, 1991:394–401

30. Matsuzawa Y. Pathogenesis of visceral obesity. Obesity Res, in press

31. Matsuzawa Y, Nakamura T, Tokunaga K. Visceral fat syndrome, a novel disease entity with multiple risk factors proposed from fat analysis by computed tomography. Proceedings of the XV International Congress of Nutrition. New York: Gordon and Breech, in press

32. Kim SH. Changing nutritional status affected by rapid economic growth of Korea. In: Proceedings of the International Symposium on Food, Nutrition, and Social Economic Development. Beijing: Chinese Academy of Preventive Medicine, 1991: 472–8

33. Popkin BM. Nutritional patterns and transitions. Popul Dev Rev 1993; 19:138–57

34. Ladda M-S, Junjana C, Puetpaiboon A. Increasing obesity in school children in a transitional society and the effect of the weight control program. Southeast Asian J Trop Med Public Health 1993; 24:590–4

35. Tamphaichitr V, Kulapogse S, Pakpeankitvatana R, Leelahhagul P, Tamwiwat C, Lochaya S. Prevalence of obesity and its associated risks in urban Thais. In: Gomura Y, Tarui S, Inoue S, Shimazu T, eds. *Progress in obesity research* 1990. London, UK: Libbey 1991:649–53

36. Gopalan C. Nutrition and developmental transition in Southeast Asia. Regional health paper, SEARO no. 21. New Delhi: WHO, 1992

37. Chadha SL, Radhakrishan S, Ramachandran K, Kaul U, Gopinath N. Epidemiological study of coronary heart disease in the urban population of Delhi. Indian J Med Res 1990; 92:424–30

38. Padmavati S. Epidemiology of cardiovascular disease in India. II. Ischemic heart disease. Circulation 1982; 25:711–17

39. Hodge A, Dowse GK, Zimmet P, Collins VR. Prevalence and secular trends in obesity in Pacific and Indian Ocean Island populations. Obesity Res, in press

40. Taylor R, Badcock J, King H, Pargeter K, Zimmet P, Fred T, Lund M, et al. Dietary intake, exercise, obesity, and non-communicable disease in rural and urban populations of three Pacific Island countries. J Am Coll Nutr 1992; 11:283–93

41. Neel JV. Diabetes mellitus: a "thrifty" genotype rendered detrimental by "progress"? Am J Hum Genet 1962; 14:353–82

42. Prior IA, Tasman-Jones C. New Zealand Maori and Pacific Polynesians. In: Trowell HC, Burkitt DP, eds. *Western diseases: their emergence and prevention.* Cambridge: Harvard University Press, 1981:227–67

43. Toor M, Katchalsky A, Agmon J, Allalouf D. Serum-lipids and atherosclerosis among Yemenite immigrants in Israel. Lancet 1957; 1:1270–3

44. Worth RM, Kato H, Rhoads GG, Kagan A, Syme SL. Epidemiologic studies of coronary heart disease and stroke in Japanese men living in Japan, Hawaii, and California: mortality. Am J Clin Epidemiol 1975; 102:481–90

45. Jamison DT, Mosley WH, Measham AR, Bobabilla JL, eds. *Disease control priorities in developing countries.* New York: Oxford University Press, 1993

46. Keyfitz N, Fileger W. *World population growth and aging: demographic trends in the late 20th century.* Chicago: University of Chicago Press, 1990

47. Popkin BM, Ge K, Zhai F, Guo X, Ma H, Zohoori N. The nutrition transition in China: a cross-sectional analysis. Eur J Clin Nutr 1993; 47:333–46

48. Lunes RF, Monteiro CA. The improvement in child nutritional status in Brazil: how did it occur? Geneva: United Nations Administrative Committee on Coordination, Subcommittee on Nutrition, 1993

49. Sichieri R, Coitinho DC, Leao MM, Recline E, Everhart JE. High temporal, geographic, and income variation in body mass index among adults in Brazil. Am J Public Health 1984; 84:793–98

50. Duncan BB. *As desiguaides socias na distribuicao de fatores de riso para doencas nao transmissiveis.* Unpublished Ph.D. dissertation, Universidade Federal do Rio Grande do Sul, 1991

51. World Bank. Brazil: the new challenge of adult health. Washington, DC, 1990

52. United Nations Administrative Committee on Coordination, Subcommittee on Nutrition. Second report on the world nutrition situation. Geneva:ACC/SCN 1992

53. Atalah ES. Analyses of the nutritional situation of the population of Santiago and some of the programs designed to improve their conditions. Archivos Latinoamericanos de Nutrition 1992; 42:22–31

54. Sinah DP, McIntosh CE. Changing nutritional patterns in the Caribbean and their implications for health. Food Nutr Bull 1992; 1488–96

55. Beckles GL, Miller GJ, Alexis SD, Price SG, Kirkwood BR, Carson DC, Byam NT. Obesity in women in an urban Trinidadian community. Prevalence associated characteristics. Int J Obesity 1985; 9:127–35

56. Trowell HC. Hypertension, obesity, diabetes mellitus, and coronary heart disease. In: Trowell HC, Burkitt DP, eds. *Western diseases: their emergence and prevention.* Cambridge: Harvard University Press, 1981:3–32

57. Bourne LT, Langenhoven ML, Steyn K, Jooste PL, Laubscher JA, Van Der Vyver E. Nutrient intake in the urban African population of the Cape Peninsula, South Africa. The BRISK Study. Cent Afr J Med 1993; 39: 238–47

58. Bourne LT, Langenhoven ML, Steyn K, Jooste PL, Nesamvuni AE, Laubscher JA. The food and meal pattern in the urban African population of the Cape Peninsula, South Africa. Cent Afr J Med 1994; 40:148–8

59. Bourne LT, Langenhoven ML, Steyn K, Katzenellenbogan J, Jooste PL, Lombard CJ, Badenhorst CJ. Urbanization and diet: an atherogenic transition.

The BRISK Study. Presented at the 12th Epidemiological Conference, Epidemiological Society of South Africa, Durban, South Africa, 1993

60. Fox FW. Diet in the urban locations as indicated by the survey. In: Janisch M, ed. *A study of African income and expenditure in 987 families in Johannesburg, January–November 1940.* Johannesburg: Radford, Adington, LTD, 1941

61. Steyn K, Joosta PL, Bourne LT, Fouris J, Badenhorst CJ, Bourne DE, Langenhoven ML, Lombard CJ, et al. Risk factors for coronary heart disease in the black population of the Cape Peninsula. The BRISK Study. South Afr Med J 1991; 79:480–5

62. World Bank 1993. World Development Report 1993: Investing in Health. New York: Oxford University Press (for the World Bank)

63. Stamler J. Editorial: epidemic obesity in the United States. Arch Int Med 1993; 153:1040–4

64. State Council. An outline for reforming and developing China's food structure in the 1990's. China Food Daily, 1993

65. Cassidy CM. The good body: when big is better. Med Anthropol 1991; 13:181–213

Chapter 2   TOBACCO

The Carcinogenic Effects of Tobacco

1. *Roffo, A. H.,* Bull. Inst. Med. Exper. of Buenos Aires, 1930, Nr. 23, p. 130.
2. *ibid:* Bull. Inst. Med. Exper. of Buenos Aires, 1930, Nr. 25, p. 1203.
3. *ibid:* Bull. Inst. Med. Exper. of Buenos Aires, Nr. 24, p. 501, 1930; cf. Krebsforschg. 1931, vol. 33, issue 4.
4. *ibid:* Bull. Inst. Med. Exper. of Buenos Aires 1931, Nr. 28, p. 545.
5. *ibid:* Bull. Inst. Med. Exper. of Buenos Aires 1931, Nr. 27, p. 277.
6. *ibid:* Bull. Inst. Med. Exper. of Buenos Aires 1936, Nr. 42, p. 287;––Dtsch. Med. Wschr. 1937, Nr. 33, p. 1267.
7. *Roffo, A. E.* (jr.): Bull. Inst. Med. Exper. of Buenos Aires 1937, Nr. 45, p. 311.
8. *Roffo, A. H.:* Bull. Inst. Med. Exper. of Buenos Aires 19 38, Nr. 47, p. 5.
9. *ibid:* Bull. Inst. Med. Exper. of Buenos Aires 1938, Nr. 48, p. 349;––Dtsch. Med. Wschr. 1939, Nr. 24 from 16 June 1939.
10. *ibid;* Bull. Inst. Med. Exper. of Buenos Aires 1939, Nr. 50 and cf. Krebsforshg. 1939, vol. 49, issue 5, p. 588.

Smoking and Lung Cancer: Recent Evidence and a Discussion of Some Questions

1. Arkin, H.: Relationship between human smoking habits and death rates. Current Med. Digest 22: 37–44, 1955.
2. Auerbach, O., Gere, J. B., Forman, J. B., Petrick, T. G., Smolin, H. J., Muehsam, G. E., Kassouny, D. Y., and Stout, A. P.: Changes in the bronchial epithelium in relation to smoking and cancer of the lung; a report of progress. New England J. Med. 256: 97–104, 1957.
3. Berkson, J.: The statistical study of association between smoking and lung cancer. Proc. Staff Meet. Mayo Clin. 30: 319–348, 1955.

4. _____: Smoking and lung cancer: Some observations on two recent reports. J. Am. Stat. Assoc. 53: 28–38, 1958.

5. Black, H., and Ackerman, L. V.: The importance of epidermoid carcinoma in situ in the histogenesis of carcinoma of the lung. Ann. Surg. 136: 44–55, 1952.

6. Blacklock, J. W. S: The production of lung tumours in rats by 3:4 benzpyrene, methylcholanthrene and the condensate from cigarette smoke. Brit. J. Cancer 11: 181–191, 1957.

7. Bock, F. G., and Moore, G. E.: Carcinogenic activity of cigarette-smoke condensate. I. Effective trauma and remote X irradiation. J. Nat. Cancer Inst. In press, 1959.

8. Breslow, L., Hoaglin, I., Rasmussen, G., and Abrams, H. K.: Occupations and cigarette smoking as factors in lung cancer. Am. J. Public Health 44: 171–181, 1984.

9. Buckwalter, J. A., Wohlwend, E. B., Colter, D. C., Tidirck, R. T., and Knowler, L.A.: ABO blood groups and disease. J. A. M. A. 162: 1210–1214, 1956.

10. Case, R. A. M.: Smoking habits and mortality among workers in cigarette factories. Nature, London 181: 84–86, 1958.

11. Case, R. A. M., and Lea, A. J.: Mustard gas poisoning, chronic bronchitis and lung cancer. Brit. J. Prev. & Social Med. 9: 62–72, 1955.

12. Chang, S. C.: Microscopic properties of whole mounts and sections of human bronchial epithelium of smokers and nonsmokers. Cancer 10: 1246–1262, 1957.

13. Cember, H., and Watson, J. A.: Bronchogenic carcinoma from radioactive barium sulfate. A. M. A. Arch. Indust. Health 17: 203–235, 1958.

14. Clemmesen, J., Nielsen, A., and Jensen, E.: Mortality and incidence of cancer of the lung in Denmark and some other countries. Acta Unio internat. contra cancrum 9: 603–635, 1953.

15. Cohart, E. M.: Socioeconomic distribution of cancer of the lung in New Haven. Cancer 8: 1126–1129, 1955.

16. Doll, R.: Etiology of lung cancer. Advances Cancer Res. 3: 1–50, 1955.

17. Doll, R., and Hill, A. B.: A study of the aetiology of carcinoma of the lung. Brit. M. J. 2: 1271–1286, 1952.

18. _____: Lung cancer and other causes of death in relation to smoking; a second report on the mortality of British doctors. Brit. M. J. 2: 1071–1081, 1956.

19. Doll, R., Hill, A. B., and Kreyberg, L.: The significance of the cell type in relation to the aetiology of lung cancer. Brit. J. Cancer 11: 43–48, 1957.

20. Dorn, H.: Tobacco consumption and mortality from cancer and other diseases. Acta Unio internal. contra cancrum. In press.

21. Dorn, H. F., and Cutler, S. J.: Morbidity from Cancer in the United States. Pub. Health Monogr. No. 29, Pub. Ser. Publ. No. 590. In press.

22. Dunn, H. F.: Lung cancer in the 20th century. J. Internat. Coll. Surgeons 23: 326–342, 1955.

23. Engelbreth-Holm, J., and Ahlmann, J.: Production of carcinoma in ST/Eh mice with cigarette tar. Acta path. et microbial. scandinav. [sic] 41: 267–272, 1957.

24. Finkner, A. L., Horvitz, D. G., Foradori, G. T., Fleischer, J., and Monroe, J.: An investigation on the measurement of current smoking by individuals.

Univ. North Carolina Inst. Statistics, Mimco Series No. 177, Chapel Hill, North Carolina, 1957.

25. Fisher, R. A.: Dangers of cigarette-smoking. Brit. M. J. 2: 297–298, 1957.

26. _____: Cigarettes, cancer and statistics. Centennial Rev. Arts and Sciences 2: 151, Michigan State University, 1958.

27. _____: Lung cancer and cigarettes? Nature, London 182: 108, 1958.

28. Gellhorn, A.: The cocarcinogenic activity of cigarette tobacco tar. Cancer Res. 18: 510–517, 1958.

29. Gilliam, A. G.: Trends of mortality attributed to carcinoma of the lung: possible effects of faulty certification of deaths due to respiratory diseases. Cancer 8: 1130–1136, 1955.

30. Graham, E. A., Croninger, A. B., and Wynder, E. L.: Experimental production of carcinoma with cigarette tar. IV. Successful experiments with rabbits. Cancer Res. 17: 1058–1066, 1957.

31. Greene, H. S. N.: Hearings before a Subcommittee of the Committee on Government Operations, House of Representatives, 85th Congress, First Session. 204–224, 1957.

32. Haag, H. B., and Hanmer, H. R.: Smoking habits and mortality among workers in cigarette factories. Indust. Ned, 26: 559–562, 1957.

33. Haenszel, W., and Shimkin, M. B.: Smoking patterns and epidemiology of lung cancer in the United States: are they compatible? J. Nat. Cancer Inst. 16: 1417–1441, 1956.

34. Haenszel, W., Shimkin, M., and Mantel, N.: A retrospective study of lung cancer in women. J. Nat. Cancer Inst. 21: 825–842, 1958

35. Haenszel, W., Shimkin, M. B., and Miller, H. P.: Tobacco smoking patterns in the United States. Pub. Health Monogr. No. 45, Pub. Health Ser. Publ. No. 426. Washington, D.C., U.S. Gov't. Print. Office, 1956, 111 pp.

36. Hammond, E. C.: Smoking in relation to lung cancer. Connecticut M. J. 18: 3–9, 1954.

37. _____: Inhalation in relation to type and amount of smoking. In press.

38. Hammond, E. C., and Horn, D.: Smoking in death rates–report on forty-four months of follow-up of 187,783 men. J. A. M. A. 166: 1159–1172 and 1294–1308, 1958.

39. Hartnett, T.: Tobacco industry scoffs at survey. New York Times, p. 44, col. 3, July 6, 1958.

40. Hilding, A. C.: On cigarette smoking, bronchial carcinoma in ciliary action. II. Experimental study on the filtering action of cow's lungs, the deposition of tar in the bronchial tree and removal by ciliary action. New England J. Med. 254: 1115–1160, 1956.

41. _____: On cigarette smoking, bronchial carcinoma in ciliary action. III. accumulation of cigarette tar upon artificially produced deciliated islands in the respiratory epithelium. Ann. Otol., Rhin and Laryng. 65: 116 130, 1956.

42. Hearings before a Subcommittee on the Committee on Government Operations, House of Representatives, 85th Congress, First Session. 1957, 795 pp.

43. Hueper, W.: A Quest into the Environmental Causes of Cancer of the Lung. Pub. Health Monogr. No. 36, Pub. Health Ser. Publ. No. 452. Washington, D. C., U. S. Gov't. Print. Office, 1956, 54 pp.

44. Kotin, P.: The role of atmospheric pollution in the pathogenesis of pulmonary cancer, *a review*. Cancer Res. 16: 375–393, 1956.

45. Kotin, P., and Falk, H.: The deposition of carcinogen-bearing particulate matter in the tracheobronchial tree in relation to particle size and effect of air pollutants and tobacco smoke on ciliary activity and mucus secretion of the respiratory epithelium. (Abstract.) Proc. Am. Assoc. Cancer Res. 2: 127–128, 1956

46. Kreyberg, L.: The significance of histological typing in the study of the epidemiology of primary epithelial lung tumours: a study of 466 cases. Brit. J. Cancer 8: 199–208, 1954.

47. Kuschner, M., Laskin, S., Cristofano, E., and Nelson, N.: Experimental carcinoma of the lung. *In* Proc. Third Nat. Cancer Conf. Philadelphia, J. B. Lippincott Co., 1956, pp. 485–495.

48. Leuchtenberger, C., Doolon, P. F., and Leuchtenberger, R.: A correlated histological, cytological, and cytochemical study of the tracheobronchial tree and lungs of mice exposed to cigarette smoke. I. *Bronchitis with atypical epithelial changes in mice exposed to cigarette smoke.* Cancer 2: 490–506, 1958.

49. Levin, M. L.: Etiology of lung cancer: present status. New York J. Med. 54: 769–777, 1954.

50. Lickint, F.: Atiologic und Prophylaxe des Lungengrebses. Dresden, T. Steinkopff, 1953, 212 pp.

51. Lilienfeld, A. M.: A study of emotional and other characteristics of cigarette smokers and nonsmokers as related to epidemiological studies of lung cancer and other diseases. J. Nat. Cancer Inst. 22: 1959, in press.

52. Little, C. C.: Hearings before a Subcommittee of the Committee on Government Operations, House of Representatives, 85th Congress, First Session. 1957, pp. 34–61.

53. Lyons, M. J., and Johnston, H. Colin Chemical investigation of the neutral fraction of cigarette smoke tar. Brit. J. Cancer 11: 554–562, 1957.

54. Macdonald, I. G.: Hearings before a Subcommittee of the Committee on Government Operations, House of Representatives, 85th Congress, First Session. 1957, pp. 224–240.

55. Mainland, D., and Herrera, L.: The risk of bias selection in forward-looking surveys with nonprofessional interviewers. J. Chron. Dis. 4: 240–244, 1956.

56. McArthur, C., Waldron, E., and Dickerson, J.: The psychology of smoking. J. Abnorm. & Social Psychol. 56: 267–275, 1958.

57. Medical Research Council: Tobacco smoking and cancer of the lung. Brit. M. J. 1: 1523–1524, 1957.

58. Mills, C. A., and Porter, M. M.: Tobacco smoking, motor exhaust fumes, and general air pollution in relation to lung cancer incidence. Cancer Res. 17: 981–990, 1957.

59. Milmore, B. K., and Conover, A. G.: Tobacco consumption in the United States, 1880–1955. Pub. Health Monogr. No. 45. Washington, D. C., U. S. Gov't. Print. Office, 1956, pp. 107–111.

60. Neyman, J.: Statistics–servant of all sciences. Science 122: 401–406, 1955.

61. Orris, L., Van Duuren, B. L., Koslak, A. I., Nelson, N., and Schmiott, F. L.: The carcinogenicity for mouse skin and the aromatic hydrocarbon content of cigarette-smoke condensate. J. Nat. Cancer Inst. 21: 557–561, 1958.

62. Passey, R. D., et al.: Cigarette smoking and cancer of the lung. Brit. Empire Cancer Campaign. Thirty-third Annual Report 1955, pp. 59–61.

63. Passey, R. D.: Carcinogenicity of tobacco tars. Brit. Empire Cancer Campaign. Thirty-fifth Annual Report, 1957, pp. 65–66.

64. Rigdon, R. H.: Hearings before a Subcommittee of the Committee on Government Operations, House of Representatives, 85th Congress, First Session. 1957, pp. 114–131.

65. Rigdon, R. H., and Kirchoff, H.: Cancer of the lung from 1900 to 1930. Internat. Abstr. Surg. 107: 105–118, 1958.

66. Rockey, E. E., Kuschner, M., Kosak, A. I., and Mayer, E.: The effect of tobacco tar on the bronchial mucosa of dogs. Cancer 11: 466–472, 1958.

67. Rosenblatt, M. B.: Letter to Surgeon General, United States Public Health Service. Hearings before a Subcommittee of the Committee on Government Operations, House of Representatives, 85th Congress, First Session. 1957, pp. 753–754.

68. Schwartz, D. and Denoix, R.: L'enquette francaise sur l'etiologic du cancer broncho-pulmonaire: rold due [sic] tabac. La Semaine des Hopitaux de Paris 33: 424–437, 1957.

69. Segi, M., Fukushima, I., Fugisaku, S., Kruihara, M., Saito, S., Asano, K., and Kamoi, M.: An epidemiologic study on cancer in Japan. Gann 48: Supp. 1957, 63 pp.

70. Shimikin, M. B.: Pulmonary tumors in experimental animals. Advances Cancer Res. 3: 223–267, 1955.

71. Society of Actuaries, Transactions, vol. 8, meeting 20, 1955 Reports of Mortality and Morbidity Experience, April, 1956.

72. Steiner, P. E.: Symposium on epidemiology of cancer of the lung; ideological implications of the geographical distribution of lung cancer. Acta Unio internat. contra cancrum 9: 450–475, 1953.

73. Stocks, P.: Report on Cancer in North Wales and Liverpool region. Brit. Empire Cancer Campaign. Thirty-third Annual Report 1957, Supp. to Part II.

74. Stocks, P., and Campbell, J. M.: Lung cancer death rates among non-smokers and pipe and cigarette smokers. Brit. M. J. 2: 923–929, 1955.

75. Smoking and Health. Joint Report of the Study Group on Smoking and Health. Science 125: 1129–1133, 1957.

76. Statistics of Smoking, Tobacco Manufacturer's Standing Committee. Paper No. 1, London (Todd, G. F., ed.) 1958.

77. Van Duuren, B. L.: Identification and some polynuclear aromatic hydrocarbons in cigarette-smoke condensate. J. Nat. Cancer Inst. 21: 1–16, 1958.

78. Vorwald, A. J., Pratt, P. C., and Urban, E. J.: The production of pulmonary cancer in albino rats exposed by inhalation to an aerosol of beryllium sulfate. Acta Unio internat. contra cancrum 11: 735, 1955.

79. Wynder, E. L., Bross, I. J., Cornfield, J., and O'Donnell, W. E.: Lung cancer in women. New England J. Med. 225: 1111–1121, 1956.

80. Wynder, E. L., Bross, I. J., and Day, E. A study of environmental factors in cancer of the larynx. Cancer 9: 86–110, 1956.

81. Wynder, E. L., Bross, I. J., and Feldman, R. M.: A study of the etiological factors in cancer of the mouth. Cancer 10: 1300–1323, 1957.

82. Wynder, E. L., and Cornfield, J.: Cancer of the lung and physicians. New England J. Med. 248: 441–444, 1953.
83. Wynder, E. L., Graham, E. A., and Croninger, A. B.: Experimental production of carcinoma with cigarette tar. Cancer Res. 13: 855–864, 1953.
84. Wynder, E. L., and Wright, G.: A study of tobacco carcinogenesis. I. The primary fractions. Cancer 10: 255–271, 1957.
85. Wynder, E. L., Wright, G., and Lam, J.: A study of tobacco carcinogenesis. V. The role of pyrolysis. Cancer. In press.

Non-smoking Wives of Heavy Smokers Have a Higher Risk of Lung Cancer:
A Study from Japan

1. Brunnemann KD, Adams JD, Ho DPS, *et al.* The influence of tobacco smoke on indoor atmospheres. II. Volatile and tobacco specific nitrosamines in main-aid sidestream smoke and their contribution to indoor pollution. In: *Proceedings of the 4th Joint Conference on the Sensitivity of Environmental Pollutants. New Orleans 1977.* Washington: American Chemical Society, 1978:876–80.
2. Brunnernann KD, Hoffmann D. Chemical studies on tobacco smoke LIX. Analysis of volatile nitrosamines in tobacco smoke and polluted indoor environments. In: Waler EA. Griciute L, Castegnaro M, eds. *Environmental aspects of N-nitroso compounds.* (IARC scientific publications No 19) *Lyons*: WHO, 1978:343–56.
3. White RJ, Froeb FH. Small-airways dysfunction in non-smokers chronically exposed to tobacco smoke. *N Engl J Med* 1980;302:720–3.
4. Hirayama T. Prospective studies on cancer epidemiology based on census population in Japan. In: *Proceedings of XI International Cancer Congress. Florence. Cancer Epidemiology and Environmental Factors, 3.* Amsterdam: Excerpta Medica. 1975:26–35.
5. Hirayama T. Epidemiology of lung cancer based on population studies. In: *Clinical implications of air pollution research.* Chicago: The American Medical Association, 1976:69–78.
6. Hirayama T. Smoking and cancer. A prospective study on cancer epidemiology based on census population in Japan. In: *Proceedings of the 3rd World Conference on Smoking and Health 1975.* Washington: Department of Health Education and Welfare. 1977:65–72. (DHEW Publication No (NIH) 77–1413.)
7. Hirayama T. Prospective studies on cancer epidemiology based on census population in Japan. In: Nieburgs H, ed. *Third International Symposium on Detection and Prevention of Cancer.* Pt 1. Vol 1. New York: Marcel, Dekter, 1977:1139–48.

Chapter 3 DENTAL HEALTH

The Conclusion of a Ten-Year Study of Water Fluoridation

1. Dean, H. T.; Arnold, F. A.; and Elove, E. Domestic Water and Dental Caries. Pub. Health Rep. 57:1155, 1942.
2. Russell, A. L.; and Elove, E. Domestic Water and Dental Caries: VII. A Study of the Fluoride-dental Caries Relationship in an Adult Population. Ibid. 66:1389, 1951.

3. Dean, H. T. Fluorine in the Control of Dental Caries. J. Am. Dent. A, 52:1, 1956.
4. Hilleboe, H. E. History of the Newburgh-Kingston Caries Fluorine Study. Ibid. Vol. 57 (Mar.), 1956.
5. Schlesinger, E. R., et al. The Newburgh-Kingston Caries-Fluorine Study: XIII. Pediatric Findings After Ten Years. Ibid. Vol. 57 (Mar.), 1956.
6. Ast, D. B., at al. The Newburgh-Kingston Caries-Fluorine Study: XIV. Combined Clinical and Roentgenographic Dental Findings After Ten Years of Fluoride Experience. Ibid. Vol. 57 (Mar.), 1956.
7. Hodge, H. C. Fluoride Metabolism: Its Significance in Water Fluoridation. Ibid. Vol. 57 (Mar.), 1956.
8a. Moulton, F.R., editor. Fluorine and Dental Health. Washington, D. C.: American Association for the Advancement of Science, 1942.
8b. _____. Dental Caries and Fluorine. Washington, D. C.: American Association for the Advancement of Science, 1946.
9. Cox, G. J.; Matuschak, M. C.; et al. Experimental Dental Caries IV. Fluorine and Its Relation to Dental Caries. J. Dent. Res. 18:481, 1939.
10. Ast, D. B. The Caries-Fluorine Hypothesis and A Suggested Study to Test Its Application. Pub. Health Rep. 58:800 57, 1943.
11. Dean, H. T. Endemic Fluorosis and Its Relation to Dental Caries. Ibid. 53:1443, 1938.
12. Zimmerman, E. R. Fluoride and Nonfluoride Enamel Opacities. Ibid. 69:1115, 1954.
13. Schlesinger, E. R.; Overton, D. E.; and Chase, H. C. Study of Children Drinking Fluoridated and Nonfluoridated Water: Quantitative Urinary Excretion of Albumin and Formed Elements. J.A.M.A. 160:20 1, 1956.

Diet and Oral Health

1. DePaola D P, Faine M P, Vogel R I. Nutrition in relation to dental medicine. In: Shils M E, Olson J, Shike M, eds. *Modern nutrition in health and disease.* Philadelphia: Lea & Febiger, 1994: 1007–1028.
2. Brunelle J A, Carlos J P. Recent trends in dental caries in U.S. children and the effect of water fluoridation. *J Dent Res* 1990 69 (Spec. Iss): 723–727.
3. Kalsbeck H. Evidence of decrease in prevalence of dental caries in The Netherlands: an evaluation of epidemiological caries surveys on 4–6 and 11–15-year-old children, performed between 1965 and 1980. *J Dent Res* 1982 61: 1321–1326.
4. Seppä L, Kärkkäinen S, Hausen H. Caries frequency in permanent teeth before and after discontinuation of water fluoridation in Kuopio, Finland. *Community Dent Oral Epidemiol* 1998 26: 256–262.
5. Stephan R M, Mellor B F. A quantitative method for evaluating physical and chemical agents which modify production of acid in bacterial plaques on human teeth. *J Dent Res* 1943 22: 45–51.
6. Imfeld T. *Identification of Low-Risk Dietary Components.* Basel, Karger, 1983.
7. Gustafson B, Quensel C, Lanke I, *et al.* The Vipeholm dental caries study: the effect of different carbohydrate intake on caries activity in 436 individuals observed for five years. *Acta Odontol Scand* 1954 11: 232–264.

8. Sreebny L M. Sugar and human dental caries. *World Review Nutr Diet* 1982 40: 19–65.

9. Walker A R P, Cleaton-Jones P E. Sugar intake and dental caries: where do we stand? *J Dent Child* 1989 56: 30–35.

10. Richardson A S, Boyd M A, Conry R F. A correlation study of diet, oral hygiene and dental caries in 457 Canadian children. *Community Dense Oral Epidemiol* 1977 5: 227–230.

11. Rugg-Gunn A J, Hackett A F, Appleton D R, Jenkins G N, Eastoe J E. Relationship between dietary habits and caries increments assessed over two years in 405 English adolescent school children. *Archs Oral Biol* 1984 29: 983–992.

12. Burt B A, Eklund S A, Morgan K J, Larkin F E, Guire K E, Brown J L O, Weintraub J A. The effects of sugar intake and frequency of ingestion on dental caries increment in a three-year longitudinal study. *J Dent Res* 1988 67: 1422–1429.

13. Lachpelle D, Couture C, Brodeur J M, Servigny J. The effects of nutritional quality and frequency of consumption of sugary foods on dental caries increment. *Canadian J Pub Hlth* 1990 81: 370–375.

14. Palin-Palokas T, Hausen H, Heinonen O. Relative importance of caries risk factors in Finnish mentally retarded children. *Community Dent Oral Epidemiol* 1987 15: 19–23.

15. Pulgar-Vidal O, Schröder U. Dental health status in Latin-American preschool children in Malmö. *Swed Dent J* 1989 13: 103–109.

16. Neiderrud J, Birkhed D, Neiderud A M. Dental health and dietary habits in Greek immigrant children in southern Sweden compared with Swedish and rural Greek children. *Swed Dent J* 1991 15: 187–196.

17. Gibson S, Williams S. Dental caries in preschool children: Association with social class, toothbrushing habit and consumption of sugar and sugar-containing foods. *Carries Res* 1999 33: 101–113.

18. Hinds K, Gregory J R. *National diet and nutrition survey: Children aged 1.5 to 4.5 years. Report of the dental survey, vol. 2.* London: HMSO, 1995.

19. Meulmeester J F. *Voedingsonderzoek bij Turkse en Marokkaanse kinderen in Nederland.* 272 p. Amsterdam, Koninklijk Instituut voor der Tropen, 1988.

20. Truin G J, KööK G, Bronkhorst E M, Frankenmolen F, Mulder J, van't Hof M A. Time trends in caries experience of 6- and 12-year-old children of different socioeconomic status in The Hague. *Caries Res* 1998 32: 1–4 and *Epidemiol Bull The Hague* 1997 32: 26–30.

21. Glass R L. Secular changes in caries prevalence in two Massachusetts towns. *Caries Res* 1981 15: 445–450.

22. Eriksen H M, Grythen J, Holst D. Is there a long-term carries-preventive effect of sugar restrictions during World War II. *Acta Odontol Scand* 1991 49: 163–167.

23. Büttner M. Wirksamkeit von zahnmedizinischen Prophylaxprogrammen bei der Schwiezer Jugend. *Dtsch Stomatol* 1991 41: 13–18.

24. König K G. Changes in the prevalence of dental caries: How much can be attributed to changes in diet? *Caries Res* 1990 24 (suppl 1): 16–18.

25. Truin G J, König K G, Bronljprst E M, Mulder J. Caries prevalence amongst schoolchildren in The Hague between 1969 and 1993. *Caries Res* 1994 28: 176–180.

26. Birkhed D, Sundin B, Westin S I. Per capita consumption of sugar-containing products and dental caries in Sweden from 1960 to 1985. *Community Dant Oral Epidemiol* 1989 17: 41–43.

27. Rolla G, Ogaard B. Reduction in caries incidence in Norway from 1970 to 1984 and some considerations concerning the reasons for this phenomenon. In: Frank R M, O'Hickey S (eds.) *Strategy for Dental Carries Prevention in European Countries According to Their Laws and Regulations.* Oxford: Information Retrieval, 1987 pp 223–229.

28. Marthaler T M. Changes in the prevalence of dental caries: How much can be attributed to changes in diet? *Caries Res* 1990 24 (suppl): 3–15.

29. König K G, Schmid P, Schmid R. An apparatus for frequency-controlled feeding of small rodents and its use in dental caries experiments. *Archs Oral Biol* 13: 13–26.

30. Storey E. Milk and dental decay. In: Storey E (ed). *Diet and Dental Disease.* Melbourne: University of Melbourne, 1982, pp 34–41.

31. Matee M I N, Mikx F H M, Maselle S Y M, van Palenstein Helderman W H. Mutans streptococci and lactobacilli in breast-fed children with rampant caries. *Caries Res* 1992 26: 183–187.

32. Gardener D E, Norwood J R, Eisenson J E. At-will breastfeeding and dental caries: Four case reports. *J Dent Child* 1977 44: 186–191.

33. Kotlow L A. Breastfeeding: A cause of dental caries in children. *J Dent Child* 1977 44: 192–194.

34. Brams M, Maloney J. 'Nursing bottle caries' in breast-fed children. *J Pediatr* 1983 103: 415–416.

35. Hackett F A, Rugg-Gunn A J, Murray J J, Roberts G J. Can breast feeding cause dental caries? *Hum Nutr Appl Nutr* 1984 38: 23–25.

36. Bibby B G. Fruits and vegetables and dental caries. *Clin Prev Dent* 1983 3–11.

37. Grobler S R. The effect of a high consumption of citrus fruits and a mixture of other fruits on dental caries in men. *Clin Prev Dent* 1991 13: 13–17.

38. Edgar W M. Bibby B G, Mundorff S, Rowley J. Acid production in plaques after eating snacks: Modifying factors in food. *J Am Dent Assoc* 1975 90: 418–425.

39. Rugg-Gunn A J, Edgar W M, Jenkins G N. The effect of eating some British snacks upon the pH of human dental plaque. *Br Den J* 1978 145: 95–100.

40. Imfeld T, Schmid R, Lutz F and Guggenheim B. Cariogenicity of Milchschnitte® (Ferrero GmbH) and apple in program-fed rats. *Caries Res* 1991 25: 253–258.

41. Graf H. Telemetrie des pH der Interdentalplaque. *Schweiz Mschr Zahnbeilk* 1969 79: 146–178.

42. Schachtele C F, Jensen M E. Human plaque pH studies: Estimating the acidogenic potential of foods. *Cereal Foods World* 1981 26: 14–18.

43. Mundorff S A, Featherstorn J D B, Bibby B G, Curzon M E J, Eisenberg A D, Espeland M A. Cariogenicity of foods. I. Caries in the rat model. *Caries Res* 1990 24: 344–355.

44. Stephan R M. Effects of different types of human foods on dental health in experimental animals. *J Dent Res* 1966 45: 1551–1561.

45. Bramstedt F, karle E, Trautner K. Preliminary results of observations on the cariogenicity of apples as between-meals (abstract). *Caries Res* 1976 10: 163–164.

46. Karle E J, Gehring F. About the cariogenicity of fruits and special sweets (abstract 20). *J Dent Res* 1976 55: D155.

47. Schweizer-Hirt C M, Schait A, Schmid R, Imfeld T, Lutz F. Erosion und Abrasion des Schmelezes. Eine experimentelle Studie. *Schweiz Mschr Zahnbeilk* 1978 88: 497–529.

48. Davis W B, Winter P J. The effect of abrasion on enamel and dentine after exposure to dietary acid. *Br Dent J* 1980 148: 253–257.

49. Lussï A, Schaffner M, Hotz P and Suter P. Dental erosion in a population of Swiss adults. *Community Dent Oral E*pid 1991 19: 286–290.

50. Järvinen V K, Rytomaa I I and Heinonen O P. Risk factors in dental erosion. *J Dent Res* 1991 70: 924–947.

51. Linke H A B, Birkenfeld L H, Moss S J. Intraoral lactic acid production following the ingestion of various starch-containing foods. *Caries Res* 1993 27: 214.

52. Pollard M A, Imfeld t, Iseli M, Borgia S and Curzon M E J. Acidogenicity of cereals and fruit using the indwelling electrode to measure plaque pH. *Caries Res* 1993 27: 215.

53. Hoover C I, Newbrun E, Metreaux G. Microflora and chemical composition of dental plaque from subjects with hereditary fructose intolerance. *Infect Immun* 1980 28: 853–859.

54. Lingström P, Imfeld T, Birkhed D. Comparison of three different models for measurement of plaque-pH in humans after consumption of soft bread and potato chips. J *Dent Res* 1993 72: 865–870.

55. Scheinin A, Mäkinen K K. Turku sugar studies. *Acta Odont Scand* 1975 33: Suppl 70.

56. Mäkinen K K, Mäkinen P-L, Pape H R, *et al.* Conclusion and review of the 'Michigan Xylitol Programme' (1986–1995) for the prevention of dental caries. *Int Dent J* 1996 46: 22–34.

57. Mäkinen K K, Mäkinen P-L, Pape H R, *et al.* Stabilisation of rampant caries: polyol gums and arrest of dentine caries in two long-term cohort studies in young subjects. *Int Dent J* 1995 45: 93–107.

58. Edgar W M. Sugar substitutes, chewing gum and dental caries—a review. *Br Dent J* 1998 184: 29–32.

59. Kandelman D. Sugar, alternative sweeteners and meal frequency in relation to caries prevention: new perspectives. *Br J Nutr* 1997 77 (Suppl 1): S121–S128.

60. Scheie A A, Fejerskov O, Danielsen B. The effects of xylitol containing chewing gums on dental plaque and acidogenic potential. *J Dent Res* 1998 77: 1547–1552.

61. Trahan L, Bourgeau G, Breton R. Emergence of multiple xylitol-resistant (Fructose PTS-negative) mutants from human isolates of mutans streptococci during growth on dietary sugars in the presence of xylitol. *J Dent Res* 1996 75: 1892–1900.

62. Uhari M, Kontiokan T, Niemela M. A novel use of xylitol sugar in preventing acute otitis media. *Pediatrics* 1998 102: 971–972.

63. Comments on[62]. *Pediatrics* 1998 102: 971–972 and 974–975.

64. Rugg-Gunn A J. The benefits of using sugar-free chewing gum: a proven anticaries effect (comment on Edgar[58]). *Br Dent J* 1998 184: 26.

65. Erickson L. Oral health promotion and prevention for older adults. *Dent Clin North Am* 1997 41: 727–750.

66. Ganss C, Schlechtriemen M, Klimek J. Dental erosions in subjects living on a raw food diet. *Caries Res* 1999 33: 74–80.

67. Rytömaa I, Meruman J, Koskinen J, *et al. In vitro* erosion of bovine enamel caused by acidic drinks and other food-stuffs. *Scand J Dent Res* 1988 96: 324–333.

68. Larsen M J, Nyvad B. Enamel erosion by some soft drinks and orange juices relative to their pH, buffering effect and contents of calcium phosphate. *Caries Res* 1999 33: 81–87.

69. Ten Cate J M, Imfeld T (eds.). Etiology, mechanisms and implications of dental erosion. *Eur J Oral Sci* 1996 104: 149–244.

70. Holm A-K. Diet and caries in high risk groups in developed and developing countries. *Caries Res* 1990 24 (Suppl 1): 44–52.

71. Löe H, Theilade E, Jensen S B. Experimental gingivitis in man. *J Periodont* 1965 36: 177–187.

72. Russell A L. International nutrition surveys: A summary of preliminary dental findings. *J Dent Res* 1963 42: 233–244.

Chapter 4   ENVIRONMENTAL HEALTH

Mortality in the London Fog Incident, 1952

1. Abercrombie, G. F. Lancet, Jan. 31, 1953, P. 234.

2. Fry, J. Ibid, p. 235.

3. Logan, W. P. D. *Ibid*, 1929, 1, 78.

The Removal of Lead from Gasoline: Historical and Personal Reflections

1. Needleman, H. L. (1998). Clamped in a straitjacket: The insertion of lead into gasoline. *Environ. Res.* 74, 5–103.

2. Robert, J. C. (1983). "Ethyl: A History of the Corporation and the People who Made It." Univ. of Virginia Press, Charlottesville.

3. Hays, S. P. (1987). "Beauty, Health and Permanence: Environmental Politics in the United States." Cambridge Univ. Press, Cambridge.

4. Wetstone, G. (1981). Chronology of events surrounding the Ethyl decision. *In* "Judicial Review of Scientific Uncertainty: International Harvester and Ethyl Cases Reconsidered" (D. L. Davis, F. R. Anderson, G. Wetstone, and Ritts, Eds.), Environmental Law Institute, Washington, DC.

5. Public Health Service Report 712, 1959.

6. Patterson, C. C. (1953). The Isotopic Composition of Meteoritic, Basaltic and Oceanic Leads, and the Age of the Earth. Report by the Subcommittee on Nuclear Processes in Geological Settings, pp. 36–40. National Academy of Sciences/National Research Council. Washington, DC.

7. Patterson, C. C. (1965). Contaminated and natural environments of man. *Arch. Environ. Health* 11, 344–360.

8. Letter, R. Kehoe to Kathryn Boucot. April 16, 1965.

9. Letter, C. Patterson to H. Needleman. Aug. 5, 1992.

10. Hearings before the Subcommittee on Air and Water Pollution, Committee on Public Works, United States Senate, June 8, 1966. U.S. Govt. Printing Office, Washington, DC.

11. Kehoe, R. A. (1964). Standards with respect to atmospheric lead. *Arch. Environ. Health* 8, 348–354.

12. Tepper, L. B. and Levin, L. S. (1975). A survey of air and population lead levels in selected American communities. *Environ. Quality Safety Suppl.* 2, 152–196.

13. Lin-Fu, J.S. (1972). Undue absorption of lead among young children: A new look at an old problem. *N. Engl. J. Med.* 286, 702–710.

14. Interview with Kenneth Bridbord, 2/25/97.

15. Goldsmith, J. R., and Hexter, A. C. (1967). Respiratory exposure to lead: Epidemiological and experimental dose-response relationships. *Science* 158, 132–134.

16. Gillette, R. (1971). Lead in the air: Industry weight on Academy panel challenged. *Science* 174, 80.

17. National Academy of Sciences/National Research Council (1972). "Lead: Airborne Lead In Perspective." Natl. Acad. Sci. Press, Washington, DC.

18. Schoenbrod, D. (1980). Why regulation of lead has failed. *In* "Low Level Lead Exposure: The Clinical Implications of Current Research" (H. L. Needleman, Ed.), pp. 259–266. Raven Press, New York.

19. Quarels, J. (1976). Cleaning UP [*sic*] America: And Insider's You of the Environmental Protection Agency. Houghton Mifflin, Boston.

20. Davis, D. L., Anderson, F. R., Wetstone, G., and Ritts. (1981). "Judicial Review of Scientific Uncertainty: International Harvester and Ethyl Cases Reconsidered." Environmental Law Institute, Washington, DC.

21. Ethyl Corp. v Environmental Protection Agency, 541 F.2d I (1976).

22. Office of Research and Development, USEPA (1977). Air Quality Criteria for Lead. EPA-600/8–77–007.

23. Yankel, A. J., and Von Lindern, I. H. (1977). The Silver Valley Lead Study: The relationship between childhood blood lead levels and environmental exposure. *J. Air Pollution Control Assoc.* 27, 763–767.

24. Lead Industries Association, Inc. Petitioner, v Environmental Protection Agency, Respondent, Nos. 78–2201, 78–2220. United States Court of Appeals, District of Columbia Circuit, June 27, 1980.

25. Interview with Joe Schwarz, Feb 3, 1998.

26. Gorsuch Promise Raises Question, *New York Times*, April 18, 1982.

27. Schwadel, F. Ethyl Corp. still defends failing product as it hunts for replacement acquisitions. *Wall Street Journal*, May 16, 1984.

28. Stein, J. (1982). Warning from health experts: Federal anti-lead drive is running out of gas. *National Journal*, June 5, 1982. pp. 1005–1007. Blanchard.

29. Needleman, H. L., Gunnor, C., Leviton, A., Peresie, H., Maher, C., and Barret, P. (1979). Deficits in psychological and classroom performance of children with elevated dentine lead levels. *N. Engl. J. Med.* 300, 689–695.

30. Perino, J., and Ernhardt, C. B. (1974). The relation of subclinical lead level to cognitive and sensorimotor impairment in black preschoolers. *J. Learning Disabilities* 7, 26–30.

31. National Research Council/Committee on Lead in the Human Environment (1980). Lead in the Human Environment. Natl. Acad. Sci. Press. Washington, DC.

32. Needleman, H. L., Geiger, S. K., and Frank, R. (1985). Lead and IQ scores: A reanalysis. *Science* 227, 701–704. [Letter]

33. US EPA/Environmental Criteria and Assessment Office (1986). Air Quality Criteria for Lead, Vol. IV, P 12–83 EPA-600/8/-83/028df, June 1986.

34. Reichelmeyer-Lais, A., and Kirschgessner, M. (1981). Depletion studies on the essential nature of lead in growing rats. *Arch. Tierahrung.* 31, 731–737.

35. Expert Committee on Trace Metal Essentiality (1983). Independent peer review of selected studies by Drs. Kirschgessner and Reichelmayer–Lais concerning the possible nutritional essentiality of lead EPA 600/8/83–028A.

36. "Lead Industry Digs in Its Heels on Gas Additive," *New York Times,* Aug. 6, 1984.

37. Agency for Toxic Substances and Disease Registry (1988). The Nature and Extent of Lead Poisoning in Children in the United States: A Report to Congress. Dept. of Health and Human Services, Atlanta, GA.

38. Brody, T. J., Pirkle, J. L., Kramer, R. A., Flegal, K. M., Matte, T. D., Gunter, E. W., and Paschal, D. C. (1994). Blood lead levels in the US population: Phase I of the Third National Health and Nutrition Examination Survey. [NHANES III, 1988 to 1991] *J. Am. Med. Assoc.* 272, 277–283.

39. Morozumi, M., Chow, T. J., Patterson, C. (1969). Chemical concentrations of pollutant aerosols, terrestrial dust, and sea salts in Greenland and Antarctic snow strata. *Geochim. Cosmochim. Acta.* 33, 1247–1204.

Global Climate Change and Infectious Diseases

1. Henle, J. On Miasmata and Contagia (translated by G. Rosen). Johns Hopkins Press, Baltimore, MD, 1938, p. 54.

2. May, J. M. Ecology of Human Disease. MD Publications, New York, 1958.

3. Knipling, E. V., and Sullivan, W. N. Insect mortality at low temperatures. J. Econ. Entomol. 50: 368–369 (1957).

4. Smith, W. W., and Love, G. J. Winter and spring survival of *Aedes aegypti* in southwestern Georgia. Am .J. Trop. Med. Hyg. 7: 309–311 (1958).

5. Centers for Disease Control. Current trends: imported dengue—United States, 1987. MMWR 38: 463–465 (1989).

6. Blake, P. A., Allegra, D. T., Snyder, J. D., Barrett, T. J., McFarland, L., Caraway, C. T., Feeley, J.C., Craig, J. P., Lee, J. V., Puhr, N. D., and Feldman, R. A. Cholera—a possible epidemic focus in the United States. N. Engl. J. Med. 302: 305–309 (1980).

7. Centers for Disease Control. Toxigenic *Vibrio cholerae* 01 infection acquired in Colorado. MMWR 38: 19–20 (1989).

8. Kaper, J. B., Bradford, H. B., Robert, N. C., and Falkow, S. Molecular epidemiology of *Vibrio cholerae* in the U.S. Gulf Coast. J. Clin. Microbiol. 16:129–134 (1982).

9. Colwell, R. R., Kaper, J., and Joseph, S. W. *Vibrio cholerae, Vibrio parahemolyticus,* and other *vibrios*: occurrence in distribution in Chesapeake Bay. Science 198: 394–396 (1977).

10. Wilson, M. L., Levine, J. F., and Spielman, A. Effect of deer-reduction on abundance of the deer tick (*Ixodes dammini*). Yale J. Biol. Med. 57: 697–705 (1884).
11. Steere, a. C., Malawista, S. E., Snydman, D. R., Shope, R. E., Andiman, W. A., Ross, M. R., and Steele, F. M. Lyme arthritis: an epidemic of oligoarticular arthritis in children and adults in three Connecticut communities. Arthritis Rheum. 20: 7–17 (1977).
12. Knudsen, D. L., and Shope, R. E. Overview of the orbiviruses. In: Bluetongue and Related Orbiviruses (T. L. Barber and M. M. Jochim, Eds.), Progress in clinical and Biological Research, Vol. 178. Alan R. Liss, Inc., New York, 1985, pp. 225–266.

Chapter 5   OCCUPATIONAL HEALTH

Mortality from Lung Cancer in Asbestos Workers

BIBLIOGRAPHY

Asbestos Industry Regulations (1931). Statutory Rules and Orders, 1931, No. 1140. H.M.S.O., London.

Boemke, F. (1953). *Med. Mschr.*, 7, 77.

Cartier, P. (1952). *Arch. industr. Hyg.*, 5, 262 (contribution to discussion).

Council of the International Organizations of Medical Sciences (1953). *Acta Un. int. Cancr.*, 9. 443.

Doll, R. (1953). *Brit. med. J.*, 2, 521.

Gloyne, S. R. (1951). *Lancet*, 1, 810.

Hueper, W. C. (1952). *Proceedings of the Seventh Saranac Symposium*. To be published.

Lynch, K. M., and Smith, W. A. (1935). *Amer. J. Cancer*, 24, 56.

Merewether, E. R. A. (1949). *Annual Report of the Chief Inspector of Factories for the Year 1947*. H.M.S.O., London.

Nordmann, M., and Sorge, A. (1941). *Z. Krebsforsch.*, 51, 168.

Smith, W. E. (1952). *Arch. industr. Hyg.*, 5, 209.

Stocks, P. (1952). *Brit. J. Cancer*, 6, 99.

Vorwald, A. J., and Karr, J. W. (1938). *Am. J. Path.*, 14, 49.

Warren, S. (1948). *Occup. Med.*, 5, 249

Diffuse Pleural Mesothelioma and Asbestos Exposure in the North Western Cape Province

BIBLIOGRAPHY

Belloni, G., and Bovo, G. (1957). *Acta med. patav.*, 17, 367.

Campbell, W. N. (1950). *Amer. J. Path.*, 26, 473.

Cartier, P. (1952). *Arch. industr. Hyg.*, 5, 262. (Contribution to the discussion.)

Doll, R. (1955). *Brit. J. industry. Med.*, 12, 81.

Frood, G. E. B. (1915). *Memorandum on the Asbestos Industry in the Cape Province*. Report of the Government Mining Engineer, Union of South Africa, pp. 76–82.

Gloyne, S. R. (1933). *Tubercle (Lond.)*, 14, 493.

Godwin, M. C. (1957). *Cancer (Philad.),* 10, 298.

Hale, C. W. (1946). *Nature (Lond.),* 157, 802.

Hall, A. L. (1930). *Asbestos in the Union of South Africa.* Memorandum no. 12. Geological Survey of South Africa.

Harington, J. S. (1959). Personal communication.

Higginson, J., and Oettle, A. G. (1957). *Acta Un. int. Cancr.,* 13, 949.

Hurwitz, M. (1959). *Proceedings of the International Conference of Experts on Pneumoconiosis.* Johannesburg, Feb. 1959. Churchill, London. (In press.)

Keasbey, L. E. (1947). *Amer. J. Path.,* 23, 871.

Klemperer, P., and Rabin, C. B. (1931). *Arch. Path. (Chicago),* 11, 385.

Lison, L. (1953). *Histochemie et Cytochimie Animales,* pp. 332–337. Gautier-villars, Paris.

Lynch, K. M., and Smith, W. A. (1935). *Amer. J. Cancer,* 24, 56.

———, McIver, F. A., and Cain, J. R. (1957). *A. M. A. Arch. industr. Hlth,* 15, 207.

Martiny, O. (1956). *Proc. Transv. Mine med. Offrs' Ass.,* 35, 63.

Maxmow, A. (1927). *Arch. exp. Zellforsch.,* 4, 1.

McCaughey, W. T. (1958). *J. Path. Bact.,* 76, 517.

Meyer, K., and Chafee, E. (1939). *Proc. Soc. Exp. Biol. (N.Y.),* 42, 797.

———, ———(1940). *J. bio. Chem.* 133, 83.

Novak, E. (1931). *Amer. J. Obstet. Gynec.,* 22, 826.

Robertson, H. E. (1924). *J. Cancer Res.,* 8, 317.

Sano, M. E., Weiss, E., and Gault, E.S. (1950). *J. thorac. Surg.,* 19, 783.

Schmähl, D. (1958). *Z. Krebsforsch.,* 62, 561.

Smart, J., and Hinson, K. F. W. (1957). *Brit. J. Tuberc.,* 51, 319.

Stout, A. P., and Murray, M. R. (1942). *Arch. Path. (Chicago),* 34, 951.

Tobiassen, G. (1955). *Acta path. microbial. scand.,* Suppl.. 105, p. 198.

van der Schoot, H. C. M. (1958). *Ned. T. Geneesk,* 102, 1124.

Vermass, F. H. S. (1952*). Trans. geol. Soc. S. Afr.,* 55, 199.

Vorwald, J. C., and Karr, J. W. (1938). *Amer. J. Path.,* 14, 49.

Wagner, J. C. (1958). *Memorandum on Pneumoconiosis Research in Europe.* Submitted to the C.S.I.R.

Willis, R. A. (1948, 1ˢᵗ ed. and 1953). *Pathology of Tumours.* Butterworth, London.

Lung Cancer in Chloromethyl Methyl Ether Workers

1. Boucot KR, Weiss W., Seidman H., et al: The Philadelphia pulmonary neoplasm research project: basic risk factors of lung cancer in older men. Am J Epidemiol 95:4–16, 1972

2. Van Duuren BL, Goldschmidt BM, Katz BS, et al: Alpha-haloethers: a new type of alkylating carcinogen. Arch Environ Health 16:472–476, 1968

3. Leong BKJ, McFarland HN, Reese WH Jr: Induction of lung adenomas by chronic inhalation of bis (chloromethyl) ether. Arch Environ 22:663–666, 1971

4. Laskin S, Kuschner M, Drew RT, et al: Tumors of the respiratory tract induced by inhalation of bis (chloromethyl) ether. Arch Environ 23:135–136, 1971

5. Van Duuren BL, Katz C, Goldschmidt BM, et al: Carcinogenicity of halo-ethers. II. structure-activity relationships of analogs of bis (chloromethyl) ether. J Natl Cancer Inst 48:1431–1439, 1972

6. Chemical suspected in six cases of lung cancer. Occup Health Saf Lett 2:6, 1972

Chapter 6   WOMEN'S HEALTH

Diagnosis of Uterine Cancer by the Vaginal Smear

1. Bourgeois, G. A. The identification of fetal squamas and the diagnosis of ruptured membranes by vaginal smear. Am. Jour. Obst. and Gyn., 44: 80–87, July, 1942.

1A. Cary, W. H. A method of obtaining endometrial smears for study of their cellular content. Am. Jour. Obst. and Gyn., 46: 422–424, September, 1943.

2. Fletcher, P. F. A study of the possible significance of the vaginal smear as an additional factor in the diagnosis of incomplete abortion. Am. Jour. Obst. and Gyn., 39: 562–575, April, 1940.

3. Frankel, L., and G. N. Papanicolaou. Growth, desquamation and involution of the vaginal epithelium of fetuses and children, with a consideration of the related hormonal factors. Am. Jour. Anat., 62: 427–451, May, 1938.

4. Papanicolaou, G. N. New cancer diagnosis. Proc. Third Race Betterment Conference, 1928. P. 528.

5. Papanicolaou, G. N. Monocytic reactions in the vagina. Anat. Record, 39 (supplement): 55–56, March, 1928.

6. Papanicolaou, G. N. The sexual cycle in the human female as revealed by vaginal smears. Am. Jour. Anat., 52 (supplement): 519–637, May, 1933.

7. Papanicolaou, G. N. Existence of a "post-menopause" sexual rhythm in women, as indicated by the study of vaginal smears. Anat. Record, 55 (supplement): 71, March, 1933.

8. Papanicolaou, G. N. Periodic activation of the histiocytes in the vaginal fluid. Anat. Record, 79 (supplement): 75–76, March, 1941.

9. Papanicolaou, G. N. A new procedure for staining vaginal smears. Science, 95: 438–439, April 24, 1942.

9A. Papanicolaou, G. N. Cytologic diagnosis of uterine cancer by examination of vaginal and uterine secretions. Am. Jour. Clin. Path. In press.

9B. Papanicolaou, G. N., and A. A. Marchetti. The use of endocervical and endometrial smears in the diagnosis of cancer and of other conditions of the uterus. Am. Jour. Obst. and Gyn., 46: 421–422, September, 1943.

10. Papanicolaou, G. N., and E. Shorr. The action of ovarian follicular hormones in the menopause, as indicated by vaginal smears. Am. Jour. Obst. and Gyn., 31: 806–831, May, 1936.

11. Papanicolaou, G. N., and H. F. Traut. The demonstration of malignant cells in vaginal smears and its relation to the diagnosis of carcinoma of the uterus. New York State Jour. Med., 43: 767–768, April 15, 1943.

11A. Papanicolaou, G. N., H. F. Traut, and A. A. Marchetti. The epithelia of woman's reproductive organs. Commonwealth Fund, New York, 1948.

12. Rubenstein, B. B., and T. Benedek. The sexual cycle in women, chap. 3, p. 31–44. Washington, D.C., National Research Council, 1942. (Psychosomatic Medicine Monographs, v. 1, no. 1–2.)

13. Shorr, E., and G. N. Papanicolaou. Action of gonadotropic hormones in amenorrhea as evaluated by vaginal smears. Proc. Soc. Exp. Biol. and Med., 41: 629–636, June, 1939.

14. Stockard, C. R., and G. N. Papanicolaou. A rhythmical "heat period" in guinea pigs. Science, 46: 42–44, July 13, 1917.

15. Traut, H. F., and G. N. Papanicolaou. Vaginal smear changes in endometrial hyperplasias and in cervical keratosis. Anat. Record, 82: 478–479, March, 1942.

Introduction of the Pill and Its Impact

1. Asbell B. The Pill: A Bibliography of the Drug that Changed the World. New York: Random House, 1995.

2. Derman R. Oral contraceptives: a reassessment. Obstet Gynecol Surv 1989;44:662–8.

3. Chasan-Taber L, Stampfer MJ. Epidemiology of oral contraceptives and cardiovascular disease. Ann Intern Med 1998;128:467–77.

4. Mishell DR Jr. Oral contraception: past, present, and future perspectives. Int J Fertil 1991;36[suppl]:7–18.

5. Ogawa N, Retherford RD. Prospects for increased contraceptive pill use in Japan. Stud Fam Plann 1991;22:378–83.

6. Sollom T, Gold RB, Saul R. Public funding for contraceptive, sterilization and abortion services, 1994. Fam Plann Perspect 1996;28:166–73.

7. Forrest JD, Samara R. Impact of publicly funded contraceptive services on unintended pregnancies and implications for Medicaid expenditures. Fam Plann Perspect 1996;28:188–95.

8. Omnibus Appropriations Bill of 1998. Public Law 105–277.

9. Westhoff CL. Oral contraceptives and breast cancer—resolution emerges. Contraception 1996;54:i–ii.

10. Gerstman BB, Gross TP, Kennedy DL, et al. Trends in the content and use of oral contraceptives in the United States, 1964–1988. Am J Public Health 1991;81:90–8.

11. Kaunitz AM. Oral contraceptive health benefits; perception versus reality. Contraception 1999;59:29S–33S.

12. Forrest JD. Contraceptive use in the United States: past, present and future. Adv Pop 1994;2:29–48.

13. Ryder NB, Westoff CF. Reproduction in the United States 1965. Princeton, NJ: Princeton University Press, 1971.

14. Piccinino LJ, Mosher WD. Trends in contraceptive use in the United States: 1982–1995. Fam Plann Perspect 1998;30:4–10, 46.

15. Dawson DA. Trends in the use of oral contraceptives—data from the 1987 National Health Interview Survey. Fam Plann Perspect 1980;22:169–72.

A Global Overview of Gender-based Violence

1. Heise L. Violence against women: global organizing for change. In: Edelson JL, Eisikovits ZC, editors. Future interventions with battered women and their families. Thousand Oaks, California: Sage Publications, 1996.

2. Heise L, Ellsberg M, Gottemoeller M. Ending violence against women. Population Reports. Baltimore: Johns Hopkins University, 1999.

3. Ellsberg M, Peña R, Herrera A, Liljestrand J, Winkvist A. Candies in hell: women's experiences of violence in Nicaragua. Soc. Sci. Med. 2000; 51:1595–1610.

4. Koss MP, Goodman LA, Browne A, Fitzgerald LF, Keita GP, Russo NF. No safe haven: male violence against women at home, at work, and in the community. Washington, DC: American Psychological Association, 1994.

5. Yoshihama M, Sorensen SB. Physical, sexual, and emotional abuse by male intimates: experiences of women in Japan. Violence Victims 1994; 9:63–77.

6. Rodgers K. Wife assault: the findings of a national survey. Juristat Serv. Bull. Can. Centre Justice Statistics 1994; 14:1–22.

7. Heise L, Moore K, Toubia N. Sexual coercion and women's reproductive health: a focus on research. New York: Population Council, 1995. p. 59.

8. World Health Organization. Violence against women: a priority health issue. WHO: Geneva 1997.

9. Weiss E, Gupta GR. Bridging the gap: addressing gender and sexuality in HIV prevention. Washington, DC: International Center for Research on Women, 1998. p. 31.

10. Heise L, Pitanguy J, Germain A. violence against women: the hidden health burden. World Bank Discussion Paper #255: Washington, DC 1994.

11. Finkelhor D. The international epidemiology of child sex abuse. Child Abuse Neglect 1994; 18:409–417.

12. Sinal SH. Sexual abuse of children and adolescents. South. Med. J. 1994; 87:1242–1258.

13. Sas LD, Cunningham AH. Tipping the balance to tell the secret: public discovery of child sexual abuse. Ontario, Canada: London Family Court Clinic, 1995.

14. Olsson A, Ellsberg M, Berglund S, Herrera A, Zelaya E, Persson L-Å. Sexual abuse during childhood and adolescence among Nicaraguan men and women: a population-based anonymous survey, submitted for publication.

15. Watkins B, Bentovim A. The sexual abuse of male children and adolescents: a review of current research. J. Child Psychol. Psychiat. 1992; 33:197–248.

16. Kendall-Tackett KA, Williams LM, Finkelhor D. Impact of sexual abuse on children: a review and synthesis of recent empirical studies. Psychol. Bull. 1993; 113:164–180.

17. Mullen PE, Martin JL, Anderson JC, Romans SE, Herbison GP. The effect of child sexual abuse on social, interpersonal and sexual function in adult life. Brit. J. Psychiat. 1994; 195:35–47.

18. Rind B, Tromovitch P. A meta-analytical review of findings from national samples on psychological correlates on child sexual abuse. J. Sex Res. 1997; 34:237–255.

19. Beitchman JH, Zucker KJ, Hood JE, daCosta GA, Akman D, Cassavia E. A review of the long-term effects of child sexual abuse. Child Abuse Neglect 1992; 16:101–118.

20. Counts DA, Brown J, Campbell J. Sanctions and sanctuary: cultural perspectives on the beating of wives. Boulder, Colorado; Westview Press, 1992.

21. Levinson D. Violence in cross cultural perspective. Newberry Park, California: Sage Publishers, 1989.

22. Heise L. Violence against women: an integrated, ecological framework. Violence Against Women 1998; 4:262–290.

23. Hotaling GT, Sugarman DB. An analysis of risk markers and husband to wife violence: the current state of knowledge. Violence Victims 1986; 1:101–124.

24. Dutton DG. The domestic assaults of women: psychological and criminal justice perspectives. Vancouver, British Columbia: University of British Columbia Press, 1995.

25. Tjaden P, Thoennes N. Extent, nature and consequences of intimate partner violence: findings from the National Violence Against Women Survey. Washington, DC: National Institute of Justice, Centers for Disease Control and Prevention, 2000. p. 72.

26. Fournier M, de los Rios R, Orpinas P, Piquet-Carneiro L. Multicenter Study on Cultural Attitudes and Norms towards Violence (ACTIVA project): methodology. Rev. Panam. Salud. Publica. 1999; 5:222–231.

27. Koeniz M, Hossain MB, Ahmed S, Haaga J. Individual and community-level determinants of domestic violence in rural Bangladesh in Hopkins Population Center Paper on Population. Baltimore: Johns Hopkins School Public Health, Department of Population and Family Health Sciences, 1999.

28. Jejeebhoy SJ. Wife-beating in rural India: a husband's right? Econo. Political Weekly (India) 1998; 23:580–862.

29. Khan ME, Townsend JW, Sinha R, Lakhanpal S. Sexual violence within marriage. New Delhi, India: Population Council, 1996.

30. Shedlin M, Hollerback PE. Modern and traditional fertility regulation in a Mexican community: the process of decision-making. Studies Family Planning 1981; 12:278–296.

31. Blanc AK, Wolff B, Gage AJ, Ezeh AC, Neema S, Ssekamatte-Sseuliba J. Negotiating reproductive outcomes in Uganda. Institute of Statistics and Applied Economics and Macro International Inc, 1996. p. 215.

32. Ezah AC. The influence of spouses over each other's contraceptive attitudes in Ghana. Studies Family Planning 1993; 24:163–174.

33. Bawah AA, Akweongo P, Simmons R, Phillips JF. Women's fears and men's anxieties: the impact of family planning on gender relations in northern Ghana. Studies Family Planning 1999; 30:54–66.

34. Folch-Lyon E, Macora L, Schearer SB. Focus group and survey research in family planning in Mexico. Studies Family Planning 1981; 12:409–432.

35. Fort AL. Investigation of the social context in fertility and family planning: a qualitative study in Peru. Int. Family Planning Perspect. 1989; 15:88–94.

36. Choque ME, Schuler SR, Rance S. Reasons for unwanted fertility and barriers to use of family planning services among urban Aymara in Bolivia. Arlington, Virginia: John Snow, Inc, 1994. p. 19.

37. Zoysa Id, Sweat MD, Denison JA. Faithful but fearful: reducing HIV transmission in stable relationships. AIDS 1996; 10:S197–203.
38. Goldstein D. The cultural, class, and gender politics of the modern disease: women and AIDS in Brazil. ABIA, ColectivoFeminista Sexualidade e Salude 1992;92.
39. Boyer D, Fine D. Sexual abuse as a factor in adolescent pregnancy. Family Planning Perspect. 1992; 24:4–11.
40. Butler JR, Burton LM. Rethinking teenage childbearing: is sexual abuse a missing link. Family Relations 1990; 39:73–80.
41. Beitchman JH, Zucker KJ, Hood JE. A review of the short term effects of child sexual abuse. Child Abuse Neglect 1991; 15:537–556.
42. Dietz PM, Spitz AM, Anda RF, et al. Unintended pregnancy among adult women exposed to abuse or household dysfunction during their childhood. J. Am. Med. Assoc. 1999; 282:1359–1364.
43. Fergusson DM, Horwood LF, Lynskey MT. Childhood sexual abuse, adolescent sexual behaviors and sexual re-victimization. Child Abuse Neglect 1997; 21:789–803.
44. Zierler S, Femgold L, Fufer D. Adolescents survivors of childhood sexual abuse and subsequent risk of HIV infection. Am. J. Public Health 1991; 81:572–575.
45. Handwerker W. Gender power differences between parents and high-risk sexual behavior by their children: AIDS/STD risk factors extend to a prior generation. J. Women's Health 1993; 2:301–316.
46. Cunningham RM, Stiffman AR, Dore P, Earls F. The association of physical and sexual abuse with HIV risk behaviors in adolescents and young adulthood: implications for public health. Child Abuse Neglect 1994; 18:233–245.
47. Felitti VJ, Anda RF, Nordenberg D, et al. Relationship of childhood abuse and household dysfunction to many of the leading causes of death in adults. The Adverse Childhood Experiences (ACE) Study. Am J. Prevent. Med. 1998; 14:245–258.
48. Johnsen LW, Harlow LL. Childhood sexual abuse linked with adult substance use, victimization, and AIDS-risk. AIDS Educat. Prevent. 1996; 8:44–57.
49. Roosa MW, Tein J-Y, Reinholtz C, Angelini PJ. The relationship of childhood sexual abuse to teenage pregnancy. J. Marriage Family 1997; 59:119–130.
50. Rotheran-Borus MJ, Mahler KA, Koopman C, Langabeer K. Sexual abuse history and associated multiple risk behavior in adolescent runaways. Am. J. Orthopsychiat. 1996; 66:390–400.
51. James J, Meyerding J. Early sexual experiences and prostitution. Am. J. Psychiat. 1977; 132:1381–1385.
52. Stevens-Simon C, Reichert S. Sexual abuse, adolescent pregnancy, and child abuse: a developmental approach to an intergenerational cycle. Arch. Pediatr. Adoles. Med. 1994; 148:23–27.
53. Yates G, MacKenzie R, Pennbridge J, Cohen E. A risk profile comparison of homeless youth involved in prostitution and homeless youth not involved. J. Adoles. Health 1991; 12:545–548.
54. Fullilove MT, Lown EA, Fullilove RE. Crack 'hos and skeezers: traumatic experiences of women crack users. J. Sex Res. 1992; 29:275–287.

55. Paone D, Chavkin W, Wilets IPF, DesJarlais D. The impact of sexual abuse: implications for drug treatment. J. Women's Health 1992; 1:149–153.
56. Sherman SG, Steckler A. "What the 'caine was tellin' me to do." Crack users' risk of HIV: an exploratory study of female inmates. Women's Health 1998; 4:117–134.
57. Bartholow BN, Doll LS, Joy D, et al. Emotional, behavioral and HIV risks associated with sexual abuse among adult homosexual and bisexual men. Child Abuse Neglect 1994; 18:747–761.
58. Strathdee SA, Patrick DM, Archibald CP, et al. Social determinants predict needle-sharing behavior among injection drug users in Vancouver, Canada. Addiction 1997; 92:1339–1347.
59. Britton BM. Gender, power and HIV: the impact of partner violence in the context of poverty on women's risk of infection in the USA (abstract #23466) in 12th World Conference on HIV/AIDS, Geneva, Switzerland 1998.
60. Richie BE, Johnsen C. Abuse histories among newly incarcerated women in a New York City jail. J. Am. Med. Womens Assoc. 1996; 51(114):7.
61. Klein H, Chao BS. Sexual abuse during childhood and adolescence as predictors of HIV-related sexual violence during adulthood among female sexual partners of injection drug users. Violence Against Women 1995; 1:55–76.
62. Brown D. In Africa, fear makes HIV an inheritance. In Washington Post 1998.
63. Ehlert U, Heim C, Hellhammer DH. Chronic pelvic pain as a somatoform disorder. Psychother. Psychosomat. 1999; 68:87–94.
64. Walker EA, Katon WJ, Hansom J, et al. Medical and psychiatric symptoms in women with childhood sexual abuse. Psychosomat. Med. 1992; 54:658–664.
65. Lee NC, Dicker RC, Rubin GL, Ory HW. Confirmation of the preoperative diagnoses for hysterectomy. Am J. Obstetr. Gynecol. 1984; 150:283–287
66. Chapman JD. A longitudinal study of sexuality and gynecologic health in abused women. Am. J. Osteopat. Assoc. 1980; 89:619–624.
67. Collett BJ, Cordle CJ, Stewart CR, Jagger C. A comparative study of women with chronic pelvic pain, chronic nonpelvic pain and those with no history of pain attending general practitioners. Brit. J. Obstetr. Gynaecol. 1998; 105:87–92.
68. Jamieson DJ, Steege JF. The association of sexual abuse with pelvic pain complaints in a primary care population. Am. J. Obstetr. Gynecol. 1997; 177:1408–1412.
69. Rapkin AJ, Kames LD, Darke LL, Stampler FM, Naliboff BD. History of physical and sexual abuse in women with chronic pelvic pain. Obstetr. Gynecol. 1990; 76:92–96.
70. Schei B. Psycho-social factors in pelvic pain. A controlled study of women living in physically abusive relationships. Acta Obstetricia et Gynecologica Scandinavica 1990; 69:67–71.
71. Schei B, Bakketeig LS. Gynaecological impact of sexual and physical abuse by spouse: a study of a random sample of Norwegian women. Brit. J. Obstetr. Gynaecol. 1989; 96:1379–1383.
72. Golding J. Sexual assault history and women's reproductive and sexual health. Psychol. Women Quart. 1996; 20:101–121.

73. Golding JM, Wilsnack SC, Learman LA. Prevalence of sexual assault history among women with common gynecologic symptoms. Am. J. Obstetr. Gynecol. 1998; 179:1013–1019.

74. Schei B. Physically abusive spouse—a risk factor of pelvic inflammatory disease? Scand. J. Primary Health Care 1991; 9;41–45.

75. Golding JM, Taylor DL. Sexual assault history and premenstrual distress in two general population samples. J. Women's Helath 1996; 5:143–152.

76. Golding JM. Sexual assault history and limitations in physical functioning in two general population samples. Res. Nursing Health 1996; 19: 33–44.

77. Golding JM, Cooper ML, George LK. Sexual assault history and health perceptions: seven general population studies. Health Psychol. 1997; 16:417–425.

78. Ballard TJ, Saltzman LE, Gazmararian JA, Spitz AM, Lazorick S, Marks JS. Violence during pregnancy: measurement issues. Am. J. Public Health 1998; 88:274–276.

79. Campbell JC. Addressing battering during pregnancy: reducing low birth weight and ongoing abuse. Semin. Perinatol. 1995; 19:301–306.

80. Curry MA, Perrin N, Wall E. Effects of abuse on maternal complications and birth in adult and adolescent women. Obstet. Gynecol. 1998; 92:530–534.

81. Gazmararian JA, Lazorick S, Spitz AM, Ballard TJ, Saltzman LE, Marks JS. Prevalence of violence against pregnant women. J. Am. Med. Assoc. 1996; 275:1915–1920.

82. Newberger EH, Barkan SE, Lieberman ES, et al. Abuse of pregnant women and adverse birth outcomes. Current knowledge and implications for practice. J. Am. Med. Assoc. 1992; 276:2370–2372.

83. Rosales J, Loaiza E. Primante D, Barberena A, Blandon Sequeira L, Ellsberg M. Encuesta Nicaraguense de demografia y salud 1998. Managua, Nicaragua: Instituto Nacional de Estadisticas y Censos, INEC, 1999.

84. El-Zanaty F, Hussein EM, Shawky GA, Way AA, Kishor S. Egypt demographic and health survey 1995. Calverton, Maryland: Macro International, 1996

85. Larrain SH. Violencia puertas adentro: la mujer golpeada. Santiago, Chile: Editorial Universitaria, 1994.

86. Johnson H. Dangerous domains: violence against women in Canada. In: Nelson, editor. Crime in Canada, Ontario, Canada: International Thomson Publishing.

87. Nelson E, Zimmerman C. Household survey on domestic violence in Cambodia. Phnom Penh, Cambodia: Ministry of Women's Affairs (MoWA) and Project Against Domestic Violence (PADV), 1996. p. 82.

88. Petersen R, Gazmararian JA, Spitz AM, et al. Violence and adverse pregnancy outcomes: a review of the literature and directions for future research. Am. J. Prev. Med. 1997; 13:366–373.

89. Dietz PM, Gazmararian JA, Goodwin MM, Bruce FC, Johnson CH, Rochat RW. Delayed entry into prenatal care: effective physical violence. Obstet. Gynecol. 1997; 90:221–224.

90. Parker B, McFarlane J, Soeken K. Abuse during pregnancy: effects on maternal complications and birth weight in adult and teenage women. Obstetr. Gynecol. 1994; 84:323–328.

91. MacFarlane J, Parker B, Soeken K. Abuse during pregnancy: associations with maternal health and infant birth weight. Nurs. Res. 1996; 45:37–42.

92. Taggart L, Mattson S. Delay in prenatal care as a result of battering in pregnancy: cross-cultural implications. Health Care Women Int. 1996; 17:25–34.

93. Valdez-Santiago R, Sanin-Aguirre LH. Domestic violence during pregnancy and its relationship with birth weight. Salud Publica Mexicana 1996; 38:352–362.

94. Valladares E, Ellsberg M, Peña R, Högberg U, Persson LÅ. Physical abuse during pregnancy: a risk factor for low birth weight, submitted for publication.

95. Berenson AB, Wiemann CM, Rowe TF, Rickert VI. Inadequate weight gain among pregnant adolescents: risk factors and relationship to infant birth weight. Am. J. Obstetr, Gynecol. 1997; 176:1220–1224.

96. Martin SL, Matza LS, Kupper LL, Thomas JC, Daly M, Cloutier S. Domestic violence and sexually transmitted diseases: the experience of prenatal care patients. Public Health Rep. 1999; 114:262–268.

97. Cokkinides VE, Coker AL, Sanderson M, Addy C, Bethea L. Physical violence during pregnancy: maternal complications and birth outcomes. Obstetr. Gynceol. 1999; 93:661–666.

98. Amaro H, Fried LE, Cabral H, Zuckerman B. Violence during pregnancy and substance use. Am. J. Public Health 1990; 80:575–579.

99. Berenson AB, Wiemann CM, Wilkinson GS, Jones WA, Anderson GD. Perinatal morbidity associated with violence experienced by pregnant women. Am. J. Obstetr. Gynecol. 1994; 170:1760–1769.

100. Bullock LF, McFarlane J. The birth-weight/battering connection. Am. J. Nurs. 1989; 89:1153–1155.

101. Dye TD, Tollivert NJ, Lee RV, Kenney CJ. Violence, pregnancy and birth outcome in Appalachia. Paediatr. Perinatal Epidemiol. 1995; 9:35–47.

102. G rimstad H, Schei B, Backe B, Jacobsen G. Physical abuse and low birth weight: a case-controlled study. Brit. J. Obstetr. Gynaecol. 1997; 104:1281–1287.

103. Schei B, et al. Does spousal physical abuse affect the outcome of pregnancy? Scand. J. Soc. Med. 1991; 19:26–31.

104. Rodriguez MA, Quiroga SS, Bauer HM. Breaking the silence: battered women's perspectives on medical care. Arch. Family Med. 1996; 5:153–158.

Chapter 7   MATERNAL CHILD HEALTH

More Folic Acid for Everyone, Now

BIBLIOGRAPHY

Boushey C. J., Beresford, S. A. A., Omenn, G. S. & Motulsky, A. G. (1995) A quantitative assessment of plasma homocysteine as a risk factor for cardiovascular disease. J. Am. Med. Assoc. 274: 1049–1057.

Brattstron, L., Lindgren, A., Israelson, B., Andersson, A. & Hultberg, B. (1994) Homocysteine and cysteine: determinants of plasma levels in middle-aged and elderly subjects. J. Intern. Med. 236: 633–641.

Centers for Disease Control and Prevention (1992) Recommendations for the use of folic acid to reduce the number of cases of spina bifida and other neural tube defects. MMWR 41 (No. RR-14):1–7.

Czizel, A. E. & Dudas, I. (1992) Prevention of the first occurrence of neural-tube defects by periconceptional vitamin supplementation. N. Engl. J. Med. 327: 1832–1835.

Dickinson, C. J. (1995) Does folic acid harm people with vitamin B-12 deficiency? Q. J. Med. 88: 357–364.

Food and Drug Administration (1973) Statement of general policy or interpretation. Subchapter B-Food and Food Products, Part 121-Food Additives, Fed. Regist. 38: 20725–20726.

Food and Drug Administration (October 14, 1993) Food Standards: Amendment of the standards of identity for in rich grain products to require addition of folic acid. Fed. Regist. 58: 53305–53312.

Hathcock, J. N. & Troendle, G. J. (1991) Oral cobalamin for treatment of pernicious anemia? J. Am. Med. Assoc. 265: 96–97.

Jacob, R. A., Wu, M. M., Henning, S. M. & Swendseid, M. E. (1994) Homocysteine increases as folate decreases in plasma of healthy men during short-term dietary folate and methyl group restriction. J. Nutr. 124: 1072–1080.

Kang, S. S., Wong, P. W. K. & Norusis, M. (1987) Homocysteinemia due to folate deficiency. Metabolism 36: 458–462.

Kirke, P. N., Molloy, A. M., Daly, L. E., burke, H., Weir, D. G & Scott, J. M. (1993) Maternal plasma folate and vitamin B-12 are independent risk factors for neural tube defects. Q. J. Med. 86: 703–708.

Lewis, C. A., Pancharujniti, N. & Sauberlich, H. E. (1992) Plasma folate adequacy as determined by homocysteine level. Ann. N.Y. Acad. Sci. 669: 360–362.

Lindenbaum, J., Rosenberg, I. H., Wilson, P. W. F., Stabier, S. P. & Allen, R. H. (1994) Prevalence of cobalamin deficiency in the Framingham elderly population. Am. J. Clin. Nutr. 60: 2–11.

MRC Vitamin Study Research Group (1991) Prevention of neural tube defects: Results of the Medical Research Council vitamin study. Lancet 338: 131–137.

O'Keefe, C. A., Bailey, L. B., Thomas, E. A., Hofler, S. A., Davis, B. A., Cerda, J. J. & Gregory, J. F. III. (1995) Controlled dietary folate affects folate status in non-pregnant women. J. Nutr. 125: 2717–2725.

Savage, D. G. & Lindenbaum, J. (1995) Folate-cobalamin interactions. In: Folate in Health and Disease (Bailey, L. B., ed.), pp. 237–285. Marcel Dekker, New York, NY.

Selhub, J., Jacques, P. F., Wilson, P. W. F., Rush, D. & Rosenberg, I. H. (1993) Vitamin status and intake as primary determinants of homocysteinemia in an elderly population. J. Am. Med. Assoc. 270: 2693–2698.

Ubbink, J. B., Vermaak, W. J. H., van der Merwe, A. & Becker, P. J. (1993) Vitamin B-12, vitamin B-6, and folate nutritional status in men with hyperhomocysteinemia. Am. J. Clin. Nutr. 57: 47–53.

A Traditional Practice that Threatens Health—Female Circumcision

1. See Lopez, A.D. Sex differentials in mortality. WHO Chronicle, 38 (5): 217–224 (1984).
2. Traditional practices affecting the health of women and children. Female circumcision, child marriage, nutritional taboos, etc. (WHO/EMRO Technical Publication No. 2). Vol. 1: Report of a Seminar (Khartoum, 1979). Alexandria WHO Regional Office for the Eastern Mediterranean, 1979. Vol. 2: Background papers to the WHO Seminar. Alexandria, WHO Regional Office for the Eastern Mediterranean, 1982.
3. To enhance acceptance of its work WHO recommended that the NGO group change its name, and in 1983 it became the Working Group on Traditional Practices that Affect the Health of Women and Children. The group was originally established under the auspices of the United Nations Commission on Human Rights.
4. *Female circumcision. Statement of WHO position and activities.* Submitted to the United Nations Commission on Human Rights, Sub-Commission on Prevention of Discrimination and Protection of Minorities, Working Group on Slavery, August 1982.
5. *The Report on a Seminar on Traditional Practices Affecting the Health of Women and Children in Africa* is available for the cost of postage from the NGO group. Please write to Ms. Margareta Linnander, 147, rue de Lausanne, 1202 Geneva, Switzerland.
6. This recommendation appears in paragraph 161 of the forward-looking strategies adopted by the World Conference to Review and Appraise the Achievements of the United Nations Decade for Women, Nairobi, 15–26 July 1985. See: The United Nations Decade for Women: an end and a beginning. *WHO Chronicle*, 39 (3): 163–170 (1985).

PART II

Chapter 8 TUBERCULOSIS

Streptomycin: A Valuable Anti-Tuberculosis Agent

1. For a review of the development of the chemotherapy of tuberculosis the lectures by Feldman (1946a, 1946b, 1946c), by Hart (1946), and by Waksman (1947) may be consulted.
2. A few months previously Rist, Bloch, and Hamon (1940) had reported independently a definite antagonistic effect of 4,4′-diaminodiphenylsulphone on tuberculosis of rabbits and guinea-pigs infected with avian tubercle bacilli.
3. The question of the action of streptomycin on tubercle bacilli *in vitro* was the subject of a recent report by Smith and Waksman (1947).
4. A report on the toxicity of streptomycin in human beings has been given by McDermott (1947).
5. A method for the determination of sensitivity of tubercle bacilli to streptomycin *in vitro* has been described by Karlson and his associates (1947).

BIBLIOGRAPHY

Baggenstoss, A. H., Feldman, W. H., and Hinshaw, H. C. (1947). *Amer. Rev. Tuberc.*, 55, 54.

Brown, H. A., and Hinshaw, H. C. (1946). *Proc. Mayo Clin.*, 21, 347.

Cantani, A. (1885). Quoted by W. H. Florey, *British Medical Journal*, 1945, 2, 635.

Council on Pharmacy and Chemistry (1947). *J. Amer. med. Ass.*, 135, 634.

Demerec, M. Quoted by F. R. Selbie (1946). *Brit. med. Bull.*, 4, 267.

Faget, G. H., Pogge, R. C., Johansen, F. H., Fite, G. L., Prejean, B. M., and Gemar, Frank (1946). *Int. J. Leprosy*, 14, 30.

Feldman, W. H. (1946a). *J. roy. Inst. publ. Hlth.*, 9, 267.

_____ (1946b). Ibid., 9, 297.

_____ (1946c). Ibid., 9, 343.

_____ and Hinshaw, H. C. (1944). *Proc. Mayo Clin.*, 19, 593.

_____ and Karlson, A. G. (1947). *Amer. Rev. Tuberc.*, 55, 435.

_____ and Mann, F. C. (1945). Ibid., 52, 269.

_____ and Moses, H. E. (1940). *Proc. Mayo Clin.*, 15, 695.

_____ Karlson, A. G., and Hinshaw, H. C. (1947). *Amer. Rev. Tuberc.*, 56, 346.

Figi, F. A., and Hinshaw, H. C. (1946). *Trans. Amer. Acad. Ophthal. Otolaryng.*, 50, 93.

Fowler, E. P., and Seligman, Ewing (1947). *J. Amer. med. Ass.*, 133, 87.

Glover, R. P., Clagett, 0. T., and Hinshaw, H. C. (1947). *Amer. Rev. Tuberc.*, 55, 418.

Hart. P. D'A. (1946). *British Medical Journal*, 2, 805, 849.

Hinshaw, H. C. (1947a). *J. Lancet*, 67, 131.

_____ (1947b). *J. Amer. med. Ass.*, 135, 641.

_____ and Feldman, W. H. (1944). *Amer. Rev. Tuberc.*, 50, 202.

_____ (1945). Proc. Mayo Clin., 20, 313.

_____ and Pfuetze, K. H. (1946). *J. Amer. med. Ass.*, 132, 778.

Karlson, A. G., Feldman, W. H., and Hinshaw, H. C. (1947). *Proc. Soc. exp. Biol.*, N.Y., 64, 6.

McDermott, Walsh (1947). *Amer. J. Med.*, 2, 491.

Molitor, Hans (1947). *Bull. N. Y. Acad. Med.*, 23, 196.

_____ Graessle, O. E., Kuna, Samuel, Mushett, C. W., and Silber, R. H. (1946). *J. Pharmacol.*, 86, 151.

O'Leary, P. A., Ceder, E. T., Hinshaw, H. C., and Feldman, W. H. (1947). *Arch. Derm. Syph.*, Chicago, 55, 222.

Pyle, Marjorie M. (1947). *Proc. Mayo Clin.*, 22, 465.

Rist, N., Bloch, F., and Hamon, V. (1940). *Ann. Inst. Pasteur*, 64, 203.

Smith, Dorothy G., and Waksman, S. A. (1947). *J. Bact.*, 54, 253.

Waksman, S. A. (1947). *J. Amer. med. Ass.*, 135, 478.

Youmans. G, P., and McCarter, J. C. (1945). *Amer. Rev. Tuberc.*, 52, 432.

_____ and Williston, Elizabeth H. (1946). *Proc. Soc. exp. Biol. N.Y.*, 63. 131.

The International Tuberculosis Campaign: A Pioneering Venture
in Mass Vaccination and Research

1. Holm J. The history of ITC. Note prepared by J. Holm, April–May 1984.
2. Final Report of The International Tuberculosis Campaign, July 1, 1948–June 30, 1951. Copenhagen: International Tuberculosis Campaign, 1951.
3. Stein KS. Report of the Danish Red Cross tuberculosis work in Poland between 1st April and 19th October 1947.
4. Charnow J. Rx for recovery. UNICEF History Project, 24 February 1986.
5. Yuan I-C, Nyboe J, Tuberculosis Research Office, WHO. Mass vaccination in Poland, 1948–49. Copenhagen: International Tuberculosis Campaign, 1950.
6. Untitled manuscript copy, 17 December 1947, Paris.
7. Letter to Dr. Brock Chisholm from Dr. Ludwic Rajchman, dated 18 December 1947.
8. Krogh T. Humanitet og Politik. Det Danske Efterkrigshjaelpearbejde 1945–51 og dets Motivbaggrund. In: Sporarkiver og historie. Copenhagen: Niels Petersen, 1987:183–201.
9. Anonymous. The Conference on European B.C.G. programmes conducted with the assistance of the Joint Enterprise, Copenhagen, Denmark, 8–12 September 1949. Annex 1. Copenhagen: The International Tuberculosis Campaign, 1950.
10. Anonymous. Mass BCG vaccination campaigns: a practical guide based upon the experience of the staff of the International Tuberculosis Campaign, July 1, 1948–June 30, 1951. Neuilly-sur-Seine, France: United Nations International Children's Emergency Fund, 1953:25–8.
11. Yuan IC, SOegaard M. Tuberculosis Research Office, World Health Organization. Mass BCG vaccination in Malta, 1950. Neuilly-sur-Seine, France: International Tuberculosis Campaign, 1951:9–10.
12. Holm J. Report to UNICEF Medical Sub-Committee, January 1949.
13. Second Annual Report of The International Tuberculosis Campaign, July 1, 1949–June 30, 1950. Issued by: UNICEF, International Tuberculosis Campaign, Copenhagen, Denmark. London: William Heinemann Medical Books, 1951:13–5.
14. Engmann H. Final Audit Report by the Third Division of the Chief Audit Department on The International Tuberculosis Campaign ("The Joint Enterprise"), Copenhagen. October 1952:1–121.
15. Minutes of Meeting of the Scandinavian Co-ordination Committee, held in Copenhagen on Saturday, December 16, 1950.
16. Palmer CE, Shaw LW, Comstock GW. Community trials of BCG vaccination. Am Rev Tuberc 1958;77:877–907.
17. Anonymous. BCG vaccination programmes, 1951–56. WHO Chron 1957; 11(5):140–6.
18. Palmer CE. Prospectus of research in mass BCG vaccination. Public Health Rep 1949;64:1250–61.
19. Publications of the Tuberculosis Research Office, World Health Organization, Copenhagen. February 1949–August 1953. Copenhagen: J. Knudsens Bogtrykkeri.

20. Edwards LB, Gelting AS. BCG-vaccine studies. 1. Effect of age of vaccine and variation in storage temperature and dosage on allergy production and vaccination lesions ten weeks after vaccination. Bull World Health Organ 1950;3:1–24.

21. Anonymous. Comparisons between Moro patch and Mantoux tests. Section C-I, Annex 4, General Introduction to Field Operations. In: Second Annual Report of The International Tuberculosis Campaign, July 1, 1949–June 30, 1950. Issued by: UNICEF, The International Tuberculosis Campaign, Copenhagen, Denmark. London: William Heinemann Medical Books, 1951:140.

22. Edwards PQ, Guld J. Tuberculin sensitivity: a study of 245 tuberculous patients. Acta Tuberculosea Scandinavica 1951;25:463–73.

23. Edwards LB, Gelting AS. BCG-vaccine studies. 2. Effect of variation in dosage of BCG vaccine on allergy production and vaccination lesions nine weeks after vaccination. Bull World Health Organ 1950; 3:279300.

24. Palmer CE, Edwards LB. Tuberculin test in retrospect and prospect. Arch Environ Health 1967;15:792–808.

25. Anonymous. Retesting programs in certain countries. In: Final Report of The International Tuberculosis Campaign, July 1, 1948–June 30, 1951. Copenhagen: International Tuberculosis Campaign, 1951: 118–9.

26. WHO Tuberculosis Research Office, Biophysics Laboratory of the University of Copenhagen. Effect of exposure of tuberculin to light. Bull World Health Organ 1955;12:179–88.

27. Edwards LB, Palmer CE, Magnus K. BCG vaccination. Studies by the WHO Tuberculosis Research Office, Copenhagen. Geneva: World Health Organization, 1953:75–81 (World Health Organization monograph series, no 12).

28. Edwards LB, Johansen B. BCG-vaccine studies. 6. Effect of exposing the vaccination site to sunlight immediately after vaccination. Bull World Health Organ 1953;9:821–7.

29. Palmer CE, Meyer SN. Research contributions of BCG vaccination programs. I. Tuberculin allergy as a family trait. Public Health Rep 1951;66:259–76.

30. Meyer SN, Jensen CM. Significance of familial factors in the development of tuberculin allergy. Am J Hum Genet 1951;3:325–31.

31. Edwards LB, Palmer CE. Geographic variation in naturally acquired tuberculin sensitivity. Lancet 1953;1:53–7.

32. Hiar AS. Long-term evaluation of mass-BCG-vaccination campaign: a study of thirty years of experience in Finland. In: Yearbook of tuberculosis and respiratory diseases. Helsinki: Finnish Anti-Tuberculosis Association, 1977:7–66.

33. Frimodt-Moller J. A community-wide tuberculosis study in a South Indian rural population, 1950–1955. Bull World Health Organ 1960;22:61–170.

The Global Tuberculosis Situation and the New Control Strategy of the World Health Organization

1. Sudre P, ten Dam G, Kocki A. 'Tuberculosis in the present tense': A global overview of the tuberculosis situation. *WHO Working Document*. (In press).

2. Murray GDL, Styblo K, Rouillon A. Tuberculosis in developing countries: Burden, intervention and class. *Bull IUATLD* 1990; 65 (1): 6–24.

3. Childhood tuberculosis and BCG vaccine. *EPI Update* Supplement. Geneva: WHO. 1989.

4. Proceedings of WHO informal meeting on assessment of TB control technologies. *WHO TUB Unit Publication*. Geneva: WHO. (In press).

5. Summer report on the WHO workshop 'Case studies for evaluation of tuberculosis control in various primary healthcare settings'. Sturbridge, Mass, USA 25–28 May 1990. *WHO TUB Unit Publication* Geneva: WHO. (In press).

6. Rieder HL, Cauthen CM, Comstock GW, Snider D Jr. Epidemiology of tuberculosis in the United States. *Epidemiol Rev* 1989; 11: 29–30.

7. Proceedings on the WHO informal meeting 'Development of guidelines for tuberculosis control in HIV epidemic countries/areas'. October 2–3 1989. *WHO TUB Unit Publication*. Geneva: WHO (In press).

8. Ninth report of the WHO expert committee on tuberculosis. *WHO Tech Rep Ser* no. 552. Geneva: WHO, 1974. [There is no corresponding number for this reference in the text, Ed.]

9. Styblo K. Tuberculosis control and surveillance. In: Flenley DC, Petty TL, Eds. *Recent Advances In Respiratory Medicine* No 4. pp. 77–108. Edinburg: Churchill Livingstone 1986.

10. Styblo K, Meijer J. Impact of BCG vaccination programmes in children and young adults on tuberculosis programmes. *Tubercle* 1976; 57: 17–43.

11. Styblo K. The elimination of tuberculosis in the Netherlands. *TSRU Prog Rep* 1999; 1: 47–65. [There is no corresponding number for this reference in the text, Ed.]

12. Kahn GR, Chang LX, Wu JS, Ma ZL. Supervised intermittent chemotherapy for pulmonary tuberculosis in rural areas of China. *Tubercle* 1985; 66: 1–7. [There is no corresponding number for this reference in the text, Ed.]

13. Abed FH. TB control programme using village health workers: some management issues. Paper prepared for the WHO meeting on 'Tuberculosis control and research strategy for the 1990s'. October 26–27 1990. *WHO TUB Unit Publication*. Geneva: WHO (In press).

14. Mori T, Kochi A. case-study on the tuberculosis control programme of the United Republic of Tanzania. *WHO TUB Unit Publication*. Geneva: WHO (In press).

15. Kochi A. Global tuberculosis situation and WHO tuberculosis control programme. *WHO TUB Unit Publication* Geneva: WHO (In press). [There is no corresponding number for this reference in the text, Ed.]

Chapter 9   HIV/AIDS

Pneumocystis Pneumonia—Los Angeles

1. Walzer PD, Perl DP, Krogstad DJ, Rawson PG, Schultz MG. *Pneumocystis carinii* pneumonia in the United States. Epidemiologic, diagnostic, and clinical features. Annm Intern Med 1974; 80:83–93.

2. Rinaldo CR, Jr, Black PH, Hirsch MS. Interaction of cytomegalovirus with leukocytes from patients with mononucleosis due to cytomegalovirus. J Infect Dis 1977; 136:667–78.

3. Rinaldo CR, Jr. Carney WP, Richter BS, Black PH, Hirsch MS. Mechanisms of immunosuppression in cytomegaloviral mononucleosis. J Infect Dis 1980; 141:488–95.

4. Drew WL, Mintz L, Miner RC, Sands M, Ketterer B. Prevalence of cytomegalovirus infection in homosexual men. J Infect Dis 1981; 143:188–92.

5. Lang DJ, Kummer JF. Cytomegalovirus in semen: observations in selected populations. J Infect Dis 1975; 132:472–3.

Cluster of Cases of the Acquired Immune Deficiency Syndrome: Patients Linked by Sexual Contact

1. Centers for Disease Control: Pneumocystis pneumonia—Los Angeles. Morbid Mortal Weekly Rep 1981; 30:250–252.

2. Centers for Disease Control: Kaposi's sarcoma and Pneumocystis pneumonia among homosexual men—New York City and California. Morbid Mortal Weekly Rep 1981; 30:305–308.

3. Gottlieb MS, Schroff R, Schanker HM, et al: Pneumocystis carinii pneumonia and mucosal candidiasis in previously healthy homosexual men. N Engl J Med 1981; 305:1425–1431.

4. Siegel FP, Lopez C, Hammer GS, et al: Severe acquired immuno-deficiency in male homosexuals, manifested by chronic perianal ulcerated herpes simplex lesions. N Engl J Med 1981; 305:1439–1444.

5. CDC Task Force on Kaposi's Sarcoma and Opportunistic Infections: Epidemiologic aspects of the current outbreak of Kaposi's sarcoma and opportunistic infections. N Engl J Med 1982; 306:248–252.

6. Centers for Disease Control: Update on Acquired Immune Deficiency Syndrome (AIDS)—United States. Morbid Mortal Weekly Rep 1982; 31:507–508, 513–514.

7. Jaffe HW, Choi K, Thomas PA, et al: National case-control study of Kaposi's sarcoma and Pneumocystis carinii pneumonia in homosexual men. Part I. Epidemiologic results. Ann Intern Med 1983; 99:145–151.

8. Centers for Disease Control: Update on Kaposi's sarcoma and opportunistic infections in previously healthy persons—United States. Morbid Mortal Weekly Rep 1982; 31:294, 300–301.

9. Centers for Disease Control: Opportunistic infections on Kaposi's sarcoma among Haitians in the United States. Morbid Mortal Weekly Rep 1982; 31:353–354, 360–1.

10. Centers for Disease Control: Pneumocystis carinii pneumonia among persons with hemophilia A. Morbid Mortal Weekly Rep 1982; 31:365–367.

11. Centers for Disease Control: Possible transfusion-associated Acquired Immune Deficiency Syndrome (AIDS)—California. Morbid Mortal Weekly Rep 1982; 31:652–654.

12. Joncas JH, DeLage G, Chad Z, LaPoite N: Acquired (or congenital) immunodeficiency syndrome in infants born of Haitian mothers (letter). N Engl J Med 1983; 308:842.

13. Centers for Disease Control: Unexplained immunodeficiency and opportunistic infections in infants—New York, New Jersey, California. Morbid Mortal Weekly Rep 1982; 31:665–667.

14. Centers for Disease Control: Immunodeficiency among female sexual partners of males with acquired immune deficiency syndrome—New York. Morbid Mortal Weekly Rep 1983; 31:697–698.

15. Friedman–Kien AE: Disseminated Kaposi's sarcoma syndrome in young homosexual men. J Am Acad Dermatol 1981; 5:468–471

16. Mantel N, Haenszel W: Statistical aspects of the analysis of data from retrospective studies of disease. JNCI 1959; 22:719–748.

17. Mantel N: Chi-square tests with one degree of freedom. J Am Stat Assoc 1963; 58:690–700.

18. Kornfeld H, Vande Stouwe RA, Lange M, Reddy MM, Griect MH: T-lymphocyte subpopulations in homosexual men. N Engl J Med 1982; 307: 729–731.

19. Lederman MM, Ratnoff OD, Scillian JJ, Jones PH, Schacter B: Impaired cell-mediated immunity in patients with classical hemophilia. N Engl J Med 1983; 308:79–83.

20. Menitove JE, Aster RH, Casper JT, et al: T-lymphocyte subpopulations in patients with classic hemophilia treated with cryoprecipitate and lypholized concentrates. N Engl J Med 1983; 308:83–86.

21. Harwood AR, Asoba D, Hofstader SL, et al: Kaposi's sarcoma and recipients of renal transplants. Am J Med 1979; 67:759–765.

22. Penn I: Kaposi's sarcoma in organ transplant recipients. Transplantation 1979; 27:8–11.

23. Centers for Disease Control: Prevention of acquired immune deficiency syndrome (AIDS): report of inter-agency recommendations. Morbid Mortal Weekly Rep 1983; 32:101–103.

AIDS—The First 20 Years

1. *Pneumocystis* pneumonia–Los Angeles. MMWR Morb Moral Wkly Rep 1981; 30:250–2.

2. UNAIDS, WHO. AIDS epidemic update: December 2000. Geneva: Joint United Nations Programme on HIV/AIDS, 2000.

3. Kaposi's sarcoma and *Pneumocystis pneumonia* among homosexual men–New York City and California. MMWR Morb Mortal Wkly Rep 1981; 30:305–8.

4. A cluster of Kaposi's sarcoma and *Pneumocystis carinii* pneumonia among homosexual male residents of Los Angeles and Orange Counties, California. MMWR Morb Mortal Wkly Rep 1982; 31:305–7.

5. Opportunistic infections and Kaposi's sarcoma among Haitians in the United States. MMWR Morb Mortal Wkly Rep 1982; 31:353–4, 360–1.

6. *Pneumocystis carinii* pneumonia among persons with hemophilia A. MMWR Morb Mortal Wkly Rep 1982; 31:365–7.

7. Update on acquired immune deficiency syndrome (AIDS)–United States. MMWR Morb Mortal Wkly Rep 1982; 31:507–9, 513–4.

8. Masur H, Michelis MA, Wormser GP, et al. Opportunistic infection in previously healthy women: initial manifestations of the community-acquired cellular immunodeficiency. Ann Intern Med; 97:533–9.

9. Acquired immune deficiency syndrome (AIDS): precautions for clinical and laboratory staff. MMWR Morb Mortal Wkly Rep 1982; 31:577–80.

10. Possible transfusion-associated acquired immune deficiency syndrome (AIDS)–California. The MMWR Morb Mortal Wkly Rep 1982; 31:652–4.

11. Unexplained immunodeficiency and opportunistic infections in infants–New York, New Jersey, California. The MMWR Morb Mortal Wkly Rep 1982; 31:665–7.

12. Immunodeficiency among female sexual partners of males with acquired immune deficiency syndrome (AIDS)—New York. MMWR Morb Mortal Wkly Rep 1983; 31:697–8.

13. Acquired immune deficiency syndrome (AIDS) in prison inmates—New York, New Jersey. MMWR Morb Mortal Wkly Rep 1983; 31:700–1.

14. Prevention of acquired immune deficiency syndrome (AIDS): report of interagency recommendations. MMWR Morb Mortal Wkly Rep 1983; 32:101–3.

15. Clumeck N, Mascart-Lemone F, de Mauberge J, Brenez D, Marcelis L. Acquired immune deficiency and black Africans. Lancet 1983; 1:642.

16. Barre-Sinoussi F, Chermann JC, Rey F, et al. Isolation of a T-lymphocyte retrovirus from a patient at risk for acquired immune deficiency syndrome (AIDS) Science 1983; 220:868–71.

17. An evaluation of acquired immune deficiency syndrome (AIDS) reported in health-care personnel—United States. MMWR Morbid Mortal Wkly Rep 1983; 32:358–60.

18. Conte JE Jr, Hadley WK, Sande M. infection-control guidelines for patients with the acquired immunodeficiency syndrome (AIDS). N Engl J Med 1983; 309:740–4.

19. Summary—cases specified notifiable diseases, United States. MMWR Morb Mortal Wkly Rep 1984; 33:4–5.

20. Gallo RC, Salahuddin SZ, Popovic M, et al. Frequent detection and isolation of psychopathic retroviruses (HTLV-III) for patients with AIDS and at risk for AIDS. Science 1984; 224:500–3.

21. Classification system for human T-lymphotropic virus type III/lymphadenopathy-associated virus infections. MMWR Morb Mortal Wkly Rep 1986; 35:334–9.

22. 1993 Revised classification system for HIV infection and expanded surveillance case definition for AIDS among adolescents and adults. MMWR Morb Mortal Wkly Rep 1992; 41 (RR-17):1–19.

23. Gottlieb MS, Schroff R, Shankar HM, et al. *Pneumocystis carinii* pneumonia and mucosal candidiasis in previously healthy homosexual men: evidence of a new acquired cellular immunodeficiency. N Engl J Med 1981; 305: 1425–31.

24. Goedert JJ, Neuland CY, Wallen WC. Amyl nitrate may alter T lymphocytes in homosexual men. Lancet 1982; 1:412–6.

25. Mavligit GM, Talpaz M, Hsia FT, et al. Chronic immune stimulation by sperm alloantigens: support for the hypothesis that spermatozoa induce immune dysregulation in homosexual males. JAMA 1984; 251:347–41.

26. Sonnabend J, Witkin SS, Purtilo DT. Acquired immunodeficiency syndrome, opportunistic infections, and malignancies in homosexual males: the hypothesis that etiologic factors in pathogenesis. JAMA 1988; 249: 2370–4.

27. Levy JA, Ziegler JL. Acquired immunodeficiency syndrome is an opportunistic infection and Kaposi's sarcoma results from secondary immune stimulation. Lancet 1983; 2:78–81.

28. Shilts R. And the band played on: politics, people, and the AIDS epidemic. New York: St. Martin's Press, 1987.

29. Waterson AP. Acquired immune deficiency syndrome. BMJ 1983; 286: 743–6.

30. Francis DP, Curran JW, Essex M. Epidemic of acquired immune deficiency syndrome: epidemiologic evidence for transmissible agent. J Nat Cancer Inst 1988; 77:1–4.

31. Hardy WD Jr, Old LJ, Hess PW, Essex M, Cotter S. Horizontal transmission of feline leukaemia virus. Nature 1973; 244:266–9.

32. Cotter SM, Hardy WD Jr, Essex M. Association of feline leukemia virus with lymphosarcoma and other disorders in the cat. J Am Vet Assoc 1975; 1966:449–54.

33. Leonidas J-R, Hyppolite N. Haiti and the acquired immunodeficiency syndrome. Ann Intern Med 1983; 98:1020–1.

34. Duesberg R, Rasnick D. The AIDS dilemma: drug diseases blamed on the passenger virus. Genetica 1998; 104:85–132.

35. The Durban Declaration. Nature 2000; 406:15–6.

36. Stewart GT, Mhlongo S, de Harven E, et al. The Durban Declaration is not accepted by all. Nature 2000; 407:286.

37. Byers VS, Levin AS, Malvino A, Waites L, Robins RA, Baldwin RW. A phase II study of effective addition of trichosanthin to the zidovudine in patients with HIV disease and failing antiretrovirals agents. AIDS Res Hum Retroviruses 1994; 10:413–20.

38. Pert CB, Hill JM, Ruff MR, et al. Octapeptides deduced from the neuropeptide receptor-like pattern of antigen T4 in brain potently inhibit human immunodeficiency virus receptor binding and T-cell infectivity. Proc Natl Acad Sci U S A 1986; 83:9254–eight.

39. Mildvan D, Buzas J, Armstrong D, et al. An open-label, dose-ranging trial of AL 721 in patients with persistent generalized lymphadenopathy and AIDS-related complex. J Acquire Immune Defic Syndr 1991; 4:945–51.

40. Schooley RT, Merigan TC, Gaut P, et al. Recombinant soluble CD4 therapy in patients with the acquired immunodeficiency syndrome (AIDS) and AIDS-related complex: a phase I-II escalating dosage trial. Ann Intern Med 1990; 112:247–53.

41. Abrams DI, Kuno S, Wong R, et al. Oral dextran sulfate (UA001) in the treatment of the acquired immune deficiency syndrome (AIDS) and AIDS-related complex. Ann Intern Med 1989; 110:183–8.

42. Pederson C, Sandström E, Peterson CS, et al. The efficacy of inosine pranobex in preventing the acquired immune deficiency syndrome in patients with human immunodeficiency virus infection. N Engl J Med 1990; 322:1757–63. [Erratum, N Engl J Med 1990; 323:1360.]

43. The HIV87 Study Group. Multicenter, randomized, placebo-controlled study of ditocarb (Imuthiol) in human immunodeficiency virus-infected asymptomatic and minimally symptomatic patients. AIDS Res Hum Retroviruses 1993; 9:83–9.

44. Thompson KA, Strayer DR, Salvato PD, et al. results of the double-blind placebo-controlled study of the double-stranded RNA drug polyI:polyC12U in the treatment of HIV infection. Eur J Clin Microbiol Infect Dis 1996; 15:580–7.

45. Gottlieb MS, Zackin RA, Fiala M, et al. Response to treatment with the leukocyte-derived immunomodulator IMREG-1 in immunocompromised patients with AIDS-related complex; a multicenter, double-blind, placebo-controlled trial. Ann Intern Med 1991; 115:84–91.

46. Arno PS, Feiden KL. Against the odds: the story of AIDS drug development, politics and profits. New York: HarperCollins, 1992.

47. Treatment issues. In: Gingell B, ed. The GMHC newsletter of experimental AIDS therapies. Vol. 2 No. 7. New York: Gay Men's Health Crisis, 1988:11–2.

48. Guidelines for the use of antiretroviral agents in HIV-infected adults and adolescents. MMWR Morb Mortal Wkly Rep 1998; 47 (RR-5):43–82. (Updated as a living document February 2001.) (See http://hivtais.org/trtgdlns .html#adultadolescent.)

49. Fischel MA, Richman DD, Grieco MH, et al. Efficacy of azidothymidine (AZT) in the treatment of patients with AIDS and AIDS-related complex: a double-blind, placebo-controlled trial. N Engl J Med 1987; 317:185–91.

50. Kolata G. After 5 years of use, doubt still clouds leading AIDS drug. New York Times. June 2, 1992:C3.

51. USPHS/IDSA guidelines for the prevention of opportunistic infections in persons infected with human immunodeficiency virus: a summary. MMWR Morb Mortal Wkly Rep 1995; 44 (RR-8):1–34.

52. Shafer RW, Seitzman PA, Tapper ML. Successful prophylaxis of Pneumocystis carinii pneumonia with trimethoprim-sulfamethoxazole in AIDS patients with previous allergic reactions. J Acquir Immune Defic Syndr 1989; 2:389–93.

53. Update: mortality attributable to HIV infection among persons aged 25–44 years—United States, 1994. MMWR Morb Mortal Wkly Rep 1996; 45:121–five.

54. Ho DD, Neumann AU, Perelson AS, Chen W, Leonard JM, Markowitz M. Rapid turnover of plasma virions and CD4 lymphocytes in HIV-1 infection. Nature 1995; 373:123–6.

55. Moore PS, Chang Y. Detection of herpesvirus-like DNA sequences in Kaposi's sarcoma in patients with and without HIV infection. N Engl J Med 1995; 332:1181–5.

56. Hammer SM, Squires KE, Hughes MD, et al. A controlled trial of two nucleoside analogues plus indinavir in persons with human immunodeficiency virus infection in CD4 cell counts as 200 per cubic millimeter or less. N Engl J Med 1997; 337:725–33.

57. Update: trends in AIDS incidence, deaths, and prevalence—United States, 1996. MMWR Morb Mortal Wkly Rep 1997; 46:165–73.

58. Mellors JW, Rinaldo CR Jr, Gupta P, White RM, Todd JA, Kingsley LA. Prognosis in HIV-1 infection predicted by the quantity of virus in plasma. Science 1996; 272:1167–70. [Erratum, science 1997; 275:14.]

59. Carr A, Samaras K, Burton S, et al. A syndrome of peripheral lipodystrophy, hyperlipidaemia and insulin resistance in patients receiving HIV protease inhibitors. AIDS 1998; 12:F51–F58.

60. Staszewski S, Morales-Ramirez J, Tashima KT, et al. Efavirenz plus zidovudine and lamivudine, efavirenz plus indinavir, and indinavir plus zidovudine and lamivudine in the treatment of HIV-1 infection in adults. N Engl J Med 1999; 431:1865–73.

61. Birmingham K. UN acknowledges HIV/AIDS as a threat to world peace. Nat Med 2000; 6:117.

62. Stolberg SG. Africa's AIDS war: pressure for affordable medicine: 'if' becomes 'when' for patients. New York Times. March 10, 2001:A1, A4.

63. Petersen M, McNeil DG Jr. Maker yielding patent in Africa for AIDS drug. New York Times. March 15, 2001:A1, A14.

64. Palella FJ Jr, Delaney KM, Moorman AC, et al. Declining morbidity and mortality among patients with advanced human immunodeficiency virus infection. N Engl J Med 1998; 338:853–60.

65. Gebo KA, Chaisson RE, Folkemer JG, Bartlett JG, Moore RD. Costs of HIV medical care in the era of highly active antiretroviral therapy. AIDS 1999; 13:963–9.

66. Chun TW, Justement JS, Moir S, et al. Suppression of HIV replication in the resting CD4+ T cell reservoir by autologous CD8+ T cells: implications for the development of therapeutic strategies. Proc Natl Acad Sci U S A 2001; 98:253–8.

67. Rosenberg T. Look at Brazil. New York Times Sunday Magazine. January 28, 2001: 26.

68. Leveton LB, Sox HC Jr, Stoto MA, eds. HIV in the blood supply: an analysis of crisis decisionmaking. Washington, D.C.: National Academy Press, 1995.

69. Food and Drug Administration. Revised precautionary measures to reduce the possible transmission of Creutzfeldt-Jacob disease (CJD) by blood and blood products: guidance document. Fed Regist 1997; 62 (184):49,694–5.

70. New medicines in development: annual summaries 1988 and 1999. Washington, D.C.: Pharmaceutical Research and Manufacturers of America, 1989, 2000.

71. Committee on the NIH Research Priority-Setting Process. Scientific opportunities and public needs: improving priority setting and public input at the National Institutes of Health. Washington, D.C.: National Academy Press, 1998.

72. Nelson KE, Celentano DD, Eiumtrakol S, et al. Changes in sexual behavior and a decline in HIV infection among young men in Thailand. N Engl J Med 1996; 335:297–303.

73. Celentano DD, Nelson KE, Lyles CM, et al. Decreasing incidence of HIV and sexually transmitted diseases in young Thai man: evidence for success of the HIV/AIDS control and prevention program. AIDS 1998; 12:F29–F36.

74. Monterroso ER, Hamburger and E., Vlahov D, et al. Prevention of HIV infection in street-recruited injection drug users: the Collaborative Injection Drug User Study (CIDUS). J Acquir Immune Defic Syndr 2000; 25:63–70.

75. Ruiz MS, ed. No time to lose: getting more from HIV prevention. Washington, D.C.: National Academy Press, 2001.

Chapter 10   VACCINE-PREVENTABLE DISEASES

Rubella during Pregnancy

1. Gregg N. McAlister: Congenital Cataract Following German Measles in the Mother. Tr. Ophth. Soc. Australia *3:* 35, 1941.
2. Fox, M. J. and Bortin, M. M.: Rubella in Pregnancy Causing Malformations in Newborn. J. A. M .A. *130:* 58, 1946.
3. Bradford Hill, A. and Galloway, T. McL: Maternal Rubella and Congenital Defects (Data from National Health Insurance Records) Lancet *1:* 299, 1949.
4. Grönvall, H. and Selander P.: Nagra virussjukdomar under graviditet och deras verkan pa fostret. Nord. Med. *37:* 409, 1946.
5. Kamerbeek, A. E. H. M.: Het rubella-probleem in het licht van Nederlandse Ervaringen. Verhandeling van het Institut voor praeventive Geneeskunde XIV. Stenfert Kroese, Leiden 1949.
6. Schick, Béla: Diaplacental Infection of the Fetus with the Virus of German Measles Despite Immunity of the Mother. Acta Paediat. *38:* 563, 94.
7. Swan, C.: Congenital Malformations Associated with Rubella and Other Infections. Modern Practice in Infectious Fevers, Vol. 2. Butterworth & CO. Ltd, London 1951.

Intussusception among Recipients of Rotavirus Vaccine—United States, 1998–1999

1. CDC. Rotavirus vaccine for the prevention of rotavirus gastroenteritis among children—recommendations of the Advisory Committee on Immunization Practices. MMWR 1999;48 (no. RR–2).
2. Committee on Infectious Diseases, American Academy of Pediatrics. Prevention of rotavirus disease: guidelines for use of rotavirus vaccine. Pediatrics 1998;102:1483–91.
3. Chen RT, Rastogi SC, Mullen JR, et al. The Vaccine Adverse Event Reporting System (VAERS). Vaccine 1994;542–50.
4. Niu MT, Salive ME, Ellenberg SS. Post-marketing surveillance for adverse events after vaccination: the national Vaccine Adverse Event Reporting System (VAERS). Food and Drug Administration Medwatch Continuing Education Article, November 1998. Available at http://www.fda.gov/medwatch/articles/vaers/vaersce.pdf. Accessed July 1, 1999.
5. Rennels MB, Parashar UD, Holman RC, Le CT, Chang H-C, Glass RI. Lack of an apparent association between intussusception and wild or vaccine rotavirus infection. Pediatr Infect Dis J 1998;17:924–5.
6. Rosenthal S, Chen R. The reporting sensitivies of two passive surveillance systems for vaccine adverse events. Am J Public Health 1995;85:1706–9.

Herd Immunity: Basic Concept and Relevance to Public Health Immunization Practices

1. Miller JD, Foege WH: Status of eradication of smallpox (and control of measles) and West and Central Africa. J Infect Dis 120:725–732, 1969
2. Miller JD: Measles control in Africa: A practical and theoretical epidemiologic challenge. Presented at the Annual Meeting of the APHA, Philadelphia, November, 1969
3. Dorland's Illustrated Medical Dictionary. Philadelphia, WB Saunders Co.1965

4. Bailey NTJ: The Mathematical Theory of Epidemics, Darien, Conn. Hafner Publishing Co. 1957
5. Serfling RE: Historical review of epidemic theory, Hum Biol 24:140 5–166, 1952
6. Abbey, H: An examination of the Reed-Frost theory of epidemics. Hum Biol 24:201–233, 1952
7. Maia J De Oliveira Costa: Some mathematical developments on the epidemic theory formulated by Reed and Frost. Hum Biol 24:167–200, 1952
8. Elveback L, Fox JP, Ackerman E., et al: Stochastic two-agent epidemic simulation models for a community of families. Amer J Epidem 93:267–280, 1971
9. Foege WH: (personal communication, 1971)
10. Scott HD: The elusiveness of measles eradication. Insights gained from three years of intensive surveillance in Rhode Island. Am J Epidem 94:37–42, 1971

Chapter 11   CANCER

Incidence of Leukemia in Survivors of the Atomic Bomb in Hiroshima and Nagasaki, Japan

1. March, H. C. Leukemia in radiologists at a twenty year period. *Am. J. M. Sc.,* 220: 282, 1950.
2. March, H. C. Leukemia in radiologists. *Radiology,* 43:275, 1944.
3. Martland, H. S. The occurrence of malignancy in radioactive persons. Am. J. Cancer, 15: 2435, 1931.
4. Sacks, M. S. and Seeman, I. A statistical study of mortality from leukemia. *Blood,* 2: 1, 1947.

Hepatocellular Carcinoma and Hepatitis B Virus

1. Szmuness W. Hepatocellular carcinoma and the hepatitis B virus: Evidence for a causal association. *Prog Med Virol* 1978; 24: 40–69.
2. Kew MC. Hepatoma and the HBV. In: Vyas GN, Cohen SN, Schmid R, eds. Viral hepatitis. Philadelphia: Franklin Institute Press, 1978: 439–50.
3. Waterhouse J, Muir C, Correa P, Powell V, eds. Cancer incidence in five continents, Vol. II. International Agency for Research on Cancer, WHO. Lyon, France, 1976.
4. MacNab GM, Urbanowicz JM, Geddes EW, Kew MC. Hepatitis B surface antigen and antibody in Bantu patients with primary hepatocellular cancer. *Br J Cancer* 1976; 33: 544–48.
5. Kaplan HS, Tsuchitani PJ, eds. Cancer in China. New York; Alan R Liss Inc, 1978.
6. Wogan GN. Aflatoxins and their relationship to hepatocellular carcinoma. In: Okuda K, Peters RL, eds. Hepatocellular carcinoma. New York: John Wiley and Sons, 1976: 25–41.
7. Lutwick L. Relation between aflatoxin, hepatitis B virus, and hepatocellular carcinoma. *Lancet* 1979; i: 755–57.
8. Smith JB, Blumberg BS. Viral hepatitis, postnecrotic cirrhosis, and hepatocellular carcinoma. *Lancet* 1969; ii: 953.
9. Simmons MJ, Yu M, Chow BK, et al. Australia antigen in Singapore Chinese patients with hepatocellular carcinoma. *Lancet* 1971; i: 1149.

10. Prince AM, Szmuness WM, Michon J, et al. A case/control study of the association between primary liver cancer and hepatitis B infection in Senegal. *Int J Cancer* 1975; 16: 376–83.

11. Simons MJ, Yap EH, Yu M, Shanmugaruatnam K. Australia antigen in Chinese patients with hepatocellular carcinoma and comparison groups: Influence of technique sensitivity on differential frequencies. *Int J Cancer* 1972; 10: 320–25.

12. Nishoka K, Hirayama T, Sekine T, et al. Australian antigen and hepatocellular carcinoma. *GANN Mono Cancer Res* 1973; 14: 167–75.

13. Melnick JL. Evidence for the association of a chronic disease (liver cancer) with persistent hepatitis virus infection. In: Stevens JG, Todaro GJ, Fox CF, eds. Persistent viruses. New York: Academic Press, 1978: 521–34.

14. Obata H, Hayashi N, Motoike Y, et al. A prospective study of the development of hepatocellular carcinoma from liver cirrhosis with persistent hepatitis B virus infection. *Int J Cancer* 1980; 25: 741–47.

15. Newberne PM, Butler WH. Acute and chronic effects of aflatoxin on the liver of domestic and laboratory animals: A review. *Cancer Res* 1969; 29: 236–50.

16. Keen P, Martin P. Is aflatoxin carcinogenic in man? The evidence in Swaziland. *Trop Geogr Med* 1971; 23: 44–53.

17. Shank RC, Gordon RC, Wogan GN, Nondasuta A, Subhamani B. Dietary aflatoxins and human liver cancer III. Field survey of rural Thai families for ingested aflatoxin. *Food Cosmet Toxicol* 1972; 10: 71–84.

18. van Rensburg SJ, van der Watt JJ, Purchase IFH, Coutino LP, Markham R. Primary liver cancer rate and aflatoxin intake in a high cancer area. *S Afr Med J* 1974; 49:1023–51.

19. Alpert ME, Hutt MSR, Wogan GN, Davidson CS. Association between aflatoxin content of food and hepatoma frequency in Uganda. *Cancer* 1971; 28: 153–59.

20. Peers FG, Linsell CA. Dietary aflatoxins and liver cancer—a population based study in Kenya. *Br J Cancer* 1975; 27: 473–85.

21. Adamson RH, Correa P, Dalgard DW. Occurrence of primary liver carcinoma in a rhesus monkey fed aflatoxin. *J Natl Cancer Inst* 1973; 50: 549–51.

22. Wei DL, Wei RD. High pressure liquid chromatogmphic determination of aflatoxins in peanut and peanut products of Taiwan. *Proc Natl Sci Counc ROC* 1980; 4:152–55.

23. Shikata T. Primary liver carcinoma and liver cirrhosis. In: Okuda K, Peters RL, eds. Hepatocellular carcinoma. New York: John Wiley and Sons, 1976: 53–71.

24. Peters RL. Pathology of hepatocellular carcinoma. In: Okuda K, Peters RL, eds. Hepatocellular carcinoma.. New York: John Wiley and Sons, 1976: 107–68.

25. Klaskin G. Persistent HB antigenemia: associated clinical manifestations and hepatic lesions. *Am J Med Sci* 1975; 279: 33–40.

Malignant Melanoma of the Skin

1. CROMBIE, I. K. Racial differences in melanoma incidence. *British journal of cancer*, 40: 185–193 (1979).

2. SOBER, A. J. ET AL. The melanin pigmentary system in man. In: Clark, W. et al., ed. *Human malignant melanoma*. New York, Grune & Stratton, 1979, pp. 3–13.

3. PATHAK, M. A. The role of natural photoprotective agents in human skin. In: Pathak, M. et al., ed. *Sunlight and man*. Tokyo, University of Tokyo Press, 1974, pp. 725–750.

4. LEE, J. A. H. Melanoma. In: Schottenfeld, D. et al., ed. *Cancer epidemiology and prevention*. Philadelphia, W. B. Saunders, 1982, pp. 984–995.

5. HOLMAN, C. D. J. ET AL. Pigmentary traits, ethnic origin, benign nevi, and family history as risk factors for cutaneous malignant melanoma. *Journal of the National Cancer Institute*, 72: 257–266 (1984).

6. BEITNER, H. ET AL. Further evidence for increased light sensitivity in patients with malignant melanoma. *British journal of dermatology*, 104: 289–294 (1981).

7. GREENE, M. H. ET AL. Acquired precursors of cutaneous malignant melanoma. *New England journal of medicine*, 312: 91–97 (1985).

8. ENGLISH, D. R. ET AL. The dysplastic naevus syndrome in patients with cutaneous malignant melanoma in Western Australia. *Medical journal of Australia*, 145: 194–198 (1986).

9. ROBBINS, J. H. ET AL. Xeroderma pigmentosum: an inherited disease with sun sensitivity, multiple cutaneous neoplasms and abnormal DNA repair. *Annals of internal medicine*, 80: 221–248 (1974).

10. SWERDLOW, A. ET AL. Benign melanocytic naevi as a risk factor for malignant melanoma. *British medical journal*, 292: 1555–1559 (1986).

11. WORLD HEALTH ORGANIZATION. *Ultraviolet radiation*. Geneva, 1979 (Environmental Health Criteria No. 14).

12. FREEMAN, R. G. Action spectrum for ultraviolet carcinogenesis. *National Cancer Institute Monograph*, 50: 27–29 (1978).

13. KRIPKE, M. L. Speculations on the role of ultraviolet radiation in the development of malignant melanoma. *Journal of the National Cancer Institute*, 63: 541–548 (1979).

14. ARMSTRONG, B. K. Melanoma of the skin. *British medical bulletin*, 40: 346–350 (1984).

15. ELWOOD, J. M. ET AL. Relationship of melanoma and other skin cancer mortality to latitude and ultraviolet radiation in the United States and Canada. *International journal of epidemiology*, 3: 325–332 (1979).

16. SWERDLOW, A. J. Incidence of malignant melanoma of the skin in England and Wales and its relationship to sunshine. *British medical journal*, 2: 1324–1327 (1979).

17. CUTCHIS, P. *On the linkage of solar ultraviolet radiation to skin cancer*. Washington, U.S. Department of Transportation, 1979 (Institute of Defence Analyses Paper, p- 1342).

18. SCOTTO, J. ET AL. Skin (other than melanoma). In: Schottenfeld, D. et al., ed. *Cancer epidemiology and prevention*. Philadelphia, W. B. Saunders, 1982, pp. 996–1011.

19. HOLMAN, C. D. J. ET AL. A theory of the etiology and pathogenesis of human cutaneous malignant melanoma. *Journal of the National Cancer Institute*, 71: 651–656 (1983).

20. HOLMAN, C. D. J. ET AL. Cutaneous malignant melanoma and indicators of total accumulated exposure to the sun: an analysis separating histogenetic types. *Journal of the National Cancer Institute*, 73: 75–82 (1984).

21. HOLMAN, C. D. J. ET AL. Relationship of cutaneous malignant melanoma to individual sunlight exposure habits. *Journal of the National Cancer Institute*, 76: 403–414 (1986).

22. ELWOOD, J. M. ET AL. Cutaneous melanoma in relation to intermittent and constant sun exposure—The Western Canada Melanoma Study. *International journal of cancer*, 35: 427–433 (1985).

23. HOLMAN, C. D. J. ET AL. The causes of malignant melanoma: results from the West Australian Lions Melanoma Research Project. *Recent results in cancer research*, 102: 18–37 (1986).

24. HEENAN, P. J. ET AL. Surgical treatment and survival from cutaneous malignant melanoma. *Australian and New Zealand journal of surgery*, 55: 229–234 (1985).

25. DAY, C. L. ET AL. Narrower margins for clinical stage I malignant melanoma. *New England journal of medicine*, 306: 479–482 (1982).

26. VERONESI, U. ET AL. Delayed regional lymph node dissection in stage I melanoma of the skin of the lower extremities. *Cancer*, 49: 2420–2430 (1982).

27. DAVIS, N. C. Cutaneous melanoma. The Queensland experience. *Current problems in surgery*, 13: 1–63 (1976).

28. LEMISH, W. M. ET AL. Survival from preinvasive and invasive malignant melanoma in Western Australia. *Cancer*, 52: 580–585 (1983).

29. CUTLER, S. J. ET AL. Trends in survival rates of patients with cancer. *New England journal of medicine*, 293: 122–124 (1975).

30. PAGE, H. S. ET AL. *Cancer rates and risks.* Washington, U.S. Department of Health and Human Services, 1985 (NIH Publication No. 65–691).

31. LITTLE, J. H. ET AL. The changing epidemiology of malignant melanoma in Queensland. *Medical journal of Australia*, 1: 66–69 (1980).

32. ARMSTRONG, B. K. ET AL. Trends in melanoma incidence and mortality in Australia. In: Magnus, K., ed. *Trends in cancer incidence. Causes and practical implications.* New York, Hemisphere Publishing Corporation, 1982, pp. 399–417.

33. HEENAN, P. J. ET AL. A histological comparison of cutaneous malignant melanoma between the Oxford Region and Western Australia. *Histopathology*, 15: 147–152 (1983).

34. GREEN, A. Incidence and reporting of cutaneous melanoma in Queensland. *Australian journal of dermatology*, 23: 105–109 (1982).

35. WATERHOUSE, J. ET AL. *Cancer incidence in five continents, Volume IV.* Lyon, International Agency for Research on Cancer, 1982.

36. ARMSTRONG, B. K. Epidemiology of cancer in Australia. *Medical journal of Australia*, 142: 124–130 (1985).

37. GORDON, D. ET AL. The epidemiology of skin cancer in Australia. In: McCarthy, W. H., ed. *Melanoma and skin cancer.* Sydney, Government Printer, 1972, pp. 23–37.

38. ISAACSON, C. Cancer of the skin in urban blacks of South Africa. *British journal of dermatology*, 100: 347–350 (1979).

39. AOKI, K. ET AL. Age-adjusted death rates for cancer by site (ICD 8th revision) in 50 countries in 1975. *Gann monographs on cancer research*, 26: 251–274 (1981).

40. MUIR, C. S. ET AL. Time trends: malignant melanoma. In: Magnus, K., ed. *Trends in cancer incidence. Causes and practical implications*. New York, Hemisphere Publishing Corporation, 1982, pp. 365–385.

41. JENSEN, O. M. ET AL. Trends in malignant melanoma of the skin. *World health statistics quarterly*, 33: 2–26 (1980).

42. GROVES, G. A. Sunburn and its prevention. *Australasian journal of dermatology*, 21: 115–141 (1980).

43. SMITH, T. The Queensland Melanoma Project—an exercise in health education. *British medical journal*, 1: 253–254 (1979).

44. SNYDER, D. S. ET AL. Ability of PABA to protect mammalian skin from ultraviolet light-induced skin tumours and actinic damage. *Journal of investigative dermatology*, 65: 543–546 (1975).

45. LYNCH, H. T. ET AL. Cancer control in xeroderma pigmentosum. *Archives of dermatology*, 113: 193–195 (1977).

46. SOBER, A. J. ET AL. Early recognition of cutaneous melanoma. *Journal of the American Medical Association*, 242: 2795–2797 (1979).

47. GREENE, M. H. ET AL. High risk of malignant melanoma in melanoma-prone families with dysplastic nevi. *Annals of internal medicine*, 102: 458–465 (1985).

Chapter 12   HEART DISEASE AND STROKE

Epidemiological Approaches to Heart Disease: The Framingham Study

1. Paul, J. R. "Epidemiology" and Green, David E., and Knox, W. Eugene (Eds.), *Research in Medical Science*. New York: McMillan, 1950. p. 53.

2. Maxcy, Kenneth F. (Ed.), *Papers of Wade Hampton Frost, M.D.* New York: Commonwealth Fund, 1941. p. 1.

3. Hill, A. Bradford, and Galloway, T. McL. Maternal Rubella and Congenital Defects. *Lancet* 256:299–301, 1949.

4. Jones, T. Duckett, *et al.* Rheumatic Fever and Rheumatic Heart Disease in *Proceedings, First National Conference on Cardiovascular Diseases*. New York: American Heart Association, 1950. pp. 66–77.

5. Mackenzie, Sir James. *The Basis of Vital Activity; Being a Review of Five Years' Work at the St. Andrews Institute for Clinical Research*. London: Faber and Gwyer, 1926.

6. Framingham Community Health and Tuberculosis Demonstration, National Tuberculosis Association, *Final Summary Report*. Framingham, July, 1924.

7. Massachusetts Medical Society, Proceedings of the Council, Annual Meeting, May 24, 1948. *New England J. Med.* 239, 4:130, 1948.

Strategy of Prevention: Lessons from Cardiovascular Disease

1. Society of Actuaries. *Build and blood pressure study 1959*. Chicago Illinois: Society of Actuaries, 1959–60.

2. Mann JI. Oral contraceptives and the cardiovascular risk. In: Oliver MF, ed. *Coronary heart disease in young women.* Edinburgh: Churchill Livingstone, 1978:184–94.

3. Veterans Administration Cooperative Study Group on Antihypertensive Agents. Effects of treatment on morbidity in hypertension. *Circulation* 1972; 45:991–1004.

4. Kannel WB, Gorton T, eds. Section 26. *Some characteristics related to the incidence of cardiovascular disease and health: Framingham Study, 16-year follow-up.* Washington, DC: US Govt Printing Office, 1970.

5. Reid DD, Hamilton PJS, McCartney P, Rose G, Jarrett RJ, Keen H. Smoking and other risk factors for coronary heart-disease in British civil servants. *Lancet* 1976;ii:979–84.

6. Committee of Principal Investigators. A co-operative trial in the primary prevention of ischaemic heart disease using clofibrate. *Br Heart J* 1978; 40:1069–1118.

Theory and Action for Health Promotion: Illustrations from the North Karelia Project

1. Hamburg D: Disease prevention: the challenge of the future. Am J Public Health 1979; 69:1026–1034.

2. Surgeon General's Report on Health Promotion—Background Papers. Washington, DC: Govt Printing Office, 1979.

3. Somers AR (ed): Promoting Health. Germantown, MD: Aspen Systems, 1976.

4. Stunkard AJ: Behavioral medicine and beyond: the example of obesity. IN: Pomerleau O, Brady J (eds): Behavioral Medicine. Baltimore, MD: Williams & Wilkins, 1979.

5. Lewin K: Field Theory in Social Science. New York: Harper, 1951.

6. Puska P: North Karelia Project: A program for community control of cardiovascular diseases. Publications of the University of Kuopio, Community Health—Series A:1, Finland, 1974.

7. Puska P, Tuomilehto J, Salonen J, *et al:* The North Karelia Project: Evaluation of a comprehensive community program for control of cardiovascular diseases in 1972–1977 in North Karelia, Finland. Monograph. WHO/EURO, Copenhagen, 1981.

8. Kirscht JP: The health belief model and illness behavior. Health Education Monographs 1974; 2:387–408.

9. Rosenstock IM: Historical origins of the health belief model. Health Education Monographs 1974; 2:328–35.

10. Jessor R, Jessor S: Problem Behavior and Psychosocial Development. New York: Academic Press, 1977.

11. Green LW, Kreuter MW, Deeds SG, Partridge KB: Health Education Planning. Palo Alto: Mayfield, 1980.

12. Kannel W.: Importance of hypertension as a major risk factor in cardiovascular disease. IN: Genest, *et al,* (eds): Hypertension. New York: McGraw-Hill Company, 1977.

13. Langfeld S: Hypertension: deficient care of the medically served. Ann Intern Med 1973; 78:19.

14. Stamler R, Stamler J Civinelli J, *et al*: Adherence and blood pressure response to hypertension treatment. Lancet 1975; 11:1227.

15. Tuomilehto J: Feasibility of the community program for control of hypertension. A part of the North Karelia Project. Publications of the University of Kuopio, Community Health—Series A: 2, Finland, 1975.

16. Nissimen A: And evaluation of the community-based hypertension program of the North Karelia Project with special reference to the awareness and treatment of elevated blood pressures and blood pressure level. A part of the North Karelia Project. Publications of the University of Kuopio, Community Health—Series original: 2, Finland, 1979.

17. Flay BR, Ditecco D, Schlegel RP: Mass media in health promotion. Health Education Quarterly, 1980:7, 127–143.

18. Katz E, Lazarsfeld PF: Personal influence. Glencoe, IL: Free Press, 1955.

19. Griffiths W, Knutson A: The role of mass media in public health. Am J Public Health 1960; 50:515–523.

20. McAllister A, Farquhar J, Throeson C, Maccoby N: Applying behavioral sciences to cardiovascular health. Health Education Monographs 1976; 4:45–74.

21. Mendelson H: Which shall it be: Mass education or mass persuasion for health? Am J Public Health 1968; 58:131–137.

22. Wikler DI: Ethical issues in governmental efforts to promote health. Washington, DC: Institute of Medicine, National Academy of Sciences, June 1978.

23. Crawford R: You are dangerous to your health: the ideology of victim blaming. Int J Health Services 1977; 7:663–680.

24. McGuire WJ: The nature of attitudes in attitude change. IN Lindsay G, Aronson E (eds): Handbook of Social Psychology. Reading, MA: Addison-Wesley, Vol III, 1969.

25. Bandura A: Principles of Behavior Modification. New York: Holt-Reinhardt, Winston, 1969.

26. Neittaanmäki L, Koskela K, Puska P, McAlister A: The role of lay workers in a community health education [*sic*] in the North Karelia Project. Scand J Soc Med 1981; 1980; 8:1–7.

27. Salonen JT: Smoking and dietary fats in relation to estimated risk of myocardial infarction before and during a preventive community program. Publications of the University of Kuopio, Community Health–Series original reports: 1, Finland, 1980.

28. Bernstein D, McAlister A: The modification of smoking behavior: progress and problems. Addictive Behavior 1976; 1:89–102.

29. Meyer AJ, Maccoby N, Farquhar JQ: The role of opinion leadership in a cardiovascular health education campaign. IN: Ruben BD (ed): Communication Yearbook I. New Brunswick: Transaction Books, 1977.

30. McKnight JL: Organizing for community health in Chicago. Science for the People 1978; 10:27–34.

31. Olsen M Jr: The Logic of Collective Action. Cambridge, MA: Harvard University Press, 1965.

32. Guskin AE, Ross R: Advocacy and democracy: the long view. Am J of Orthopsych 1971; 41:43–57.

33. Perlman JE: Grass-rooting the system. Social Policy 1976; 7:4–20.

34. Glasunov I, Dowd J, Jaksic Z, *et al*: Method logical aspects of the design and conduct of preventive trials in ischemic heart disease. Int J Epidemiol 1973; 2: 137–143.

35. Salonen JT, Puska P, Mustainin H: Changes in morbidity and mortality during a comprehensive community program to control cardiovascular diseases during 1972–1977 in North Karelia. Br Med J 1979; 2:1178–1183.

36. Puska P, McAlister A Koskela K, *et al*: A comprehensive television smoking cessation program in Finland. In J Health Educ (supplement) 1979; 22:1 26.

37. Farquhar J, Maccoby N, Wood P, *et al*: Community education for cardiovascular health. Lancet 1977; 1: 1192–1195.

PART III

Chapter 13   MEDICAL AND PREVENTIVE CARE

Uncertainty and the Welfare Economics of Medical Care

1. This point has been stressed by I. M. D. Little [19, pp. 71–74]. For the concept of a "persuasive definition," see C. L. Stevenson [27, pp. 210–17].

2. The separation between allocation and distribution even under the above assumptions has glossed over problems in the execution of any desired redistribution policy; in practice, it is virtually impossible to find a set of taxes and subsidies that will not have an adverse effect on the achievement of any optimal state. But this discussion would take us even further afield than we have already gone.

3. The basic theorems of welfare economics alluded to so briefly above have been the subject of voluminous literature, but no thoroughly satisfactory statement covering both the theorems themselves and the significance of exceptions to them exists. The positive assertions of welfare economics and their relation to the theory of competitive equilibrium are admirably covered in Koopmans [18]. The best summary of the various ways in which theorems can fail to hold is probably Bator's [6].

4. There are further minor conditions, for which see Koopmans [18, pp. 50–55].

5. For a more precise statement of the existence conditions, see Koopmans [18, pp. 56–60] or Debreu [12, Ch. 5].

6. The theory, in variant forms, seems to have been first worked out by Allais [2], Arrow [5], and Baudier [7]. For further generalization, see Debreu [11] and [12, Ch. 7].

7. It should also be remarked that in the presence of uncertainty, indivisibilites that are sufficiently small to create little difficulty for the existence and viability of competitive equilibrium may nevertheless give rise to a considerable range of increasing returns because of the operation of the law of large numbers. Since most objects of insurance (lives, fire hazards, etc.) have some element of indivisibility, insurance companies have to be above a certain size. But it is not clear that this effect is sufficiently great to create serious obstacles to the existence and viability of competitive equilibrium in practice.

8. One form of production of information is research. Not only does the product have unconventional aspects as a commodity, but it is also subject to increasing returns in use, since new ideas, once developed, can be used over and over without being consumed, and to difficulties of market control, since the cost of reproduction is usually much less than that of production. Hence, it is not surprising that a free enterprise economy will tend to underinvest in research, see Nelson [21] and Arrow [4].

9. An important current situation in which normal market relations have had to be greatly modified in the presence of great risks is the production and procurement of modern weapons; see Patch and Scherer [23, pp. 581–82] (I am indebted for this reference to V. Fuchs) and [1, pp. 71–75].

10. For an explicit statement of this view, see Baumol [8]. But I believe this position is implicit in most discussions of the functions of government.

11. Since writing the above, I find that Buchanan and Tulloch [10, Ch. 13] have argued that all redistribution can be interpreted as "income insurance."

12. For an illuminating survey to which I am much indebted, see S. Mushkin [20].

13. In governmental demand, military power is an example of a service used only irregularly and unpredictably. Here too, special institutional and professional relations have emerged, though the precise social structure is different for reasons that are not hard to analyze.

14. Even with material commodities, testing is never so adequate that all elements of implicit trust can be eliminated. Of course, over the long run, experience with the quality of product of a given seller provides a check on the possibility of trust.

15. See [22, p. 463]. The whole of [22, Ch. 10] is the most illuminating analysis of the social role of medical practice; though Parsons' interest lies in different areas from mine, I must acknowledge here my indebtedness to his work.

16. I am indebted to Herbert Klarman of Johns Hopkins University for some of the points discussed in this and the following paragraph.

17. The belief that the ethics of medicine demands treatment independent of the patient's ability to pay is strongly ingrained. Such a perceptive observer as René Dubois has made the remark that the high cost of anticoagulants restricts their use and may contradict classical medical ethics, as though this were an unprecedented phenomenon. See [13, p. 419]. "The time *may come* when medical ethics will have to be considered in the harsh light of economics" (emphasis added). Of course, this expectation amounts to ignoring the scarcity of medical resources; one has only to have been poor to realize the error. We may confidently assume that price and income do have some consequences for medical expenditures.

18. A needed piece of research is the study of the exact nature of the variations of medical care received and medical care paid for as income rises. (The relevant income concept also needs study.) For this purpose some disaggregation is needed; differences in hospital care which are essentially matters of comfort should, in the above view, be much more responsive to income than, e.g., drugs.

19. This role is enhanced in a socialist society, where the state itself is actively concerned with illness in relation to work; see Field [14, Ch. 9].

20. About 3 per cent of beds were in proprietary hospitals in 1958, against 30 per cent and voluntary nonprofit, and the remainder in federal, state, and local hospitals; see [26, Chart 4–2, p. 60].

21. C. R. Roren has pointed out to me from further factors in this analysis. (1) Given the social intention of helping all patients without regard to immediate ability to pay, economies of scale would dictate a predominance of community-sponsored hospitals. (2) Some proprietary hospitals will tend to control total costs to the patient more closely, including the fees of physicians, who will therefore tend to prefer community-sponsored hospitals.

22. Without trying to assess the present situation, it is clear in retrospect that at some point in the past the actual differential knowledge possessed by physicians may not have been much. But from the economic point of view, it is the subjective belief of both parties, as manifested in their market behavior, that is relevant.

23. The degree of subsidy in different branches of professional education is worthy of a major research effort.

24. Strictly speaking, there are four variables in the market for physicians; price, quality of entering students, quality of education, and quantity. The basic market forces, demand for medical services and supply of entering students, determine two relations among the four variables. Hence, if the nonmarket forces determine the last two, market forces will determine price and quality of entrants.

25. The supply of Ph.D.'s is similarly governed, but there are other conditions in the market which are much different, especially on the demand side.

26. Today only the Soviet Union offers an alternative lower level of medical personnel, the feldshers, who practiced primarily in the rural districts (the institution dates back to the 18th century). According to Field [14, pp. 98–100, 132–33], there is clear evidence of strain in the relations between physicians and feldshers, but it is not certain that the feldshers will gradually disappear as physicians grow in numbers.

27. The law does impose some limits on risk-shifting in contracts, for example, its general refusal to honor exculpatory clauses.

28. There may be an identification problem in this observation. If the failure of the market system is, or appears to be, greater in medical care than in, say, food an individual otherwise equally concerned about the two aspects of others' welfare may prefer to help in the first.

29. See [16, pp. 118–37]. The calculations involve many assumptions and must be regarded as tenuous; see the comments by C. Reinold Noyes in [16, pp. 407–10].

30. It might be argued that the existence of racial discrimination in entrance has meant that some of the rejected applicants are superior to some accepted. However, there is no necessary connection between an increase in the number of entrants and a reduction in racial discrimination; so long as there is excess demand for entry, discrimination can continue unabated and new entrants will be inferior to those previously accepted.

31. One problem here is that the tax laws do not permit depreciation of professional education, so that there is a discrimination against this form of investment.

32. To anticipate later discussion, this condition is not necessarily fulfilled. When it comes to quality choices, the market may be inaccurate.

33. It is assumed that there are two classes, rich and poor; the price of medical services to the rich is twice that to the poor, medical expenditures by the rich are 20 per cent of those by the poor, and the elasticity of demand for medical services is 0.5 for both classes. [The remainder of this footnote has been removed to save space, Ed.]

34. A striking illustration of the desire for security in medical care is provided by the expressed preferences of émigrés from the Soviet Union as between Soviet medical practice and German or American practice; see Field [14, Ch. 12]. Those in Germany preferred the German system to the Soviet, but those in the United States preferred (in a ratio of 3 to 1) the Soviet system. The reasons given boil down to the certainty of medical care, independent of income or health fluctuations.

35. It is a popular belief that the Chinese, at one time, paid their physicians when well but not when sick.

36. Francis Bator points out to me that some protection can be achieved, at a price, by securing additional opinions.

37. The situation is very reminiscent of the crucial role of the focal point in Schelling's theory of tacit games, in which two parties have to find a common course of action without being able to communicate; see [24, esp. pp. 225 ff.].

38. How well they achieve this end is another matter. R. Kessel points out to me that they merely guarantee training, not continued the performance of medical technology changes.

REFERENCES

1. A. A. ALCHIAN, K. J. ARROW, and W. M. CAPRON, An Economic Analysis of the Market for Scientists and Engineers, RAND RM-Z190-RC. Santa Monica 1958.

2. M. ALLIS, "Géneralisation des théories de l'équilibre économique général et du rendement social au cas du risque," in Centre National de la Recherche Scientifique, Econometrie, Paris 1953, pp. 1–20.

3. O. W. ANDERSON AND STAFF OF THE NATIONAL OPINION RESEARCH CENTER, Voluntary Health Insurance in Two Cities. Cambridge, Mass. 1957.

4. K. J. ARROW, "Economic Welfare and the Allocation of Resources for Invention," in Nat. Bur. Econ. Research, The Role and Direction of Inventive Activity: Economic and Social Factors, Princeton 1902. pp. 609–25.

5. _____, "Les rôle des valeurs boursières pour la répartition la meilleure des risques," in Centre National de la Recherche Scientifique. Econometrie, Paris 1953, pp. 41–46.

6. F. M. BATOR, "The Anatomy of Market Failure," Quart. Jour. Econ. Aug. 1958, 72, 351–79.

7. E. BAUDIER, "L'introduction du temps dans la théorie de l'équilibre général," Les Cahiers Economiques, Dec. 1959, 9–16.

8. W. J. BAUMOL, Welfare Economics and the Theory of the State. Cambridge, Mass. 1952.

9. K. BORCH, "The Safety Loading of Reinsurance Premiums," Skandinavisk Aktuariehdskrift, 1960, pp. 163–84.

10. J. M. BUCHANAN AND G. TULLOCK, *The Calculus of Consent*. Ann Arbor 1962.
11. G. DEBREU, "Une économique de l'incertain," *Economie Appliquée*,1960, 13, 111–16.
12. _____, *Theory of Values*. New York 1959.
13. R. Dunos, "Medical Utopias," *Daedalus*, 1959, 88, 410–24.
14. M. G. FIELD, *Doctor and Patient in Soviet Russia*. Cambridge, Mass. 1957.
15. MILTON FRIEDMAN, "The Methodology of Positive Economics," in *Essays in Positive Economics*, Chicago 1953, pp. 3–43.
16. _____AND S. S. KUZNETS, *Income from Independent Professional Practice*. Nat. Bur. Econ. Research, New York 1945.
17. R. A. KESSEL, "Price Discrimination in Medicine," *Jour. Law and Econ.*, 1958, 1, 20–53.
18. T. C. KOOPMANS, "Allocation of Resources and the Price System," in *Three Essays on the State of Economic Science*, New York 1957, pp. 1–120.
19. I. M. D. LITTLE, *A Critique of Welfare Economics*. Oxford 1950.
20. SELMA MUSHKIN, "Towards a Definition of Health Economics," *Public Health Reports*, 1958, 73, 785–93.
21. R. R. NELSON, "The Simple Economics of Basic Scientific Research," *Jour. Pol. Econ.*, June 1959, 67, 297–306.
22. T. PARSONS, *The Social System*. Glencoe 1951.
23. M. J. PECK AND F. M. SCHERER, *The Weapons Acquisition Process: An Economic Analysis*. Div. of Research, Graduate School of Business, Harvard University, Boston 1962.
24. T. C. SCHELLING, *The Strategy of Conflict*. Cambridge, Mass. 1960.
25. A. K. SHAPIRO, "A Contribution to a History of the Placebo Effect," *Behavioral Science*, 1960, 5, 109–35.
26. H. M. SOMERS AND A. R. SOMERS, *Doctors, Patients, and Health Insurance*. The Brookings Institution, Washington 1961.
27. C. L. STEVENSON, *Ethics and Language*. New Haven 1945.
28. U. S. DEPARTMENT OF HEALTH, EDUCATION AND WELFARE, *Physicians for a Growing America*, Public Health Service Publication No. 709, Oct.1959.

Small Area Variations in Health Care Delivery

1. For example, see J. P. Bunker, *N. Engl. J. Med.* 282, 135 (1970); A. M. Burgess, Jr., T. Cotton, O. L. Peterson, *ibid.* 273, 533 (1965); C. E. Lewis, *ibid.* 281, 880 (1969); L. S. Reed and W. Carr, *Soc. Sec. Bull.* 31, 12 (1968); S. Shapiro, L. Weiner, P. M. Densen, *Amer. J. Public Health* 48, 170 (1958); Department of Health, Education, and Welfare, Social Security Administration, *Reimbursement by County and State; Medicare 1970* (Government Printing Office, Washington, D. C., 1972).
2. Each data set has been modified into a standard format and code system for individual physicians, diagnoses, procedures, and other key variables. Since 1969, hospital discharge abstracts have been collected for all patients discharged from the 18 short-term, voluntary hospitals in the state and for Vermont residents discharged from referral hospitals in New Hampshire and New York. Patient information from hospitals participating in the Professional Activities Study (PAS) was obtained from the Commission on

Professional and Hospital Activities, Ann Arbor, Michigan. Four smaller, non-participating hospitals were surveyed directly by the staff. Although hospitalization of Vermonters outside these areas has not been reported, the resultant underreporting is estimated to be less than 3 percent for all classes of admission. Nursing home admission files and home health agency files have been obtained through staff surveys of each institution and agency in the state. Medicare Part B information has been obtained from the third-party carrier responsible for reimbursement. Problems of data accuracy are bound to arise in multi-institutional studies. Despite extensive consistency checks made by PAS and by the staff, the reliability of certain items of information is primarily dependent upon the initiators of the record form. This applies particularly to diagnosis and cause of death, where the criteria are unspecified and the extensive diagnostic workup highly variable. Simple facts such as sex, age, date, place, and procedures appear to be recorded with a reasonable degree of accuracy, based on independent reabstracting of samples of records from several institutions. An age-specific rate relates to the events in the population within a particular age category. An age-adjusted rate is the weighted average of age-specific rates within a given group. It is designed to account for differences in age structure among populations and to permit direct comparisons between areas and groups. In this article, the weights are the proportions of persons in each 5-year age group in the entire state. Since many of the occurrences under consideration are highly age-dependent, we have used age-adjusted rates whenever the relevant data were available to us.

3. In contrast to highly urbanized centers, the hospital service areas of Vermont tend to be relatively discrete and seldom overlap. Over 85 percent of all hospitalizations for Vermont residents in 1969 took place in the service area of residence. Maternity patients, patients requiring general surgery, and most patients with medical conditions that comprise the majority of admissions are usually hospitalized in their own area. Patients with conditions requiring specialized services were more often referred to other areas. In the community hospital areas, about two-thirds of the admissions for neoplasms were treated locally and one-third treated in referral hospitals. Neoplasm was the major diagnosis in 5 percent of hospital admissions.

4. The major effect of the allocation procedure on estimated that supply was to distribute one-third of the 587 beds of the referral hospital to the other hospital service areas in and outside of the state. In four areas, the number of allocated beds was lower than the number of resident beds, reflecting overlap at service boundaries. In none of the community hospital service areas did the allocated number of beds differ from the resident beds by more than 20 percent.

5. Significance level for simple regression coefficient with 11 degrees of freedom: r: .55=5 percent; .68=1 percent.

6. Unpublished report prepared by the Northern New England Regional Medical Program for the Connecticut Valley Health Compact, Springfield, Vermont, 1971.

7. Blendon's classification of level of difficulty of surgical procedures was used [R. J. Blendon, thesis, Johns Hopkins University (1969)].

8. Cochrane has recently summarized technical and organizational problems encountered in appraising the effectiveness and efficiency of health services.

Failure to subject particular medical actions to randomized, controlled trials is, in his opinion, the major reason for uncertainty about the value of many common preventive, therapeutic, and diagnostic activities [A. L. Cochrane, *Effectiveness and Efficiency* (Nuffield Provencial Hospital Trust, London, 1972)].

9. Modified from *Vermont State Plan for Construction and Modernization of Hospital and Medical Facilities* (Vermont State Health Department, Burlington, 1971).
10. Partially supported by Public Health Service grant PHS-RM0303. We gratefully acknowledge the help of W. Gifford, R. Gillim, P. Hickox, K. Provost, and J. Senning in the work leading to the development of this article.

Quantifying the Burden of Disease: The Technical Basis for Disability-adjusted Life Years

1. Murray CJL, Lopez AD. Global and regional cause of death patterns in 1990. *Bulletin of the World Health Organization*, 1994, 72: 447–480.
2. Murray CJL, Lopez AD. Quantifying disability: data, methods and results. *Bulletin of the World Health Organization*, 1994, 72: 481–494.
3. Murray CJL, Lopez AD, Jamison DT. The global burden of disease in 1990: summary results, sensitivity analysis and future directions. *Bulletin of the World Health Organization*, 1994, 72: 495–509.
4. Power M. Linear Index Mortality as a measure of health status (Letter). *International journal of epidemiology*, 1989, 18: 282.
5. Sullivan DF. *Conceptual problems in developing an index of health*. US Public Health Service Publication Series No. 1000. Vital and Health Statistics Series 2. No. 17. Bethesda, MD, National Center for Health Statistics, 1966.
6. Sullivan DF. A single index of mortality and morbidity. *Health reports*, 1971, 86: 347–354.
7. Holland WW, Ipsen J, Kostrzewski J. *Measurement of levels of health*. Copenhagen, WHO Regional Office for Europe, 1979.
8. Jones–Lee MW. *The value of life: an economic analysis*. London, Martin Robertson, 1976.
9. Rawls J. *A theory of justice*. Cambridge, Harvard University Press, 1971.
10. Garber AM, Phelphs CE. *Economic foundations of cost-effectiveness analysis*. Cambridge, MA, 1992 (National Bureau of Economic Research Working Paper 4164).
11. Max W, Rice DP, MacKenzie EJ. The lifetime cost of injury. *Inquiry*, 1990, 27(4): 332–343.
12. Rice DP, Kelman S, Miller LS. Estimates of economic costs of alcohol and drug abuse and mental illness 1985 and 1988. *Public health reports*, 1991, 106(3): 280–292.
13. Daniels N. *Just health care*. New York, Cambridge University Press, 1985.
14. Dempsey M. Decline in tuberculosis. The death rate fails to tell the entire story. *American review of tuberculosis*, 1947, 56: 157–164.
15. Murray CJL, Lopez AD. *The global burden of disease and injury*. Geneva, World Health Organization (in preparation).
16. Romeder JM, McWhinnie JR. Potential years of life lost between ages 1 and 70: an indicator of premature mortality for health planning. *International journal of epidemiology*, 1977, 6: 143–151.

17. Greville TNE. Decline in tuberculosis: the death rate fails to tell the entire story. *American review of tuberculosis*, 1948, 57: 417–419 (comments on M. Dempsey's articles).

18. Haenszel W. A standardized rate for mortality defined in units of lost years of life. *American journal of public health*, 1950, 40: 17–26.

19. Dickinson FG, Welker EL. What is the leading cause of death? Two new measures. *Bulletin of the Bureau of Medical Economics of the American Medical Association*, 1948, 64: 1–25.

20. Robinson HL. Mortality trends and public health in Canada. *Canadian journal of public health*, 1948, 39(2): 60–70.

21. Kohn R. An objective mortality indicator. *Canadian journal of public health*, 1951, 42: 375–379.

22. Murray CJL. The infant mortality rate, life expectancy at birth and a linear index of mortality as measures of general health status. *International journal of epidemiology*, 1987, 16(4): 101–107.

23. Feachem R et al. *The health of adults in the developing world*. Oxford, Oxford University Press (for the World Bank), 1992.

24. Anonymous. Leads from the MMWR. Years of potential life lost before age 65—United States, 1987. *Journal of the American Medical Association*, 1989, 261: 823–827.

25. Ghana Health Assessment Project Team. A quantitative method of assessing the health impact of different diseases in less developed countries. *International journal of epidemiology*, 1981, 10: 73–80.

26. Drummond MF, Stoddard GL, Torrance GW. *Methods for the economic-evaluation of health care programmes*. Oxford, Oxford Medical Publications, 1987.

27. Jamison DH et al., eds. *Disease control priorities in developing countries*. Oxford, Oxford University Press (for the World Bank), 1993.

28. Ruzicka LT, Lopez AD, eds. *Sex differentials in mortality: trends, determinants and consequences*. Canberra, Australian National University, 1983.

29. Heligman L. Patterns of sex differentials in mortality in less developed countries. In: Ruzicka LT, Lopez AD, eds. *Sex differentials in mortality: trends, determinants and consequences*. Canberra, Australian National University, 1983: 7–32.

30. United Nations. *World population prospects, 1992 assessment*. New York, United Nations, 1992.

31. Wilkens R, Adams O, Brancker A. Changes in mortality by income in urban Canada from 1971 to 1986. *Health reports*, 1989, 1(2): 137–174.

32. Pressat R. Surmortalite biologique et surmortalite sociale. *Revue frangaise de sociologie*, 1973, 14: 103–110.

33. Prost A, Prescott N. Cost-effectiveness of blindness prevention by the Onchocerciasis Control Programme in Upper Volta, *Bulletin of the World Health Organization*, 1984, 62: 795–802.

34. Barnum H. Evaluating healthy days of life gained from health projects. *Social science and medicine*, 1987, 24: 833–841.

35. Clearing House on Health Indexes. Bibliography on health indexes. Hyattsville, MD, National Centre for Health Statistics, 1993, issue #3.

36. Chiang CL. *An index of health: mathematical models.* (Public Health Services Publications 1000 Series 2. No. 5). Washington, DC, National Centre for Health Statistics, 1965.

37. Fanshel S, Bush JW. A health-status index and its application to health services outcomes. *Operations research*, 1970, 18: 1021–1066.

38. Patrick DL, Bush JW, Chen MM. Methods for measuring levels of well-being for a health-status index. *Health services research*, 1973, 8: 228–245.

39. Berg RL. Weighted life expectancy as a health status index. *Health services research*, 1973, 8: 153–156.

40. Koplan JP. Health promotion, quality of life, and QALYS: a useful interaction. In: *Challenges for public health statistics in the 1990s. Proceedings of the 1989 Public Health Conference on Records and Statistics.* Bethesda, Department of Health and Human Services, 1989: 294–298 (Publication No. PHS 90–1213).

41. Torrance G, Thomas WH, Sackett DL. A utility maximization model for evaluation of health care programmes. *Health services research*, 1972, 7: 118–133.

42. Weinstein M, Stason WB. *Hypertension: a policy perspective.* Cambridge, Harvard University Press, 1976.

43. Zeckhauser R, Shephard D. Where now for saving lives? *Law and contemporary problems*, 1976, 40(b): 5–45.

44. Kaplan RM, Bush JW, Berry CC. Health status: types of validity and the index of well-being. *Health services research*, 1976, 11: 478–507.

45. Torrance GW. Measurement of health state utilities for economic appraisal: a review. *Journal of health economics*, 1986, 5: 1–30.

46. Nord E. Methods for quality adjustment of life years. *Social science and medicine*, 1992, 34: 559–569.

47. Boyle MH, Torrance GW. Developing multiattribute health indexes. *Medical care*, 1984, 22: 1045–1057.

48. Williams AH. Economics of coronary artery bypass grafting. *British medical journal*, 1985, 291: 326–329.

49. Lohr KN, Ware JE Jr, eds. Proceedings of the advances in health assessment conference. *Journal of chronic disease*, 1987, 40(suppl 1): 1S–191S.

50. Lohr KN, ed. Advances in health status assessment: conference proceedings. *Medical care*, 1989, 27(suppl): S1–S294.

51. Lohr KN. Advances in health status assessment: fostering the application of health status measures in clinical settings. Proceedings of a conference. *Medical care*, 1992, 30(5) supplement: MS1–MS293.

52. Greenfield S, Nelson EC. Recent developments and future issues in the use of health status assessment measures in clinical settings. *Medical care*, 1992, 30(5) supplement: MS23–MS41.

53. *International classification of impairment, disability and handicap.* Geneva, World Health Organization, 1980.

54. Réseau Espérance de Vie en Santé. *Statistical world yearbook.* Retrospective 1993 issue. Montpellier, INSERM, 1993.

55. Robine JM, Mathers CD, Bucquet D. Distinguishing health expectancies and health-adjusted life expectancies from quality-adjusted life years. *American journal of public health*, 1993, 83: 797–798.

56. Oregon Health Services Commission. *Prioritization of health services: A report to the Governor and Legislature.* Portland, State of Oregon, 1991.

57. Hadorn DC. Setting health care priorities in Oregon: cost-effectiveness meets the Rule of Rescue. *Journal of the American Medical Association,* 1991, 265: 2218–2225.

58. Dasgupta P, Marglin S, Sen A. *Guidelines for project evaluation.* New York, United Nations, 1972.

59. Lind R. *Discounting for time and risk in energy policy.* Baltimore, Johns Hopkins University Press, 1982.

60. Little I, Mirrlees J. *Project appraisal and planning for developing countries.* London, Heinemann, 1974.

61. Hartman RW. One thousand points of light seeking a number: A case study of CBO's search for a discount rate policy. *Journal of environmental economics and management,* 1990, 18: S3–S7.

62. Martens LLM, van Doorslaer EKA. Dealing with discounting. *International journal of technology assessment in health care,* 1990, 6: 139–145.

63. Fuchs V. *The health economy.* Cambridge, Harvard University Press, 1986.

64. Fuchs V, Zeckhauser R. Valuing health—a priceless commodity? *American economic review,* 1987, 77: 263–268.

65. Hammit J. Discounting health increments. *Journal of health economics,* 1993, 12: 117–120.

66. Krahn M, Gafna A. Discounting in the economic evaluation of health care interventions. *Medical care,* 1993, 31: 403–418.

67. Olsen J. On what basis should health be discounted. *Journal of health economics,* 1993, 12: 39–53.

68. Viscusi WK, Moore M. Rates of time preference and valuations of the durations of life. *Journal of public economics,* 1989, 38: 297–317.

69. Johannesson M. On the discounting of gained life years in cost-effectiveness analysis. *International journal of technology assessment in health care,* 1992, 8: 359–364.

70. Anonymous. Discounting health care: only a matter of timing? *Lancet,* 1992, 340: 148–149.

71. Parsonage M, Neuberger H. Discounting and health benefits. *Health economics,* 1992, 1: 71–76.

72. Cairns J. Discounting and health benefits: another perspective. *Health economics,* 1992, 1: 76–79.

73. Messing SD. Discounting health: the issue of subsistence and care in an underdeveloped country. *Social science and medicine,* 1973, 7: 911–916.

74. Ganiats TG. On sale: future health care. The paradox of discounting. *Western journal of medicine,* 1992, 156: 550–553.

75. Keeler E, Cretin S. Discounting of life-saving and other nonmonetary effects. *Management science,* 1983, 29: 300–306.

REFERENCES

[a] Murray CJL. Mortality measurement and social justice. Paper presented at the Annual Conference of the Institute of British Geographers, 5 January 1986, Reading, England.

b Murray CJL. The determinants of health improvement in developing countries. Case-studies of St. Lucia, Guyana, Paraguay, Kiribati, Swaziland, and Bolivia. Oxford University D. Phil. thesis, 1988.

c Rothenberg R. Application of years of life lost to the elderly: demographic influences on a composite statistic. Presented at 46th Annual Scientific Meeting of the American Geriatrics Society, Boston, MA, 1989.

d Piot M, Sundaresan TK. A linear programme decision model for tuberculosis control. Progress report on the first test-runs. Unpublished WHO document No. WHO/TB/Techn. Information/67.55, 1967.

e See footnote d.

f Wood PHN. Classification of impairments and handicaps. Unpublished WHO document No. WHO/lCD9/REV.CONF/75.15, 1975.

g See footnote d.

h Note that in a continuous discount function r is not precisely the same as r in the discrete form. The formula for the discrete form is simply $1/(1+r)'$. If the discount rate in the discrete formula is r, then the equivalent result is achieved with a continuous discount rate of $ln\ (l+r)$.

Chapter 14   MEDICAL ETHICS AND HUMAN RESEARCH

Ethics and Clinical Research

1. Pope Pius XII. Address. Presented at the First International Congress on Histopathology of Nervous System, Rome, Italy, September 14, 1952.

2. Platt (Sir Robert), 1st bart. *Doctor and Patient: Ethics, morals, government.* 87 pp. London: Nuffield provincial hospitals trust, 1963. Pp. 62 and 63.

3. Pappworth, M. H. Personal communication.

4. Beecher, H. K. Consent in clinical experimentation: myth and reality. J.A.M.A. 195:34, 1966.

5. Great Britain, Medical Research Council. *Memorandum,* 1953.

Thalidomide and the Titanic: *Reconstructing the Technology Tragedies of the Twentieth Century*

1. Hawthorn J. *Cunning Passages: New Historicism, Cultural Materialism, and Marxism in the Contemporary Literary Debate.* London, England: Arnold; 1996.

2. Beesley L, Gracie A, Lightoller C, Bride H. *The Story of the Titanic as Told by Its Survivors.* Mineola, NY: Dover Publications Inc; 1960: 94.

3. Bernstein A. Formed by thalidomide: mass torts as a false cure for toxic exposure. *Columbia Law Review.* 1997; 97:2153–2176.

4. Insight Team of the Sunday Times of London. *Suffer the Children: The Story of Thalidomide.* New York, NY: Viking Press; 1979.

5. Dally A. Thalidomide: was the tragedy preventable? *Lancet.* 1998; 351: 1197–1199.

6. Lenz W. Klinische Misbildungen nach Medikament: einnahme Wahrend der Graviditat? *Dtsch Med Wochenschr.* 1961; 86:2555–2565.

7. McBride WG. Thalidomide and congenital abnormalities. *Lancet.* 1961; 2:1358–1363.

8. Newman CGH. The thalidomide syndrome: risks of exposure and spectrum of malformations. *Clin Perinatol.* 1986; 13:555–573.
9. Smithells RW, Newman CHG. Recognition of thalidomide defects. *J Med Genet.* 1992; 29:716–723.
10. Elias SE, Annas GJ. *Reproductive Genetics and the Law.* St. Louis, Mo: Mosby-Yearbook; 1987:207.
11. Koren G, Pastusak A, Shinya I. Drugs in pregnancy. *N Engl J Med.* 1998; 338:1126–1137.
12. Castilla EE, Ashton-Prolla P, Barreda-Megia E, et al. Thalidomide: a current teratogen in South America. *Teratology.* 1996; 54:273–277.
13. Stolberg SG. Thalidomide wins FDA's approval. *New York Times.* July 17, 1998:1.
14. Food and Drug Administration. *FDA Talk Paper on Thalidomide.* Washington, DC: Public Health Service; July 16, 1998.
15. Jacobson JM, Greenspan JS, Spritzler J, et al. Thalidomide for the treatment of oral aphthous ulcers in patients with human immunodeficiency virus infection. *N Engl J Med.* 1997; 336: 1487–1493.
16. Shulman SR. The broader message of Accutane. *Am J Public Health.* 1989; 79:1565–1568.
17. *Roe v Wade,* 410 U.S. 113 (1973).
18. Garrow DJ. *Liberty & Sexuality: The Right to Privacy and the Making of Roe v. Wade.* New York, NY: Macmillan; 1994: 285–289.
19. Annas GJ. Fetal protection and employment discrimination—the Johnson Controls case. *N Engl J Med.* 1991; 325:740–743.
20. American College of Obstetricians and Gynecologists. *Statement on Thalidomide.* Washington, DC: American College of Obstetricians and Gynecologists; August 27, 1997.
21. Stolberg SG. Their devil's advocate: thalidomide returns with an unlikely ally—a group of its original victims. *New York Magazine.* January 25, 1998:24.
22. Moore TJ. Time to act on drug safety. *JAMA.* 1998; 279: 1571–1573.
23. Sharpe R. Med Watch system comes under fire: FDA defends drug monitoring as physicians, advocates are cautious. *Wall Street Journal.* June 24, 1998:B5.
24. Hopkinson N. Advocacy group petitions FDA to ban diabetes drug troglitazone. *Wall Street Journal.* July 28, 1998:B6.
25. Daws G. *Holy Man: Father Damien of Molokai.* Honolulu, Hawaii: University of Hawaii Press; 1973.

Kidneys, Ethics, and Politics: Policy Lessons of the ESRD Experience

1. G. B. Kolata, "Dialysis After Nearly a Decade," *Science* 208 (2 May 1980): 473–476.
2. Ibid., p. 473.
3. *Congressional Record,* October 12, 1977, p. 161.
4. See James W. Childress, "Rationing of Medical Treatment," *The Encyclopedia of Bioethics,* Vol. 4, ed. W. T. Reich (New York: The Free Press, 1978).
5. See A. L. Caplan, "Ethical Engineers Need Not Apply: The State of Applied Ethics Today," *Science, Technology, and Human Values* 6 (Fall 1980): 24–32.
6. The invalidity of this assumption is persuasively shown in Renee C. Fox and Judith P. Swazey, *The Courage to Fail,* Chapter 3, 2nd ed. (Chicago: University of Chicago Press, 1978).

7. J. K. Iglehart, "Kidney Treatment Problem Readies HEW for National Health Insurance," *National Journal* 8 (26 June 1976): 895–900; and B. D. Colen, "The Life and Death Cost of Health," *The Washington Post,* 22 July 1977.

8. It is a matter of both health policy concern and empirical fact that health care wants, demands, and needs do not always overlap. See M. H. Cooper, *Rationing Health Care* (New York: John Wiley & Sons, 1975). It is also a matter of empirical fact that not all health care needs can be met at any given time. For the purposes of this paper, health care wants are any subjectively desired physical or mental state or service for obtaining such a state; health care demands are articulated health care wants; health care needs are assessments by health care professionals of what is required for health; and supply is a mode of medical therapy for meeting a health care need.

9. Those persons directly concerned with current dialysis policy and planning are less likely to subscribe to the five myths cited here. But numerous policy analysts not directly concerned with dialysis or transplant subscribe to most or all of these myths. Even more believers can be found in the ranks of physicians, nurses, philosophers, social scientists, theologians and legislators who have cavalierly attempted to put the ESRD experience to use to support particular political or policy agendas.

10. As Renee Fox among many authors has argued, "Dialysis became increasingly available to a larger number of people even before the passage of the Public Law, but the extensive financial coverage that the legislation made possible is the major factor that accounts for the dramatic change in accessibility of dialysis," *Essays in Medical Sociology* (New York: John Wiley & Sons, 1970), p. 139. See also "Competition in Kidney Dialysis" *Regulation,* January/February, 1981, pp. 9–12.

11. Thomas Szasz defends this myth as true of every mode of supply in health care at some length in Chapter 9 of his book, *The Theology of Medicine* (Baton Rouge: Louisiana State University Press, 1977).

12. See Victor W. Sidel, "The Right to Health Care: An International Perspective," in *Bioethics and Human Rights,* ed. Elsie L. Bandman and Bertram Bandman (Boston: Little, Brown, and Co., 1978), pp. 341–349. See also the discussion of patient selection among nephrologists in V. Parsons and P. Lock, "Triage and the Patient With Renal Failure," *Journal of Medical Ethics* 6 (December 1980): 173–176.

13. D. Rennie, "Home Dialysis and the Costs of Uremia," *New England Journal of Medicine* 298 (16 February 1978): 399–400. See also L. B. Berman, "Nephrology," *Journal of the American Medical Association* 245 (5 June 1981): 2199–2200. S. H. Altman and R. Blendon, eds., *Medical Technology: The Culprit Behind Health Care Costs?* (Washington, D.C.: Government Printing Office, 1979). DHEW Publication No. PHS 79–3216.

14. Richard A. Rettig, "Health Care Technology: Lessons Learned From The End-Stage Renal Disease Experience," *The Rand Paper Series* P–5820 (November 1976), pp. 1–36.

15. Ibid., p. 4.

16. As reported in Fox and Swazey, *The Courage to Fail,* pp. 202–3.

17. The terms acute and chronic are used by physicians to describe the time period involved from the initial onset of a disease to its final outcome. Chronic

conditions are generally ailments or diseases that reach and maintain a persistent level of disability for more than a day or two.

18. Rettig, "Health Care Technology," pp. 11–13.

19. Richard Rettig, "Valuing Lives: The Policy Debate on Patient Care Financing ForVictims of End-Stage Renal Disease," *Rand Paper Series* P–5672 (March 1976) pp 20–21.

20. Ibid., pp. 30–31.

21. Louis B. Russell, *Technology in Hospitals* (Washington, D.C.: Brookings, 1979), p. 111.

22. See for example H. S. Abram and W. Wadlington, "Selection of Patients For Artificial and Transplanted Organs," *Annals of Internal Medicine* 69 (September 1968): 615–620; H. K. Beecher, "Scarce Resources and Medical Advancement," *Daedalus* 98 (Spring 1969): 275–313; N. Rescher, "The Allocation of Exotic Medical Lifesaving Therapy" *Ethics* 79 (April 1969): 173–186.

23. Rettig, "Valuing Lives," pp. 24–25.

24. Ibid., pp. 13–16.

25. In addition to dialysis in a medical center and renal transplants, possible alternative treatments included home dialysis, peritoneal dialysis, and dietary management. See E. A. Freidman, et al., "Pragmatic Realities in Uremia Therapy" *New England Journal of Medicine* 298 (16 February 1978): 368–371, and L. B. Russell, *Technology in Hospitals*, Appendix D.

26. H. F. Klarman, J. O. Francis, and G. D. Rosenthal, "Cost Effectiveness Analysis Applied to the Treatment of Chronic Renal Disease," *Medical Care* 6 (January/February 1968): 48–54.

27. Rettig uses this term to describe the decision of the Gottschalk Committee, "Valuing Lives," p. 16.

28. U. S. Bureau of the Budget, *Report of the Committee on Chronic Kidney Disease*, (Washington, D. C.: Government Printing Office, September 1967), pp. 2–4.

29. Thomas Manis and Eli A. Friedman, "Dialytic Therapy For Irreversible Uremia," *New England Journal of Medicine* 301 (13 December 1979): 1321–1328.

30. Ibid., pp. 1323–1326.

31. L. B. Russell, *Technology in Hospitals*, p. 111. In 1979, 46,000 patients were receiving dialysis. See G. B. Kolata, "Dialysis After Nearly a Decade," p. 473.

32. Ibid. (as quoted), p. 473.

33. Ibid., p. 474.

34. Rescher, "The Allocation of Therapy." Also, Paul Ramsey, *The Patient As Person* (New Haven: Yale, 1970); J. Childress, "Who Shall Live When Not All Can Live? ," *Soundings* 43 (Winter 1970): 339–362; L. R. Adams, "Medical Coverage For Chronic Renal Disease: Policy Implications," *Health and Social Work* 3 (3 November 1978 41–53; M. D. Basson, "Choosing Among Candidates For Scarce Medical Resources," *Journal of Medicine and Philosophy* 4 (September 1979): 313–333.

35. Fox and Swazey, *The Courage to Fail*, pp. 346–351.

36. It is interesting to note the relevance to policy outcomes of having *identified* as opposed to *statistical* lives at risk. Rather than place a measure of value on individual lives, or deny treatment to specific individuals, government officials found it politically opportune to permit blanket reimbursements for

dialysis. It was politically impossible to follow either a policy of "weighing worthy lives" (a process the first kidney selection committees found easier to conduct behind closed doors), or one which denied aid to specific, identifiable persons. Such situations have parallels in the willingness of government to spend large sums of money to save the victims of mine disasters or earthquakes, but, not to lower 'statistical' deaths in areas such as auto safety. See M. Bayles and A. L. Caplan, "Medical Fallibility and Malpractice," *Journal of Medicine and Philosophy* 3 (NO.3 1978): 169–186.

37. D. Rennie, "Home Dialysis," p. 399.
38. Robert J. Wineman, "Federal Legislation and Agency Actions Concerning Self-Care Dialysis," *Journal of Dialysis* 2 (NO.1, 1978): 103–109.
39. Quoted in M. H. Cooper, *Rationing Health Care* (New York: John Wiley & Sons, 1975) p. 92.
40. *Proceedings of the European Dialysis and Transplant Association* 13 (Hamburg: Pitman Medical, 1976), p. 18.
41. V. Parsons, "The Ethical Challenges of Dialysis and Transplantation," *The Practitioner* 220 (June 1978): 872–877.
42. Ibid., p. 872. The same concerns about affordability and efficacy are reflected in a prescient statement by a French nephrologist concerning this same period in the evolution of dialysis technology:

> "If the problem of treating chronic renal failure on a large scale is to be solved, home hemodialysis must be developed. It would be unreasonable to consider the unlimited creation of dialysis centers requiring large numbers of doctors and especially nurses for the treatment of chronic conditions. . . . If they were meant mainly to train patients for hemodialysis, the present centers in France could handle all patients."
> J. Mion, "Renal Dialysis," *Progress in Nephrology* (1973), p. 72.

43. Ibid., p.872.
44. A. J. Nicholls, et al., "Integrated Dialysis and Renal Transplantation: Small Is Beautiful," *British Medical Journal,* 21 June 1980, pp. 1516–1517.
45. E. Bergsten, et al., "A Study of Patients on Chronic Haemodialysis," *Scandinavian Journal of Social Medicine,* Supplement No. 11 (1977), p. 7.
46. Ibid.
47. During a recent trip to the Netherlands, I learned that nephrologists there have informally agreed upon a cut-off age of roughly 65 for administering dialysis despite the availability of government reimbursements. Severe diabetes and hypertension are also felt to be contraindications for dialysis among the elderly, as they are in the United Kingdom and Sweden.
48. E. G. Knox, "Principles of Allocation of Health Care Resources," *Journal of Epidemiology and Community Health* 32 (March 1978): 309; and Stephen Roberts, et al., "Cost-Effective Care of End-Stage Renal Disease: A Billion Dollar Question," *Annals of Internal Medicine* 92 (February 1980): 243–248.
49. New therapies for renal failure in poor countries involve dietary management in conjunction with oral sorbents and diarrhea therapy. The prohibitive costs of dialysis make these supply modes attractive in these settings. Cf. Manis and Friedman, "Dialytic Therapy for Irreversible Uremia," p. 1326.

50. This ignorance has had costly results in other areas. See Robert A. Solo, "The Saga of Synthetic Rubber," *The Bulletin of the Atomic Scientists* 36 (April 1980): 31–36.

51. Nicholas Rescher's recent book, *Scientific Progress* (Pittsburgh: University of Pittsburgh Press, 1978), for example, falls into the error of not analyzing specific cases of technological evolution. He claims that the cost of progress in science and technology necessarily increases since it become[s] harder and harder to learn more and more about the world. But this view obscures the important costs of advertising or mastering a new technology—costs not related to the costs of acquiring new knowledge.

Chapter 15 GLOBAL HEALTH

1. WHO News. Prize goes to authors of Public Health Classic. *Bull WHO* 2002;80(12): 991. Dilip Mahalanabis, Nathaniel Pierce, Norbert Hirschborn, and David Nalin, who together pioneered oral rehydration therapy, have been awarded the first Pollin Prize for Paediatric Research. Their discovery was hailed by the *Lancet* as "the most important medical discovery of the 20th century". It was reported by Mahalabis et al. in the *Johns Hopkins Medical Journal* in January 1973, and reprinted by the *Bulletin* as a Public Health Classic in May 2001 *(Bulletin* 79: 471-9). The treatment is credited with saving 40 million lives in the last 30 years.

2. The Lalonde Report was presented in the House of Commons on April 1, 1974. The paper identifies two main health-related areas: the health care system, and the prevention of health problems as well as the promotion of good health. It proposes integrating these two aspects in health care policy development and details 5 main strategies and 74 proposals to meet this objective.

A Review of Major Influences on Current Public Health Policy in Developed Countries in the Second Half of the 20th Century

1. US Department of Health, Education and Welfare. Healthy People: The Surgeon General's Report On Health Promotion and Disease Prevention. Washington DC: US Department of Health Education and Welfare, 1979. Available online at: profiles.nlm.nih.gov/NN/B/B/G/K/_/nnbbgk.pdf (accessed 5 December 2005)

2. Fielding J. Public Health in the Twentieth Century: Advances and Challenges. *Ann Rev Public Health* 1999; 20: xiii–xxx

3. World Health Organization. Constitution of the World Health Organization. New York: World Health Organization, 1946. Available online at: whqlibdoc. who.int/hist/official_records/constitution.pdf (accessed 5 December 2005)

4. Japanese Government. The Constitution of Japan. Tokyo: Japanese Government, 1946. Available online at: www.ndl.go.jp/constitution/e/etc/c01.html (accessed 5 December 2005)

5. Nakahara T. Public Health Policies and Strategies in Japan. In: Detels R, Holland W, McEwen J, Omenn G, editors. Oxford Textbook of Public Health. Third edition. Oxford: Oxford University press, 1997. pp. 323–9

6. Lalonde M. A New Perspective on the Health of Canadians: Working Document. Ottawa: Canadian Ministry of Health and Welfare, 1974. Available

Online at: www.hc-sc.gc.ca/hcs-sss/alt_formats_e.pdf (accessed 5 December 2005) [URL not functional, Ed. See: http://www.hc-sc.gc.ca/hcs-sss/alt-formats/hpb-dgps/pdf/pubs/1974-lalonde/lalonde-eng.pdf (accessed 15 April 2009)]

7. Glouberman S. Towards a New Perspective on Health Policy. Ottawa: Canadian Policy Research Networks, 2001. Available online at: www.healthandeverything.org/pubs/TNP.pdf (accessed 5 December 2005) [URL not functional, Ed. See: http://www.hpclearinghouse.ca/downloads/Canada_towards_a_new_perspective_on_health_policy.pdf (accessed 15 April 2009)]

8. Colgrove J. The McKeown Thesis: A historical controversy and its enduring influence. *Am J Public Health* 2002; 92 (5):725-729

9. Hancock T. Lalonde and beyond: looking back at 'A New Perspective on the Health of Canadians.' *Health Promot* 1986; 1(1): 93-100

10. World Health Organization. Formulating Strategies for Health for all by the Year 2000. Geneva: World Health Organization, 1979. Health for all series, No. 2

11. World Health Organization. Declaration of Alma-Ata. International Conference on Primary Health Care; 6-12 September 1978, Alma-Ata, USSR. Geneva: World Health Organization, 1978. Available online at: http://www.who.int/hpr/NPH/docs/declaration_almaata.pdf (accessed 5 December 2005)

12. Green L. Health education's contributions to public health in the twentieth century: A glimpse through health promotion's rear-view mirror. *Ann Rev Public Health* 1999; 20:67-68

13. Breslow L. Musings on sixty years in public health. *Ann Rev Public Health* 1998; 19:1-15

14. Black D. Inequalities in Health. London: Department of Health and Social Security, 1980

15. World Health Organization. Health for All Targets: The Health Policy for Europe Updated Edition September 1991. Copenhagen: World Health Organization, 1993

16. Van de Water H, van Herten L. Health Policies on Target? Review of Target and Priority-Setting in 18 European Countries. Leiden: TNO Prevention and Health, Public Health Division, 1998

17. Ritsatakis A. Experience in setting targets for health in Europe. *European J Public Health* 2000; 10 (4 supplement):7-10

18. World Health Organization. Ottawa Charter for Health Promotion. 1st International Conference on Promotion; 21 November 1986, Ottawa, Canada. Ottawa: World Health Organization, 1986. Available online at: http://www.who.int/hpr/NPH/docs/ottawa_charter_hp.pdf (accessed 5 December 2005)

19. World Health Organization. Healthy Cities Network. Geneva: World Health Organization, 2005. Available online at: www.who.dk/healthy-cities (accessed 5 December 2005) [URL not functional, Ed. See: http://www.euro.who.int/document/e82653.pdf (accessed 15 April 2009)]

20. World Health Organization. The Adelaide Recommendations. 2nd International Conference on Health Promotion; 5-9 April 1988, Adelaide, South Australia. Copenhagen: World Health Organization, 1988. Available online at: www.who.int/hpr/NPH/docs/Adelaide_recommendations.pdf (accessed 5 December 2005)

21. World Health Organization. The Jakarta Declaration on Leading Health Promotion into the 21st Century. 4th International Conference on Promotion: 21–25 July 1997, Jakarta, Indonesia. Geneva: World Health Organization, 1997. Available online at: www.who.int/hpr/NPH/docs/jakarta_declaration_en.pdf (accessed 5 December 2005)

22. Atchison D. Independent Inquiry into Inequalities in Health Report. London: HMSO, 1998. Available online at: http://www.archive.official-documents. co.uk/document/doh/ih/ih.htm (accessed 5 December 2005)

23. Health 21. An Introduction to the Health for All Policy Framework for the WHO European Region. Copenhagen: World Health Organization, 1998

24. Health 21. The Health for All Policy Framework for the WHO European Region. Copenhagen: World Health Organization, 1999

25. van Herten L, van de Water H. New global Health for All targets. *BMJ* 1999; 319(7211):700–3

26. Treaty on European Union. Maastricht, The Netherlands: The European Union; 1992. Available online at: www.hri.org/docs/Maastricht92/ (accessed 5 December 2005) [URL not functional, Ed. See http://www.eurotreaties.com/maastrichtec.pdf (accessed 15 April 2009)]

27. Treaty of Amsterdam. Amsterdam, The Netherlands; The European Union; 1997. Available online at: europa.eu.int/eur-lex/en/treaties/selected/livre545. html (accessed 5 December 2005) [URL not functional, Ed. See http://www. europarl.europa.eu/topics/treaty/pdf/amst-en.pdf (accessed 15 April 2009)]

Mortality by Cause for Eight Regions of the World: Global Burden of Disease Study

1. World Bank. World development report 1993: investing in health. Oxford: Oxford University Press, 1993.

2. Murray CJL, Lopez AD, eds. Global comparative assessments in the health sector. Disease burden, expenditures and intervention packages. Geneva: WHO, 1994.

3. Murray CJL, Lopez AD, eds. The global burden of disease: a comprehensive assessment of mortality and disability from diseases, injuries, and risk factors in 1990 and projected to 2020. Cambridge: Harvard University Press, 1996.

4. Murray CJL, Lopez AD. Global health statistics: a compendium of incidence, prevalence and mortality estimates for over 200 conditions. Cambridge: Harvard University Press, 1996.

5. Murray CJL, Lopez AD. Global health statistics: a compendium of incidence, prevalence and mortality estimates for over 200 conditions. Cambridge: Harvard University Press, 1996.

6. Murray CJL. Quantifying the burden of disease: the technical basis for disability-adjusted life years. *Bull World Health Organ* 1994; 72: 429–45.

7. Anand S, Hansen K. Disability-adjusted life years: a critical review. *J Health Economics* (in press).

8. Murray CJL, Yang G, Qiao X. Adult mortality: levels, patterns and causes. In: Feachem RGA, Kjellstrom T, Murray CJL, Over M, Phillips MA, eds. The health of adults in the developing world. New York: Oxford University Press, 1992: 23–112.

9. Omran AR. The epidemiological transition: a theory of the epidemiology of population change. *Milbank Q* 1971; 49: 509–38.

10. United Nations. World Population prospects 1992 assessment. New York: United Nations, 1992.

11. Hill K, Yazbeck A. Trends in child mortality 1960–90: estimates for 84 developing countries. The World Bank World Development Report 1993: investing in health. Background Paper Series, no 6.

12. Timaeus I. Adult mortality. In: Feachem RGA, Jamison DT, eds. Disease and mortality in sub-Saharan Africa. New York: Oxford University Press, 1991.

13. Preston SH. Mortality patterns in national populations. New York: Academic Press, 1976.

14. Stehbens WE. An appraisal of the epidemic rise of coronary heart disease and its decline. *Lancet* 1987; i: 606–11.

15. Campbell M. Death rate from diseases of the heart: 1876–1959. *BMJ* 1963; ii: 528–35.

16. Robb-Smith AHT. The enigma of coronary heart disease. Chicago: Year Book Medical Publishers, 1967.

17. Lozano R, Murray CJL, Lopez AD. The French paradox revisited: undercoding of ischemic heart disease mortality. Massachusetts: Harvard Center for Population and Development Studies Working Papers 1996.

18. Office of Registrar General, Government of India. Medical certification of causes of death. Annual report 1991. New Delhi: Ministry of Home Affairs, 1992.

19. Office of Registrar General, Government of India. Survey of causes of death (rural). Annual report 1991. New Delhi, Ministry of Home Affairs, 1992.

20. Hakulinen T, Hansluwka H, Lopez D, Nakada D. Global and regional mortality patterns by cause of death in 1980. *Int J Epidemiol* 1986; 15: 226–33.

21. Hull TH, et al. A framework for estimating causes of death in Indonesia. *Majalah Demografi Indonesia* 1981; 15: 77–125.

22. Lopez AD, Hull TH. A note on estimating the cause of death structure in high mortality populations. *Pop Bull United Nat* 1983; 14: 66–70.

23. Garenne M, Leroy O, Beau J-P, Sene I. Child mortality after high-titre measles vaccines: prospective study in Senegal. *Lancet* 1991; 338: 903–07.

24. de Francisco A, Schellenberg JA, Hall AJ, Greenwood AM, Cham K, Greenwood BM. Comparison of mortality between villages with and without primary health care workers in Upper River Division, The Gambia. *J Trop Med Hygiene* 1994; 97: 69–74.

25. Ghana VAST Study Team. Vitamin A supplementation in northern Ghana: effects on clinic attendances, hospital admissions, and child mortality. *Lancet* 1993; 342: 7–12.

26. Omondi-Odhiambo, ban Ginneken JK, Voorhoeve AM. Mortality by cause of death in a rural area of Machakos district, Kenya in 1975–78. *J Biosoc Sci* 1990; 22: 63–75.

27. Adult Mortality and Morbidity Project Team. Policy implications of adult morbidity and mortality: a preliminary report of the adult morbidity and mortality project, Tanzania. Dar es Salaam: AAMP, 1993.

28. Parkin DM, Pisani P, Lopez AD, Masuyer E. At least one in seven cases of cancer is caused by smoking. Global estimates for 1985. *Int J Cancer* 1994; 59: 494–504.

29. Barker DJP, Martyn CN. The maternal and fetal origins of cardiovascular disease. *J Epidemiol Community Health* 1992; 46: 8–11.
30. Frenk J. Health transition in middle-income countries: new challenges for health care. *Health Policy Planning* 1989; 4: 29–39.
31. Parkin DM, Muir CS. Cancer incidence in five continents. Comparability and quality of data. *IARC Sci Publ.* 1992; (120): 45–173.

Global Health—The Gates–Buffett Effect

1. Gottret P, Schieber G. Health financing revisited: a practitioner's guide. Washington, DC: World Bank, 2006.
2. Specter M. What money can buy. The New Yorker. October 24, 2005.

INDEX

With page numbers, f refers to figure; t refers to table.

ABOUT THE EDITORS

Dona Schneider is professor and associate dean at the Edward J. Bloustein School of Planning and Public Policy at Rutgers, The State University of New Jersey. The recipient of multiple teaching and service awards, she has taught various classes in epidemiology and public health to several thousand students.

David E. Lilienfeld is an internationally known physician, epidemiologist, and medical historian. A winner of the Society for Epidemiologic Research's Professors' Prize in the History of Epidemiology, he has published extensively on the history of epidemiology and public health.